Medical-Legal Aspects of Alcohol

Fourth Edition

Edited by James C. Garriott

Contributing Authors

William H. Anderson
Barbara Basteyns
Yale H. Caplan
Kurt M. Dubowski
Bruce A. Goldberger
Patrick Harding
William C. Head
A. W. Jones
Graham R. Jones
Jerry Landau
Barbara R. Manno
Joseph E. Manno
Morton F. Mason
Bill H. McAnalley
Boris Moczula
Herbert Moskowitz
Richard F. Shaw
Theodore F. Shults

 Lawyers & Judges Publishing Company, Inc.

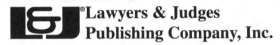

Lawyers & Judges Publishing Company, Inc.

P.O. Box 30040 • Tucson, AZ 85751-0040
(800) 209-7109 • FAX (800) 330-8795
e-mail: sales@lawyersandjudges.com

Library of Congress Cataloging-in-Publication Data

Medical-legal aspects of alcohol / edited by James C. Garriott ;
contributing authors, William H. Anderson ... [et al.].-- 4th ed.
    p. cm.
Includes bibliographical references and index.
  ISBN 1-930056-69-9 (hardcover)
  1. Alcohol in the body--Measurement. 2. Alcohol--Law and legislation.
3. Drunk driving--Investigation. I. Garriott, James C. II. Anderson,
William H. (William Henry), 1940-
  RA1061.5.M42 2003
  614'.1--dc22

                    2003018906

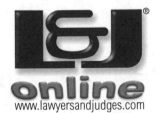

www.lawyersandjudges.com

ISBN 1-930056-69-9
Printed in the United States of America
10 9 8 7 6 5 4 3

Contents

17. Prosecuting Driving-under-the-Influence Cases
Jerry Landau

18. Defending Driving-under-the-Influence Cases
William C. Head

19. The Role and Responsibilities of an Expert Witness
Theodore F. Shults, J.D. and Yale H. Caplan, Ph.D.

20. Alcohol Testing in the Workplace
Kurt M. Dubowski, Ph.D. and Yale H. Caplan, Ph.D.

Preface

Forensic alcohol analysis is without question the most frequently performed of all analyses in forensic laboratories, and likewise is the most commonly used laboratory result in courts of law. Alcohol-related litigation most frequently pertains to arrests of drinking drivers, but also includes industrial accidents as well as aircraft and public transport accidents.

Approximately 2.21 gallons of ethanol per person are consumed annually in the United States based on the population aged fourteen and older. This is about one and two thirds regular beers or glasses of wine daily per person, if one excludes the approximately one-third of the population who abstain from alcohol consumption (National Institute on Alcohol Abuse and Alcoholism, 2002). It is therefore not surprising that alcohol has a great impact on society. There were 42,000 motor vehicle-related deaths and 2 million disabling injuries in the United States in 1993 with an half or more being alcohol-involved, the latest data available at the last printing of this book in 1996. In 2000, 41,821 motor vehicle deaths occurred with 16,653, or 40 percent, involving alcohol, while over 3 million disabling injuries occurred in the same year (MWMR, 2001). It is assumed that stricter drinking and driving laws, improved enforcement of these laws, and the recent trend toward lower blood alcohol limits have been responsible for the lowering alcohol involved traffic fatality rates, keeping in mind the ever increasing number of vehicles on the road. Studies of homicides, suicides, or victims of other forms of violent death generally show that greater than half involve alcohol. Alcohol misuse is one of nine factors responsible for half of all deaths among U.S. residents, and accounted for 100,000 deaths (5 percent) in 1993.

In death investigation, an alcohol analysis is often the first and sometimes sole chemical analysis performed. All fifty states of the United States, as well as most countries of Western Europe and other parts of the world, have statutes regulating driving a motor vehicle while under the influence of alcohol and other laws govern use of alcohol under other circumstances, such as public intoxication and use of alcohol in the workplace. Thus, testing for use of alcohol in living or deceased individuals under a variety of circumstances is nearly universal. Whether such testing is performed on body fluids or organ tissues taken at autopsy, or on blood, urine, or breath in living individuals, it is often extremely important that the alcohol analyses be performed accurately and correctly and that the results are properly interpreted. Forensic toxicologists and pathologists are often called upon to interpret alcohol concentrations found in autopsy specimens or in mishandled blood specimens. We must sometimes conclude that the results are meaningless or have been misinterpreted due to factors discussed in the ensuing chapters. Alcohol litigation may involve attorneys, pathologists, physicians, toxicologists or other laboratory specialists. A reference work dedicated to the forensic science of alcohol, to include its disposition in the body, measurement in blood, breath and other body specimens, postmortem influences, legal considerations, and many other facets is often needed and sought by these experts.

This fourth revised edition of the original text, *Medicolegal Aspects of Alcohol in Biological Specimens*, is designed to provide up-to-date and authoritative information on alcohol in all aspects of its involvement in the forensic sciences and in litigation. Many of the eighteen authors are those who originally contributed to the first edition and have been retained because of their unique and valuable expertise in this field. Dr. A. W. Jones has shared his unique expertise by contributing a second chapter, "Disposition and Fate of Alcohol" to supplement his earlier one on "Biochemistry and Physiology . . ." and Dr. Herbert Moskowitz joins with a review of studies, many of which are his own, on alcohol and its effects on driving. The study of alcohol and its kinetics in man began with the classic research of Erik Widmark in the 1920s and 1930s, and his work and discoveries are still valid today. Likewise, a few chapters such as the review of breath testing by Drs. Kurt Dubowski and Morton F. Mason have been retained as originally published.

J.C.G.

References

Morbidity and Mortality Weekly Report, Centers for Disease Control and Prevention, v.5 #47, 2001.

National Institute on Alcohol Abuse and Alcoholism, Division of Biometry and Epidemiology, September, 2002.

National Highway Traffic Safety Administration, 2001.

Chapter 1

The Chemistry of Alcoholic Beverages

Bill H. McAnalley, Ph.D.

Significant technological advances in the science of alcoholic beverages coupled with increasing regulatory requirements have enabled manufacturers to explore the concept of beverage "fingerprints." New accurate instrumentation has allowed companies to produce more consistent and more desirable products and meet new regulations, especially in regard to agricultural chemicals and trace metal residues potentially remaining in finished beer and wine (Dowhanick and Russell, 1993). Beverage "fingerprints" have enabled companies to identify the desired components and reproduce them at considerable savings to the consumer. All beverage constituents other than ethyl alcohol are called congeners.

Alcoholic beverages include wines, beers, and spirits. Wines are made from fermenting fruits, berries, honey, and even milk. Beers are produced from fermenting grains, and spirits are distilled from wines and beers. Ethyl alcohol is the alcohol of "alcoholic" beverages. It is also known as drinking alcohol, grain alcohol and ethanol. Fermentation of sugars by yeast is the oldest synthetic organic chemical produced by man (Morrison and Boyd, 1983).

During fermentation, sugar is converted to drinking alcohol, and carbon dioxide is released as gas bubbles, for example, as in carbonated drinks. This chemical change was a great mystery to ancient man because the mixture appeared to be boiling without heat. Knowledge resulting from the study of wine fermentation was a major contributor to the early development and progress of the modern sciences of microbiology and biochemistry. Understanding the "mysteries" that baffled the artisan winemaker began in the 1860s when Louis Pasteur discovered that alcoholic fermentation could occur only in the presence of small living "ferments" or, as they are known today, yeasts.

In 1897, Edward Buchner reported that yeasts could be broken up and that the cell-free yeast juice could ferment sugar. Later, the yeast juice was found to contain enzymes which are responsible for the conversion of sugars to alcohol and carbon dioxide.

The learning process of mankind is exemplified by beverage making. The natural course of events in acquiring knowledge begins with "magic" which, with more understanding, becomes an art, and with further understanding, a science.

1.1 A Description and History of Common Alcoholic Beverages

The liquor industry is almost as old as mankind. A description of alcoholic beverages and some knowledge of their history are useful in understanding their chemical makeup. The first beverages were made from fruits (wine) or grains (beer). Later, distillation was developed and utilized in beverage production in order to achieve a more potent drink.

"For nearly 10,000 years of known Western history, beer and wine, not water, were the major daily thirst quenchers, consumed by all ages" (Vallee, 1994). Not until the nineteenth century were humans able to produce water suitable for consumption.

Wine is the term used for an alcoholic beverage that is made from fruits, herbs, berries, milk, or even from flowers, but generally refers to products made from fermented grapes. Wines are classified according to color—red, rosé (pink), and white. Contrary to popular belief, white or red grapes can be used to make red or white wines. Both red and white grapes have color pigments (white grapes produce dark seedless raisins). The length of time the grape skins are left in the fermenting must (grape juice) determines the color of the wine. In general, red wines are produced by fermenting the must with the skins; for a rosé wine the skins are left in for part of the fermentation; the skins are removed before fermentation for white wine.

The taste is classified as sweet or dry with varying degrees of each. Sweet wines are higher in sugar content than dry wines. Also, high acidity may contribute to the dryness of a wine.

Wines are also classified as table, sparkling, or fortified wines. In table wines the alcohol content ranges from about 7 percent to 15 percent and they may be white, rosé, or red. Sparkling wines are usually white but may be red or rosé with an alcohol content similar to table wines. Fortified wines may be red or white with a higher average alcohol content ranging from 16 percent to 25 percent. The higher alcohol content is provided by adding brandy or some distilled spirit. Fortified wines with added flavoring are called aromatic wines.

Paleontologists have found evidence of grape stems and skins that apparently were from grapes crushed by prehistoric man. Egyptians credit Osiris and the Greeks credit Dionysius with the gift of wine, but the Hebrews claim that Noah first introduced it. Numerous references in the Bible indicate that not only wine but stronger beverages were made. Different Hebrew words were used to describe the wines—*yayin* for common wine, *homer* for fresh, unmixed wine, *tiros* for strong wine, *meseg* for mixed wine, and *sekhor* for strong drink.

Indeed, the church had the single greatest influence on the development of wines. The priests needed wine for the sacramental functions and their major efforts were directed toward improving the vines and the quality of the wine. Padre Junipero, a Dominican missionary, planted the first vines in California, bringing them from Spain. Today, wine is defined as the fermented juice of grapes and other fruits.

Beer is a malted and hopped (the addition of hops, an herb) somewhat bitter beverage. Malt can be made from cereal grains such as rice and wheat, but barley is the main cereal used. Barley is dried until the moisture content is 12 percent to 14 percent and then stored for at least four weeks to overcome its natural dormancy and to render it suitable for uniform germination. Gibberellic acid may be added to speed up the germination rate, and potassium bromate may be added to restrict rootlet formation, which means less sugar energy is used in root production.

During germination, enzymes convert the starches to sugars which are required for fermentation. The maltster knows when to stop the germination process and grind the plant embryo into malt which can then be used to produce beer. The art of brewing is as old as recorded history—over 7,000 years. Archaeologists have found hieroglyphics which represent brewing. Also, from analysis of beer jugs, they have found that barley has been used to produce beer for centuries. The Egyptians made beer from corn, the Chinese made *samshu* and the Japanese made *sake* from rice, while the Russians made *quass* or *kvass* from rye.

William Penn was probably the first to operate a large commercial brewery in America. Beer played an important part in American history. The Pilgrims on the Mayflower would have continued their journey to Virginia but instead landed at Plymouth Rock because, as recorded in their journal, "We could not now take time or further search and considerations, our victuals being spent, especially our beer" (Grossman and Lembeck, 1983).

Distilled spirits are alcoholic beverages in which the concentration of ethyl alcohol has been increased above that of the original fermented mixture. The principle of alcohol distillation is based upon the different boiling points of alcohol (173.3°F or 78.5°C) and water (212°F or 100°C). When the alcohol-containing mixture is heated above 173.3°F, the alcohol begins to vaporize and can be separated from the water.

Distilled spirits have fewer congeners than beer or wine because many substances will not vaporize in the distillation process and are left behind. However, some of the volatile congeners with low boiling points will be concentrated much like the ethyl alcohol.

The first mention of distillation is attributed to Albukasen, an Arabian alchemist of the tenth century. It probably originated with the Arabs or Saracens, as they gave us the words *alcohol* and *alembic*, the latter meaning "still." Distilled spirits are called ardent spirits which comes from the Latin *adere*, meaning "to burn." A popular Spanish brandy is called *aguardiente* (burning water). The following are common examples of distilled spirits.

Absinthe was developed by Dr. Ordinaire, a French physician and pharmacist, while he was exiled in Switzerland. It was one of the most potent alcoholic beverages, with an alcoholic content of 68 percent by volume. Oil of wormwood was the chief flavoring ingredient and other minor ingredients included licorice, hyssop, fennel, aniseed, and star anise. Henry Louis Pernod purchased the formula from Dr. Ordinaire and it was first produced commercially in 1797. It was yellowish-green in color and turned to a cloudy opalescent white when mixed with water. Wormwood came to be considered dangerous because it was thought to cause hallucinations, mental deterioration, and sterility. Switzerland, in 1908, and France, in 1915, prohibited the sale of absinthe. Other countries soon followed suit. Today, similar beverages, lower in alcohol content and without wormwood, are sold under trade names such as Pernod and Ricard.

Aquavit is a clear to pale yellow, dry liquor ranging in alcohol content from 42 percent to 45 percent by volume. It is distilled from fermented potato or grain mash and then redistilled in the presence of various flavoring agents to extract their flavors. Flavoring agents include lemon and orange peel, caraway or cumin seed, cardamom, and aniseed. In Sweden the beverage is call *snops* and the equivalent Danish product is called *schnapps*.

Brandy is an alcoholic liquor distilled from wine or various fermented fruit juices. Reportedly, the best brandies are the cognac and armaqnac, named for the two French regions where they are produced. Most spirits today are distilled in continuous stills. True cognac comes from the traditional pot-still type of distillation. In this process, the first and last runs of brandy are discarded and only the middle or heart is retained. The history of brandy making can be traced to a Dutch shipmaster who hit upon the idea of concentrating wine to reduce freight charges. His plan was to concentrate wine by eliminating the water in France and transporting the spirit to Holland where it could be diluted with water. The Dutch liked the taste of the concentrate, however, and decided it would be a waste of water to try to return it to its original state. The new product was called *brandewyn*, a Dutch word for "burned wine."

Gin is a distilled liquor usually made from grain and flavored principally with the juniper berry which is responsible for its name. Juniper in French is *genièvre*. The name was altered by the Dutch to *genever* and shortened by the English to *gin*. Gin producers use botanicals such as orris, angelica, licorice root, caraway, coriander, cardamom, anise, fennel, and orange and lemon oils to provide a unique flavor to their product. Franciscus Sylvius, a professor of medicine at the University of Leyden in Holland, invented gin. His objective was a medicinal product. He felt that by redistilling pure alcohol with the juniper berry he could obtain the natural diuretic properties of the plant in an inexpensive form. In the seventeenth century, English soldiers, returning home, brought back gin and in no time it became the national drink of England, a position it stills holds today.

Vodka is a clear beverage without much taste or flavor of its own and an alcohol content of 33 percent to 45 percent by volume. Potatoes are frequently used in Russia and Poland to produce vodka while cereal grains are more frequently used in the United States. Vodka combines well with other beverages without imparting much flavor of its own. This makes vodka drinks such as the "screwdriver," made with orange juice, and the "bloody Mary," made with tomato juice, very popular. Some vodkas are flavored with buffalo grass, lemon peel, berries, peppercorns, or caraway. Vodka originated in Russia during the fourteenth century. *Vodka* means "little water" in Russian.

Liqueurs are flavored and sweetened distilled beverages with an alcohol content ranging from 24 percent to 60 percent by volume. Liqueurs are usually produced by combining a basic spirit such as brandy with herb and fruits and sweetening them with a syrup at a concentration of 2.5 percent or more by volume. Fruit liqueurs are produced by the infusion method whereby fruit is steeped in the spirit, which absorbs the color, flavor, and aroma.

Plant liqueurs are made by percolating or distilling a beverage in the presence of plants, seeds, roots, or herbs. In the percolator the plant material is placed in the top section and the bottom section holds the beverage. The process is much the same as that of percolating coffee.

Popular liqueur flavors are apricot, pineapple, crème de cacao, mint and coffee (Kahlua). *Ocha* is a Japanese liqueur flavored with green tea. The British make Drambuie with a Scotch whiskey base. Cherry Heering (made from cherries) comes from Denmark, Triple Sec and Grand Marnier (both made from orange peel) are produced in the Cognac region of France, and Galliano is made in Italy; the United States produces Creme Yvette and Forbidden Fruit, among others.

Okolehao, also referred to as **Oke**, is a product of Hawaii. Okolehao was first made about 1790 by an Australian, William Stevenson, who cooked the sacred ti root and allowed the mash, rich in fructose, to ferment in the bottom of a canoe. Next, he distilled the fermented mash using the ship's cooking

pot and a water-cooled gun barrel for a coil. Today, a modern distillery is used. Okolehao is not aged but is filtered through charcoal.

Pulque is the fermented juice of the mezcal plant, which is a species of Agave. It is distilled to make a brandy called maguey. In Mexico a species of Agave (*A. atrovirens*) is known as *maguey*. The best mescal is grown near Tequila, Mexico, and it is used to make the pulque which is distilled to make tequila, named for the city near which the natural plant is grown.

Rum is any alcoholic beverage made from distillates of sugar cane, molasses, or other sugar cane products. It has been made in the West Indies for more than 300 years. Aroax is a rum produced in Java and owes many of its characteristics to the wild yeast, *Saccharomyces vordermanni* which is used in its production.

The word **whiskey** comes from the Scottish and Irish word *usquebaugh* (pronounced "us kwibo"), meaning "water of life." Scotch whiskey is obtained primarily from barley. The grain is soaked in water and when the sprouts are about three quarters of an inch long they are transferred to a kiln. The green malt, as the sprouts are called, is placed on a screen directly above a peat fire which provides the acrid and oily smoke which gives Scotch whiskey part of its unique flavor. Until 1853, Scotch whiskeys were either straight malt or straight grain whiskeys. Then Andrew Usher and Company began the practice or blending malt and grain, achieving blended Scotch whiskey. A Scotch whiskey blend can easily contain thirty to forty malt whiskeys with five or more grain whiskeys. The secret of fine Scotch whiskey lies in the art of the blender. The depth of color is governed by the amount or caramel and burned sugar used to produce a uniform color.

Two different yeasting processes are currently used in America: sour mash and sweet mash. In the sour-mash process, at least one quarter of the fermenting mash comes from a previous distillation which is mixed with fresh mash and allowed to ferment from seventy-two to ninety-six hours. Sweet mash, also known as a yeast mash, is processed totally from fresh mash and allowed to ferment from thirty-six to fifty hours. The acid pH of sour mash inhibits bacterial contamination, making it easier to control than sweet mash, which must be processed above 80°F to help avoid contamination.

Canadian whiskey, contrary to popular belief, is not a rye whiskey but is made from corn, rye, wheat, and barley, with no one grain making up more than 50 percent of the whole.

Scotch whiskey gets its smoky flavor from peat, a partially carbonized vegetable matter, usually mosses, found in bogs. Irish whiskey has a similar barley malt character without the smoky flavor. Scotch and Irish whiskeys are lighter in body than American straight whiskeys because they are aged longer—seven to twelve years. Maturation in previously used cooperage, wooden containers, requires a longer period. American whiskeys are charred in new oak cooperage which makes an earlier maturation possible. However, the longer maturation period practiced in Ireland and Scotland allows for formation or more esters which provide greater depth of flavor.

1.2 Fermentation

In general, alcoholic beverages can be produced from any substance that contains sufficient sugar or starch. Beverages fall into three basic categories: (1) fermented beverages which are made from agricultural products such as grapes or other fruits and grains, (2) distilled or spirituous beverages, and (3) compounded beverages which are made by combining fermented and distilled beverages with flavoring substances (Grossman et al., 1983). The chemical process or fermentation was formulated by Gay-Lussac in 1810; one molecule of sugar (glucose) was shown to result in two molecules of ethanol and two molecules of carbon dioxide. This equation can be written as

$$(C_6H_{12}O_6) \rightarrow 2(CH_3CH_2OH) + 2(CO_2) .$$

Theoretically, 180 grams of glucose should produce 92 grams of ethanol and 88 grams of carbon dioxide which would yield 51.1 percent of the weight of sugar fermented as ethanol. The actual yield is only 48 percent because the yeast uses energy to produce a series of compounds other than alcohol, and some sugar is used to synthesize new yeast cells. Byproducts include acetaldehyde, higher molecular weight alcohols (fusel oil), and other fermentation and flavoring chemicals.

The conversion of sugar to alcohol requires at least a dozen enzymes in a sequence of chemical reactions called the Embden-Meyerhof pathway. The 6-carbon sugars are converted to fructose-1, 6-diphosphate which is split into two 3-carbon triose phosphates. These are dihydroxyacetone phosphate and glyceraldehyde-3-phosphate, which are converted to two molecules of pyruvic acid. The pyruvic acid is converted to acetaldehyde and carbon dioxide as gas bubbles. The acetaldehyde is converted to ethanol, drinking alcohol. Some glycerin is produced in every wine fermentation, ranging from 0.2 percent to 1.5 percent. More may be produced in the presence of high amounts of bisulfite. Glycerol is slightly sweet and contributes to the "body" of wine. Some pyruvic acid is converted to alanine, an amino acid, and a small amount of pyruvic acid is changed to lactic acid. A portion of the acetaldehyde is converted to acetic acid (vinegar). Undesirable bacterial contamination can result in too much acetic acid and ruin the wine.

It is the minor constituents that are of major importance to the flavor and aroma of alcoholic beverages. These important esters and other aromatic components determine the quality and distinctive characteristics of the various beverages. Fusel oils, including 5-carbon or amyl alcohols, 4-carbon butanols, and 3-carbon propyl alcohols compose less than 0.01 percent of wine. Also, some yeast cells die and "leak" or break up (autolyze) and contribute constituents to the solution. In addition to yeast, other microorganisms produce flavor substances.

As an alternative to sugar, beverages can be made from grains rich in starch, which converts to sugar, the grains are allowed to sprout which results in an enzyme called amylase. This phenomenon was first understood in the 1930s and the enzyme was then called diastase, from the Greek *diastasis* meaning "separation." Today, in the beverage industry, amylase and diastase are used interchangeably. Amylase acts to separate large starch molecules into the simple sugar maltose. Once this step has occurred, the sugar can be converted to alcohol by the familiar process of fermentation. This process is illustrated schematically in Figure 1.1.

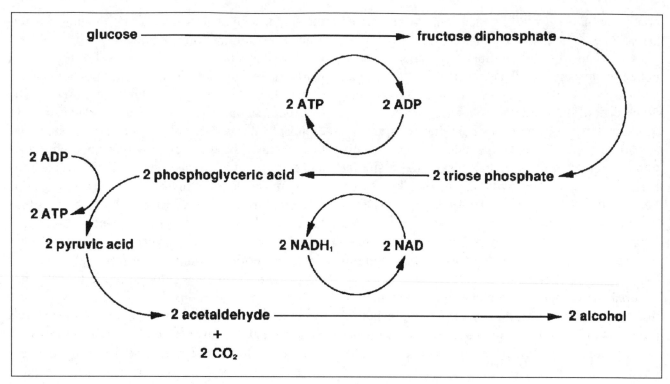

Figure 1.1 Diagram of fermentation

A. Yeasts

The flavor composition of beverages is markedly altered by the yeast fermentation process. Generally, the dominant beverage flavor constituents are formed during yeast fermentation (Schreier, 1979). The yeast species can affect the flavor and chemical composition considerably. For example, the amount of D(–)-lactic acid depends on the yeast species. Saccharomyces rose forms relatively small amounts of lactic acid (about 100 mg/L) whereas the formation of lactic acid is much higher (about 1,800 mg/L) when *S. veronae* is used. The common beverage yeasts are *S. carlsbergensis* (lager beer), *S. cerevisiae* (ale), and the sulfur dioxide-resistant *S. ellipsoideus* (California wine).

B. Bacterial contamination

The alcohol fermentation process must be carefully guarded against undesirable microorganisms which can impair the quality of or even spoil the beverage. Bacteria such as *Enterobacteriaceae*, originating in the intestine of warm-blooded animals, have been found in beverages (Van Vuuren et al., 1981). These microorganisms can affect the congener content by producing different chemical substances which, in turn, can be used to detect bacterial contamination. For example, D(–)-lactic acid is formed by yeasts but L(+)-lactic acid is produced by bacteria (Schreier, 1979). High amounts of acetic acid also indicate spoilage, usually by *Acetobacter* (Kupina et al., 1982).

1.3 Nutritional Value of Alcoholic Beverages

There is general agreement among nutritionists that the modern Western diet contains too much alcohol (Chatton and Ullman, 1984). Americans consumed 2.43 gallons of absolute ethanol per person in 1989 (Williams and DeBakey, 1992). Alcohol provides seven calories per gram compared to nine calories per gram for fats and four calories per gram for protein and carbohydrates. The caloric values of some common beverages are provided in Table 1.1.

Some people survive almost completely on alcoholic beverages. Excessive intake can contribute to malnutrition in several ways. It may depress appetite, displace food, or affect gastrointestinal absorption or digestion. Through its effect on the liver, it can alter the utilization of nutrients.

**Table 1.1
Caloric Content of
Some Common Alcoholic Beverages**

Beverage	Calories
Beer (8 oz)	110
Ale (8 oz)	150
Gin (1 oz)	
80 proof	65
86 proof	88
Rum (1 oz)	70
Whiskey (1 oz)	80
Wine (3 oz)	
Red	145
White	90
Vermouth, sweet (1 oz)	50
Manhattan (3 oz)	165
Martini (3 oz)	140

From Guthrie, 1983

As a general rule, distilled beverages contain few, if any, vitamins and minerals, but beers and wines can contain significant amounts.

A. Carbohydrates

Distilled beverages do not contain carbohydrates unless they are added after distillation because sugars do not vaporize during the distillation process. Beers and wines contain varying amounts of carbohydrates.

Approximately 50 percent of the energy obtained from the average American diet comes from carbohydrates (Guthrie, 1983). It is now recommended that this amount be decreased to 40 percent with dietary fat and protein each providing 30 percent of the remaining calories (Chatton and Ullman, 1984).

The average adult consumes approximately 300 grams of carbohydrates each day. This is the amount of carbohydrates contained in approximately fifteen quarts of beer or wine that is 2 percent carbohydrate. A quart of one of the very sweet liqueurs contains approximately 300 grams of carbohydrate. The carbohydrate content of several types of beverages is given in Table 1.2.

B. Proteins

The recommended daily allowance of protein for the average adult is 44 grams for women and 56 grams for men. Little of this can be obtained from alcoholic beverages because alcohol causes protein to precipitate. In wines and beers this precipitate is usually filtered out during bottling. Protein is not volatile and therefore is not found in distilled beverages. Wines contain 0.1 to 2.0 g/L and beers from 0.63 to 6.2 g/L of protein (Pirola, 1978).

This means that an adult would need to consume several gallons of beer or wine each day to get the recommended daily allowance (RDA) of protein. For example, a man would need to drink from 9 to 90 quarts of beer daily. As you can see, beer is not rich in protein, and wine and other alcoholic beverages usually contain even less. For this reason many alcoholics are protein-deficient which can severely restrict the immune system and other natural functions of the human body.

C. Fats

The fruits and grains used to make beverages are very low in fat. They are selected for their carbohydrate content and for this reason most alcoholic beverages contain little or no fat. Beer contains the most

**Table 1.2
Carbohydrate Content of Selected Beverages**

Beverage	Total Carbohydrate (%)	Source
Beers	2.1–8.3	Pirola, 1978
Wines	2.0–12.0	Ondus et al., 1983
Sprite	10.3	Ondus et al., 1983
Cola	12.3	Ondus et al., 1983
Apple juice	10.4	Ondus et al., 1983
Liqueurs	2.5–35	Grossman and Lembeck, 1983

fat with an average fat content of 0.06 percent (Watt and Merill, 1963).

D. Vitamins and minerals

Only beers and wines contain vitamins. They are not usually found in distilled beverages. The RDA for various vitamins can be compared to their content in selected beverages by referring to Tables 1.3 and 1.4. The reader will note that beers contain more B vitamins than wines in most cases, but nicotinic acid is the only vitamin that is in sufficient quantity to meet the RDA. Both wines and beers contain extremely variable amounts of minerals. Many lay reports state that various beverages are high in some vitamins or minerals, but one cannot rely on obtaining vitamins or minerals from alcoholic beverages.

1.4 Antimicrobial Properties of Alcoholic Beverages

Both antibiotic (Asmus et al., 1983) and antiviral properties (Konowalchuk and Speirs, 1976) have been attributed to nondistilled alcoholic beverages. Lincomycin is a medium-spectrum antibiotic that is produced during fermentation of beers and wines. A mixture of lincomycin A and lincomycin B is produced with a reported total concentration ranging

Table 1.3
Vitamin Content of Wines and Beers (mg/L)

Vitamins	Wines[1]	Beers[1]	Recommended Daily Allowance (mg)[2]
Thiamine (vitamin B$_1$)	0–240	20–60	1.0–1.5
Riboflavin (vitamin B$_2$)	60–220	300–1200	1.2–1.7
Pantothenic acid	70–450	400–900	4.0–7.0
Pyridoxine (vitamin B$_6$)	220–820	400–900	1.7–2.0
Nicotinic acid	410–960	5,000–20,000	1.3–1.9
Cobalamin (vitamin B$_{12}$)	0.009–0.025		0.002
Folic acid	15–21		0.2
Biotin	0.6–4.6	0–15	.05–0.1

[1] From Pirola, 1978

[2] RDA-10th Rev. 1990 NTL-AC.Science

Table 1.4
Mineral Content of Wines and Beers (mg/L)

Mineral	Wines[1]	Beers[1]	RDA (mg)
Chloride	10–80		1,700–5,100
Calcium	29–99	20–70	800–1,200
Copper	0–9	T–0.40	1.5–3.0
Iron	0–20	T–0.64	10–15
Potassium	180–1,620	130–1,040	1,875–5,625
Sodium	10–200	68–550	1,100–3,300
Fluoride	1–10	0.1–0.9	1.5–4.0
Phosphate	30–900	50–300	800–1,200
Magnesium	10–350	50–300	270–350
Manganese	T–51	—	2.5–5.0
Iodide	T[2]	—	0.15
Chromium		0.5–22.0 mg/L	0.05–0.2
Selenium		0.2–2.50 mg/L	0.04–0.007

[1] From Pirola, 1976; Zee et al., 1983; Robberecht et al., 1984

[2] RDA = recommended daily allowance; T = trace amounts

from 340 to 10,020 m/L in alcoholic beverages (Asmus, 1983).

The recommended oral dose of lincomycin for adults is 500 mg every six to eight hours (Weinstein, 1975). A comparison of the recommended oral dose with the reported fermentation concentrations supports the anecdotal reports that certain alcoholic beverages may have antibiotic properties.

Lincomycin was first isolated from soil collected near Lincoln, Nebraska, and the drug was first reported in the literature in 1962. The adverse effects are diarrhea, nausea, vomiting, skin rashes, and vaginitis (Weinstein, 1975). Because of the possible unwanted effects, there are few if any valid reasons to use lincomycin (Sonde and Mandell, 1980).

Antiviral activity has been demonstrated in a variety of wines, and in grape juice the activity was demonstrable in fractions of juice varying in molecular weight from 1,000 to 30,000 as determined by membrane filtration (Konowalchuk and Speirs, 1976).

This area of study is fascinating and further research could explain some of the varying effects observed in different individuals. For example, as many as 20 percent of patients who take lincomycin orally have diarrhea as a side effect (Weinstein, 1975), and many beverage drinkers report having diarrhea from drinking certain alcoholic beverages. These studies also support the practice of the Egyptian warriors who were instructed to mix wine with their drinking water to disinfect it and reduce illness.

1.5 Cancer and Alcohol

Epidemiologic studies find that alcoholics are at higher risk of getting cancer (Hoeft and Obe, 1983). Some tests implicate acetaldehyde as the mutagen (Obe, 1980). Some of the nonvolatile residues have been shown to induce mutations (Hoeft and Obe, 1983).

The high incidence of esophageal cancer in certain areas has been correlated with the mutagenic activity of acrolein, butyrolactone, furfural, and glycidol, usually found in certain brandies (Loquet et al., 1981). The Institute of Public Health in the Netherlands found that beer was the major source of nitrosamine, contributing, in the late 1970s, 71 percent of the average daily intake (Stephany and Schuller, 1980). As a result of concern over this carcinogenic activity, the beverage manufacturers have taken steps to remove the suspected carcinogens or reduce them to acceptable levels.

1.6 Ethyl Alcohol Content

By definition, any drinkable liquid containing from 0.5 percent to 95 percent ethyl alcohol is an alcoholic beverage. Before scientific methods, beverage strength was measured by mixing equal amounts of spirit and gunpowder. When ignited, if the mixture did not burn it was too weak. If it burned too rapidly it was too strong; an even blue flame meant the beverage was proved. Today, we know this concentration to be about 50 percent alcohol, and the term proof is used to describe the strength of alcoholic beverages. Proof is just about twice the percentage of the alcohol concentration of a beverage. For example, 50 percent alcohol by volume equals approximately 100 proof. (Since alcohol causes water to contract, fifty parts alcohol + 53.73 parts H_2O gives not 103.73 parts mixture, but 100. Proof is slightly more than double.) The ethyl alcohol content of some selected beverages is provided in Table 1.5.

1.7 Congeners

Ethyl alcohol is the major physiologically active component of most alcoholic beverages. Together with water, it makes up the greater part of the alcoholic drink. The remaining fraction is collectively made up of compounds called congeners. Although quantitatively small, congeners play a crucial and often overlooked role in the social use and abuse of alcoholic beverages.

Congeners may be highly volatile (easily evaporated) compounds consisting of a variety of alcohols (in addition to ethanol), acids, aldehydes, ketones, and esters. Other components of alcoholic beverages, sometimes also termed congeners, include carbohydrates, tannins, phenols, metals, coloring agents, vitamins, minerals, histamine, and other pharmacologically active agents. Current data indicate that the congener content of commercial alcoholic beverages differs significantly for each type of beverage (Greizerstein, 1981).

Table 1.5
Ethyl Alcohol Content of Selected Beverages

Beverage	Percent
Beers (lager)	3.2–4.0
Ales	4.5
Porter	6.0
Stout	6.0–8.0
Malt liquor	3.2–7.0
Sake	14.00–16.0
Table wines	7.1–14.0
Sparkling wines	8.0–14.0
Fortified wines	14.0–24.0
Aromatized wines	15.5–20.0
Brandies	40.0–43.0
Whiskies	40.0–75.0
Vodkas	40.0–50.0
Gins	40.0–48.5
Rum	40.0–95.0
Aquavit	35.0–45.0
Okolehao	40.0
Tequila	45.0–50.5

From Grossman and Lembeck, 1983

Congeners are responsible for the variable taste, aroma, and color of different beverages. Some have nutrient and medicinal effects and others may have toxic effects, even though quantities may be small. Some congeners are derived from primary plant materials, some from the fermentation process, and others come from the aging process, for example, by contact with wooden containers.

Consumers of alcoholic beverages have noticed for years that certain beverages appear to have a more pronounced effect than others, immediately upon consumption as well as in the post-drinking period. Before 1958, no literature existed concerning the analysis of alcoholic beverages by gas liquid chromatography (Carrol, 1970). In the 1960s, with new analytical techniques and with increased knowledge of the effects of alcoholic beverages, the questions of the relationship between the congeners and the effects of the beverage became subject to experimental inquiry. The nature of these congeners and other components of alcoholic beverages is the subject of this chapter.

1.8 Classification of Congeners

Hundreds of different chemicals have been detected in alcoholic beverages (Schreier, 1979). With today's advanced analytical equipment, thousands of congeners can be identified in beverages, but full understanding of their significance will take many years of research.

The congeners can be classified in accordance with the analytical methods used for their analysis. They can be divided into acid, basic and neutral fractions designated as volatile, semivolatile and nonvolatile. The nonvolatile fractions can be divided into minerals, vitamins, carbohydrates and proteins.

Modern analytical methods can be used to identify congeners responsible for the taste and quality of a beverage (Marais et al., 1981), and its chemical components can be used to identify the geographic region in which the beverage was produced (Brown and Clapperton, 1978; Marais et al., 1981).

In this section only the major volatile congeners and those having the greatest impact on the quality and character of the beverage will be discussed.

A. Volatile congeners

The many volatile congeners which, in addition to ethyl alcohol, make up an alcoholic beverage are responsible for its taste and aroma and many of them can have pharmacologic effects.

While thousands of different volatile congeners may be found in various beverages at one time or another, several have been found to be consistently present. Acetaldehyde, ethyl acetate, ethyl formate, and the small aliphatic alcohol make up the major volatile congener content of beers, wines, and distilled spirits.

B. Alcohols

In addition to ethyl alcohol, more than forty-five different alcohols have been identified in alcoholic beverages (Schrier, 1979). When starch is the sugar source, a mixture of primary alcohols is produced, consisting mostly of isopentyl alcohol with smaller amounts of n-propyl alcohol, isobutyl alcohol, and normal butyl alcohol. This mixture is commonly called fusel oil from the German *Fusel*, meaning inferior liquor (Morrison and Boyd, 1983).

Methyl alcohol is the simplest, lowest molecular weight alcohol, yet it is the most toxic of all, due to its metabolic products. Methyl alcohol is also known as methanol, wood spirit, carbinol, wood alcohol, methylol and colonial spirit. Severe poisoning and death have occurred primarily from ingestion of beverages adulterated with methyl alcohol.

Typically, within eighteen to forty-eight hours after ingestion, the victim develops acidosis, nausea, abdominal pain, headache, shortness of breath, and blurred or double vision. Severely poisoned individuals become comatose and may die, and those who recover can be left blind (Proctor and Hughes, 1978). In the body, methanol is oxidized to formaldehyde and formic acid. Both of these metabolites are very toxic (Cleland and Kingsbury, 1977). Ethyl alcohol competes with methyl alcohol for the alcohol metabolizing system. For this reason, ethyl alcohol is given in the treatment of methyl alcohol poisoning. The best treatment so far is a combination of hemodialysis to remove the methanol, and the administration of ethanol to inhibit the metabolism of methanol and reduce the rate of production of the more toxic metabolite. Sodium bicarbonate is used to correct the acidosis.

Ethyl alcohol (ethanol, ethyl hydroxide, grain alcohol, methyl carbinol) is an irritant to the eyes and mucous membranes, and causes CNS depression. The second smallest alcohol next to methanol, it is a clear, colorless, flammable liquid with a burning taste. Ethyl alcohol is rapidly oxidized in the body and converted to carbon dioxide and water. It has also been found in public drinking water samples in concentrations of 5 mg/L. The Environmental Protection Agency (EPA) has established 26 mg/L as the estimated permissible concentration in drinking water (Cleland and Kingsbury, 1977).

N-propyl alcohol (ethylcarbinol, propanol) is a potent narcotic similar to ethyl alcohol. It is slightly more toxic than isopropyl alcohol and at very high dosages has produced cancer in rats. Public drinking water samples have been shown to contain 1.0 mg/L; the EPA has established 6.9 mg/L as the estimated permissible concentration in water (Cleland and Kingsbury, 1977).

Isobutyl alcohol (isobutanol, 2-methyl-1-propanol) is a clear, sweet-smelling liquid. It acts as a narcotic at high concentrations, and is more toxic than n-butanol alcohol. Isobutyl alcohol, like ethyl alcohol, causes central nervous system (CNS) depression. The EPA has established as the estimated permissible concentration in drinking water 2.07 mg/L (Cleland and Kingsbury, 1977).

N-butyl alcohol, also known as n-butanol, is a colorless volatile liquid; the estimated permissible concentration for drinking water is 2.07 mg/L (Cleland and Kingsbury, 1977).

Isopentyl alcohol (isoamyl alcohol, isobutyl carbinol) has a disagreeable, pungent odor. Like the other alcohols, it causes CNS depression. The EPA has set 5.0 mg/L as the estimated permissible concentration in drinking water (Cleland and Kingsbury, 1977).

Fermentation has been taking place since yeast first appeared on the earth, and, as mentioned above, many of the alcohols are found in drinking water supplies. It is interesting to compare the EPA criteria to the actual concentrations found in alcoholic beverages (Table 1.6). Many beverages exceed the recommended water limits for the congeners.

Table 1.6
Alcohol Content of Beverages Compared to EPA Water Criteria (mg/L)

Beverages	Ethyl Alcohol	Methyl Alcohol	N-Propyl Alcohol	Isopropyl Alcohol	N-Butyl Alcohol	Isopentyl Alcohol
Beers	33,000–40,000	6–27	16–124	15–109	1–6	44–248
Wines	88,000–144,000	96–329	96–329	54–109	2–15	115–166
Distilled spirits	153,000–392,000	3.3–220	1–122	1–296	1–17	1–381
EPA[1]	26.0	3.6	6.9	2.07	2.07	5.0

[1] EPA's estimated permissible concentration in drinking water (Cleland and Kingsbury, 1977). Current EPA recommendations do not list these alcohols (EPA National Recommended Water Quality Criteria: 2002). From Greizerstein, 1981.

C. Aldehydes

Only a few aldehydes have been detected in alcoholic beverages. Probably, because of the sulfur dioxide treatment, many of the aldehydes are converted to bisulfite addition products which, because of their high water solubility, escape detection. Twenty-seven aldehydes have been identified in grapes (Schreier, 1979).

Acetaldehyde (acetic aldehyde, ethanal, ethyl aldehyde) is colorless with a fruity aroma and is found in most alcoholic beverages. Like drinking alcohol, acetaldehyde is a CNS depressant. It has been found in public drinking water supplies at concentrations of 0.0001 mg/L; the EPA's estimated permissible concentration in drinking water is 2.45 mg/L (Cleland and Kingsbury, 1977).

Only trace amounts of the other aldehydes have been reported in beverages. Cinnamaldehyde, which is used commercially as a flavoring agent, has been detected in wines (Schreier, 1979).

D. Esters

The aroma of beverages is strongly influenced by esters developed during the yeast fermentation. Predominantly, ethyl, isobutyl, and isopentyl esters have been detected, but the list of identified esters surpasses 100 (Schreier, 1979). Some common esters with their reported concentrations are given in Table 1.7. Ethyl acetate and ethyl formate are potentially pharmacologically active.

Table 1.7
Common Esters Found
in Alcoholic Beverages (mg/L)

Compound	Concentration Range
Ethyl formate	T–166.0
Ethyl acetate	T–285.0
Isobutyl acetate	T–0.2
Isopentyl acetate	T–8.0
Hexyl acetate	0.1–2.0
2-Phenethyl acetate	T–2.6
Ethyl propionate	T–1.2
Ethyl 2-hydroxypropanoate	10–400
Ethyl hexanoate	0.1–2.0
Ethyl octanoate	0.2–1.5
Ethyl laurate	T–0.4
Diethyl succinate	0.8–20.0

Ethyl acetate (acetic ester, ethyl ethanoate) has a potent fruity odor. It causes extreme depression of the CNS and in high doses induces narcosis.

Ethyl formate (formic ether, ethyl methanoate) is used as a solvent for cellulose nitrate, in synthetic flavors, and as a fumigant. It also causes CNS depression.

E. Alcohols, aldehydes and esters

Up to the present, most alcohol research has been conducted on ethyl alcohol since it is the alcohol found in beverages in the highest concentration However, people do not drink pure ethyl alcohol. Alcoholic beverages contain other alcohols as well as aldehydes and esters that have effects similar to ethyl alcohol.

Generally speaking, these can produce gastric irritation when swallowed and, in higher doses, cause headache, nausea and vomiting. The higher molecular weight alcohols are absorbed more slowly than ethyl alcohol so their effects are felt later than those of ethyl alcohol. Also, the body cannot eliminate these alcohols as quickly as it eliminates ethyl alcohol so their effects last longer. This helps explain the common complaint of some drinkers that when they drink a particular beverage, they wake up drunk the next day.

The individual and total congener content of some common beverages is provided in Table 1.8. Because of their volatility, congeners are evaporated along with ethyl alcohol during distillation, giving distilled beverages the highest concentration of congeners compared with other beverages. However, by taking into account the standard drink sizes for beers (12 ounces), wines (four ounces), and distilled beverages (1.5 ounces), beers and wines contain the highest congener content on a per drink basis.

This is consistent with studies showing that beer and wine produce the most severe hangovers (Haag et al., 1959), and that the severity of the hangover is greater after drinking whiskey than after consuming equivalent amounts of vodka (Chapman, 1970), which contains less congeners.

The threshold limit values (TLVs) are provided at the bottom of Table 1.8 to help evaluate the relative potency of the congeners. It will be noted that ethyl alcohol is the least hazardous alcohol, based on

Table 1.8
Congener and Ethanol Content per Standard Drink of Beer (mg/12 oz), Wine (mg/4 oz) and Distilled Spirits (mg/1.5oz)

	Total Congener Content	Acetaldehye	Ethyl Formate	Ethyl Acetate	Methanol	N-propanol	Isobutanol	N-butanol	Isopentanol	Ethanol
Beers										
Budweiser	142.5	12.2	13.9	6.8	6.7	42.3	37.1	0.6	22.9	13,600
Michelob	48.6	3.5	9.2	2.6	2.3	8.0	5.4	1.6	16.0	13,600
Miller	64.3	4.6	14.1	3.0	9.2	5.4	5.0	1.7	21.3	13,000
Genesse	55.1	4.7	7.6	3.3	6.2	8.5	9.6	0.2	15.0	12,300
Genesee Cream	76.9	7.5	11.3	3.1	2.4	12.0	13.1	1.2	26.4	11,900
Michelob Lite	120.1	4.5	4.0	1.1	2.1	8.1	13.9	1.9	84.5	11,300
Wines										
Taylor Tawny Port	93.7	14.1	7.5	3.4	36.5	6.1	6.8	0.4	18.9	16,400
Widmer port	115.8	29.6	4.1	10.0	37.4	7.2	10.8	1.7	15.0	16,400
Martini Rossi dry vermouth	108.4	26.0	17.8	2.8	33.2	7.6	7.2	0.7	13.1	15,900
Cinzano sweet vermouth	58.6	7.7	2.9	1.7	14.2	6.1	9.6	1.1	15.3	14,000
Gallo Burgundy	62.9	8.1	4.0	1.2	17.2	5.3	6.1	0.2	20.8	10,900
Almaden rose	77.3	9.0	18.9	2.0	10.9	7.2	12.4	0.5	16.4	10,000
Distilled spirits										
Smirnoff vodka 100°	8.5	0.4	0.7	0.2	1.6	2.1	3.3	0.1	0.2	16,700
J & B scotch	20.3	1.2	0.6	0.8	2.4	2.6	5.8	0.1	6.8	14,100
Coronet Brandy	36.5	1.1	0.9	0.4	9.4	3.4	4.4	0.7	16.2	13,900
Gordon's Dry Gin	6.8	0.5	0.9	0.3	1.0	3.4	0.1	0.1	0.7	13,800
Smirnoff vodka 60°	15.7	0.4	1.9	0.2	1.6	4.4	7.0	0.1	0.2	13,600
Bacardi light rum	16.8	0.6	0.8	0.3	5.6	3.4	2.5	0.1	3.6	13,500
Chex vodka 60°	9.2	0.3	0.7	0.3	0.8	3.3	0.1	0.1	3.8	13,400
Hiram Walker whiskey	11.5	1.9	2.6	0.4	1.5	1.2	1.5	0.1	2.4	13,400
Dewar's scotch	48.6	1.1	1.5	0.4	2.4	5.2	12.6	0.2	25.2	13,300
Schnapps	12.8	0.2	0.5	0.1	0.7	2.4	5.7	0.1	3.2	10,200
Amaretto liqueur	13.2	0.7	0.9	0.1	1.1	0.1	10.5	0.1	0.1	6,500
TLV mg/m³		360	300	1400	260	500	300	450	360	1,900

TLV = threshold limit values; see text. From Greizerstein, 1981.

the TLVs. For example, the average adult inhales ten cubic meters of air in eight hours (Cleland and Kingsbury, 1977), and the TLV of ethanol is 1,900 mg/m³. Thus in eight hours an average adult could consume 1,900 mg/m³ × 10 m³ per eight hours = 19,000 milligrams per eight hours. This is a little over 0.5 ounce in eight hours, and would result in no detectable effects.

Threshold limit values are the concentration limits set by the National Institute for Occupational Safety and Health as permissible exposure limits (Proctor and Hughes, 1978). The TLV for ethanol (1,900 mg/m³) is four to seven times higher than that for other congeners, which reflects their higher toxicity.

The total amount of congener per drink, as shown in Table 1.8, varies from 6.8 mg/L to 48.6 mg/L in distilled beverages and from 48.6 mg/L to 142.5 mg/L for beers and wine. Many investigators feel that the effects of these congeners need to be considered when assessing health problems caused by excessive alcoholic beverage consumption (Greizerstein, 1981).

F. Common Acids

Over 130 different acids have been identified in alcoholic beverages. The predominant acids in grapes are malate, tartrate, and citrate acids, with malate and tartrate acids accounting for over 90 percent of the total acid content. Many acids are natural byproducts of alcohol fermentation.

Acetic acid is a normal by-product of yeast metabolism during the early stages of alcohol fermentation. It is found in good wines and may range in concentration from 300 mg/L to 500 mg/L. Higher concentrations indicate spoilage by microorganisms, usually *Acetobacter*. This can make the wine undrinkable. The legal limit of volatile acidity in California is 1,200 mg/L for red wine and 1,100 mg/L for white wine (Kupina et al., 1982).

Generally, the dominant flavor constituents of wine are formed during yeast fermentation with the formation of the volatile acids. The acid content of wine is used to differentiate between species or varieties of grapes, fruits, and growing conditions. Naturally occurring acids such as transgeranoic acid that are not produced or changed by fermentation are used for this purpose (Schreier, 1979). Some common acids in alcoholic beverages are listed in Table 1.9.

G. Ketones

3-Hydroxy-2-butanone (acetoin) and the diketones are produced during the fermentation process. The acetoin concentration is usually in the range of approximately 2 to 32 mg/L but sherry can contain up to 350 mg/L (Schreier, 1979). Mainly they contribute flavor to the beverages but they can have pharmacologic properties. Acetone, for example, like ethyl alcohol, depresses the CNS.

Table 1.9
Common Acids in Alcoholic Beverages (mg/L)

Compound	Biogenesis	Concentration
Acetic acid	F, B	T–1,000
Succinic acid	F	100–2,000
Malic acid	G	500–5,000
Tartaric acid	G	1,000–2,000
Citric acid	G	130–400
Pyruvic acid	F	8–50
2-Hydroxpropenoic acid	B	0.1–3000
Gluconic acid	D	T–2,500
Galacturonic acid (0-coumaric)	F, D	10–2,000
Lactic acid	beers	500–800

F = yeast fermentation, B = bacterial origin, G = grapes, D = other origin, T = traces. From Schreier, 1979; Pirola, 1978.

H. Phenols

Both volatile and nonvolatile phenols have been detected in alcoholic beverages (Lehtonen, 1983b). Phenols produce a smoky aroma in alcoholic drinks and other foods. Scotch whisky owes some of its smoky character to phenolic compounds (Lehtonen, 1983a).

The nonvolatile phenolic compounds enter distilled beverages during the aging process by alcoholysis of lignin in the oak barrels. Lignin dissolves in the beverage and then decomposes into many phenolic compounds (Otsuka and Imai, 1964).

The volatile phenols found in beverages include phenol, *o*-cresol, *m*-cresol, *p*-cresol, guaiacol, *p*-ethylphenol, *p*-ethylguaiacol, eugenol, and *p*-(*n*-propyl)-guaiacol in concentrations ranging from 0 to 2 mg/L (Lehtonen, 1983a). Lehtonen also found that the cresols occurred only in Scotch, Spanish, and Japanese whiskeys as a consequence of the raw materials used, especially peated malt. Also, *p*-(*n*-propyl)-guaiacol was found only in dark rum.

The nonvolatile phenols in distilled alcoholic beverages have been detected in concentrations ranging from 0 to 11 mg/L. Gallic acid and syringaldehyde were the main components (Lehtonen, 1983b). In addition, vanillic acid, syringic acid, vanillin, and ferulic acid were the minor phenolic compounds detected. High concentrations of nonvolatile phenols have been detected in wines in ranges of 0 to 123.9 mg/L with catechin, epicathechin, and caftaric acid making up the major phenolics, while gallic acid, couteric acid, astilbin, and engeletin were the minor phenols.

As little as 10 grams of phenol may be lethal (Proctor and Hughes, 1991). Symptoms of phenol poisoning include anorectic weight loss, weakness, and liver and kidney damage. The cresols have approximately the same toxicity as phenol, causing CNS depression, mental confusion, and liver and kidney damage. Also, certain individuals become hypersensitive to cresol (Proctor and Hughes, 1991). It is apparent that phenolics can play a significant role in the effects of congeners from different alcoholic beverages.

1.9 Vasoactive Congeners

A. Tyramine

Some alcoholic beverages contain tyramine (Lovenberg, 1974) and histamine (Schreier, 1979). Both are vasoactive and can affect blood pressure. The enzyme monoamine oxidase metabolizes primary amines such as adrenaline in the body. Drugs that inhibit monoamine oxidase were the first antidepressants. Severe hypertensive reactions have occurred in patients treated with such drugs who then consumed tyramine in certain wine (e.g., Chianti) (Goth, 1978). Tyramine levels range from 2 to 10 mg/L in beer, and from 0 to 25 mg/L in wine (Lovenberg, 1974).

B. Histamines

Selected alcoholic beverages can exert potent histamine activity (Ough, 1971; Trethewie, 1979; Parodi et al., 1980). As little as 0.1 milligram of histamine phosphate injected intravenously causes a sharp decline in blood pressure, tachycardia, elevation of the cerebrospinal fluid pressure, flushing of the face, and headache (Goth, 1978). In asthmatics it may precipitate a severe asthmatic attack. Histamine taken by mouth is less effective because much of it is metabolized before it can enter the main blood stream.

The headache and flushing sometimes experienced after ingestion of some alcoholic drinks may be partly due to their histamine content. As a general rule, a histamine headache is not produced when the histamine level in beverages is less than 2 mg/L, even in subjects prone to migraine (Trethewie, 1979). Wine containing 8 mg/L has been shown to cause headaches (Shinohara and Watanabe, 1981; Trethe-wie, 1979). The histamine content of some alcoholic beverages is shown in Table 1.10.

Maturing wine in wood can reduce histamine content. For example, an Australian red wine matured in wood contained negligible histamine levels, whereas the same wine not matured in wood contained 5 mg/L of histamine (Trethewie, 1979).

C. Toxic metals

Both the type and amount of metal must be considered in evaluating its toxicity. A small amount may be essential and excessive amounts can be toxic. For

Table 1.10
Histamine Content of Selected Alcoholic Beverages

	Histamine (mg/L)		
	Range	Average	No. of Samples
Chilean wines	0.0–2.20	-	100
French wines	0.1–30.0	5.4	60
California wines	0.1–15.5	-	300
Fruit wines	-	0.56	
Dessert wines	-	2.60	
Chianti Becchi	-	2.60	3
Bourgueil wine	-	15.10	2
Moselle wine	-	0.04	1
Swedish beer	2.6–4.7	3.8	6
Danish beer	3.2–15.0	7.8	5
Brandy	-	0.0	
Scotch whisky	-	0.0	

From Ough, 1971

example, marginal chromium deficiency leads to impaired glucose and lipid metabolism.

In one study, 12 ounces (355 milliliters) of ordinary beer would supply 7 percent of the minimum recommended safe and adequate intake of chromium (Anderson, 1983). In another study of seventy-four different beers, approximately twelve ounces, contained 5 percent of the chromium and 1 percent of the selenium recommended as the minimum safe and adequate intake (Robberecht et al., 1984).

Food and drink account for the major portion of man's daily intake of lead and arsenic. The maximum allowable limit has been gradually reduced as scientists learn more about the health effects of these two metals. The EPA has set 0.05 mg/L as the drinking water limit for lead and 0.1 mg/L for arsenic, and the Australian National Health and Medical Research Council has reduced the lead and arsenic maximal residue limits in wine to 0.2 mg/L and 0.1 mg/L, respectively (Handson, 1984).

In a recent survey of twenty-seven table wines, the average concentrations of lead and arsenic were 0.31 mg/L and 0.08 mg/L, respectively, for wines from vineyards that had used a lead arsenate compound for caterpillar control, and 0.03 mg/L (lead) and 0.01 mg/L (arsenic) in control vineyards (Handson, 1984). Wine samples that contained 50 mg/L have been implicated in arsenic poisoning in

humans (Houser and Vitek, 1979; Gerhardt et al., 1980).

Since moonshine (illegally distilled whiskey) is still consumed in many areas of the United States and other parts of the world, the potential for toxicity from trace elements in this beverage is very real. In a recent study of twelve samples, lead and arsenic were found in potentially toxic concentrations (Gerhardt et al., 1980).

1.10 Congeners from Spices and Herbs

"Secret" herbs and spices are used to give alcoholic beverages the variety of flavors unique to each. Just as water is used to extract flavoring chemicals from coffee and tea, alcohol and water are used to extract chemicals from herbs and spices in concentrations that water alone would not extract.

The congeners extracted from many herbs and spices in alcoholic beverages are reported to have pharmacologic effects. The beverage consumer may not know that a beverage contains these natural products which can affect his health in many different ways. Some of these agents are listed here along with some of the health effects associated with them. The chemical composition of many herbs and spices is not known and the effect of many of the known chemical constituents is unknown. The information on flavoring agents is abstracted from a pharmacognosy text (Tyler et al., 1981).

Angelica (gin). A volatile oil constitutes 5 percent of angelica. It is used medically as a bronchial tonic, a diaphoretic (an agent that increases perspiration), a diuretic, and in the treatment of rheumatism. Both the dried fruit and the root are used but the chemical composition of angelica is unknown.

Anise or **aniseed** (gin, aquavit) is one of the oldest known medicinal plants, mentioned by Dioscorides of Anazarbos, Pliny and Theophrastus. It contains 1 percent to 3 percent volatile oil consisting of 80 percent to 90 percent anethole. It is used as a carminative (an agent that relieves flatulence) and for the relief of colic and griping. Its most common use is as a flavoring agent. Anethole is (E)-*p*-propenylanisole, but the Japanese anise is very poisonous and contains a toxin called hananomin.

Cacao (liqueurs) is made from the seeds of *theobroma cacao*, a tropical American tree (*theobroma* is Greek for "food of the gods"). The seeds contain 35 percent to 50 percent fixed oil, about 15 percent starch, 15 percent protein, 1 percent to 4 percent theobromine, and 0.07 percent to 0.36 percent caffeine. Theobromine is a diuretic and smooth muscle relaxant. It is used in the treatment of cardiac edema and angina pectoris. The usual dose is 200 milligrams three times a day. Caffeine is also a diuretic, but also has a stimulant effect.

Caraway (gin, aquavit, vodka) is used for its flavor and as a carminative. The volatile oil is about 50 percent (+)-carvone and 50 percent (+)-limonene.

Cardamom (gin, aquavit) is also used as a carminative. The volatile oil contains 26 percent to 40 percent cineole, 28 percent to 34 percent (+)-terpinyl acetate, 14 percent limonene, 3 percent to 5 percent sabinene, and 8 percent linalyl acetate.

Coriander oil (gin) is used, like caraway and cardamom, a flavoring agent and carminative. The oil contains (+)-linalool, limonene, α-pinene, γ-terpinene, *p*-cymene.

Fennel (gin) is also a carminative and the oil contains 50 percent to 60 percent anethole, (+)-fenchone and (+)-fenchone and (+)-pinene.

Hops (beer) contain *b*-myrcene and esters of myrcenol and linalool. In addition, they contain humulon and lupulon, which are resins with bacteriostatic properties. Hops also have sedative properties, which are attributed to humulon and lupulon.

Hyssop (absinthe) is described in the Bible and has been used in folk medicine for fever, rheumatism, and to remove the discoloration from a black eye. Hyssop contains cadinene, pinene, (-)pino-camphenol, and pinocamphone.

Juniper (gin) is used to flavor beverages and in the over-the-counter (OTC) drug market as a diuretic. It contains pinene, myrcene, limonene, and terpineol.

Licorice or **glycyrrhiza** (gin, liqueurs) contains glycyrrhizin which is fifty times sweeter than sugar. Other constituents include liquiritin, rhomnoisoliquiritin, and the coumarin derivatives herminarin and umbelliferon. Licorice is a demulcent and expectorant. It is used in dermatology for its anti-inflammatory properties. Glycyrrhizin can increase sodium and fluid retention. Therefore persons with cardiac problems should avoid consumption of significant amounts of licorice.

Nutmeg (eggnog) contain myristicin and elemicin. Myristicin has been used to help control diarrhea. Large doses can cause flushing of the skin, tachycardia, dry mouth, and have an hallucinogenic effect.

Wormwood (absinthe) has a long history of use for indigestion, flatulence, and as a diaphoretic. It was used to flavor absinthe, a beverage thought to cause acute and chronic toxicity. It contains thujone which causes trembling, stupor, convulsions, dementia, and even death. Today, most countries prohibit its use (Grossman and Lembeck, 1983).

1.11 Semivolatile Congeners

In reviewing the literature, it seems that the semivolatile congeners have been largely overlooked. Samples of beers, wines, and distilled spirits were examined, using the method described in the Appendix. Only the major peaks were identified and they are listed in Tables 1.11 through 1.16.

The significance of these congeners remains to be determined. The content and concentration of the semivolatile constituents are as variable as the volatile and nonvolatile congeners or alcoholic beverages.

continued on page 20

Table 1.11
Semivolatile Congeners in Selected Wines (mg/L)

Compound	Paul Masson	Rosé Gallo	Nectarose	Taylor
Cyclohexane	70	81	105	72
3-Methyl-1-butanol	883	789	401	851
Diethylene glycol	103	138	497	171
1-Hexanol	28	20	-	15
Methyl hexanol	28	31	33	-
Heptanoic acid	18	-	-	11
Hexadienoic acid	321	317	-	110
Benzeneethanol	188	266	697	37
Diethyl succinate	249	182	146	294
Caprylic acid	33	23	-	47
Ethyl caprylate	15	-	-	16
β-Phenylethyl isobutanoate	17	32	54	59
2,3-Butanediol	-	19	52	40
3-Methylthio + propanol	-	-	35	-

Compound	Paul Masson	Chablis Chablis Fer Cru	Taylor	Almaden
Cyclohexane	81	94	T	85
2,2-Dimethylhexane	22	-	T	-
3-Methyl-1-butanol	956	1542	98	991
Diethylene glycol	106	146	18	108
1-Hexanol	32	48	T	17
Methyl hexanol	26	-	-	-
Heptanoic acid	63	55	T	67
Hexadienoic acid	295	-	32	331
Benzeneethanol	210	762	24	140
Diethyl succinate	118	425	17	196
Caprylic acid	36	-	T	38
Ethyl caprylate	24	33	T	23
β-Phenylethyl isobutanoate	25	38	-	35
2,3-Butanediol	-	-	T	-

Compound	Paul Masson	Burgundy Thomas Taylor	Freres	Gallo
Cyclohexane	T	84	82	64
2,2-Dimethylhexane	T	17	17	26
3-Methyl-1-butanol	45	389	1,081	174
Diethylene glycol	43	492	674	163
1-Hexanol	T	46	26	37
Methyl hexanol	T	57	54	68
Heptanoic acid	T	-	-	T
Hexadienoic acid	-	216	-	10
Benzeneethanol	43	418	353	334
Diethyl succinate	11	68	T	155
Caprylic acid	-	-	-	178
β-Phenylethyl isobutanoate	-	23	20	25
2,3-Butanediol	T	112	109	74
3-Methylthio + propanol	-	35	-	-

T = trace

Table 1.12
Semivolatile Congeners in Selected Bourbons (mg/L)

Compound	Jim Beam	Jack Daniels	Weller
Cyclohexane	73	-	-
3-Methyl-1-butanol	569	61	849
Benzeneethanol	T	300	738
Ethyl caprylate	98	25	84
Ethylester of dodecanoic acid (mol wt 228)	42	-	40
Ethylester of dodecanoic acid (mol wt 220)	116	51	152
Diethoxy ethane	T	63	383
2-Methyl propanol	73	403	241
Urea	-	-	T
Furaldehyde	-	48	86

T = trace

Table 1.13
Semivolatile Congeners in Tequila (mg/L)

Compound	Azteca	Cuervo
3-Methyl-1-butanol	2,056	107
Benzeneethanol	105	-
Ethyl caprylate	51	T
Ethylester of dodecanoic acid (mol wt 228)	39	17
Ethylester of dodecanoic acid (mol wt 220)	173	27
Diethoxy ethane	33	-
2-Methyl propanol	66	-
Dimethoxy methane	435	-

T = trace

Table 1.14
Semivolatile Congeners in Selected Gins (mg/L)

Compound	Tanqueray	Beefeater	Gordon's	Gilbey's	Seagram's
Cyclohexane	-	-	-	T	-
3-Methyl-1-butanol	66	-	-	-	-
Benzeneethanol	86	111	90	T	137
Heptonic acid	-	-	-	T	-
Ethyl caprylate	63	13	T	T	18
Ethylester of dodecanoic acid (mol wt 228)	-	-	-	T	-
Ethylester of dodecanoic acid (mol wt 220)	30	11	40	-	41
Diethoxy ethane	-	-	-	T	-
2-Methyl propanol	-	-	-	T	-
4-Carene (or similar terpine)	193	488	206	T	525

T = trace

Table 1.15
Semivolatile Congeners in Selected Scotch Whiskies (mg/L)

Compound	Johnny Walker	Cutty Sark	J&B	Chivas Regal	Usher's
Cyclohexane	25	-	-	-	-
3-Methyl-1-butanol	504	1076	1796	906	1222
Benzeneethanol	112	128	278	86	108
Ethyl caprylate	166	106	123	76	85
Ethylester of dodecanoic acid (mol wt 228)	99	111	57	36	42
Ethylester of dodecanoic acid (mol wt 220)	267	241	263	129	173
β-Methyl histamine	-	25	83	17	32
Diethoxy ethane	338	38	62	40	14
2-Methyl propanol	169	56	91	195	243
Pentyl ester of acetic acid	40	39	31	-	-

Table 1.16
Semivolatile Congeners in Selected Beers (mg/L)

Compound	Carta Blanca	Pilsner Urquell	Dos Equis	Budweiser	Michelob Lite	Guiness Stout	Heineken Dark	Heineken Light
3-Methyl-1-butanol	82	90	137	103	T	137	58	78
Benzeneethanol	98	51	T	78	-	T	98	68
β-Methyl histamine	-	-	T	T	-	T	-	T
Pentyl ester of acetic acid	-	T	T	T	-	T	-	T

T = trace

1.12 Xenobiotics in Alcoholic Beverages

The United States maximum limit for lead in drinking water was reduced from 0.05 to 0.005 mg/L in 1991. The mean concentration in Australian wines in approximately 0.04 mg/L which is below their 0.2 mg/L limit for lead in beverages. However, it is approximately ten times the new drinking water limit in the United States (Chen et al., 1993). Methyl-2-benzimidazolecarbamate (MBC) was found in ninety-eight of 134 red and white wine samples recently tested. MBC is a fungicide used in Europe and it is a major breakdown product of benomyl, a fungicide used widely in the United States (Bushway et al., 1993). MBC has been shown to cause cancer in laboratory animals. Increasing regulatory requirements and public awareness result in an increasing need to better understand the chemistry of alcoholic beverages which is rapidly turning the art of beverage manufacturing into a science.

References

Anderson, B.M. Separation of alpha and beta and iso gamma acids in hop products and beer by high performance liquid chromatography. *J. Chromatogr.* 262:448–450, 1983.

Asmus, P.A., Landis, J.B. and Vila, C.L. Liquid chromatographic determination of lincomycin in fermentation beers. *J. Chromatogr.* 264:241–248, 1983.

Brown, D.G. and Clapperton, J.F. Discriminant analysis of sensory and instrumental data on beer. *J. Inst. Brewers* 84:318–323, 1978.

Bums, H.G. and Gump, H.B. Technological advances in the analysis of wines. ACS Symposium Series: 5 3 6:1–12, 1993.

Carroll, R.B. Analysis of alcoholic beverages by gas-liquid chromatography. *Q. J. Stud. Alcohol* 5:6–19, 1970.

Chapman, L.F. Experimental induction of hangover. *Q. J. Stud. Alcohol* 5:67–86, 1970.

Chatton, M.J. and Ullman, P.M. Nutrition: Nutritional and metabolic disorders. In: Krupp, M.A. and Chatton, M.J. (eds.), *Current Medical Diagnosis and Treatment*. Los Altos, CA: Lange Medical Publications, 1984, pp. 790–791.

Chen, G.N., Scollary, G.R. and Vicente-Beckett, V. Determination of lead in eine by stripping potentiometry. *Journal of the Grape & Wine Industry* 352:7–11, 1993.

Cleland, J.G. and Kingsbury, G.L. Multimedia environmental goals for environmental assessment. U.S. Environmental Protection Agency publication No. 600/7-77-136b, Nov. 1977, pp. E29-450.

Committee on Dietary Allowances Food and Nutrition Board, *Recommended Dietary Allowances*, 9th ed. Washington, DC: National Academy of Sciences, pp. 1–185, 1980.

Dowhanick, T.M. and Russell, I. Advances in detection and identification methods applicable to the brewing industry. In: Gump, B.H and Pruett, D.J. (eds.), *Beer and Wine Production Analysis, Characterization, and Technological Advances*, ACS Symposium Series 536. Washington, DC: American Chemical Society, pp. 13–31, 1993.

Gerhardt, R.E., Crecelius, E.A. and Hudson, J.B. Trace elements content of moonshine. *Arch. Environ. Health* 35:332–334, 1980.

Goth, A. *Medical Pharmacology*. St. Louis: C.V. Mosby, 1978, pp. 103–104.

Greizerstein, H.B. Congener contents of alcoholic beverages. *J. Stud. Alcohol* 42:1030–1037, 1981.

Grossman, H.J. and Lembeck, H. *Grossman's Guide to Wines, Beers, and Spirits*. NY: Charles Scribner's, 1983.

Guthrie, H.A. *Introductory Nutrition*. St. Louis: C.V. Mosby, 1983, pp. 41–42.

Haag, H.G. et al. Studies on the acute toxicity and irritating properties of the congeners in whiskey. *Toxicol. Appl. Pharmacol.* 1:618–627, 1959.

Handson, P.D. Lead and arsenic levels in wines produced from vineyards where lead arsenate sprays are used for caterpillar control. *J. Sci. Food Agric.* 35:215–218, 1984.

Hoeft, H. and Obe, G. SCE-inducing congeners in alcoholic beverages. *Mutation Research.* 121:247–251, 1983.

Houser, W.C. and Vitek, R.K. Arsenic intoxication. *Postgrad. Med.* 66:225–226, 1979.

Konowalchuk, J. and Speirs, J.I. Virus inactivation by grapes and wines. *Appl. Environ. Microbiol.* 32:757–763, 1976.

Kupina, S.A., Kutschinski, J.L., Williams, R.D. et al. A refined gas chromatographic procedure for the measurement of acetic acid in wines and its comparison with the distillation method. *Am. J. Enol. Vitic.* 3 3:67–74, 1982.

Lehtonen, M. Gas liquid chromatographic determination of volatile phenols in matured distilled alcoholic beverages. *J. Assoc. Off. Anal. Chem.* 66:62–70, 1983a.

Lehtonen, M. High performance liquid chromatographic determination of nonvolatile phenolic compounds in matured distilled alcoholic beverages. *J. Assoc. Off. Anal. Chem.* 66:71–78, 1983b.

Loquet, C., Toussaint, G. and Le Talaer, J.Y. Studies in mutagenic constituents of apple brandy and various alcoholic beverages collected in western France, a high incidence area for esophagal cancer. *Mutat. Res.* 88:155–164, 1981.

Lovenberg, W. Psycho- and vasoactive compounds in food substances. *J. Agric. Food Chem.* 22:23–26, 1974.

Marais, J., Van Rooyen, P.C. and Duplessis, C.S. Differentiation between wines originating from different red wine cultivars and wine regions by the application of stepwise discriminate analysis to gas chromatographic data. *S. Afr. J. Enol. Vitic.* 2:19–23, 1981.

Morrison, R.T. and Boyd, R.N. *Organic Chemistry.* Boston: Allyn & Bacon, 1983, pp. 463–464.

Obe, G. Mutagenic activity of ethanol. In: Eriksson, K., Sinclair, J.D. and Kiiamnaa, K. (eds.), *Animal Models in Alcohol Research.* NY: Academic Press, 1980, pp. 377–391.

Ondus, M.G., Wenzel, J. and Zimmerman, G.L. Sugar determination in foods with a radially compressed high performance liquid chromatography column. *J. Chem. Education* 60:776–778, 1983.

Otsuka, K. and Imai, S., *Agric. Biol. Chem.* 28:356–362, 1964.

Ough, C.S. Measurement of histamine in California wines. *J. Agric. Food Chem.* 19:241, 1971.

Parodi, A., Guarrera, M. and Rebora, A. Flushing in rosacea: An experimental approach. *Arch. Dermatol. Res.* 269:269–273, 1980.

Pirola, R.C. *Drug Metabolism and Alcohol.* Baltimore: University Park Press, 1978, pp. 123–129.

Proctor, N.H. and Hughes, J.P. *Chemical Hazards of the Work Place.* NY: Van Nostrand Reinhold, 1991.

Robberecht, H., Van Schoor, O. and Deelstra, H. Selenium and chromium content of European beers as determined by AAS. *J. Food Sci.* 49:300–301, 1984.

Schreier, P. Flavor composition of wines: A review. *CRC Crit. Rev. Food Sci. Nutri.* 59:1–121, Nov. 1979.

Shinohara, T. and Watanabe, M. Gas chromatographic analysis of volatile esters of wines. *Agric. Biol. Chem.* 45:2903–2905, 1981.

Sonde, M.A. and Mandell, G.L. Miscellaneous antibacterial agents: Antifungal and antiviral agents. In: Gilman, A.G., Goodman, L.S. and A. Gilman, A. (eds.), *Goodman & Gilman's The Pharmaco-*

logical Basis of Therapeutics, 6th ed. NY: MacMillan, 1980, p.1225.

Stephany, R.W. and Schuller, P.L. Daily dietary intakes of nitrate, nitrite, and volatile N-nitrosamines in the Netherlands using the duplicate portion sampling technique. *Oncology* 37:203–210, 1980.

Trethewie, E.R. Wines and headaches. *Med. J. Aust.* 6:94–95, 1979.

Tyler, V.E., Brady, L.R. and Robbers, J.E. *Pharmacognosy.* Philadelphia: Lea & Febiger, 1981, pp. 103–472.

Vallee B.L. Alcohol in human history. In: Jansson, B. et al. (eds.) *Toward a Molecular Basis of Alcohol Use and Abuse.* Basel, Switzerland: Birkhauser Verlag, 1994, pp.1–8.

Van Vuuren, H.J.J. et al. The identification of Enterobacteriaceae from breweries: Combined use and comparison of API 20 E system, gel electrophoresis of proteins and gas chromatography of volatile metabolites. *J. Appl. Bacteriol.* 51:51–65, 1981.

Watt, B.K. and Merrill, A.L. *Composition of Foods,* Publication No. 8. Government Printing Office, 1963, pp. 75–76.

Weinstein, L. Miscellaneous antibacterial agents: Antifungal and antiviral agents. In: Goodman, L.S. and Gilman, A. (eds.), *Goodman & Gilman's The Pharmacological Basis of Therapeutics*, 5th ed. NY: MacMillan, 1975, pp. 1227–1228.

Williams, G.D. and DeBakey, S.E. Changes in levels of alcohol consumption in the United States, 1983–1989. *Brit. J. Addiction* 87:643–648, 1992.

Zee, J.A. et al. Elemental analysis of Canadian European and American wines by photon-induced x-ray fluorescence. *Am. J. Enol. Vitic.* 34:152–156, 1983.

Chapter 2

Pharmacology and Toxicology of Ethyl Alcohol

James C. Garriott, Ph.D.

Ethyl alcohol is so common in western societies that it is usually thought of as a social beverage, and we often lose sight of the fact that it is a drug, comparable in many ways to more highly respected therapeutic and "recreational" drugs such as tranquilizers, narcotics, sedatives, and hypnotics. Alcoholic beverages are so strongly associated with society that fermentation is thought to have developed in parallel with civilization. However, until recent history and the development of distillation processes, beverages containing alcohol were of low concentration. Since it is not controlled as a drug, but is available without restriction to all persons of legal age, it comes as a surprise to many that it has pharmacological properties very similar to narcotic drugs such as morphine and heroin. Alcohol and narcotic drugs alike: (1) are euphorigenic, (2) are central nervous system (CNS) and respiratory depressants, (3) induce tolerance and (4) physical dependence (addiction). Probably the major distinctions between the two are the strong analgesic effects of narcotics versus the very weak pain-killing action of alcohol, and the generally weaker potency of alcohol, requiring tens of grams for effectiveness rather than a few milligrams.

Due to the low potency of ethyl alcohol, high concentrations must be present in the body to be effective, and consequently it affects virtually all organ and biochemical systems of the body.

This chapter consists primarily of an overview of the effects of alcohol on the body—its pharmacology and toxicology—with emphasis on the CNS effects, which are of most concern to forensic scientists.

2.1 Skin

Alcohol in higher concentrations acts as a protein precipitant, as it dehydrates protoplasm and is an irritant to denuded surfaces and mucous membranes. This is known as an **astringent** effect. Since it cools the skin as it evaporates and acts as a bactericidal agent, it may be used as a skin rubbing agent or **rubefacient**, especially in bedridden patients to prevent bedsores. Concentrations of about 70 percent are the most effective for antibacterial action (Ritchie, 1980).

Ingestion of alcohol in moderate doses induces a marked dilation of the blood vessels of the skin, resulting in a feeling of warmth and redness or flushing of the face and other parts of the body. Sweating may occur, and heat is lost more rapidly causing lowered body temperature after higher doses. Very large doses, resulting in high blood concentrations of alcohol (e.g., greater than 0.30 to 0.40 g/dL) impair general circulation and the skin may be cold and pale. Studies of deaths from hypothermia have indicated that alcohol is a major risk factor in these occurrences due to loss of body heat via the skin (Kortelainen, 1991).

2.2 Gastrointestinal Tract

The effects of ethyl alcohol on the gastrointestinal (GI) tract are influenced by many factors, such as the presence or absence of food, the type of food present, the degree of tolerance for alcohol, and the presence or absence of GI disease. As with other mucous membranes, alcohol acts as an irritant to the GI tract in higher concentrations (above 40 percent) and can cause hyperemia, gastritis, and erosion. It has been estimated that one out of three heavy drinkers suffers from chronic gastritis (Ritchie, 1980).

The presence of food in the stomach tends to dilute the alcohol, thus alleviating irritation, and delaying absorption due to the mixing with alcohol and physical interactions with alcohol by some food types. In lower concentrations, alcohol stimulates gastric secretions, both by a direct action on the stomach and by reflex. Beverages with about 10 percent alcohol concentration result in a gastric secretion rich in acid, while the psychic reflex secretion is rich in pepsin. As the concentration rises above 20 percent, however, these secretions are inhibited and the stomach may secrete mucous as a protection against the irritation.

Although an indirect effect, alcohol regularly induces nausea and vomiting in nontolerant individuals. This is believed to be the result of a direct stimulation of the chemoreceptor trigger zone of the CNS.

This action occurs when alcoholic beverages are consumed rapidly and when the blood concentration reaches about 0.12 g/dL. It also occurs when alcohol is administered intravenously (IV), thus proving it to be a central effect rather than a direct effect on the GI tract (Newman, 1954).

Continuous use of large amounts of alcohol causes a spectrum of deleterious effects on the GI and hepatic functions. Esophageal varices, resulting from impaired hepatic circulation in cirrhosis, and gastric lesions and ulceration are commonly seen in alcoholics. Hemorrhage from these lesions may be life threatening. Acute and chronic pancreatitis occurs often in alcoholism, and may be due to a stimulation of pancreatic secretions combined with obstruction of pancreatic ducts (Wallgren and Barry, 1970). Approximately 70 percent of pancreatitis in the U.S. is associated with alcoholism. Mortality approaches 70 percent in chronic alcoholic pancreatitis within twenty years, and pancreatic cancer develops in about 4 percent of cases (Tsirambidis et al., 2003).

Alcohol may have some beneficial effects on GI function in small or moderate doses and lower concentrations by stimulating the secretion of gastric digestive juices, if ingested in combination with meals. Chronic or heavy alcohol consumption, however, is markedly detrimental—by irritation of the gastric lining, suppression of digestive functions, and nausea and vomiting; and after chronic heavy use by induction of severe organ system damage such as cirrhosis, esophageal varices with risk of hemorrhaging; and acute or chronic pancreatitis.

2.3 Cardiovascular System

Moderate doses of alcohol cause a slight increase in pulse rate and blood pressure and increase plasma high-density lipoprotein (HDL) levels, which are associated with lower coronary artery disease rates. Thus, low to moderate alcohol consumption may have a beneficial effect on the heart. Epidemiology studies have demonstrated that the risk of coronary artery disease and myocardial infarction decreases with moderate alcohol consumption. One to three drinks per day may result in a 10 to 40 percent decreased risk of coronary heart disease, compared to abstainers (Goldstein, 1983; Lavy et al., 1994; Gaziano et al., 1993; Srivastava et al., 1994). The bioflavinoids present in red wines may play an extra role in protecting low-density lipoproteins (LDL) from oxidative damage, which leads to atherosclerosis (Fleming et al. 2000). Resveratrol (trans-3,5,4'-trihydroxy-stilbene), a potent antioxidant found largely in the skins of red grapes, has demonstrated benefits in cardiovascular disease and cancer (Bertelli et al., 1996; Jang, 1997).

The most prominent effect with higher doses, however, is a depression of cardiovascular functions. This depression is probably a combination of central vasomotor and respiratory depression, and a direct depression of the heart muscle.

Chronic use of high doses of alcohol, as in chronic alcoholism, results in intracellular myocardial lesions, probably associated with congestive heart failure and hypertension (Regan, 1971; Ferrans, 1966). Alcoholic cardiomyopathy from excessive consumption of alcohol is a well-established syndrome. Cardiac dysfunction, heart muscle disease or both occur in about one-third of alcoholics. This is not due to impaired nutritional status, but appears to a direct toxic effect of alcohol on the heart muscle (Liang et al., 1999). Fibrosis, edema, enlarged and distorted mitochondria, and lipid accumulation in the heart muscle cells are characteristic of alcoholic cardiomyopathy (Goldstein, 1983).

2.4 Liver

Alcohol-induced liver disease is a very common condition. Cirrhosis now ranks as the eighth most common cause of death by disease in the United States killing 25,000 people, and is the fourth leading cause of death in some urban areas (National Digestive Diseases Information Clearinghouse, 2000; Lieber, 1997). Chronic alcohol consumption is its most common cause. It is estimated that 8 percent to 20 percent of chronic alcoholics eventually develop cirrhosis. It is therefore apparent that factors other than alcohol consumption are involved in the etiology of cirrhosis, but these are as yet unknown (Mezey, 1979). The incidence of cirrhosis has significantly declined since the mid-1970s, when it was ranked as the fourth leading cause of death. Contributing factors to the decline may include changes in dietary habits, prevention efforts, and reduced exposure to other predisposing factors, such as smoking and vitamin deficiencies (Smart, 1991).

Fatty infiltration of the liver occurs readily after the ingestion of alcohol. This effect is due to an overloading of the liver's metabolic functions by alcohol, and the resultant storage of unmetabolized fatty acids (Goldstein, 1983). However, this is a reversible condition, and is not thought to result directly in cirrhosis. The deposition of excess collagen in the liver initiates hepatic fibrosis which becomes irreversible, developing into cirrhosis. The resultant progressive deterioration in liver function may culminate with liver failure, hepatic coma, and death. Alcoholic liver disease is usually associated with consumption of over 80 g/dL (about six ounces of 100-proof whiskey or six beers), but has been linked with consumption of three to four drinks per day in men and as few as two to three drinks per day in women. The incidence of cirrhosis increases dramatically when consumption exceeds 160 g/dL, either regularly or in "binges," over a ten-to-fifteen-year period (Marshall et al., 1979; National Digestive Diseases Information Clearinghouse, 2000).

2.5 Kidney

The principal effect of ethyl alcohol on the kidney is that of a diuretic. This appears to be a direct effect, exerted by virtue of a decrease in renal tubular reabsorption of water. It is assumed that alcohol causes this diuresis by inhibiting the secretion of antidiuretic hormone in the hypophyseal system. The diuretic effect appears to be directly proportional to the blood alcohol concentration and occurs when the blood alcohol concentration is rising, but not when it is stable or falling (Wallgren and Barry, 1970; Goldstein, 1983). No deleterious effect on the kidneys or renal function has been attributed to alcohol.

2.6 Endocrine System

Acute alcohol administration induces a stress effect on the adrenal cortex. Thus plasma levels of cortisol and other corticosteroids are increased in a dose-related response to alcohol. Ethanol essentially mimics the adrenocorticotropic hormone (ACTH) by stimulating the adrenal production of steroids (Goldstein, 1983).

In addition, alcohol produces an immediate increase in the excretion of epinephrine and norepinephrine. This release may be responsible for a transient hyperglycemia, pupillary dilatation, and a slight rise in blood pressure that occurs during early stages of alcohol intoxication (Ritchie, 1980).

The disinhibiting effect of alcohol may initially lead to increased libido and sexual desire. However, ethyl alcohol decreases plasma testosterone due to inhibition of testicular synthesis of the sex hormone and stimulation of androgen metabolism, while the hypothalamic pituitary response to low levels of circulating testosterone is decreased (Goldstein, 1983). Impotence, sterility, testicular atrophy, gynecomastia and general feminization may occur in alcoholic men. It has also been demonstrated that alcohol significantly decreases penile tumescence and vaginal pressure, thus decreasing sexual responsiveness in both men and women (Rall, 1990). This negative effect of alcohol on sexual performance has long been recognized, as Shakespeare's Porter told Macduff (*Macbeth*, Act II, Scene I) "Drink, sir, is a great provoker of three things—nose-painting, sleep, and urine. Lechery, sir, it provokes the desire, but it takes away the performance."

2.7 Central Nervous System
A. General
The central nervous system (CNS) is the bodily system most severely affected by alcohol, and since this system is the source of any behavioral aberrations due to alcohol, these effects are the most important to consider for medicolegal interpretation of alcohol related situations.

The intensity of the CNS effects of alcohol is proportional to the concentration of alcohol in the blood. These general effects are outlined in relation to alcohol concentrations in Table 2.1 (Dubowski, 1997). However, the effects are considerably more pronounced when the blood level is rising than when falling. This is known as the Mellanby effect and is believed to result from so-called acute (functional) tolerance to alcohol, achieved during the course of the intoxication (Mellanby, 1919; Moskowitz et al., 1977; Goldstein, 1983; Nicholson et al., 1992; Bennet et al., 1993; Wang et al., 1993). It was previously proposed that a portion of this effect is due to

the higher alcohol concentrations in the brain during the rising or absorptive phase of the blood alcohol curve due to rapid equilibration of the brain with arterial blood. Aside from this distributional artifact, however, it has been shown that rats are about twice as tolerant to a moderate alcohol dose at a given brain level sixty minutes after as compared to ten minutes after the injection (LeBlanc et al., 1975). In humans, the magnitude of the effect is probably a function also of the rate the alcohol is consumed. It was observed that the more rapid the rate of drinking, the greater the degree of performance decrements at the same blood alcohol concentration (BAC) (Moskowitz et al., 1977). A recent study demonstrated that breath measurements were higher than blood in the earlier phases, and that the results of the acute tolerance studies varied according to which analysis was used. In breath testing, acute tolerance was demonstrated for light drinkers at doses of 0.5 and 1.0 kilogram, while moderate drinkers showed the effect only with the higher dose (Hiltunen, 1997). An extreme example of acute tolerance was reported in a human patient in whom a maximum blood alcohol level of 0.78 g/dL was found. When the patient reached a level of 0.30 g/dL, she was, by clinical observations, sober (Hammond et al., 1973).

The general CNS effects of alcohol and relation to locus of action are illustrated in Figure 2.1. The frontal lobes are sensitive to low concentrations of alcohol, resulting in alteration of thought and mood. The early effects of alcohol are often considered stimulant actions, mediated by depression of the reticular activating system, and thereby releasing the cortex from selective control and inhibition. Increased confidence, a more expansive and vivacious personality, mood swings, garrulousness, and increased social interactions are characteristic (Wallgren and Barry, 1970; Majchrowicz and Barry, 1979). These effects are actually due to depression of the inhibitory central mechanisms. Thus the intoxicated individual may act in ways or perform acts he would not ordinarily do. He may become more aggressive and even violent, due to pent-up hostilities, or express abnormal desires and drives normally kept under control. He may become overcon-

Table 2.1
Stages of Acute Alcoholic Influence and Intoxication

Blood-Alcohol Concentration (grams/100 mL)	Stage of Alcoholic Influence	Clinical Signs and Symptoms
0.01–0.05	subclinical	Influence or effects not apparent or obvious Behavior nearly normal by ordinary observation Impairment detectable by special tests
0.03–0.12	euphoria	Mild euphoria, sociability, talkativeness Increased self-confidence, decreased inhibitions Diminution of attention, judgment, and control Some sensory-motor impairment Slowed information processing Loss of efficiency in critical performance tests
0.09–0.25	excitement	Emotional instability, loss of critical judgment Impairment of perception, memory, and comprehension Decreased sensory response, increased reaction time Reduced visual acuity, peripheral vision and glare recovery Sensory-motor incoordination, impaired balance Drowsiness
0.18–0.3	confusion	Disorientation, mental confusion, dizziness Exaggerated emotional states (fear, rage, grief, etc.) Disturbances of vision (diplopia, etc.) and of perception of color, form, motion, dimensions Increased pain threshold Increased muscular incoordination, staggering gait, slurred speech Apathy, lethargy
0.25–0.4	stupor	General inertia, approaching loss of motor functions Markedly decreased response to stimuli Marked muscular incoordination, inability to stand or walk Vomiting, incontinence of urine and feces Impaired consciousness, sleep or stupor
0.35–0.5	coma	Complete unconsciousness, coma, anesthesia Depressed or abolished reflexes Subnormal temperature Impairment of circulation and respiration Possible death
0.45+	death	Death from respiratory arrest

Copyright by Kurt M. Dubowski, University of Oklahoma College of Medicine, Oklahoma City, OK, 1997

fident and take dangerous risks he would not ordinarily take (e.g., speeding and reckless driving).

First affected are processes that depend on previous training and experience and that govern self-restraint and inhibition. Memory, fine discrimination, and concentration functions are dulled as the blood alcohol level rises, as vision (occipital lobe) and co-ordination (cerebellum) also become impaired. All bodily functions and abilities governed by the brain are impaired progressively. With acute intoxication (blood levels in excess of 0.40 g/dL), even autonomic (automatic) functions governed by the medulla and the brain stem are affected. At these levels,

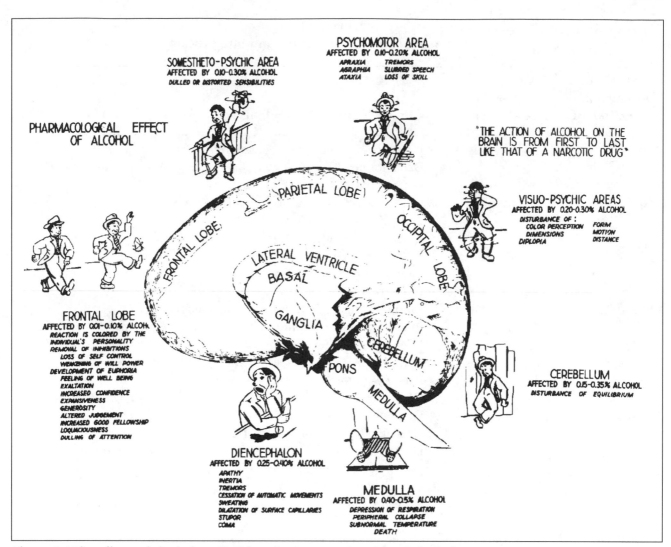

Figure 2.1 *The effects of alcohol on CNS functioning at various blood alcohol concentrations (0.10% = 0.10 g/dL). Reproduced courtesy of S.R. Gerber, M.D., Coyahoga County, Cleveland, Ohio.*

there is considerable risk of death from depression of the respiratory centers (Dubowski, 1997).

B. Chronic CNS effects

Chronic excessive ingestion of alcohol is directly associated with neurologic and mental disorders related to brain damage. An increased risk of seizures occurs in regular drinkers, and is dose-related. Nutritional and vitamin deficiencies from poor nutrition or from impaired gastrointestinal and hepatic function cause neuropsychiatric syndromes. Wernicke's encephalopathy, a triad of acute mental confusion, ataxia and ophthalmoplegia, and Korsakoff's psychosis, characterized by profound impairment of recent memory, are two conditions characteristic of al-

coholism. Intravenous thiamine administration may be ameliorative. Alcohol itself is neurotoxic, however, regardless of its impact on nutritional status. Chronic alcohol abuse causes shrinkage of the brain due to loss of both white and gray matter (Kril and Halliday, 1999). Delirium tremens (uncontrollable tremors), tonic-clonic seizures and alcoholic hallucinosis (persistent hallucinations) may occur within about three days after withdrawal from alcohol in alcohol dependency. The withdrawal syndrome can be fatal without treatment, but if the patient does not die, recovery may occur in five to seven days. Disturbed brain function may persist for many months, however (Jaffe, 1990).

2.8 Impairment of Specific Functions Related to Driving Ability

A. Vision

A number of studies have been performed to test the effects of ethyl alcohol on vision, with conflicting results. Several early studies reported little or no effect, but doses were unusually low, in most cases ranging from 0.2 to approximately 0.7 g/kg (Marquis et al., 1957; Miles, 1924; Blomberg and Wassen, 1959). Mortimer (1963) reported only a 3-percent visual decrement at a blood alcohol concentration of 0.06 g/dL.

However, studies in which more substantial and socially realistic doses of alcohol were used have substantiated significant decrements of visual acuity after alcohol ingestion. With blood alcohol levels varying between 0.06 and 0.22 g/dL (average 0.115 g/dL), visual acuity was impaired in 54 percent of subjects with levels between 0.06 and 0.10 g/dL, and in 85 percent of the subjects with levels between 0.101 and 0.125 g/dL (Newman and Fletcher, 1941). Other early studies have shown that alcohol may diminish the sensitivity, persistence, or speed of response to visual stimulation (Suzuki et al., 1957; Lewis et al., 1969; Idestrom and Cadenius, 1968).

Some studies have shown that alcohol slows adaptation to both darkness and light, and lowers resistance to glare at blood alcohol levels ranging from 0.09 to 0.15 g/dL (Wallgren and Barry, 1970). Impairment of discrimination of colors has been observed after alcohol doses of 0.7 g/kg (Schmidt and Bingel, 1953; Wallgren and Barry, 1970). Mergler et al. (1988) studied the relationship between alcohol consumption and color discrimination capacity in 136 subjects. He found that the prevalence of dyschromatopsia increased with alcohol intake in all age categories, and that heavy drinkers (greater than 751 grams or fifty-plus alcoholic drinks per week) consistently presented with dyschromatopsia. Color loss was primarily in the blue-yellow range, but some subjects showed impairment of red-green color discrimination. In another study (Zrenner et al., 1986) subjects with BACs from 0.07 to 0.16 g/dL exhibited a specific impairment on the function of blue-sensitive cones and their interaction with longer wavelength-sensitive cones.

Brecher et al. (1955) demonstrated impairment of alcohol on binocular coordination by measuring fusion speed or focusing ability on two light sources. Decrements were seen with blood alcohol levels as low as 0.03 g/dL, and in up to 89 percent of subjects with levels of 0.18 g/dL.

Diplopia (double vision) is a well-recognized symptom of alcohol intoxication. Miller al (1991) found measurable effects on fusion latency with blood alcohol levels as low as 0.05–0.06 g/dL. Fusion latency is described as the time required to fuse a binocularly visible target. This effect of alcohol is the source of the well-known "double vision" effect.

In a study of alcohol effects on vision, tracking, and division of attention, it was found that when either visual or tracking functions were examined in complex situations requiring simultaneous visual and tracking responses, as occur in actual driving situations, large performance decrements occurred at low blood alcohol concentrations of as low as 0.02 g/dL with nearly all subjects exhibiting effects at 0.08 g/dL (Moskowitz, 1974; Moskowitz and Sharma, 1974). Of studies performed measuring visual skills after low doses of alcohol, twelve of twenty-eight found impairment at blood concentrations of 0.05 g/dL or less (Moskowitz and Robinson, 1988). These studies were in the area of oculomotor control, dealing with eye movement and fusion ability. See also Moskowitz (Chapter 13) for further discussion of studies of the visual effects of alcohol.

In summary, studies performed to specifically measure the effects of alcohol on driving-related visual skills in which more than simple visual skills were studied showed that its effect is significant. Impairment may occur in some individuals at blood concentrations as low as 0.02 g/dL, and marked impairment occurs in nearly all individuals at concentrations greater than 0.08 g/dL (Honneger et al., 1970; Newman and Fletcher, 1941; Moskowitz, 1974; Mortimer, 1963).

B. Auditory discrimination

The auditory sense seems to be more resistant to the effects of alcohol than most other senses. Auditory acuity is not generally affected in humans at low blood alcohol levels (less than 0.10 g/dL). Pihkanen and Kauko (1962) reported impairment in two out of three tests performed to measure auditory capability at average blood levels of 0.10 g/dL). A large decrement in discrimination between volumes and intensity of sounds but a less clear effect on ability to detect faint sounds has been reported (Jellinik and McFarland, 1940).

C. Other sensory effects

Olfactory and taste sensibilities are affected at low doses of alcohol (0.1–0.2 g/kg). These senses may be affected at blood levels of 0.04 g/dL or greater (Wallgren and Barry, 1970).

D. Reaction time

Many studies have demonstrated that alcohol has a detrimental effect on reaction time. In general, blood levels in excess of 0.07 g/dL consistently impair reaction responses. Blood levels of alcohol ranging from 0.012 to 0.12 g/dL increased simple reaction time by 5 percent to 17 percent (Blum et al., 1964; Boyd et al., 1962; Buffard 1959; Carlson et al., 1934). In other studies, blood levels of from 0.05 to 0.15 g/dL lengthened reaction time in 42 percent to 82 percent of subjects (Huber, 1955; Izard and Saby, 1962; Moureau, 1957). An increase in reaction time of 40 percent to 55 percent was reported by Starck (1953) at blood levels of from 0.13 to 0.18 g/dL.

In slightly more complicated tasks, in which subjects perform more than one attentive task at one time, alcohol doses of 1.0 to 1.2 g/kg, with alcohol levels averaging 0.11 g/dL, increased reaction time by more than 200 percent (Gruner, 1955; Gruner and Ptasnik, 1953). This situation relates more closely to the effects of alcohol on driving skills, since the driver must control the speed and position of the vehicle, as well as monitor outside signals such as traffic lights and signs. The additional demands on the driver's attention and judgment appear to greatly enhance the detrimental effects of alcohol. Bjerver and Goldberg (1950) reported increased time required to perform certain driving skills ranging from 3 percent for a single task to 72 percent for a more complicated test of parking an automobile, at blood levels averaging 0.05 g/dL. Many similar tests have demonstrated effects of alcohol at low to moderate blood levels detrimental to driving-related skills. West et al. (1993) found that a moderate dose of alcohol (0.05

g/dL BAC) increased mean time to respond to hazards from 2.5 seconds with no alcohol to 3.2 seconds after this dose of alcohol. The speed, as measured by time required to drive a timed course, was not affected. A recent and comprehensive study of the effects of alcohol on information processing and reaction time has now clearly shown that low levels of alcohol (BAC 0.05 g/dL) impair both simple and complex reaction time (Tzambazis and Stough, 2000).

E. Review of research on alcohol impairment of driving and piloting skills

1. Motor vehicle

In a review of 177 studies of alcohol related impairment, 158 reported impairment of one or more behavioral skills at one or more BACs (Moskowitz and Robinson, 1988; Moskowitz, Chapter 13). In thirty-five studies, impairment was found at BACs of 0.04 g/dL or less, and the majority found impairment below 0.07 g/dL. It was considered that, since the majority of the studies examined only one blood level of alcohol, these results must represent an underestimation of the level at which impairment begins. The studies were categorized into nine behavioral categories: (1) reaction time, (2) tracking, (3) vigilance or concentrated attention, (4) divided attention (5) information processing, (6) visual function, (7) perception, (8) psychomotor skills and (9) actual driving skills on the road or in a simulator.

The area showing the greatest impairment effect of alcohol was **divided attention performance**, with decrements demonstrated at BACs of less than 0.02 g/dL. The second fastest rise in impairment was found with tracking performance, at or below 0.05 g/dL. Driving has been described as a time sharing task made up of two major types of activity: compensatory tracking and visual search. It is the requirement for divided attention which is particularly sensitive to the effects of alcohol. In one study of the effect of low BACs on driving skills performance, divided-attention and information processing tasks, impairment began at levels as low as 0.015 mg/dL and increased with increasing BACs through 0.06 g/dL, the maximum studied (Moskowitz et al., 1985; see also Moskowitz, Chapter 13).

Although few of the studies examined performance effects at alcohol levels less than 0.05 g/dL, there was sufficient evidence to demonstrate that BACs of 0.05 g/dL and above produce impairment of the major components of driver performance, to include reaction time, tracking, divided attention performance, information processing, oculomotor functions, perception and other aspects of psychomotor performance. Tolerance to some of the impairment parameters of alcohol can occur to some extent. Studies designed to compare impairment in experienced versus light drinkers have been performed, and results vary with the type of test parameters and with different studies (see review, Cheser and Greely, 1992). In a recent on-road study of the effects of alcohol on driving skills in light and heavy drinkers, serious impairment occurred in all subjects at BAC levels of 0.10 g/dL and higher in all subjects (Laurell et al., 1990). There was no evidence of any difference between the two groups. Another study compared the performance of alcoholics, heavy drinkers and social drinkers on cognitive tasks while sober and intoxicated (Rosen and Lee, 1976). The social drinkers showed gross signs of intoxication at BACs of 0.10 g/dL and above, while the heavy drinkers and alcoholics showed almost none of these symptoms. However, all groups were equally impaired on the cognitive performance measures. The groups also had equivalent performance levels while sober, negating any chronic deficits in the alcoholic subjects.

Low blood alcohol levels were associated with increased driver responsibility rates in a multistate driver fatality study. Whereas drug- and alcohol-free drivers were responsible in 67.7 percent of cases, drivers with blood alcohol concentrations of 0.05–0.07 g/dL were responsible in 80.6 percent, and those with 0.08–0.10 g/dL in 94.4 percent of cases (Terhune et al., 1992).

2. Motorcycle

A few studies that looked at the relationship between alcohol impairment and motorcycle operation suggest an even stronger impact than that associated with car/truck drivers. Performance decrements were noted as BAC increased from 0.038–0.059 g/dL in a motorcycle simulator experiment (Robinson et al., 1990). An assessment of operating performance of experienced motorcyclists using a motorcycle simulator revealed positive correlations between potentially fatal errors and breath alcohol levels well below the usually accepted legal limit of intoxication of 0.10 g/dL (Colburn et al., 1993). In a survey of motorcycle fatalities, 58 percent were positive for alcohol, but nearly half of those were under 0.10 g/dL. Of motorcycle arrestees for driving while intoxicated (DWI), those positive for alcohol had significantly lower levels than a comparable group of car and truck drivers (Watson et al., 1992). Of all operators involved in motorcycle or motor vehicle accidents admitted to a trauma center in New Jersey, 33 and 35 percent had measurable blood alcohol. The mean for the two groups was 0.124 g/dL and 0.18 g/dL, respectively (Sun et al., 1998). A considerably greater risk of injury and death after drinking for motorcycle drivers than for motor vehicle drivers is implied, likely reflecting the need for greater coordination and balance when operating a two-wheeled vehicle. See also Manno and Manno, Chapter 14, for additional studies of alcohol involvement in motorcycle fatalities.

3. Aviation

Another area of concern for alcohol impairment is in general and military aviation. The effects of alcohol on specific piloting skills have been evaluated extensively, and impairment has been demonstrated at low BACs (Modell and Mountz, 1990). Concentrations as low as 0.015 g/dL may reduce the ability to perform complex psychomotor tasks during the absorptive phase after alcohol ingestion. Concentrations in the range of 0.03 to 0.05 g/dL have been associated with impairment in tracking of radio-frequency signals, airport-traffic-control vectoring, traffic observation and avoidance, and aircraft descent (Ross and Mundt, 1988), as well as impairment of short-term memory, decreases in tracking performance during whole-body motion, target tracking, measures of flight coordination and configuration and complex coordination (Tang and Rosenstein, 1967; Ryback, 1970).

In thirty actual flights, each including four approaches in a single-engine aircraft using an instrument landing system, approximately twice as many major procedural errors and one episode of loss of aircraft control were observed with mean blood alcohol concentrations of 0.04 g/dL (Billings et al., 1973). Current Federal Aviation Administration regulations prohibit any crew member of a civil aircraft from flying within eight hours after the consumption of any alcoholic beverage, while under the influence of alcohol, or while having 0.04 percent by weight or more alcohol in the blood (Modell and Mountz, 1990). Results of performance studies clearly demonstrate piloting skills impairment at and below the permissible limit.

Yesavage and Leirer (1986) reported pilot performance impairment even after complete clearance of alcohol from the blood. They demonstrated a "hangover effect" fourteen hours after alcohol ingestion to reach a BAC of 0.10 g/dL or greater which resulted in poorer piloting skills performance in all tests administered. The tests were designed to test emergency response by pilots during takeoff and landing procedures.

In summary, most testing for alcohol-related impairment of performance on driving and flying-related skills shows distinct impairment at levels of 0.05 g/dL or even lower. Although few studies have examined the effects at higher levels (>0.15 g/dL), one can logically expect increases in reaction time of several hundred percent as blood concentrations exceed 0.2 and 0.3 g/dL, as well as drastic impairment of other driving-related senses and skills. Surveys of average blood alcohol levels in motor vehicle fatalities range from 0.16 g/dL upward (Cimbura et al., 1982; Fell and Nash, 1989; Garriott, 1977). Psychomotor performance effects as related to driving and flying skills are further discussed in Chapters 14 and 15.

2.9 Effects of Alcohol in Combination with Other Drugs

Ethyl alcohol has some degree of interaction with a wide spectrum of other drugs. Classically, it exerts a potentiation or synergistic effect when ingested in the presence of other drugs having CNS depressant effects. When alcohol is ingested in the presence of other drugs having a depressant effect on the CNS, such as sedatives, hypnotics, anticonvulsants, antidepressants, tranquilizers, some analgesics, and opiates, a greatly enhanced depressant effect may occur. Pharmaceutical package inserts and other drug infor-

mation circulars warn physicians and patients of the dangers of concomitant use of drugs in the above classes and alcohol.

The enhanced intoxication effect of drugs can occur with low levels of alcohol. This effect can be profound, and numerous deaths have occurred resulting from "mixing alcohol and drugs". The severe intoxication that can occur in this manner also may be a significant factor in the incidence of motor vehicle accidents as studies of arrested or killed drivers have shown (Garriott and Latman, 1976; Garriott et al., 1977, Cimbura et al., 1982). Of 1,882 fatally injured drivers from seven states, drug and alcohol combinations were detected in 11.4 percent (Terhune et al., 1992). These drugs were predominantly cocaine, marihuana, benzodiazepines, and amphetamines. Drugs in combination, other than cocaine which had no effect, increased responsibility in crash causation significantly only with low (less than 0.10 g/dL) blood alcohol concentrations.

Chronic alcohol use also affects the body's disposition of other drugs. Many drug half-lives are significantly reduced in alcoholics, or by prior alcohol consumption, when compared with controls. The mean half-life of meprobamate was decreased by half after four weeks of ethanol consumption, from a mean control value of 16.7 to 8.1 hours (Rubin and Lieber, 1971). Other drugs similarly affected are pentobarbital, phenobarbital, phenytoin, warfarin, diazepam, propranolol and probably many others (Kater et al., 1969; Iber, 1971; Mello and Mendelson, 1970; Lieber, 1997). This effect results from hypertrophy of liver smooth endoplasmic reticulum, which contains a variety of drug-metabolizing enzymes. Thus a given dose of various drugs may have a reduced effect in drinking individuals as compared with nondrinkers, and thereby require higher prescription doses to reach the desired effect (Lieber et al., 1971).

Alcohol may also interact with numerous drugs of other classes as well. These interactions may occur with agents including antidepressants, salicylates, antidiabetics (oral hypoglycemic agents), insulin, anticonvulsants and even certain food substances, such as mushrooms, among others (Iber, 1971; Wier and Tyler, 1960; Hills and Venable, 1982). Such interactions may result in enhanced effects, reduced effects (antagonism), or severe toxic effects (Seixas, 1975).

A. Acetaminophen

Even therapeutic amounts of acetaminophen (2.5–4 grams per day) can cause hepatic injury in alcoholics. Ethanol induces cytochrome P450, enhancing metabolism of acetaminophen while inhibiting the synthesis of reduced glutathione which is necessary in the conjugation and detoxification of toxic intermediate metabolites of acetaminophen. With depleted stores of glutathione, these intermediate metabolites bind with sulfhydryl groups of hepatic cells resulting in necrosis of the liver (Lieber, 1997). Massive and complete hepatic failure leading to death can occur rapidly (Wooten, 1990).

B. Amphetamines

Amphetamines and other CNS stimulants may antagonize the depressant effect of alcohol to some degree, but do not effectively counteract the impaired motor function induced by alcohol (Martin, 1971).

C. Analgesics and narcotics

Analgesics with CNS depressant properties may have this effect increased by alcohol. Thus alcohol significantly enhances the depressant effects of narcotics such as codeine, morphine, propoxyphene, and other synthetic narcotics, increasing the risk of respiratory depression and death.

Co-ingestion of alcohol in heroin users greatly increases the risk of death from respiratory depression, and a large proportion of fatal heroin overdose victims are also intoxicated with alcohol (Garriott, 1994). Studies of heroin deaths suggest that alcohol (and other depressant drugs) may be *the* most important risk factor in heroin deaths and that fatalities involving only heroin constitute a minority of ascribed "heroin" overdoses (Darke and Zador, 1996; Sporer, 1999; Melent'ev and Novikov, 2002). Salicylates (aspirin), when taken in the presence of alcohol, increase the probability of gastric hemorrhage (Martin, 1971).

D. Antidepressants

The tricyclic antidepressants (TCADs) potentiate sedation with alcohol, causing enhanced CNS depres-

sion and hypothermic coma in high doses. In addition, inhibition of intestinal movement and fatty changes in the liver may result from this interaction (Griffin and D'Arcy, 1975).

Driving skills are adversely affected if one ingests alcohol during therapy with tricyclic antidepressants. This effect may not persist after the first few days of therapy, and doxepin hydrochloride (Sinequan) plus alcohol may be less likely to impair driving performance than the other tricyclics (Landauer et al., 1969; Milner and Landauer, 1973; Lery et al., 1982). Tricyclic antidepressants are now a leading cause of deaths from drug overdose, and often these deaths involve concomitant alcohol ingestion.

Other antidepressants such as the serotonin selective receptor inhibitor (SSRI) group may have a considerably reduced toxicity when used with alcohol in comparison with the TCAs (Lau and Horowitz, 1996; Barbey and Roose, 1998). Therapeutic doses of paroxetine (20 milligrams) and 1 milligram of lorazepam were studied in combination with and without 0.6 g/kg alcohol (Kerr et al., 1992). Paroxetine had little to no effect on most of the tests, while lorazepam produced sedation and disrupted performance. Paroxetine, on the other hand, had a slight antagonistic effect on alcohol induced sedation.

E. Barbiturates

All barbiturates, but especially the rapid-acting ones, enhance the CNS depressant effects of alcohol, and vice versa, in a synergistic manner. Alcohol and barbiturates in combination have resulted in numerous deaths. With even low doses of both agents, reaction time is lengthened and judgment is impaired.

An interesting paradoxical relationship exists between alcohol and barbiturates. A metabolic cross-tolerance occurs so that a chronic alcohol drinker can metabolize barbiturates faster than a nondrinker, and some barbiturates (e.g., phenobarbital) appear to enhance the metabolism of alcohol, resulting in lowered blood levels. Yet, acute intoxication with alcohol inhibits the metabolism of barbiturates, resulting in higher barbiturate blood levels and therefore a greater combined effect. For example, the half-life of pentobarbital was doubled in the presence of alcohol (Hansten, 1976; Rubin and Lieber, 1971; Lery et al., 1982). The lethal combination of alcohol and barbiturate sleeping pills (most commonly secobarbital and amobarbital) resulted in so many deaths in past years that these drugs are rarely prescribed today. As a result, combined barbiturate and alcohol deaths are now rare in most localities (Garriott et al., 1982; Caplan, 1985).

F. Benzodiazepines

Although earlier studies using low doses of alcohol with chlordiazepoxide or diazepam demonstrated little or no enhancement of effects (Forney and Hughes, 1968), more recent observations have documented additive or synergistic detrimental effects of diazepam and alcohol (Linnoila and Hakkinen, 1974; Linnoila et al., 1974; Linnoila and Mattila, 1973; Lery et al., 1982). It is probable that moderate, therapeutic doses of benzodiazepines to which one is accustomed do not markedly add to the effect of low or moderate alcohol concentrations (Forney and Hughes, 1968). However, as the dosage of either or both drugs increases, the combined effect is more marked. Circumstantial evidence for this exists from observations of drivers arrested for "driving under the influence." In one study, 22 percent of drivers with drugs present had diazepam detected in their blood, and about half of these had benzodiazepines and alcohol in combination (Garriott and Latman, 1976). The interactions of benzodiazepines with alcohol lead to a pronounced association of the combination with drug-induced deaths, clinical drug overdoses, and traffic and other accidents.

A mechanism for synergism or enhanced effects with diazepam and alcohol may be the higher blood levels of diazepam when taken with alcohol. Peak blood levels were often twice as high when diazepam was ingested in an ethyl alcohol suspension than when ingested with water (Hayes et al., 1977). Peak plasma levels of triazolam were about 33 percent higher in subjects given 0.9 gm/kg of ethanol one hour before and additional doses to maintain a BAC of about 0.08 to 0.10 g/dL (Dorian et al., 1985). In addition, the subjects on the triazolam-ethanol combination had greater psychomotor impairment than with either drug alone. This phenomenon of enhanced and more rapid absorption of drugs from the

GI tract may be applicable to many other drugs and may account for the increased lethality of other drugs, such as tricyclic antidepressants, when ingested with alcoholic beverages. In addition, moderate doses of alcohol (0.8 g/kg) given to human volunteers significantly impair the clearance of benzodiazepines from the blood, resulting in higher blood levels and longer half lives (Hoyumpa, 1984). Clearance of chlordiazepoxide, diazepam, and lorazepam was inhibited 37 percent, 24 percent, and 18 percent, respectively.

The effects of alprazolam, a current highly popular benzodiazepine tranquilizer, were studied in forty-eight human volunteers given 1 milligram alone, and in combination with 0.5 g/kg of alcohol and then challenged with psychological testing. Alprazolam caused subjective sedation, unsteadiness, dizziness, fatigue, and impaired performance on all tasks studied. Although the effects of the combination were greater than those using either alone, they were generally additive, and no more than would be predicted (Bond, A. et al., 1991; Bond et al., 1992).

Midazolam, a short acting, potent benzodiazepine commonly used in induction of anesthesia during surgery, was studied for its possible adverse interactions with alcohol in patients who might drink after receiving anesthetic doses during surgery (Lichtor, 1991). Four hours after receiving anesthetic doses of midazolam (0.1 mg/kg) intravenously, the subjects ingested 0.7 g/kg of alcohol after which psychomotor performance and mood were assessed. No significant interactions (potentiation of one by the other) between the two drugs were found. This lack of effect was believed to be due to the dissipation of the effects of the short-acting benzodiazepine within a few hours of its administration.

G. Caffeine

Since caffeine-containing beverages are often ingested to "sober up" after drinking, studies have been performed to determine if this drug can antagonize the effects of alcohol. Earlier reports found no counteraction of alcohol effects in animal or human experiments, and one study reported greater impairment when alcohol was combined with caffeine than with alcohol alone (Forney and Hughes, 1968). One study investigating the effects of alcohol and caffeine, separately or in combination, on reaction time in human subjects reported a synergistic interaction of caffeine with alcohol on reaction time (Osborne and Rogers, 1983).

More recent studies have elicited the expected counteractive effect of caffeine on alcohol, however. The impaired reaction time and slowed rapid information processing task rate induced by 0.7 g/kg (expected BAC 0.10 g/dL) of ethanol were effectively counteracted by doses of 3.3 mg/kg of caffeine, in a computer controlled study using rapid information processing tasks (Hasenfratz et al., 1993). Caffeine in doses equivalent to one or two cups of coffee lessened alcohol's detrimental effects on alertness and peripheral responses, including compensatory tracking, divided attention, and critical tracking test (Burns and Moskowitz, 1989–90). Only moderate doses of alcohol, yielding blood concentrations up to 0.12 g/dL, were studied, and some parameters of driving performance were unaffected. When caffeine effects on subjects with 0.08 g/dL were studied, alertness and reaction time were improved, but impairment was not completely counteracted (Liguori and Robinson, 2001). The evidence suggests that the popular use of coffee to "sober up" after use of alcohol may be of some benefit, at least after moderate alcohol consumption.

H. Cocaine

Combined use of cocaine and alcohol is widespread in the United States, with over 90 percent of those who report cocaine use also reporting current alcohol use (Higgins et al., 1992). Cocaine concentrations are increased in plasma when alcohol is used concomitantly, resulting in an enhanced euphoric effect, greater increase in heart rate, and reduced alcohol-induced sedation (Farre et al., 1997).

Alcohol has a unique interaction with cocaine when both are used concomitantly. A new metabolite, cocaethylene (ethylbenzoylecgonine) is formed resulting from transesterification in the liver (Hearn, 1991a). Cocaethylene is longer acting than cocaine, and enhances the euphoria associated with alcohol and cocaine use. It is also more toxic than cocaine, resulting in a higher incidence of death (Hearn et al., 1991b).

An increase in death due to liver toxicity has been observed in mice pretreated with alcohol and then given low doses of cocaine. The alcohol treatment was thought to result in a higher production of toxic products of cocaine metabolism (Hoyumpa, 1984; Smith et al., 1981).

While alcohol's impact on behavior and performance is due to its CNS depressant actions, cocaine is a strong CNS stimulant, and can counteract some of the behavioral impairment induced by alcohol. Cocaine consistently antagonizes the learning deficits, psychomotor performance deficits and driving performance deficits induced by alcohol (Pennings et al., 2002). In a study designed to measure the behavioral effects of cocaine and alcohol on human learning and performance, the combined doses of cocaine (4 to 96 mg/kg) and alcohol (0 to 1.0 g/kg) attenuated the effects observed with alcohol and cocaine alone (Higgins et al., 1992). Both doses of cocaine studied, when combined with alcohol, reduced errors in acquisition (learning) to placebo levels. Likewise, the percentage of errors in performance was consistently reduced below that observed with similar doses of alcohol alone. Thus, cocaine may be an effective antagonist to the depressant effects of alcohol, at least in the moderate alcohol dose ranges as used in this study.

The combination of cocaine and alcohol tends to raise levels of cocaine in the blood, and increases heart rate greater than in an additive manner, resulting in a potentiation of cardiotoxicity also induced by cocaethylene. It is likely that the combination of cocaine and alcohol potentiates the tendency toward violence (Pennings et al., 2002). This relationship is supported by a medical examiner survey of drug use in homicide cases in which a high incidence of cocaine use with alcohol was found (Garriott, 1993).

I. Inhibition by histamine$_2$-receptor antagonists

Individuals taking H$_2$-receptor antagonists, such as ranitidine or cimetidine (Zantac and Tagamet, two popular drugs commonly used as treatment for peptic ulcer or stomach hyperacidity), have been found to be more susceptible to alcohol effects. These drugs inhibit gastric alcohol dehydrogenase, increasing the bioavailability of ingested alcohol. After pretreatment with 150 milligrams of ranitidine the area under the curve (AUC), a measure of the body burden of alcohol, was increased by 41 percent after a low dose (0.3 g/kg) of oral ethanol, and resulted in BACs similar to those obtained with intravenous administration. No change was produced by ranitidine after intravenous alcohol administration. The calculated quantity of ethanol entering the blood increased by 17 percent, decreasing first pass metabolism from 70 ± 10 to 31 ± 9 mg/kg. Cimetidine, another common H_2-receptor antagonist, increased peak alcohol level by 96 percent and the AUC by 96 percent (DiPadova et al., 1992). It should be noted that the maximum BAC's achieved in the treated group were only approximately 0.01 g/dL greater than the untreated group. The maximum level after cimetidine, however, increased from about 0.023 to 0.055 g/dL. Cimetidine is also known to bind liver cytochrome P450, and consequently impair drug metabolism. This has potential impact on the MEOS, which comes into play primarily at high BACs. A potentially adverse impact on metabolism during acute alcohol intoxication could result from impaired clearance (DiPadova et al., 1992). A recent review of available literature on the subject concludes, however, that there is no interaction between H_2-antagonists and alcohol at doses of 0.3 g/kg and above, and no interactions at doses that would impair psychomotor skills (above 0.025 g/dL) (Fraser, 1998). See also discussion of H_2 antagonist effect in Chapter 4.

J. Marihuana

Tetrahydrocannabinol, the active component of marihuana, and its metabolites have been detected in several studies of impaired motor vehicle drivers (Zimmerman, 1983) or fatalities (Garriott, 1986; Mason and McBay, 1984; Cimbura, 1990; Terhune et al., 1992), often in combination with alcohol. Marihuana, itself, induces impairment of some skills in road driving simulation experiments, especially divided attention tasks, while alcohol impairs psychomotor performance on virtually all driving related skills (Heishman et al., 1989). Since the effects of the two drugs are different, the effect of marihuana in combination with alcohol appears to be primarily additive (Cheser, 1986). In one study, mari-

huana alone did not impair driving performance, but when alcohol was given in combination, the interaction resulted in greater impairment in driving performance than with alcohol alone (Sutton, 1983). Peck et al. (1986) found significant effects of both alcohol and marihuana on driving performance, with even greater effects under treatment with both drugs.

2.10 Antagonists to Alcohol and Pharmacotherapeutic Agents for Alcoholism

Due to the frequent admission of acutely intoxicated alcohol drinkers to hospitals for treatment of injuries suffered as the result of alcohol-induced impairment or of alcoholic coma, an extensive search has long been under way for agents that may antagonize the effects of alcohol or accelerate the metabolism of alcohol. No effective "antidote" has yet been discovered, although caffeine and other respiratory stimulants are frequently used in hospitals. These may be mildly effective in counteracting some of the depressant actions of alcohol.

Fructose long ago was discovered to enhance the metabolism of alcohol. In some animal studies, the rate of disappearance was increased from 120 percent to 150 percent. However, doses of fructose must be high to be effective, and practical effectiveness in humans is questionable. In a double-blind study, intoxicated subjects were given IV 100 grams of fructose or glucose in 1,000 milliliters of water over a one-hour period. No differences in alcohol metabolism could be discerned between the two groups, and the authors recommended that fructose not be used for this purpose (Iber, 1977; Levy et al., 1977). A dramatic reduction in lethality in mice was observed when dimethylsulfoxide (DMSO) was administered concomitantly with alcohol. In a limited human experiment, the alcohol was observed to be metabolized slightly faster with DMSO treatment, although psychomotor impairment was greater than with alcohol alone (Mallach and Etzler, 1965).

A. Disulfiram (Antabuse) and other acetaldehyde antagonists

The classic disulfiram-alcohol reaction results from the inhibition of metabolism of acetaldehyde by inhibiting the actions of acetaldehyde dehydrogenase.

Thus acetaldehyde blood levels are increased, resulting in severe toxic effects. Even a few milliliters of ethanol can produce a reaction in a person taking disulfiram. Flushing, throbbing in the head and neck, throbbing headache, nausea, vomiting, sweating, palpitations, syncope, vertigo, blurred vision, confusion and convulsions may occur. Decreased blood pressure and respiratory depression can lead to shock and even death if the person is not treated (Rall, 1990). This effect, while toxic and potentially lethal, is the basis for its use in selective treatment of chronic alcoholism. The patient must be fully advised of the dangers of ingestion of alcohol while taking disulfiram (Antabuse).

A number of other agents can induce a similar, disulfiram-like reaction when consumed in the presence of alcohol. These include chloramphenicol, furazolidone, griseofulvin, quinacrine hydrochloride, metronidazole, procarbazine hydrochloride, sulfonylureas (oral antidiabetics), and some edible mushrooms, such as *Coprinus atramentarius* (inky cap) and *Clitocybe clavipes*, and certain industrial chemicals, such as oximes, amides, carbamates, dithiocarbamates, among others (Forney and Hughes, 1968; Griffin, 1975; Weir and Tyler, 1960; Hills and Venable, 1982; Lieber, 1997).

Naloxone hydrochloride (a commonly used narcotic antagonist) has been reported to arouse patients from alcoholic coma and to prevent the impairment of psychomotor performance induced by low levels of alcohol (MacKenzie, 1979; Jeffcoate et al., 1979; Sorensen and Mattison, 1978). Naltrexone, a narcotics antagonist which blocks opiate receptors and is used in treatment of opiate addiction, has been found to reduce alcohol drinking in monkeys (Myers et al., 1986) and in rats, and blocks the post-stress drinking of alcohol observed in rats (Volpicelli at al, 1986). In two separate reports, alcoholics were treated with conventional methods utilizing psychotherapies combined with either naltrexone or placebo (Volpicelli et al., 1992; O'Malley et al., 1992). In both studies, naltrexone proved superior to placebo as measured by relapse rate and other alcohol-related problems. Relapse in both studies occurred in only half the number of patients taking naloxone as it did in those on placebo. Naltrexone was approved by the FDA for treatment of alcoholism in 1994 (Fleming et al., 2000).

B. Other agents used in treatment of alcoholism

Acamprosate, an analog of gamma-aminobutyric acid (GABA) is used widely in Europe for treatment of alcoholism. It decreased drinking frequency and reduces relapse drinking in abstinent alcoholics, with an efficacy similar to naltrexone. Ondansetron, a serotonin receptor antagonist and antiemetic, reduces alcohol consumption in laboratory animals and is currently being tested in human subjects. Drugs such as selective serotonin reuptake inhibitors (SSRI) and lithium have also been shown to reduce alcohol consumption in alcoholics (Schaffer and Naranjo, 1998; Fleming et al., 2000).

20.11 Tolerance

Drug tolerance may be defined as a diminution of effectiveness after a period of continuous or large-dose administration of the drug. This effect does not include individual variations in sensitivity to an agent, such as species, sex, age, genetic background, or other predetermined factors. Tolerance arises only after exposure to the drug or to a closely related drug. Tolerance occurring after exposure to another drug is known as cross-tolerance.

Tolerance may result from two separate mechanisms: dispositional (or metabolic) and functional. In metabolic tolerance, the drug is metabolized or inactivated at an increased rate after chronic administration. Thus a given dose produces lower blood levels after tolerance has developed. With functional tolerance, an actual change in the sensitivity of an organ or system to the drug occurs, so that with repeated administration, higher doses and higher blood levels are required to elicit the same effect.

Few studies have been performed to assess the actual ability of ethanol to stimulate its own metabolism. Well-controlled studies are difficult to perform in humans, due to the extreme variations in habits and genetics. However, what work has been done suggests that this form of tolerance to alcohol does occur. For example, in alcoholic volunteers and normal controls, alcohol metabolism rates increased 36 percent and 72 percent, respectively, after a period of chronic alcohol consumption (Mendelson et al., 1965).

In comparisons of blood alcohol biological half-life between controls and still-drinking alcoholics, the drinking alcoholics' half-lives ranged from about thirty to 100 minutes versus nonalcoholic control half-lives of eighty to 250 minutes (Iber, 1971). Researchers comparing rates of blood alcohol elimination in nondrinkers, social drinkers, and alcoholics found marked differences in the three groups. The mean rates were: 12 ± 4 mg/dL/h in nondrinkers; 15 ± 4 mg/dL/h in social drinkers; and 30 ± 9 mg/dL/h in alcoholics (Winek and Murphy, 1984). A group of fifteen patients admitted to a treatment facility for alcohol dependency had serial blood alcohols performed on admission. The average initial blood alcohol concentration was 0.24 g/dL. The average rate of decline was 26.6 ± 7.0 mg/dL/h (range 15.9–43.0 mg/dL/h) (Clothier et al., 1985). These rates are considerably greater than the rates of 15 to 18 mg/dL/h, often considered as representing the "average" rate of alcohol metabolism (American Medical Association, 1968; Ritchie, 1980).

It has also been shown that the rate of metabolism varies in the individual according to the blood alcohol concentration. In fourteen subjects, ethanol metabolism rates averaged 21.9 ± 7.2 mg/dL/h for patients after acute alcohol intoxication with maximum concentrations of 336 ± 114 mg/dL. When doses leading to levels of 42 ± 11 mg/dL were ingested at a later time, the rates were 14.6 ± 4.8 mg/dL/h (Bogusz et al., 1977). A sixteen-year-old male was admitted to a hospital in status epilepticus, having consumed a large amount of alcohol on a dare some three hours earlier. His BAC on admission was 0.757 g/dL. Prior to treatment with hemodialysis, his clearance rate was 54 mg/dL/h (from BAC 0.757 to 0.407 g/dL), 84 mg/dL/h during hemodialysis, and four hours post hemodialysis at BAC ranges of 0.139–0.084 g/dL, the clearance had fallen to 21 mg/dL/h (Morgan et al., 1995). An earlier case report (Hammond et al., 1973) documented a very high clearance rate of 53 mg/dL/h, after admission to a hospital of an acutely intoxicated woman (initial BAC of 0.78 g/dL). This was over three times the metabolism rate considered to be average in humans.

See also Jones (Chapter 4) for discussion of alcohol metabolism rates.

Functional or constitutional tolerance has been more easily demonstrated. Goldberg (1943) studied alcohol impairment in heavy drinkers, moderate drinkers, and abstainers. He found that the tolerance for alcohol was nearly twice that for habitual drinkers as compared to nondrinkers. In animal studies, tolerance to the effects of alcohol can be induced within one to two weeks; tolerance was lost within two weeks when exposure ceased (LeBlanc et al., 1975; Goldstein, 1983; Mello and Mendelson, 1970). Male social drinkers who ingested either 0.75 or 1.0 g/kg body weight of alcohol over five consecutive days developed chronic tolerance to alcohol's effects, measured by eye-hand coordination motor task after each drink, within four days (Bennett et al., 1993). Jones (1999) examined eighty-one drinking drivers who had blood alcohol concentrations of 0.40 g/dL or greater. The range measured was 0.40 to 0.545 g/dL, expected to fall in stage-6 "coma" of acute alcoholic influence/intoxication (Table 2.1). Disappearance rates from the blood averaged 0.023 ± 0.01 g/dL per hour, with a range of 0.013 to 0.061 g/dL/h, reflecting metabolic as well as extreme functional tolerance in these drivers.

References

American Medical Association, Committee on Medicolegal Problems. *Alcohol and the Impaired Driver*. American Medical Association, Chicago, 1968, pp. 21–22.

Barbey, J.T. and Roose, S.P. SSRI safety in overdose. *J. Clin. Psychiatr.* 59 Suppl 15:42–48, 1998.

Bennett, R.H., Cherek, D.R. and Spiga, R. Acute and chronic alcohol tolerance in humans: Effects of dose and consecutive days of exposure. *Alcohol Clin. Exp. Res.* 17:740–745, 1993.

Bertelli A.A. et al. Antiplatelet activity of cisresveratrol. *Drugs Exp. Clin. Res.* 22:61–3, 1996.

Billings, C.E. et al. Effects of ethyl alcohol on pilot performance. *Aerosp. Med.* 44:379–382, 1973.

Bjerver, K. and Goldberg, L. Effect of alcohol ingestion on driving ability: Results of practical road tests and laboratory experiments. *Q. J. Stud. Alcohol* 11:1–30, 1950.

Blomberg, L.-H. and Wassen, A. Preliminary report on the effect of alcohol on dark adaptation determined by an objective method. *Acta Ophthalmol.* 37:2, 1959.

Blum, B., Stern, M.H. and Melville, K.I. A comparative evaluation of the actions of depressant and stimulant drugs on human performance. *Psychopharmacologia* 6:173–177, 1964.

Bogusz, M., Poch, J. and Stasko, W. Comparative studies on the rate of ethanol elimination in acute poisoning and in controlled conditions. *J. Forensic Sci.* 22:446–451, 1977.

Bond, A., Silveira, J.C. and Lader, M. Effects of single doses of alprazolam and alcohol alone and in combination on psychological performance. *Human Psychopharmacol.* 6:219–228, 1991.

Bond, A., Silveira, J.C. and Lader, M. The effects of alprazolam alone and combined with alcohol on central integrative activity. *Clin. Pharmacol.* 42:495–498, 1992.

Boyd, E.S., Morken, D.A. and Hodge, H.C. A psychomotor test to demonstrate a depressant action of alcohol. *Q. J. Stud. Alcohol* 23:34–39, 1962.

Brecher, G.A., Hartman, A.P. and Leonard, D.D. Effect of alcohol on binocular vision. *Am. J. Ophthalmol.* 39:44–52, 1955.

Buffard, S. Study of the psychomotor reactions of 22 subjects after ingestion of a moderate quantity of alcohol. *Ann. Med. Leg.* 39:124–128, 1959.

Burns, M. and Moskowitz, H. Two experiments on alcohol-caffeine interaction. *Alcohol, Drugs and Driving* 5,6:303–315, 1989–90.

Caplan, Y.H. et al. Drug and chemical related deaths: Incidences in the stated of Maryland, 1975–1980. *J. Forensic Sci.* 30:1012–1021, 1985.

Carlson, A.J. et al. *Studies on the Possible Intoxicating Action of 3.2 Percent Beer.* University of Chicago Press, Chicago, 1934.

Chesher, G.B. Effects of alcohol and marihuana in combination: A review. *Alcohol, Drugs and Driving* 2:105–119, 1986.

Chesher, G. and Greeley, J. Tolerance to the effects of alcohol. *Alcohol, Drugs and Driving*, 8:93–106, 1992.

Cimbura, G. et al. Incidence and toxicological aspects of drugs detected in 484 fatally injured drivers and pedestrians in Ontario. *J. Forensic Sci.* 27:855–867, 1982.

Cimbura, G. et al. Incidence and toxicological aspects of cannabis and ethanol detected in 1394 fatally injured drivers and pedestrians in Ontario (1982–1984). *J. Forensic Sci.* 35:1035–1041, 1990.

Clothier, J. et al. Varying rates of alcohol metabolism in relation to detoxification medication. *Alcohol* 2:443–445, 1985.

Colburn, N. et al. Should motorcycles be operated within the legal alcohol limits for automobiles. *J. Trauma* 35:183–186, 1993.

Darke, S. and Zador, D. Fatal heroin "overdose": A review [Review]. *Addiction* 91:1765–72, 1996.

Dorian, P. et al. Triazolam and ethanol interaction: Kinetic and dynamic consequences. *Clin. Pharmacol. Ther.* 37:558–562, 1985.

Dubowski, K.M. *Stages of Acute Alcoholic Influence/Intoxication*, The University of Oklahoma College of Medicine, Oklahoma City, 1997.

Farre, M. et al. Cocaine and alcohol interactions in humans: Neuroendocrine effects and cocaethylene metabolism. *J. Pharmacol. Exp. Ther.* 283:164–76, 1997.

Fell, J.C. and Nash, C.E. The nature of the alcohol problem in U.S. fatal crashes. *Health Education Quarterly* 16:335–343, 1989.

Ferrans, V.J. Alcoholic cardiomyopathy. *Am. J. Med. Sci.* 252:89–104, 1966.

Fleming, M., Mihic, S.J. and Harris, R.A. Ethanol. In: Hardman, J.L., Limbird, L.E. and and Gilman, A.G. (eds.), *Goodman & Gilman's The Pharmacological Basis of Therapeutics,* 10th ed. McGraw-Hill, New York, 2000.

Forney, R.B. and Harger, R.N. Toxicology of ethanol. *Annu. Rev. Pharmacol.* 9:379–392, 1969.

Forney, R.B. and Hughes, F.W. *Combined Effects of Alcohol and Other Drugs.* Charles C Thomas, Springfield, Ill. 1968.

Fraser, A.G. Is there an interaction between H2-antagonists and alcohol? [Review]. *Drug Metabolism & Drug Interactions* 14:123–145, 1998.

Garriott, J.C. and Latman, N. Drug detection in cases of driving under the influence. *J. Forensic Sci.* 21: 398–415, 1976.

Garriott, J.C., DiMaio, V.J.M. and Petty, C.S. Death by poisoning: A ten-year survey of Dallas County. *J. Forensic Sci.* 27:868–879, 1982.

Garriott, J.C. et al. Incidence of drugs and alcohol in fatally injured motor vehicle drivers. *J. Forensic Sci.* 22:383–389, 1977.

Garriott, J.C. Forensic toxicology for the general pathologist. *Advances in Pathology and Laboratory Medicine* 7:313–357, 1994.

Garriott, J.C. Drug use among homicide victims: Changing patterns. *Am. J. Forens. Med. Pathol.* 14:234–237, 1993.

Gaziano, J.M. et al. Moderate alcohol intake, increased levels of high-density lipoprotein and its subfractions, and decreased risk of myocardial infarction. *N. Engl. J. Med.* 329:1829–34, 1993.

Goldberg, L. Quantitative studies on alcohol tolerance in man. *Acta Physiol. Scand.* 5 (suppl. 16):1–128, 1943.

Goldstein, D.B. *Pharmacology of Alcohol.* Oxford University Press, New York, 1983, p. 80.

Griffin, J.P., and D'Arcy, P.F. *A Manual of Adverse Drug Interactions.* John Wright & Sons, Bristol, England, 1975, p. 57.

Gruner, O. Alkohol und Aufmerksamkeit. Ihre Bedeutung im motorisierten Verkehr. *Dtsch. Z. Ges. Gerichtl. Med.* 44:187–195, 1955.

Gruner, O., and Ptasnik, H. Zur Frage der Beeinflussung alkoholbedingten Leistungsabfalles durch Laevulosegaben. *Münch. Med. Wochenschr.* 95: 931–933, 1953.

Hammond, K.B., Rumack, B.H. and Rodgerson, D.O. Blood ethanol: A report of unusually high levels in a living patient. *JAMA* 226:63–64, 1973.

Hansten, P.D. *Drug Interactions,* 3rd ed. Lea & Febiger, Philadelphia, 1976, pp. 156–161.

Hasenfratz, M. et al. Antagonistic effects of caffeine and alcohol on mental performance parameters. *Pharmacol. Biochem. Behav.* 46:463–5, 1993.

Hayes, S.L. et al. Ethanol and oral diazepam absorption. *N. Engl. J. Med.* 296: 186–189, 1977.

Hearn, W.L. et al. Cocaethylene: A unique cocaine metabolite displays a high affinity for the dopamine transporter. *J. Neurochem.* 56:698–701, 1991a.

Hearn, W.L. et al. Cocaethylene is more potent than cocaine in mediating lethality. *Pharmacol. Biochem. and Behav.* 39:531–533, 1991b.

Heishman, S.J., Stitzer, M.L. and Bigelow, G.E. Alcohol and marijuana: Comparative dose effect profiles in humans. *Pharmacology, Biochemistry, and Behavior* 31:649–655, 1989.

Higgins, S.T. et al. Effects of cocaine and alcohol, alone and in combination on human learning and performance. *J. Experiment. Anal. of Behavior* 58:87–105, 1992.

Hills, B.W. and Venable, H.C. The interaction of ethyl alcohol and industrial chemicals. *Am. J. Indust. Med.* 3:321–333, 1982.

Honneger, H., Kampschulte, R. and Klein, H. Storung der Sehscharfe fur bewegte Objekte durch Alkohol. *Blutalkohol* 7:31–44, 1970.

Hiltunen, A.J. Acute alchol tolerance in social drinkers: Changes in subjective effects dependent on the alcohol dose and prior alcohol experience. *Alcohol*, 14:373–376, 1997.

Hoyumpa, A.M. Alcohol interactions with benzodiazepines and cocaine. *Advances in Alc. and Subst. Abuse* 3:21–34, 1984.

Huber, O. Untersuchungen uber die Veranderung der Fahrtuchtigkeit von Kraftradfahrern nach massigem Alkoholgenuss. *Dutsch. Z. Ges. Gerichtl. Med.* 44:559–577, 1955.

Iber, F.L. Increased drug metabolism in alcoholics. In: Roach, M.K, McIsaac W.M. and Creavan, P.J. (eds.), *Advances in Mental Science*, vol. 3, *Biological Aspects of Alcohol*. University of Texas Press, Austin, 1971, pp. 94–110.

Iber, F.L. The effect of fructose on alcohol metabolism. *Arch. Intern. Med.* 137:1121, 1977.

Idestrom, C.-M., and Cadenius, B. Time relations of the effects of alcohol compared to placebo. *Psychopharmacologia* 13:189–200, 1968.

Izard, A., and Saby, G. Contribution a l'etude du comportement psychomoteur de l'homme apres absorption de doses moyennes d'alcool. *Arch. Mal. Prof.* 23, 854–858, 1962.

Jaffe, J.H. Drug addiction and drug abuse. In: A.G. Gilman, A.G. et al. (eds.), *The Pharmacological Basis of Therapeutics*, 8th ed. Pergamon Press: New York, 1990, pp. 373–374.

Jang M. et al. Cancer chemopreventive activity of resveratrol, a natural product derived from grapes. *Science* 275:218–20, 1997.

Jeffcoate, W.J. et al. Prevention of effects of alcohol intoxication by naloxone. *Lancet* 2:1157–1159, 1979.

Jellinek, E.M. and McFarland, R.A. Analysis of psychological experiments on the effects of alcohol. *Q. J. Stud. Alcohol* 1:272–371, 1940.

Jones, A.W. The drunkest drinking driver in Sweden: Blood alcohol concentration 0.545 % w/v. *J. Stud. Alc.* 60:400–406, 1999.

Kater, R.M., Carulli, N. and Iber, F.L. Differences in the rate of ethanol metabolism in recently drinking alcoholic and non-drinking subjects. *Am. J. Clin. Nutr.* 22:1608–1617, 1969.

Kerr, J.S. et al. The effects of paroxetine, alone and in combination with alcohol on psychomotor performance and cognitive function in the elderly. *Int. Clin. Psychopharmacol.* 7:101–108, 1992.

Kortelainen, M.L. Hyperthermia deaths in Finland in 1970–86. *Am. J. Forensic Med. Pathol.* 12:115–118, 1991.

Kril, J.J. and Halliday, G.M. Brain shrinkage in alcoholics: A decade on and what have we learned? *Prog. Neurobiol.* 58:381–387, 1999.

Landauer, A.A., Milner, G. and Patman, J. Alcohol and amitriptyline effects on skills related to driving behavior. *Science* 163:1467–1468, 1969.

Lau, G.T. and Horowitz, B.Z. Sertraline overdose. *Academic Emergency Medicine* 3:132–136, 1996.

Laurell, H., McLean, A.J. and Kloeden, C.N. *The Effect of Blood Alcohol Concentration on Light and Heavy Drinkers in a Realistic Night Driving Situation.* NH&MRC Road Accident Research Unit, University of Adelaide, South Australia. Research Report 1/90, 1990.

Lavy, A. et al. Effect of dietary supplementation of red or white wine on human blood chemistry, hematology and coagulation: Favorable effect of red wine on plasma high-density lipoprotein. *Ann. Nutr. Metab.* 38:287–294, 1994.

LeBlanc, A.E., Kalant, H. and Gibbins, R.J. Acute tolerance to ethanol in the rat. *Psychopharmacologia* 41:43–46, 1975.

Lery, N. et al. Interactions between alcohol and drugs. *Vet. Hum. Toxicol.* 24:427–443, 1982.

Levy, R., Elo, T. and Hanenson, I.B. Intravenous fructose treatment of acute alcohol intoxication. *Arch. Intern. Med.* 137:1175–1177, 1977.

Lewis, E.G., Dustman, R.E. and Beck, E.C. The effect of alcohol on sensory phenomena and cognitive and motor tasks. *Q. J. Stud. Alcohol* 30:618–633, 1969.

Liang, Q. et al. A transgenic model of acetaldehyde overproduction accelerates alcohol cardiomyopathy. *J. Pharmacol. Exper. Ther.* 291:766–72, 1999.

Lichtor, J.L. et al. Alcohol after midazolam sedation: Does it really matter? *Anesth. Analg.* 73:829–30, 1991.

Lieber, C.S., Rubin, E. and deCarli, L.M. Interactions of ethanol, drug, and lipid metabolism: Adaptive changes after ethanol consumption. In: Roach, M.K, McIsaac W.M. and Creavan, P.J. (eds.), *Advances in Mental Science,* vol. 3, *Biological Aspects of Alcohol.* University of Texas Press, Austin, 1971, pp. 138–167.

Lieber, C.S. Ethanol metabolism, cirrhosis and alcoholism. *Clinica Chimica Acta* 257:59–84, 1997.

Liguori, A. and Robinson, J.H. Caffeine antagonism of alcohol-induced driving impairment. *Drug and Alcohl Dependence* 63:123–9, 2001.

Linnoila, M. and Hakkinen, S. Effects of diazepam and codeine, alone and in combination with alcohol, on simulated driving. *Clin. Pharmacol. Ther.* 15:368, 1974.

Linnoila, M., and Mattila, M.J. Drug interaction on psychomotor skills related to driving: Diazepam and alcohol. *Eur. J. Clin. Pharmacol.* 5:186–194, 1973.

Linnoila, M., Saario, I. and Maki, M. Effect of treatment with diazepam or lithium and alcohol on psychomotor skills related to driving. *Eur. J. Clin. Pharmacol.* 7:337–342, 1974.

MacKenzie, A.I. Naloxone in alcohol intoxication. *Lancet* 2:733–734, 1979.

Mallach, H.J. and Etzler, K. Tierexperimentelle Untersuchungen uber die gemeinsame Wirkung von Dimethylsufoxid und Aethylalkohol. *Arzneimittelforsch.* 15:1305–1308, 1965.

Marquis, D.G. et al. Experimental studies of behavioral effects of meprobamate in normal subjects. *Ann. N. Y. Acad. Sci.* 67:701–711, 1957.

Marshall, J.P. et al. Biochemistry of hepatic coma in alcohol-induced liver diseases and other types of hepatic dysfunction. In: Majchrowicz, E. and Noble, E.P. (eds.), *Biochemistry and Pharmacology of Ethanol*, vol. 1. Plenum Press, New York, 1979, pp. 479–499.

Martin, E.W. Table of Drug Interactions. In: Alexander, S.F, Hassan, W.E. and Farage, D.J (eds.), *Hazards of Medication.* J.B. Lippincott, Philadelphia, p. 415, pp. 430–437, 1971.

Mehar, G.S., Parker, J.M. and Tubas, T. Interaction between alcohol, minor tranquilizers and morphine. *Int. J. Clin. Pharmacol.* 9:70–74, 1974.

Melent'ev, A.B. and Novikov, P.I. [Role of alcohol in heroin overdose]. *Sudebno-Meditsinskaia Ekspertiza.* 45:12–17, 2002.

Mellanby, E. *Alcohol: Its Absorption into and Disappearance from the Blood Under Different Conditions.* Medical Research Committee, Special Report Series, No. 31, 1919.

Mello, N.K. and Mendelson, J.H. Experimentally induced intoxication in alcoholics: A comparison between programmed and spontaneous drinking. *J. Pharmacol. Exp. Ther.,* 173:101–116, 1970.

Mendelson, J.H., Stein, S. and Mello, N.K. Effects of experimentally induced intoxication on metabolism of ethanol-1-Cl4 in alcoholic subjects. *Metab. Clin. Exp.* 14:1255–1266, 1965.

Mergler, D. et al. Colour vision impairment and alcohol consumption. *Neurotoxicol. Teratol.* 10:255–260, 1988.

Mezey, E. Ethanol and hepatic fibrogenesis. In: Majchrowicz, E. and Noble, E.P. (eds.), *Biochemistry and Pharmacology of Ethanol*, vol. 1. Plenum Press, New York, 1979, pp. 459–479.

Miles, W.R. *Alcohol and Human Efficiency*. Carnegie Institute publication No. 333, Pittsburgh, 1924.

Miller, R.J. The effect of ingested alcohol on fusion latency at various viewing distances. *Percept. Psychophysiology*. 50:575–583, 1991.

Milner, G. and Landauer, A.A. The effects of doxepin, alone and together with alcohol, in relation to driving safety. *Med. J. Aust.* 1:837, 1973.

Modell, J.G. and Mountz, J.M. Drinking and flying: The problem of alcohol use by pilots. *NEJM* 323: 455–461, 1990.

Morgan, D.L. et al. Severe ethanol intoxication in an adolescent. *Am. J. Emerg. Med.* 13:416–418, 1995.

Mortimer, R.G. Effect of low blood alcohol concentrations in simulated day and night driving. *Percept. Mot. Skills* 17:399–408, 1963.

Moskowitz, H. Alcohol influences upon sensory motor function, visual perception, and attention. In: *Alcohol, Drugs, and Driving,* publication HS 801-096. National Highway Traffic Safety Administration, U.S. Dept. of Transportation, Mar. 1974, pp. 49–69.

Moskowitz, H., Daily, J. and Henderson, R. The Mellanby effect in moderate and heavy drinkers. *Proc. Seventh Int. Conf. on Alc. Drugs and Traffic Safety*, Melbourne, 23–28 Jan., 1977.

Moskowitz, H. and Sharma, S. Effects of alcohol on peripheral vision as a function of attention. *Hum. Factors*, 16:174–180, 1974.

Moskowitz, H., Burns, M.M. and Williams, A.F. Skills performance at low blood alcohol levels. *J. Stud. Alc.* 46:482–485, 1985.

Moskowitz, H. and Robinson, C.D. *Effects of Low Doses of Alcohol on Driving-Related Skills: A Review of the Evidence,* DOT HS 807-280. SRA Technologies, Inc., U.S. Department of Commerce. National Technical Information Service, Springfield, VA 22161, 1988.

Moureau, P. Tendances de la legislation belge en ce qui concerne l'intoxication alcoolique et les accidents de roulage. *Rev. Alcoolisme* 4:178–180, 1957.

MMWR. Deaths and hospitalizations from chronic liver disease and cirrhosis: United States, 1980–1989. *Morb. Mortal. Wkly. Rep.* 41:969–973, 1993.

Myers, R.D., Borg, S. and Mossberg, R. Antagonism by naltrexone of voluntary alcohol selection in the chronically drinking macaque monkey. *Alcohol* 3:383–388, 1986.

National Digestive Diseases Information Clearinghouse (NIDDK). *Cirrhosis of the Liver*, NIH Publication 00-1134, April 2000.

Newman, H.W. and Fletcher, E. The effect of alcohol on vision. *Am. J. Med. Sci.* 202:723–731, 1941.

Newman, H.W. Emetic action of ethyl alcohol. *Arch. Intern. Med.* 94:417–419, 1954.

Nicholson, M.E. et al. Variability in behavioral impairment involved in the rising and falling BAC curve. *J. Stud. Alcohol* 53:349–356, 1992.

O'Malley, S.S. et al. Naltrexone and coping skills therapy for alcohol dependence: A controlled study. *Arch. Gen. Psychiatry* 49:881–887, 1992.

Osborne, D.J. and Rogers, Y. Interactions of alcohol and caffeine on human reaction time. *Aviat. Space Environ. Med.* 54:528–534, 1983.

Peck, R.C. et al. The effects of marijuana and alcohol on actual driving performance. *Alcohol, Drugs, and Driving* 2:135–154, 1986.

Pennings, E.J., Leccese, A.P. and Wolfe, F.A. Effects of concurrent use of alcohol and cocaine. [Review] *Addiction* 97:773–783, 2002.

Pihkanen, T.A. and Kauko, O., The effects of alcohol on the perception of musical stimuli. *Ann. Med. Exp. Fenn.* 40:275–285, 1962.

Rall, T.W. Hypnotics and sedatives: Ethanol. In: Gilman, A.G. et al. (eds.), *The Pharmacological*

Basis of Therapeutics, 8th ed. Pergamon Press, New York, 1990, pp. 373–374.

Regan, T.J. Ethyl alcohol and the heart. *Circulation* 44:957–963, 1971.

Ritchie, M. The aliphatic alcohols. In: Gilman, A.G., Goodman, L.S. and Gilman, A. (eds.), *Goodman & Gilman's The Pharmacological Basis of Therapeutics*, 6th ed. MacMillan, New York, 1980, p. 72, pp. 376–390.

Robinson, A.et al. Effect of ethyl alcohol on reaction times as measured on a motorcycle simulator. (Abst) *Clin. Chem.* 36:1170, 1990.

Rosen, L.J. and Lee, C.L. Acute and chronic effects of alcohol use on organizational processes in memory. *J. Abnor. Psychol.* 85:309–317, 1976.

Ross, L.E. and Mundt, J.C. Multiattribute modeling analysis of the effects of a low blood alcohol level on pilot performance. *Hum. Factors* 30:293–304, 1988.

Rubin, E. and Lieber, C.S. Alcoholism, alcohol, and drugs. *Science* 172:1097–1102, 1971.

Ryback, R.S. Effects of alcohol on memory and its implications for flying safety. *Aerosp. Med.* 41:1193–1195, 1970.

Schmidt, L. and Bingel, A.G.A. *Effect of Oxygen Deficiency and Various Other Factors on Color Saturation Thresholds.* U.S.A.F. School of Aviation Medicine Project Reports: Project No. 21-31-002 1953.

Schaffer, A. and Naranjo, C.A. Recommended drug treatment strategies for the alcoholic patient. [Review.] *Drugs* 56:571–585, 1998.

Seixas, F.A. Alcohol and its drug interactions. *Ann. Intern. Med.* 83:86–92, 1975.

Smart, R.G. Factors in recent reductions in liver cirrhosis deaths. [Review.] *J. Stud. Alc.* 52:232–40, 1991.

Smith, A.C., Freeman, R.W. and Harbison, R.D. Ethanol enhancement of cocaine-induced hepatotoxicity. *Biochem. Pharmacol.* 30:453–458, 1981.

Sorensen, S.C. and Mattison, K.W. Naloxone as an antagonist in severe alcohol intoxication. *Lancet* 2:688–689, 1978.

Sporer, K.A. Acute heroin overdose. [Review.] *Ann. Int. Med.* 130:584–90, 1999.

Srivastava, L.M. et al. Relation between alcohol intake, lipoproteins and coronary heart disease: the interest continues. [Review.] *Alc. Alcohol.* 29:11–24, 1994.

Starck, H.J. Untersuchungen uber die Verkehrssicherheit alkoholgewohnter Kraftfahrer bei Blutalkoholwerten um 1.5 g-%. *Dtsch. Z. Ges. Gerichtl. Med.* 42:155–161, 1953.

Sutton, L.R. The effects of alcohol, marihuana and their combination on driving ability. *J. Stud. Alc.* 44:438–445,1983.

Sun, S.W., Kahn, D.M. and Swan, K.G. Lowering the legal blood alcohol level for motorcyclists. *Accident Analysis and Prevention* 30:133–136, 1998.

Suzuki, K. et al. Effects of injection of analgetics and alcohol drinking on values of electric flicker. *Tohoku J. Exp. Med.* 66: 327–331, 1957.

Tang, P.C. and Rosenstein, R. Influence of alcohol and dramamine, alone and in combination, on pilot performance. *Aerosp. Med.* 38:818–821, 1967.

Terhune, K.W. et al. *The Incidence and Role of Drugs in Fatally Injured Drivers,* DOT HS 808-065. U.S. DOT, National Highway Traffic Safety Administration, Oct. 1992.

Tsirambidis, J.V., Conwell, D.L. and Zuccaro, G. Chronic pancreatitis. *Medscape General Medicine,* 5(1), 2003.

Tzambazis, K. and Stough, C. Alcohol impairs speed of information processing and simple and choice reaction time and differentially impairs higher-order cognitive abilities. *Alcohol & Alcoholism* 35:197–201, 2000.

Volpicelli, J.R. et al. Naltrexone in the treatment of alcohol dependence. *Arch. Gen. Psychiatry* 49:876–880, 1992.

Volpicelli, J.R., Davis, M.A. and Olin, J.E. Naltrexone blocks the post-shock increase of ethanol consumption. *Life Sci.* 38:841–847, 1986.

Wallgren, H. and Barry, H. III. *Actions of Alcohol,* vol. 1, *Biochemical Physiological, and Psychological Effects.* Elsevier, New York, 1970, p. 287.

Wang, M.Q., Nicholson, M.E. and Mahoney, B.S. The effects of high and low BACs on the Hoffman reflex. *J. Neurol. Sci.* 117:107–110, 1993.

Watson, W.A. and Garriott, J.C. Alcohol and motorcycle riders: A comparison of motorcycle and car/truck DWI's. *Vet. Hum. Toxicol.* 34:213–215, 1992.

West, R. et al. Effect of low and moderate doses of alcohol on driving hazard perception latency and driving speed. *Addiction* 88:527–532, 1993.

Wier, J.K. and Tyler, V.E. An investigation of Coprinus atramentarius for the presence of disulfiram. *J. Am. Pharmacol. Assoc.* 49:426–429, 1960.

Winek, C.L. and Murphy, K.L. The rate and kinetic order of ethanol elimination. *Forensic Sci. Int.* 25:159–166, 1984.

Wooten, F.T. and Lee, W.M. Acetaminophen hepatotoxicity in the alcoholic. *Southern Medical Journal,* 83:1047–1049, 1990.

Yesavage, J.A. and Leirer, V.O. Hangover effects on aircraft pilots 14 hours after alcohol ingestion: A preliminary report. *Am. J. Psychiatry* 143:1546–1550, 1986.

Zimmerman, E.G. et al. Measurement of delta 9-tetrahydrocannabinol (THC) in whole blood samples from impaired motorists. *J. Forens. Sci.* 28:957–962, 1983.

Zrenner, E. et al. Effects of ethyl alcohol on the electrooculogram and color vision. *Doc. Ophthalmol.* 463:305–312, 1986.

Chapter 3

Disposition and Fate of Ethanol in the Body

A.W. Jones, Ph.D., D.Sc.

3.1 Introduction

The disposition and fate of ethanol in the body have been studied extensively since the 1930s following the pioneering work and publications of Erik M.P. Widmark (Widmark, 1932; Andréasson and Jones, 1996). The chapter dealing with disposition of alcohol in man appearing in the previous (third) edition of this book (Garriott, 1996) focused heavily on the experimental work and results reported in Widmark's 1932 monograph (Baselt, 1981).

Disposition relates to what happens to a drug after it enters the body and is therefore closely linked to absorption and other pre-systemic processes as well as the events occurring after the drug reaches the blood circulation, particularly its distribution and elimination through metabolism and excretion (Benet et al., 1990). Knowledge about the disposition and fate of ethanol in the body predates that of all other drugs and xenobiotics thanks to the early availability of a reliable quantitative method for measuring ethanol in blood and other biological fluids (Widmark, 1922). A micro-method, which utilized only 100 μL of fingertip blood for a single determination, allowed scientists to track the concentration-time profiles of ethanol after healthy volunteers drank moderate amounts of alcohol (Widmark, 1922; Widmark, 1932).

The subject of **pharmacokinetics** deals with the way that drugs are absorbed, distributed and eliminated from the body and how these processes can be described in quantitative terms (Gabrielsson and Weiner, 2000; Wagner, 1993). Kinetics comes from the Greek word *kinesis*, which means "motion," so pharmacokinetics means the movement or time-course of a drug (in Greek, *pharmacon*) in the body. The mathematical relationships that best describe the way that drug-concentrations (or amounts) change as a function of time after intake forms the basis of clinical pharmacokinetics (Greenblatt and Koch-Weser, 1975a,b; Rowland and Tozer, 1980). By contrast, the term **pharmacodynamics** relates to the mechanism of action of drugs and how they alter a person's behavior and normal body functioning and also any dose-response and concentration-effect relationships (Ross, 1990). These two important terms closely related to the fate of a drug in the body, namely pharmacokinetics and pharmacodynamics, are distinguished in Figure 3.1.

Comprehensive reviews dealing with disposition and metabolism of ethanol mostly appear in articles and textbooks devoted to biomedical alcohol research rather than the forensic sciences (Wilkinson, 1980; Von Wartburg, 1989; Kalant, 1996b; Lands, 1998; Matsumoto and Fukui, 2002; Ramchandani et al., 2001). Indeed, the overview by Kalant (1996b), which updated his previous treatise on the topic of absorption, distribution and elimination of alcohol, is highly recommended (Kalant, 1971). Some of the journals specializing in clinical pharmacology publish comprehensive reviews of adverse drug-alcohol interactions and various aspects of ethanol pharma-

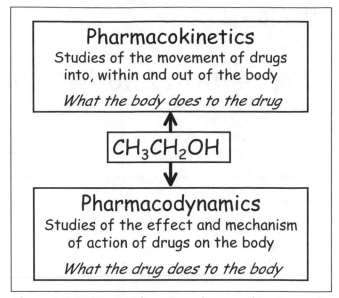

Figure 3.1 *Distinction between pharmacokinetics and pharmacodynamics, key concepts when considering the disposition and fate of drugs in the body*

cokinetics (Holford, 1987; Fraser, 1997; Norberg et al., 2003).

Medicolegal aspects of alcohol, the subject of this book, are closely related to the analysis of ethanol in body fluids (blood, breath, urine) from both living and dead and the interpretation of the results, for example, in connection with driving under the influence of alcohol (DUI) and other alcohol-related crimes (Dubowski, 1985; Garriott, 1996; Jones, 2000c; Langford et al., 1999). The reliability of forensic alcohol analysis and the problems and pitfalls encountered when the results are interpreted have been reviewed elsewhere (Hume and Fitzgerald, 1985; Batt, 1989; Khanna et al., 1989; Ferner, 1996). In this connection the book by Cooper et al. (1979) put major emphasis on the kind of questions and calculations commonly encountered in forensic casework when drunk drivers are prosecuted (Breen et al., 1998; Langford et al., 1999). The book by Walls and Brownlie (1985) entitled *Drink, Drugs and Driving* covered forensic aspects of alcohol specifically targeted to the British legal system. Ley (1997) wrote a book devoted to drink driving law and practice in UK, and gave an extensive review of case law as well as a survey of the many defense challenges arising over the years (Jones, 1991b). Likewise, the law and science of drunk-driving litigation has been extensively covered from the U.S. perspective

(Erwin, 1991; Cohen and Green, 1995; Fitzgerald, 2001). These works often run into several volumes and are regularly updated with special supplements. The target readers are obviously lawyers and law firms specializing in defending drinking drivers who need to keep abreast of developments in case law as well as the pros and cons of a multitude of defense challenges (Lewis, 1986b; Jones, 1991b; Ferner and Norman, 1996; Langford et al., 1999). A book by Rockerbie (1999) focused on the forensic pharmacology of ethanol and other matters related to driving under the influence of alcohol and drugs.

Forensic alcohol research has developed alongside biomedical alcohol research and is tightly linked to the fate of alcohol in the body and the analysis of ethanol in body fluids and how the results should be interpreted in a legal context (Jones, 1996a; Jones, 2000c). The literature pertaining to the disposition and fate of ethanol in the body is extensive and many specialist alcohol research journals exist including an online database called ETOH, which is produced and maintained by the U.S. National Institute on Alcohol Abuse and Alcoholism (NIAAA). Noteworthy too are many articles dealing with forensic aspects of alcohol written in the German language. The leading journal is *Blutalkohol* (blood alcohol), which first appeared in 1961 and is still going strong. Unfortunately, much of the research reported in *Blutalkohol* is little known outside German-speaking countries and the articles are rarely cited in international peer-reviewed journals. The book by Cooper (1979) focused heavily on the older German literature, which makes it a useful reference source for those without access to *Blutalkohol* or who don't understand the German language.

In this chapter, the disposition and fate of ethanol in the body are reviewed based on information gleaned from articles and reviews published in forensic science and biomedical research journals. It is not my intention here to update the chapter by Baselt (1996), which appeared in the third edition of this book. Instead, I present a fresh appraisal of the subject based on the current state of knowledge and my own experiences from many years of working in the field of experimental alcohol research (Jones, 1996a). Much of the original material used for this presentation comes from controlled drinking studies conducted by our research group in Sweden or together with collaborators in other countries. The involvement in the design, planning and execution of human studies including participating in the actual research and evaluating the results for publication helps to boost confidence in the conclusions reached.

3.2 Analytical Considerations

Peng and Chiou (1990) discussed the importance of standardized protocols and the availability of accurate, precise and specific methods for analysis of drugs in studies of their absorption, distribution and metabolism in the body (Tagliaro et al., 1992).

Different countries have their own legal traditions and standards of proof in drunk-driving legislation. This is reflected not only in the various threshold alcohol limits for driving but also in the methods of analysis used, the biological specimens recommended and the way the concentrations of ethanol are reported to the courts. The punishable alcohol limits for driving are reported as g/100 mL (U.S.A.), mg/100 mL (UK and Ireland), g/L (France, Spain and most of continental Europe) or g/kg (Germany) or mg/g (Nordic countries). This sometimes causes confusion when articles from different scientific journals are compared and contrasted. The concentration units used to report BAC values have ramifications for the pharmacokinetic parameters of ethanol, such as β-slope and *rho*, which are widely used when making forward or backward estimations of BAC (Lewis, 1986a; Stowell and Stowell, 1998).

The peak concentration reached in blood (C_{max}), the rate of elimination of ethanol from the bloodstream (k_o or β) as well as the apparent volume of distribution of ethanol (V_d or *rho*) will differ depending on whether mass/mass or mass/volume concentration units are used. Even more importantly, whether the specimen analyzed was whole blood as opposed to plasma or serum needs consideration because ethanol is not evenly distributed into the various constituents of blood. The red cells or erythrocytes are ~70 percent w/w water, plasma ~93 percent w/w water whole blood ~80 percent w/w water (Lentner, 1981; Rosenfeld, 1996). Some of the articles appearing in general medical journals mention measuring blood-alcohol concentration but after reading the text it becomes obvious that serum or plasma were the specimens used for the assay (Raufman et al., 1993; Al-lanqawi et al., 1992).

When the first methods of blood-ethanol analysis appeared in the 1920s, the aliquots of blood used for analysis were weighed on a torsion balance, because this operation could be accomplished more accurately than measuring a fixed volume of blood with a pipette (Widmark, 1922). Accordingly, the results of the measurements were reported as mass/mass units (e.g., mg/g or g/kg), which are not the same as mass/volume units (g/L or g/100 mL). The difference depends on the specific weight of whole blood, which on the average is 1.055 (Lentner, 1981). All Widmark's publications reported the concentrations of ethanol as mass/mass units (mg/g) and this needs to be considered when his kinetic parameters (β and rho) are compared with values reported today when weight/volume units are the norm (g/L, mg/dL or g/100 mL). Accordingly, a C_{max} of 1.0 mg/g, a β-slope of 0.15 mg/g/h and a rho of 0.68 as reported by Widmark are equivalent to 1.055 g/L (C_{max}), 0.16 g/L/h (β) and 0.66 L/kg (rho), respectively. Furthermore, many articles published in biochemical journals report concentrations of ethanol as mmol/L and therefore the molecular weight of ethanol (46.05) needs to be introduced into the calculation to express the result as mass/volume; thus 22.7 mmol/L is the same as 1.0 g/L. Inter-relationships between the various units used to report concentrations of ethanol measured in whole blood and plasma/serum are given in Table 3.1.

For the analysis of ethanol in biofluids such as saliva, urine and cerebrospinal fluid the difference between w/w and w/v is negligible because the specific gravity of these liquids is close to unity (Lentner, 1981). Furthermore, in autopsy work the water content of blood and its density can vary widely depending on different circumstances and various postmortem artifacts (Jones, 2000b). Making an adjustment for differences between w/w and w/v, as is customary with fresh whole blood from living individuals, is more complicated and probably unnecessary in medical examiner cases. The reliability of blood-alcohol analysis in autopsy specimens depends on many factors (e.g., sampling site, postmortem diffusion and neoformation) as discussed in other chapters in this book and elsewhere (O'Neal and Poklis, 1996; Jones, 2000b).

Breath-alcohol instruments are being increasingly used in pharmacokinetic studies of alcohol and drug-alcohol interactions and great care is needed to ensure correct calibration of the units and other quality assurance aspects necessary to increase confidence in the results (O'Connor et al., 1998; Gullberg, 2000).

Table 3.1
Inter-relationships between Ethanol Concentrations Measured in Plasma or Serum Compared with Those Present in Whole Blood when the Results are Reported in Different Concentration Units

The mean plasma/blood ratio was taken as 1.15:1 and the molecular weight of ethanol as 46.05.

Plasma or serum, mmol/L	Plasma or serum, g/L[1]	Whole blood, mmol/L[2]	Whole blood, mg/mL or g/L[3]	Whole blood, mg/g or g/kg[4]
5	0.23	4.34	0.20	0.189
10	0.46	8.69	0.40	0.379
20	0.92	17.4	0.80	0.758
30	1.38	26.1	1.20	1.14
50	2.3	43.5	2.00	1.89

[1] (mmol/L × 46)/1000
[2] (mmol/L plasma or serum)/1.15
[3] (mmol/l blood × 46)/1,000
[4] (g/L/1.055)

3.3 Disposition and Fate of Ethanol in the Body

For a drug to exert its pharmacological effect it must enter the body in sufficient amounts to reach the site of action, whether this is the brain for psychotropic substances or receptor sites located at other target organs or tissue (Ross, 1990; Benet et al., 1990). Compared with most drugs of abuse alcohol is a relatively weak pharmacological agent and large quantities must be ingested to bring about the feeling of euphoria and inebriation (Goldstein, 1983). However, the therapeutic index for ethanol is fairly narrow with ED_{50}/LD_{50} ratios of only about 1:8. After drinking a small dose of ethanol to produce a peak BAC of 0.5 g/L, which would probably cause mild euphoria in most people, drinking a much larger dose to produce a BAC of 4 g/L causes gross intoxication, stupor, coma and probably death (Jones and Holmgren, 2003).

The blood-alcohol concentration reached after drinking depends not only on the amount or the dose of ethanol consumed but also on the speed of drinking, and the rates of absorption, distribution, and metabolism in the body. Figure 3.2 lists many of the variable factors involved in the disposition of ethanol in the body, which makes it easy to appreciate the reason for large inter- and intra-individual variations in the BAC profiles observed in experimental studies.

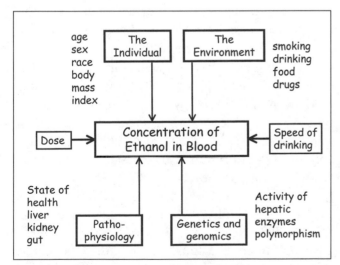

Figure 3.2 *Summary of the multitude of factors that influence the concentration of ethanol in blood after drinking*

3.4 Absorption of Ethanol

Absorption is the process by which a drug enters the blood circulation after administration by any extravascular route (e.g., oral, intramuscular, intradermal, sublingual, or rectally) (Benet et al., 1990; Rowland and Tozer, 1980). The uptake of the compound from the site of administration to the systemic circulation is also part of the absorption process (Benet et al., 1990). Alcohol can be administered to the human body in a number of different ways including by the intravenous route (injection or continuous IV infusion) and *per rectum*.

A. Inhalation of ethanol vapors

Small amounts of alcohol can theoretically be absorbed into the blood by inhalation of ethanol vapors through the lungs. However, studies have shown that the vapor concentrations of ethanol needed are so high that the person being exposed cannot tolerate them (Lester and Greenberg, 1951). One well-designed study showed that if subjects were exposed to ethanol vapors in an environmental chamber after they had been drinking, the elimination of ethanol already in the bloodstream was slowed down appreciably. It seems that the amounts inhaled balanced the amounts metabolized during the exposure (Kruhoffer, 1983). However, in practice much will depend on the size of the room, whether there were open windows, the exposure time, the concentration of ethanol in the air breathed and the degree of lung ventilation during the exposure (Lewis, 1985; Mason and Blackmore, 1972). The results from these human studies are in conflict with animal models using mice and rats in which inhalation of alcohol vapor is a standard method to induce tolerance and dependence on the drug (Goldstein and Zaechelein, 1983). It should be noted that small rodents have a higher minute volume (lung ventilations per minute) than humans and cannot complain about the disagreeable high concentrations of alcohol vapor they are being exposed to.

B. Absorption through skin

There is no solid evidence that ethanol can be absorbed via the unbroken skin, which probably stems from the low lipid solubility of ethanol (Kalant, 1971; Goldstein, 1983). However, if there are cuts and abrasions on the exposed surface and also open blood vessels, measurable amounts can be absorbed (Jones and Rajs, 1997). It appears that the rate and extent of uptake of ethanol through the lungs or percutaneously is always much less than the overall rate of metabolism (~6–8 g/h), making it virtually impossible to achieve an increasing BAC by these routes of administration (Anderson et al., 1991; Pendlington et al., 2001).

3.5 Dosage Forms

The dosage form of a drug designates the physical form in which the substance is administered or ingested and is comparable with the drug delivery system, whether as solution, tablets, capsules, coated tablets, syrups and so on (Rowland and Tozer, 1980). The choice of dosage form can markedly influence the rate of absorption after oral intake of certain drugs (Rowland and Tozer, 1980). For ethanol the kind of beverage consumed, whether beer, wine, spirits, or cocktails, can be considered the dosage form of alcohol as opposed to ingesting pure ethanol solvent diluted with water. Besides ethanol and water many alcoholic beverages contain trace amounts of other low-molecular substances, known as the congeners, which help to impart the taste and flavor to the drink (Iffland and Jones, 2003). Spirits are often diluted with various soft drinks containing CO_2 which might enhance stomach emptying. Many beers as well as the now so popular "alco-pops" contain varying amounts of carbohydrates, which can delay emptying of the stomach and slow the rate of uptake of alcohol into the bloodstream (Kalant, 1996b; Goldberg et al., 1979).

3.6 Absorption from the Gut

For all practical purposes alcohol is taken by mouth (*per os*), and enters the gastrointestinal tract where absorption begins partly through the stomach wall (~20 percent), but mainly from the duodenum and small intestine (~80 percent). Absorption occurs by a diffusion process in accordance with Fick's law and should therefore depend on the concentration gradient across the gastric lumen (Berggren and Goldberg, 1940). After drinking alcoholic beverages, whether in the form of beer, wine or spirits, the alcohol they contain reaches the stomach and absorption

begins both during drinking and for some time after finishing the drink (Cooke and Birchall, 1969; Cooke, 1970). Figure 3.3 illustrates the sites of absorption of ethanol from the stomach and the resulting shape of the BAC curve for slow compared with rapid gastric emptying.

3.7 Gastric Emptying

The mechanisms regulating gastric motility and thereby stomach emptying via the pyloric sphincter are crucially important for determining the rate of uptake of alcohol into the bloodstream. This follows because of the much larger surface area in the duodenum and jejunum compared with the stomach (Kalant, 1996b; Jones, 1996a). Inter- and intra-individual differences in gastric emptying account for much of the variability in the absorption profiles as reflected in large differences in C_{max} and t_{max} when individual blood-alcohol curves are compared. In an interesting approach to resolve the importance of gastric emptying on rate of ethanol absorption, volunteers were administered a fat emulsion or saline as control treatment directly into the ileum (McFarlane et al., 1986). This maneuver avoided an interaction between ethanol and the food in the stomach, which otherwise would complicate interpretation of the results. Absorption of 0.5 g/kg ethanol was slowed appreciably after treatment with lipids, which prevented emptying of the stomach into the duodenum; the C_{max} was lower and the entire absorption phase was more prolonged lasting for several hours. Similarly, a delayed absorption of ethanol was reported when the lipids were infused into the duodenum.

A multitude of experimental variables can alter gastric emptying and this topic is of concern in the field of gastroenterology when upper abdominal problems are being investigated (Rose, 1979; Vantrappen, 1994). Perhaps the most important variable in this connection is the presence of liquid or solid food in the stomach before alcohol is consumed (Sedman et al., 1976b; Wilkinson et al., 1977a; Jones and Jönsson, 1994b; Watkins and Adler, 1993; Jones and Neri, 1991; Singh, 1999). Also the amount and composition of the food and its calorific value as well as the relative proportions of fat, carbohydrate, and protein should be considered (Ramchandani et al., 2001a). However, the size of

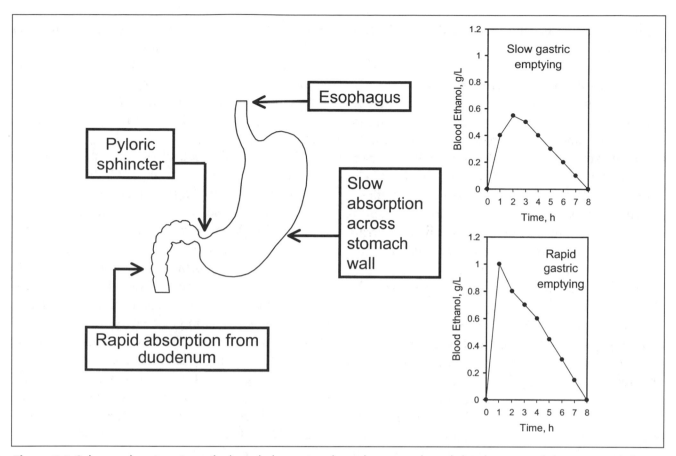

Figure 3.3 *Scheme showing sites of ethanol absorption from the stomach and duodenum and the expected shapes of the blood-ethanol profiles for rapid and slow emptying of the stomach*

the meal and closeness to the time of drinking the alcohol seems more important for slowing absorption into the blood than the composition of the meal in terms of its macronutrients (Jones et al., 1997c; Horowitz et al., 1989). Under some circumstances, when alcohol is taken after a meal it might require several hours to become fully absorbed into the bloodstream, owing to binding of ethanol with the food components and thus preventing or delaying direct contact with the absorption surface in the stomach (Cortot et al., 1986; Shultz et al., 1980; Horowitz et al., 1989).

In several studies, it was shown that eating a meal increased the clearance rate of ethanol from blood even when the alcohol was administered intravenously and that carbohydrate content was more important than fat and protein (Rogers et al., 1987; Hahn et al., 1994). This points to food-induced increases in activity of alcohol metabolizing enzymes or perhaps the liver blood flow was increased after

the food thus causing a more effective hepatic clearance of ethanol (Bode, 1978; Bosron et al., 1984; Host et al., 1996; Dedrick and Forrester, 1973).

Medications that alter gastric motility, such as the prokinetic drug cisapride, metoclopramide or erythromycin, which speed up stomach emptying, also accelerate the absorption of ethanol into the bloodstream (Edelbroek et al., 1993; Kechagias et al., 1997; Kechagias et al., 1999; Oneta et al., 1998). Gastric emptying appears to be faster in the morning compared with the evening, although this might depend on diurnal variations in blood-glucose concentration (Lötterle et al., 1989; Schvarcz et al., 1995; Goo et al., 1987). Accordingly, the time of day when alcohol is consumed is another variable to consider when absorption profiles of ethanol are interpreted. Smoking cigarettes was shown to delay gastric emptying resulting in a slower uptake of alcohol into the bloodstream and accordingly a lower C_{max} and later

t_{max} in venous blood (Hanson and Lilja, 1987; Johnson et al., 1991).

3.8 Drinking on an Empty Stomach

Drinks taken on an empty stomach (e.g., after an overnight ten-hour fast) are generally absorbed rapidly because under these conditions gastric emptying is quicker when the ethanol molecules reach the much larger absorption surface area in the duodenum (Jones, 1984). However, some people might experience a pyloric spasm after they drink neat spirits on an empty stomach. This is caused by local irritation of emptying mechanisms or contractions of the stomach and leads to a much slower absorption of ethanol into the blood and a lower C_{max} and later t_{max} (Jones, 1984).

The shape of the BAC profiles when gastric emptying is rapid resemble the curves seen when the ethanol is administered by constant rate intravenous infusion (Alha, 1951; Wilkinson et al., 1976; Jones and Hahn, 1997; Davidson et al., 1997). After an unusually rapid absorption of ethanol an overshoot peak is often observed (see Figure 3.3) and for a short time C_{max} is higher than expected for the amount (dose) of alcohol consumed. However, the excess ethanol rapidly dissipates and the C_{max} is followed by a diffusion plunge during which time the alcohol in the central compartment (blood) distributes throughout the total body water (Hahn et al., 1997). The diffusion plunge appears to be an exponential function with a half-life of ~7 minutes (Hahn et al., 1995). Accordingly, it should take about 35 minutes (5 × half-life) for the blood-alcohol concentration to drop to the concentration expected for complete equilibration with the total body water.

The existence of an overshoot peak was recently demonstrated when women who had undergone gastric bypass surgery for morbid obesity consumed a bolus dose of ethanol (Klockhoff et al., 2002). The C_{max} was higher in the operated women compared with controls but by thirty-five minutes post-dosing, the BAC curves were not significantly different between the two groups of women. Whether other medical problems in the upper gastrointestinal tract, such as ulcers, dyspepsia, gastritis, *helicobacter pylori* infections or gastroesophageal reflux affect the speed of alcohol absorption remains to be studied

(Salmela et al., 1994; Lieber, 1997b; Simanowski et al., 1998). Indeed, other disease states such as diabetes mellitus, hyperthyroidism and anorexia nervosa are likely to alter gastric emptying, rate of absorption of ethanol and the resulting C_{max} and t_{max} for a given dose (Nowak et al., 1995; Kong and Horwitz, 1999).

The dose and speed of drinking are important considerations when the peak BAC, the time of its occurrence, and variability in areas under the BAC profiles are discussed in forensic situations (O'Neill et al., 1983; Winek et al., 1996; Wilkinson et al., 1977b). In general, the larger the dose of alcohol and the faster the rate of drinking the higher is the BAC and impairment of the individual is more pronounced. Small doses of ethanol are absorbed faster than larger doses as might be expected. Moreover, after low doses (< 0.3 g/kg) some of the alcohol is metabolized during the first passage of blood through the gut and liver, which is known as first pass metabolism (FPM). This presystemic clearance of ethanol is especially marked when small doses of alcohol are ingested after eating food (Wagner, 1986; Oneta et al., 1998). Variability in absorption profiles and C_{max} are less if the dose of alcohol is administered per kilogram body water instead of per kilogram body weight. This follows because of the different proportions of adipose tissue in different individuals with the same body weight (Wang et al., 1992; Graham et al., 1998). Moreover, the percentage of water in the body decreases in the elderly (Schoeller, 1989) and the blood-alcohol concentration for a given dose is expected to be somewhat higher in the aged, especially in men (Jones and Neri, 1985; Mirand and Welye, 1994). A lower proportion of body water per kilogram body weight is the primary reason for women reaching a higher peak blood-alcohol concentrations than men after the same dose and pattern of drinking (Roche et al., 1996; Thomasson, 1995; Davies et al., 1999; Lucey et al., 1999).

After absorption from the gut, ethanol enters the portal venous blood and is transported first to the liver and then to the heart via the hepatic vein before reaching all parts of the body (Kalant, 1971). Alcohol (ethanol) mixes with water in all proportions and a quantitative relationship exists between the dose (amount) of alcohol consumed and the resulting blood-ethanol concentration (Wilkinson et al., 1977a; O'Neill et al., 1983). Alcohol easily penetrates the blood-brain barrier and starts to exert its untoward effects on the central nervous system immediately after start of drinking.

3.9 Beverage Type and Alcohol Absorption

The concentration of alcohol in the drink and whether this was in the form of spirits (40 percent v/v) or beer (5 percent v/v) is likely to influence the absorption profiles of alcohol and both C_{max} and t_{max} (Roine et al., 1991).

Figure 3.4 shows the results of experiments done many years ago in Finland to compare the shapes of BAC profiles after subjects drank either brandy or beer in a crossover design study, with each subject acting as his own control (Takala et al., 1957). The beer curves showed a slower rise and a lower and slightly later occurring peak BAC compared with brandy. But by 120 minutes post-dosing the curves

ran close together and stayed this way for the rest of the time that the measurements were made (Takala et al., 1957). The drinks were consumed on an empty stomach and under these conditions one can expect the beverage with the highest concentration of ethanol to be absorbed faster, in accordance with Fick's law (Springer, 1972). However, the carbohydrates in beer might delay the absorption of ethanol, which is supported by the fact that the difference between the average curves was greatest during the first 60 minutes—that is, during the absorption phase. The differences between different beverages are less marked when drinking occurs after a meal and under these conditions, ethanol in the form of beer was paradoxically absorbed faster compared with drinking ethanol in the form of whisky (Roine et al., 1993).

Sex differences in the absorption rate of ethanol have not been thoroughly investigated and many factors need to be considered including sex differences in blood-glucose concentration, hormonal influ-

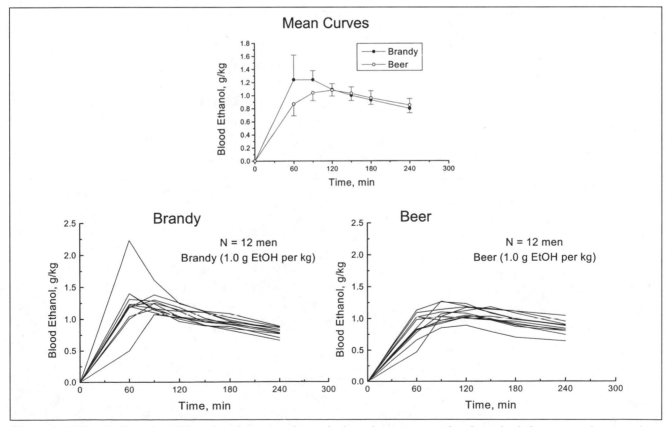

Figure 3.4 *Blood-ethanol profiles after the same dose of ethanol was ingested as brandy (left trace) or beer (right trace) after an overnight fast, with the mean curves shown above (redrawn from Takala et al., 1957)*

ences, phase of menstrual cycle and whether women are taking oral contraceptive steroids (Baraona et al., 2001; Brick et al., 1986; Gill, 1997; Mumenthaler et al., 1999; Mumenthaler et al., 2000). To what extent these factors account for variability in rate of alcohol absorption or elimination from the body needs further investigation with larger numbers of subjects (Wang et al., 1992; Lammers et al., 1995). Regarding the distribution of ethanol, there is general agreement that the lower volume of distribution in women is the major reason for the sex-related differences found in practice (Breslin et al., 1997; Mumenthaler et al., 2000; Thomason, 1995; Davies et al., 1999; Cowan et al., 1996). Females have a smaller aqueous volume owing to more fat and less body water per kilogram total body weight (Edelman and Leibman, 1959; VanLoan, 1996). Also women have a slightly larger liver mass per kilogram lean body weight than men and this probably explains the swifter rate of disappearance of alcohol from the bloodstream (steeper β-slope) in females (Kwo et al., 1998; Thomasson, 2000).

The absorption stage of ethanol disposition is undoubtedly the most variable part of the blood-ethanol curve (Holt, 1981; Pikaar et al., 1988; Friel et al., 1995a) and more attention should be given to the factors influencing gastric emptying and first pass metabolism (see later sections) when forensic scientists and others engage in theoretical calculations of BAC expected for a given intake of alcohol. Lack of attention to factors impacting on absorption probably accounts for many conflicting reports, such as the effects of drugs on the pharmacokinetics of ethanol (Gibbons and Lant, 1975; Holt et al., 1980; Pikaar et al., 1988; Jones et al., 1999; Gentry, 2000a and 2000b). It is important not to confuse an altered absorption profile and a lower, higher or more delayed C_{max} with a change in the distribution or elimination rate of ethanol in the body (Hahn et al., 1992).

Table 3.2 lists many of the variable factors that might lead to fast or slow absorption of ethanol.

A marked retardation of ethanol absorption occurs if there is food in the stomach and this was well documented in a rat model by removing the stomachs and analysis of ethanol remaining at various times post-dosing (Schultz et al., 1980). Both C_{max} and AUC were vastly different from the unfed con-

Table 3.2
Factors Influencing the Absorption of Ethanol from the Gut

Slow rate of absorption

- food in the stomach
- various carbohydrates and amino acids (fructose, glycin)
- smoking cigarettes
- drugs that delay gastric emptying (anticholinergic agents, propantheline)
- beers with high carbohydrate content
- trauma, shock and blood loss

Fast rate of absorption

- drinking on empty stomach (overnight fast)
- more concentrated alcohol beverages (e.g., undiluted spirits)
- drugs that accelerate gastric emptying (e.g., cisapride, metoclopramide, erythromycin)
- surgery to the gut (e.g., gastrectomy or gastric bypass)

trol animals and it was suggested that alcohol was bound to components of the food and that this bound fraction was retained in the stomach for many hours even after the BAC curve had peaked and was in the descending phase. The bound alcohol could have been metabolized in the stomach or during first passage of blood through the liver. An appreciably lower C_{max} and smaller AUC were reported when the amino acid glycine (2 g/kg) was administered to rats prior to them receiving a large dose of ethanol (Iimuro et al., 1996). Care is needed when results from animal studies are extrapolated to humans, owing to differences in basal metabolic rate, hepatic enzyme activity, blood and body water distribution and stomach emptying mechanisms.

3.10 Gastric First-Pass Metabolism
A. General
In the 1980s considerable interest was aroused in the notion that a substantial part of the ethanol consumed might undergo metabolism already in the stomach in a process known as gastric first-pass me-

tabolism (FPM) of ethanol (Rowland and Tozer, 1980; Lieber, 1997b). The strongest proponents for gastric FPM of ethanol were Dr. Charles Lieber and his research group from New York. These investigators published scores of articles dealing with, among other things, the effects of sex, ethnicity, age, alcoholism as well as various commonly prescribed drugs such as aspirin, cimetidine and ranitidine (Roine et al., 1990; Caballeria et al., 1989a; Caballeria, 1989b; DiPadova et al., 1992). The evidence supporting the importance of gastric ADH in FPM of ethanol included the following.

- Identification by histochemical methods of several forms of alcohol dehydrogenase (primarily class-IV or sigma ADH) in the human gastric mucosa (Cabelleria et al., 1989a; Moreno and Pares, 1991).
- The fact that about 20 percent of the dose of ethanol is absorbed directly through the stomach wall and therefore gets exposed to the gastric ADH enzyme (Kalant, 1971).
- The area under the BAC time curve is always less when ethanol is administration by mouth (peroral) compared with the same dose given intravenously, thus indicating a lower systemic availability (Baraona et al., 1994).
- First pass metabolism is reduced after concomitant use of certain drugs (e.g., aspirin, cimetidine, ranitidine) known to inhibit gastric ADH enzymes in vitro (Roine et al., 1990; DiPadova et al., 1992; Gentry et al., 1999).
- First pass metabolism is less pronounced in subjects with smaller gastric mass (e.g., after gastrectomy) (Caballeria et al., 1989b).
- Gastric first-pass metabolism is diminished or absent in Japanese subjects many of whom apparently lack gastric ADH enzymes (Baraona et al., 1991).

There is general consensus that some part of the dose of ethanol a person consumes fails to reach the systemic circulation, but whether this FPM occurs predominantly in the stomach or the liver is still unsettled (Levitt and Levitt, 1994; Levitt and Levitt, 2000b). Some investigators favor the stomach as the site of FPM and suggested that gastric ADH served

as a protective barrier against the toxic effects of ethanol and its metabolite acetaldehyde (Frezza et al., 1990). Early studies of FPM were criticized because its impact was assessed from the ratio of AUC after oral and intravenous administration of the same dose (Levitt and Levitt, 1998; Levitt and Levitt, 2000a). No attention was given to the fact that ethanol is a drug eliminated by Michaelis-Menten (MM) kinetics and AUC therefore increases more than proportionately with increasing dose (Wagner, 1993). Levitt and Levitt (2000a) maintained that a two-compartment model was necessary to describe the absorption and elimination kinetics of ethanol to enable a proper understanding of FPM and the role of gut versus liver. These workers became strong advocates of the liver as the major site for FPM with a negligible contribution from gastric ADH (Levitt and Levitt, 1998). Furthermore, the percentage differences in AUC after oral and intravenous administration was greater the smaller the dose of ethanol (0.15 > 0.25 > 0.30 g/kg). FPM was especially marked when alcohol was consumed one hour after volunteers had eaten a fat-rich meal, which is known to slow absorption rate of ethanol (Fraser, 1998).

Whether the site of FPM was primarily the stomach or the liver proved difficult to resolve and strong differences of opinion were ventilated in the literature (Levitt et al., 1994; Gentry et al., 1994). In an elegant experiment designed to determine the bioavailability of ethanol, investigators used a deuterium labeled analogue (0.3 g/kg), which was given perorally and unlabeled ethanol (0.3 g/kg) was given at the same time intravenously (Ammon et al., 1996). To sidestep FPM occurring in the stomach ethanol was also given intraduodenally in one set of experiments. A careful evaluation of the BAC profiles obtained for the various routes of administration, led the authors to conclude that FPM could only account for a few percent of the total dose of 0.6 g/kg administered. They also found that sex-related difference in FPM were small or negligible. From an evaluation of the various routes of administration of ethanol, this research group seemed to favor the liver as the primary site for FPM of ethanol and others have echoed these views (Fraser, 1997; Levitt, 1994; Levitt and Levitt, 2000b).

Most of the studies on FPM and gastric ADH were done after subjects drank very small doses (< 0.3 g/kg) of ethanol about one hour after a meal and these conditions favor slow and intermittent gastric emptying (Wagner, 1986; Amir et al., 1996). After giving moderate doses of ethanol (0.50–0.80 g/kg) on an empty stomach, the first-pass metabolism was negligible or absent and, indeed, the ethanol-dilution technique can be used to estimate total body water (Jones et al., 1992) giving results in good agreement with isotope-dilution methods (Endres and Grüner, 1994). Because of the saturable kinetics of ethanol metabolism, the AUC is highly dependent on the dose and speed of gastric emptying (Wagner, 1986; Fraser et al., 1992; Levitt and Levitt, 1994). Low concentrations of ethanol in the portal venous blood are effectively cleared during the first contact of blood with the hepatic metabolizing enzymes and AUCs are thereby diminished (Fraser et al. 1995; Oneta et al., 1998).

A multitude of factors need to be considered when FPM of ethanol is quantitated and Levitt and Levitt (2000b) have provided convincing evidence that the liver is the primary site for FPM to occur. Among other things the amount of ADH enzyme in the gastric mucosa is only a fraction of that in the liver (Levitt and Levitt, 1994). Another confounding factor is the effect of food on hepatic blood flow, which increases the rate of exposure to metabolizing enzymes (Host et al., 1996; Lautt and Macedo, 1997). If ethanol is rapidly absorbed, the concentrations in the liver rise quickly and the ADH is saturated with substrate and hepatic FPM is no longer possible. Gastric residence time is therefore a key variable in any discussion of FPM of ethanol and the longer the drug remains in the stomach the more opportunity for oxidation by gastric ADH (Oneta et al. 1998). Clearly the rate of absorption is a key consideration not only for determining C_{max} but also AUC and indirectly FPM (Levitt et al., 1997; Levitt and Levitt, 2000b). Gastric ADH activity and consequently gastric FPM was less pronounced in many Japanese subjects who seemed to lack class-IV ADH in the stomach (Baraona et al., 1991). Neither were there any diurnal variations in gastric FPM of ethanol (Sharma et al., 1995).

B. Effects of drugs on first-pass metabolism

Considerable interest in FPM and gastric ADH was aroused when it was shown that commonly prescribed drugs, such as H_2-receptor antagonists (ranitidine and cimetidine) and aspirin inhibited gastric ADH in vitro. Many studies by Lieber and his group went on to show that concomitant use of these drugs with ethanol resulted in higher C_{max}, which they attributed to drug-induced inhibition of gastric ADH in-vivo. Many other research groups attempted to replicate this kind of drug-alcohol interaction but without much success. Indeed, the study by Toon et al (1994) was particularly convincing because they used a randomized crossover design and 0.5 gram ethanol per kilogram body weight was given in the morning, at midday and in the evening both on an empty stomach and one hour after subjects had eaten a meal. These investigators failed to find any significant effect of pretreatment with ranitidine on C_{max}, t_{max} and AUC but a significant change in these parameters was found after the subjects had eaten a meal before drinking (Toon et al., 1994). Similar negligible effects of ranitidine were reported after twenty-four men received doses of 0.15, 0.30 and 0.60 g/kg body weight with or without pretreatment with the drug (Bye et al., 1996). A very small rise in BAC (higher C_{max}) was observed after the smallest dose of ethanol but this might just as well have been caused by the drug altering gastric emptying, independent of any inhibition of gastric ADH. A thorough well balanced overview of the effects of H_2-antagonists on gastric ADH and FPM of ethanol was presented by Fraser (1998). He concluded that an effect of these drugs on C_{max} and AUC was small or negligible and only evident after very small ethanol doses (0.15 g/kg) so this interaction lacked any clinical or forensic significance (Fraser, 1998). Westenbrink (1995) gave examples of forensic cases when co-ingestion of ethanol and cimetidine was used as a defense argument in a drunk driving case.

The main supporters of gastric ADH and its role in FPM maintained that bolus dose studies were not appropriate for investigating this type of drug-alcohol interaction and instead advocated use of repetitive intake of alcoholic beverages (Gupta et al., 1995; Arora et al., 2000; Baraona, 2000; Lieber, 2000). Higher C_{max} after pretreatment with cimetidine was confirmed after four separate doses of ethanol (0.15 g/kg each) were consumed every fifteen minutes for two hours and FPM was evaluated with a more sophisticated pharmacokinetic model (Gupta et al., 1995). Similarly, pretreatment with ranitidine (150 mg twice daily for seven days) followed by repetitive drinking of alcohol (4 × 0.15 g/kg per dose) also resulted in a higher C_{max} and AUC, which was attributed to drug-induced inhibition of gastric ADH. The magnitude of FPM was assessed by calculating the difference between the amount of ethanol reaching the blood after IV and oral administrations of the same dose using an integrated form of the MM equation to calculate V_{max} and k_m parameters (Arora et al., 2000).

Another criticism of research on gastric ADH and its inhibition by drugs is that almost all the studies were done in healthy volunteers and not patient groups suffering from gastritis or other upper GI ailments that require this kind of medication. This was remedied in a study with elderly patients diagnosed with atrophic gastritis who received 0.225 g/kg ethanol both orally and intravenously (Pedrosa et al., 1996). Gastric ADH activity was significantly lower in atrophic gastritis patients compared with controls but the main determinant of FPM was the rate of gastric emptying. Neither atrophic gastritis nor treatment with tetracycline had any impact on FPM of ethanol as judged by comparing C_{max} and AUC in male and female patients (Pedrosa et al., 1996). After a four-hour fast and pretreatment with cimitidine (400 mg twice daily) there was no evidence for any effect of this drug on FPM when two different doses of ethanol (0.15 g/kg and 0.45 g/kg) were compared (Clemmesen and Sestoft, 1997). These results tallied with another fasting study in which 0.8 g/kg was administered to twelve volunteers after pretreatment with cimetidine, ranitidine or omeprazole (Jönsson et al., 1992).

When evaluating studies dealing with the effect of exogenous factors (e.g., food, drugs and smoking) on C_{max} and AUC, it is important to recall that the values obtained can never be higher than those expected for an instantaneous and 100 percent absorption of the dose. The only exception is the kind of overshoot peak seen after rapid gastric emptying and this lasts no longer than thirty-five minutes post-dos-

ing (Klockhoff et al., 2002). A meta-analysis of papers dealing with the effect of H_2-receptor antagonists on C_{max} and AUC concluded that small increases in these parameters were possible after cimetidine and ranitidine but not after famotidine and nizatidine (Weinberg et al., 1998). With larger numbers of participants in the experiments, it was less likely to find such differences in C_{max} and AUC. It was also concluded that relative to accepted legal definitions of intoxication, the effect of these drugs on BAC is unlikely to be clinically relevant.

3.11 Hepatic First-Pass Metabolism

The principal enzyme involved in the metabolism of ethanol, namely class-I ADH, has a low k_m for ethanol as substrate and therefore quickly becomes saturated even after a one or two drinks (Wilkinson, 1980; Wilkinson et al., 1980; Kalant, 1996b; Norberg et al., 2003). Ethanol is a drug that exhibits a dose-dependent elimination kinetics and this can best be described by the Michaelis-Menten (MM) equation, whereby the reaction velocity depends on the concentration of the substrate at the active enzyme sites (Lundquist and Wolthers, 1958; Norberg et al., 2003; Gabrielsson and Weiner, 2000; Wagner and Patel, 1972; Wagner et al., 1989; Rangno et al., 1981).

The equation for a Michaelis-Menten kinetic model with saturable metabolism is usually represented as follows.

Rate of metabolism

$$-dc/dt = (V_{max} \times C_s)/(K_m + C_s)$$

$$-dc/dt = V_{max}/(K_m/C_s + 1)$$

where V_{max} is the maximum velocity of the enzymatic reaction, C_s is the concentration of the substrate (ethanol) and K_m is the Michaelis constant for the enzyme, which is the concentration of ethanol when the rate of reaction is half the maximum value (Wilkinson, 1980; Kalant, 1996b). The K_m for ethanol with class-I ADH is about 0.05 g/L so when BAC exceeds 0.1 g/L ($2 \times K_m$) the enzymes are close to being saturated and working at maximum velocity. The above equations also show that when C_s is high compared with K_m the rate of elimination of ethanol from blood ($-dc/dt$) becomes equal to V_{max} because K_{max}/C_s is now close to zero. Similarly, when C_s is much smaller than K_m the elimination rate ($-dc/dt$) is equal to $(V_{max}/K_m) \times C_s$ and effectively being directly proportional to C_s, which implies first order elimination kinetics. The existence of polymorphic forms of the ADH enzymes with different V_{max} and K_m and also contributions from microsomal P450 enzymes on reaching high BAC gives an indication of the highly complex nature of the pharmacokinetics of ethanol (see Norberg et al., 2003 for a review).

Another consequence of saturable metabolism of ethanol is that the area under the BAC-time curve does not increase proportionally with increase in the dose of ethanol administered (Wagner, 1986). After very small doses of ethanol, the concentrations of ethanol in the portal venous blood remain low and the hepatic enzymes are not saturated so the ethanol is effectively cleared during the first passage of blood through the liver. This leads to a lower bioavailability of ethanol, which becomes more pronounced when there is food in the stomach before drinking or when other factors delay gastric emptying (Welling et al., 1977).

The operation of Michaelis-Menten kinetics also means that after large doses of ethanol are consumed as occurs in most forensic situations, the elimination kinetics of ethanol approximates to a zero-order elimination process until very low BACs are reached (Wagner, 1993; Gabrielsson and Weiner, 2000; Norberg et al., 2003). This means that the classic Widmark one-compartment model still remains valid for most applications required in routine forensic casework, such as prosecution of drunk drivers (Widmark, 1932; Kalant, 1996b; Wallgren, 1970; Barbour, 2001; Gullberg and Jones, 1994; Forrest, 1986). The operation of Michaelis-Menten kinetics helps to explain the large variability observed in BAC profiles after drinking very small doses (< 0.3 g/kg) (Norberg et al., 2003). Others have suggested that multicompartment models are needed to describe the pharmacokinetics of ethanol and it is evident that the disposition and fate of ethanol in the body is more complicated than many people are prepared to admit (Wedel et al., 1991; Smith et al., 1993).

3.12 Type of Beverage and Rate of Ethanol Absorption

Roine et al. (1991) investigated whether the concentration of ethanol in the drink consumed could alter the shape of the BAC profiles, especially C_{max}, t_{max} and AUC. To five volunteers, they gave the same dose of ethanol (0.3 g/kg ethanol) as 4-percent, 16-percent or 40-percent v/v solutions in water, which was finished in ten minutes. When the alcohol was ingested on an empty stomach, the C_{max} and AUC were about the same regardless of the concentration of ethanol in the drink. However, when eight other subjects drank 4-percent v/v or 40-percent v/v one hour after eating a standardized (rather fatty) breakfast, the C_{max} and AUC were significantly higher after the more dilute alcoholic drink. The difference in the BAC profiles was most striking during the absorption period and by 120–150 minutes post-dosing the two curves met. In the post-prandial state these results are in conflict with expectations based on absorption of ethanol according to concentration gradients and Fick's law (Berggren and Goldberg, 1940).

The results suggest an interaction between the concentration of ethanol in the drink and the prandial state, which somehow alters the emptying rate of the stomach depending on the ethanol concentration in the drink. In a follow-up study, Roine et al. (1993) compared BAC profiles after eleven men ingested 0.3 g/kg ethanol in the form of either beer (4.3 percent v/v) or whisky (40 percent v/v). When the drinks were taken one hour after breakfast or at the same time as eating breakfast, the peak BAC and AUC were higher after the beer compared with the whisky. In the fasting state, whisky gave a higher BAC and AUC, although the time needed to reach the peak BAC was not significantly different. The authors speculated about first-pass metabolism of ethanol in the stomach depending on the concentration of ethanol in the drink consumed (Roine et al., 1993). Whatever the mechanism, the very small dose of ethanol administered and the short drinking time makes it unwise to extrapolate these results to real world conditions when much higher doses and prolonged drinking times are the norm.

3.13 Distribution of Ethanol

Distribution is the processes by which a drug spreads out once it enters the body and after it reaches the systemic circulation (Benet et al., 1990). Drugs move either by simple diffusion or instead might require an active transport from intravascular space to extravascular space (body tissue). The drug is distributed into one or more so-called volumes or spaces. Regardless of whether absorption occurs from the stomach or the intestine, the ethanol molecules enter the portal venous blood and reach the liver before passing into the hepatic vein and via the heart and lungs get distributed throughout all body fluids and tissues. During and shortly after drinking the concentrations of ethanol in the portal vein and arterial blood are higher than that in the venous blood returning to the heart from the peripheral organs and tissues and an arterial-venous concentration difference can be measured (Martin et al., 1984; Mather, 2001). A-V differences in concentrations of ethanol are especially marked for resting skeletal muscles, owing to the low ratio of blood flow to tissue mass for this anatomical region (Guyton, 1986; Mather, 2001).

A. Arterial-venous differences in ethanol concentration

The existence of A-V differences in ethanol concentration is illustrated in Figure 3.5, which shows the concentration-time profiles of ethanol in blood drawn from two different parts of the vascular system, namely a radial artery at the wrist and a cubital vein at the elbow on the same arm (Jones et al., to be published). The single male subject drank 0.6 g/kg body weight of ethanol in fifteen minutes before blood was drawn nearly simultaneously with the aid of indwelling catheters. During the absorption phase shortly after the end of drinking, the arterial BAC is higher than venous BAC and the two curves crossed at about ninety minutes post-dosing, which probably indicates a time when absorption and distribution processes end. At all later times, provided no more alcohol is consumed, there is a redistribution of ethanol from the skeletal muscles back into the central compartment for metabolism in the liver. After the A-V crossover point, the venous BAC exceeds arterial BAC for the rest of the time that alcohol is in the

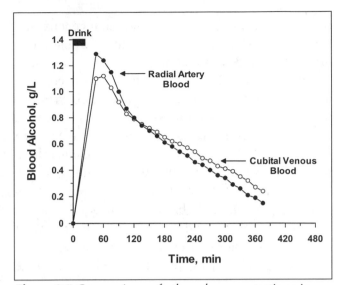

Figure 3.5 *Comparison of ethanol concentrations in blood samples from radial artery and cubital vein after a single male subject drank 0.6 gram of ethanol per kilogram of body weight in fifteen minutes (Jones et al., to be published)*

body and consequently the β-slope is steeper for arterial blood compared with venous blood. In this example, the areas under BAC curves for venous and arterial blood showed no significant differences. Similar BAC difference, albeit less pronounced, were observed when capillary blood alcohol was compared with venous blood alcohol (Sedman et al., 1976a; Jones et al., 1989). The concentration of blood gases, glucose and ethanol in capillary blood samples can be considered midway between that of venous and arterial blood specimens (Chiou, 1989).

The rate of distribution of alcohol depends on the blood flow to organs and tissues so brain, kidney and lungs, with a high ratio of blood flow to tissue mass rapidly reach equilibrium with the concentration of ethanol in arterial blood. The resting skeletal muscles on the other had have a low ratio of blood flow to tissue mass and more time is needed for complete equilibrium with the concentration of ethanol in arterial blood. This time can be shortened by muscular activity or other physical excretion during and after the drinking period (Guyton, 1986).

B. Concentrations of ethanol in plasma and whole blood

Whole blood is a complex fluid consisting mainly of water (~80 percent) containing red and white cells, proteins, lipids and a host of other endogenous substances. Because the water content of whole blood differs from red cells and plasma the concentrations of ethanol will also differ. Whole blood contains about 45–55 percent red cells or erythrocytes and this number is referred to as the blood hematocrit, which is slightly lower for women than men (Lentner, 1981). The plasma fraction contains about 92 percent water and as such will contain about 92/80 or 15 percent more ethanol compared with an equal volume of whole blood. The red cells contain mainly hemoglobin and about 66–70 percent water so the concentration of ethanol in erythrocytes will be correspondingly lower compared with whole blood. The alcohol distribution relationships expected theoretically have been confirmed empirically in many studies involving analysis of ethanol in plasma/serum and whole blood (Winek and Carfagna, 1987; Jones et al., 1990; Charlebois et al., 1996; Iffland et al., 1999).

Figure 3.6 shows an example of the concentration-time profiles of ethanol for whole blood and plasma from two male subjects who drank 0.3 g/kg on an empty stomach. The average curves for nine subjects are shown above the individual traces (Jones, unpublished work). Plasma-ethanol concentrations were always higher than whole blood during the absorption, the distribution and the elimination

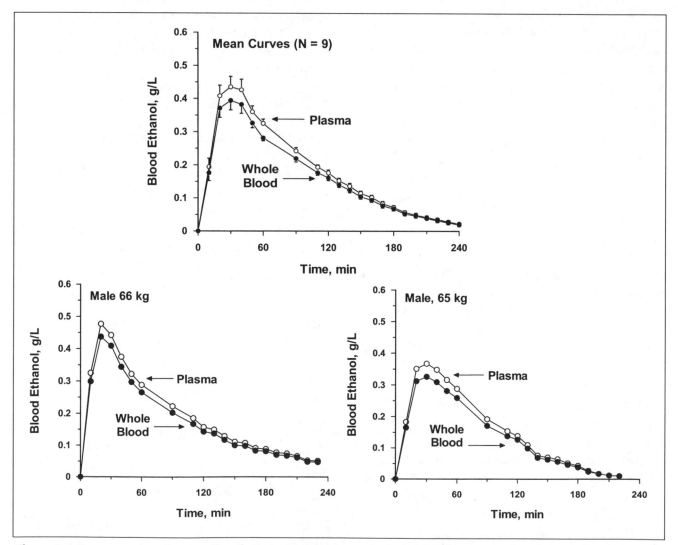

Figure 3.6 *Concentration-time profile of ethanol in plasma and whole blood in two male subjects after they drank 0.3 gram of ethanol per kilogram of body weight on an empty stomach, with the mean curves for N = nine subjects shown above*

phases as expected from the difference in water content. Theoretically, one can expect a difference of 12–15 percent based on water content determined by freeze-drying or desiccation and the distribution ratios of ethanol are in good agreement with expectations (Winek and Carfagna, 1987). A percentage difference means that at very low concentrations of ethanol (i.e., as the BAC curves approach zero) the absolute differences in ethanol concentration are very small (Figure 3.6).

Iffland et al. (1999), reviewed many previous studies of the serum/whole blood distribution ratios of ethanol (N = 835) and reported an overall mean value of 1.16:1 and in 96 percent of cases this ranged from 1.13 to 1.19. Charlebois et al. (1996) found a mean serum/blood ratio of 1.14 with standard deviation 0.041 (N = 235) and a range from 1.04–1.26. The corresponding mean distribution ratio of ethanol between erythrocytes and whole blood (N = 167) was 0.965 with a range from 0.66 to 1.00. The lower distribution ratio for red cells is mainly a consequence of the water content difference (~70 percent) compared with the whole blood (~80 percent). Hak et al. (1985) took two near simultaneous blood specimens from 134 volunteers after they had consumed alcohol. One of the specimens was centrifuged to separate serum and the concentrations of ethanol were determined by gas chromatography. The mean serum/whole blood ratio was 1.15 with standard deviation 0.02 and an experimental range of 1.10 to 1.25. The mean concentrations of ethanol were 1.05 g/L for whole blood (range 0.21–1.54 g/L) and 1.20 g/L for serum (range 0.25–1.83 g/L).

Drunk driving legislation and the punishable concentration of ethanol refer to whole blood specimens and not plasma or serum (e.g., that portion of the blood remaining after the erythrocytes are removed by centrifugation). This means that measurements of ethanol concentration in plasma or serum, which are the fluids normally used at hospital clinical laboratories, will be systematically higher than the corresponding concentration in whole blood. For all practical purposes, dividing the concentration of ethanol measured in plasma or serum by a factor of 1.2 provides a conservative estimate of the coexisting ethanol concentration in whole blood.

3.14 Widmark's Factor *rho*
A. General
Widmark developed an equation to allow forensic scientists and others to calculate the amount of alcohol in the body from the concentration measured in a specimen of blood (Barbour, 2001; Cowan et al., 1996; Baselt, 1981). This calculation requires knowledge about the way alcohol distributes between the body and the blood and he defined this ratio as a factor *r* or *rho*, which is more commonly referred to today as the volume of distribution. Because alcohol is not soluble in bone and fatty tissues and distributes only in the water fraction of the body and the blood, the *rho* factor must obviously be less than unity, roughly being about 60/80 or 0.75 for a person with a total body water of 60 percent and a blood water content of 80 percent.

During an evaluation of BAC profiles when subjects drank moderate amounts of ethanol, Widmark back extrapolated the linear post-absorptive phase to the time of starting to drink. The y-intercept was called C_0 and this represented the BAC expected if absorption and distribution of the entire dose had occurred instantaneously without any alcohol being metabolized. The factor "*r*" was needed to lower the person's body weight (*reducierade körpermass*) so that the measured BAC (mg/g) or C_0 was the same as the dose of alcohol administered in g/kg, that is $C_0 = g/(kg \times r)$. In this way, Widmark arrived at an equation relating the amount of alcohol absorbed and distributed in the body (A), to the person's body weight in kilograms (p) and the concentration of ethanol measured in a specimen of whole blood (C):

$$A = r \times p \times C$$

where A = amount of alcohol equilibrated in all body fluids at time of blood sampling; r = reduction or Widmark factor (the ratio of alcohol in the body to alcohol in the blood), being approximately 0.7 for men and 0.6 for women; p = the person's body weight in kilograms, and C = the concentration of alcohol measured in a specimen of whole blood expressed in units of mg/g or g/kg.

Because total body water is 50–60 percent of body weight and water content of whole blood is fairly constant at 78–83 percent, the Widmark factor

r can only take certain values (e.g., 50/83 or 0.60 and 60/78 or 0.77) for an average person. Individual variations will depend on factors influencing body water and blood water and the main variable is the proportion of fat-to-lean tissue in the body, which in turn depends on age, sex and obesity as reflected in body mass index. The value of *rho* for women can be expected to be less than for men for the simply reason that women have less body water and also slightly more water in their blood, owing to a lower hematocrit value (packed cell volume) (Lentner, 1981; VanLoan, 1996).

Widmark (1932) derived his distribution factor r from drinking experiments with twenty men and ten women, and found the following average values, standard deviation (SD) and coefficients of variation (CV):

Men   0.68 (SD ± 0.085, CV 13%)
              with range from 0.55 to 0.86
Women   0.55 (SD ± 0.055, CV 10%)
              with range from 0.47 to 0.65

Another early study from Sweden expanded Widmark's work to include another twenty women and ten men who drank 0.5–0.9 g/kg ethanol as brandy or vodka on an empty stomach (Österlind et al., 1944). The values of β and *rho* obtained were in good agreement with those reported by Widmark except for finding a slightly larger *rho* factor in women of 0.61 ± 0.072 (± SD) with a range from 0.48–0.75 compared with 0.70 ± 0.071 for men with a range from 0.60–0.82. These two early studies meant that the *rho* factors used for forensic calculations of BAC versus amount consumed were taken as 0.7 for men and 0.6 for women. Note that the *rho* factor is not the same as the proportion of water in the human body because ethanol is measured in whole blood, which contains about 15 percent of solid matter. If ethanol had been determined in the water fraction of whole blood as obtained by precipitation of proteins and the resulting concentration-time plots used to derive a *rho* factor from the ratio dose (g/kg)/C_0 this would be the same as the fraction of water in the body.

In any attempt to verify Widmark's *rho* values, it is essential to observe the strictly controlled condi-tions under which his experiments were performed. For example, he measured and reported BAC in mg/g and the dose of alcohol was given as g/kg so the ratio of dose/C_0 is without dimensions. If, instead, the BAC had been reported in units of g/L and dose in g/kg then the ratio dose/C_0 will have the units L/kg. These two ratios are not the same because the density of whole blood is greater than unity, being on the average 1.055 (Lentner, 1981). This difference needs to be considered whenever Widmark's *rho* values are compared with those reported today.

Breath-alcohol instruments should not be used to estimate blood-ethanol concentration if the aim is to verify the Widmark factors, because the BAC/BrAC ratio is a moving target and depends on many factors (see later). These include the person's pre-exhalation breathing pattern and the instrument sampling parameters used to ensure obtaining deep-lung alveolar air as well as the underlying blood-alcohol concentration and the stage of ethanol metabolism (Jones and Andersson, 1996b). In most studies comparing venous blood- and breath-alcohol concentration, the common finding is that BAC is underestimated by about 10 percent on the average when a 2,100:1 factor is used and when the tests are made in the post-absorptive period (Jones and Andersson, 2003). In Widmark's experiments the volunteer subjects had fasted overnight before they drank the alcohol, which is not the same as dosing two to three hours after lunch or together with a sandwich or bar snack as is often the case.

Furthermore, Widmark dosed his subjects with neat spirits (e.g., brandy, whisky or vodka) and this was taken as a bolus dose in a drinking time of five to fifteen minutes (Jones, 1984). Deviation from these experimental conditions can often explain failures to confirm the values of β and *rho* found by Widmark. An updating of Widmark's work is however justified because the body composition of people in the 1920s and 1930s in Sweden is probably not representative of the average person today in terms of obesity, body mass index or proportions of fat-to-lean tissue. Obesity is a worldwide problem even among younger age groups and children and this impacts on the distribution of alcohol between body compartments and the blood (Yanovski and Yanovski, 2002; Flegal et al., 2002).

In textbooks devoted to pharmacology the term closely related to Widmark's *rho* factor is the volume of distribution of the drug (V_d), calculated by dividing the dose administered by the concentration measured in blood or plasma extrapolated to the time of starting to drink (C_0) (Rowland and Tozer, 1980; Gabrielsson and Weiner, 2000). In this connection, the value of C_0 will depend to some extent on the kind of body fluid analyzed, whether whole blood, plasma or serum or saliva and so on, because these biofluids don't have the same amounts of water. Thus the V_d or *rho* factor for ethanol will accordingly be lower if plasma or serum was analyzed compared with whole blood, owing to the steeper slope of the post-absorptive elimination phase.

A valid forensic application of the Widmark equation is to estimate the amount of alcohol absorbed and distributed in the body fluids and tissues at the time of sampling the blood from the measured BAC. Any ethanol from the recent drink that remains unabsorbed in the stomach is not within the systemic circulation so the amount of alcohol consumed is underestimated by applying this kind of calculation. Furthermore, alcohol starts to become metabolized from the start of drinking even as the BAC curve is rising so some of the alcohol is eliminated by the time the blood sample is taken. If the time of starting to drink is known the amount of alcohol removed by metabolism needs to be added to the amount in the body at the time of sampling blood as the following equation shows.

$$\text{Amount consumed} = (BAC \times rho \times kg) + (B_{60} \times t)$$

The *BAC* represents concentration of ethanol in blood at time of sampling, *rho* is Widmark's factor, *kg* is body weight of the individual in kilograms, B_{60} is the rate of elimination of alcohol from the whole body, assumed to be 0.1 g/kg/h independent of sex, and *t* is number of hours elapsed from time of starting to drink up until the time of sampling blood. An alternative approach is to back extrapolate BAC assuming a certain rate of ethanol elimination from blood (e.g., 0.15 g/L/h) and then converting the value obtained into the amount of alcohol in the body using the Widmark formula ($A = BAC \times rho \times$

kg) and if necessary the number of drinks consumed can easily be calculated.

Theoretical calculations of this nature are less reliable for making prospective estimate of BAC—that is, the concentration expected in the blood some time after drinking started. Such calculations are suspect even when absorption and distribution are complete owing to the possibility that first-pass metabolism has taken place in the stomach or liver or both organs. The systemic availability of ethanol during social drinking is never 100 percent and the difference can sometimes be appreciable, for example after long periods of continuous drinking and especially after eating a meal (Zink and Reinhardt, 1984; Jones and Neri, 1985).

B. Updating the Widmark ρ factor

In 1981 investigators from New Zealand (Watson et al., 1981) published a well-cited paper in which they attempted to update the Widmark equation by considering a person's total body water (TBW) from information about age, weight and height. They presented multiple regression equations with total body water as the outcome variable (*y*-variate) and anthropometric values (age, weight and height) as the predictor variables. Equations were given for men and women separately along with the standard deviations of the estimates of TBW.

For men (N = 458) aged 17–86 years, their age (years) and body weight (kilograms) were the most important variables:

$$\text{TBW (liters)} = 20.03 - 0.1183 \text{ age (years)} + 0.3626 \text{ weight (kilograms)}$$

Using this equation the standard deviation of the TBW obtained was ± 3.86 liters.

For women (N = 265) aged 17–84 years, their body weight was the most important variable:

$$\text{TBW (liters)} = 14.46 + 0.2549 \text{ weight (kg)}$$

Using this equation the standard deviation of the TBW obtained was ± 3.72 liters.

A strong motivation for adopting the above equations in DUI litigation is that they are tailored to each particular individual and information about age, weight and height are readily available and can be easily checked. This tends to boost confidence in BAC calculations compared with using a population average value for the distribution factor *rho*. Moreover, Widmark's *rho* was derived from experiments with Swedes in the 1930s and body composition for the average male and female drinker has changed considerably in terms of obesity (Borkan and Norris, 1977). The TBW values derived according to the above equations need to be divided by the water content of blood (0.8 g/g or 0.85 g/mL) to give the *rho* factors comparable with those of Widmark. Recently Gabe (1997) made a reappraisal of the original Watson et al. (1981) formulae and pointed to some small deficiencies in the calculations, such as the need to use mass/volume units for blood-water content if the BAC is reported in such units.

For a man with body weight of 75 kilograms, height 180 centimeters and age thirty-five years, TBW according to the above equation is 43 liters, which corresponds to 57 percent of the body weight. By dividing percent TBW (57 percent) by percent of water in whole blood (80 percent w/w) this gives 0.71 as the ratio of water in whole body to water in blood, which is the definition of Widmark's *rho* factor. This value is slightly higher than the average for men found by Widmark, but agrees well with the mean ± SD of his data, namely 0.68 ± 0.085.

More recently, Seidl et al. (2000) attempted to update the Widmark equation with the aim of avoiding the need to accept an arbitrary absorption deficit (e.g., a lower C_0 than expected for the dose administered). They proposed the following equations to estimate *rho* factors for men (r_m) and women (r_w) based on measurements of TBW from noninvasive bioelectrical impedance analysis and the blood-water content, which was determined by desiccation.

For men,
$$r_m = 0.31608 - 0.004821 \text{ weight (kg)} + 0.004632 \text{ height (cm)}.$$

For women,
$$r_w = 0.31223 - 0.006446 \text{ weight (kg)} + 0.004466 \text{ height (cm)}.$$

These equations were verified by drinking experiments taking into consideration age, sex, body weight, and height of the individual and also their TBW. With the same 75-kilogram man, height 180 centimeters and age thirty-five years, the above equation gives r_m of 0.788, a value considerably greater than 0.71 determined according to Watson et al. (1981) and 0.68 according to Widmark (1932). Many others have offered formulae and nomograms to compute *rho* factors from anthropometric data for use in BAC calculations (Forrest, 1986; Barbour, 2001).

3.15 Elimination of Ethanol

Of the total amount of alcohol that enters the bloodstream approximately ~94 percent is eliminated by oxidative metabolism and the remainder is excreted unchanged in breath, sweat and urine (Kalant, 1996b). A very small fraction (< 0.1 percent) of the dose undergoes nonoxidative metabolism in the liver in a phase-II conjugation reaction to produce a water-soluble metabolite ethyl glucuronide, which is then excreted in the urine (Schmitt et al., 1995; Schmitt et al., 1997; Seidl et al., 2000). Ethyl glucuronide is a specific metabolite of ethanol and has found applications in forensic and clinical medicine as a biochemical marker of recent drinking (Droenner et al., 2002). Acetaldehyde, which is the primary oxidative metabolite of ethanol, is not easy to analyze in blood owing to the small amounts present and the tendency for some of the ethanol to be converted to acetaldehyde in-vitro after sampling.

The conjugation metabolite of ethanol, ethyl glucuronide (EtG), has a different pharmacokinetic profile compared with ethanol. The concentration of EtG in blood increases more slowly than ethanol and reaches a later peak and the whole curve is displaced considerably in time (Droenner et al., 2002). Moreover, EtG can be measured in blood and urine for long after ethanol is no longer detectable. This means that assay of EtG can serve to disclose recent drinking after ethanol has left the body. Another application of EtG in forensic toxicology has been to test whether a blood specimen might have been contaminated with ethanol, such as, from the swab used to disinfect the skin prior to venepuncture. Also whether ethanol might have been produced in the body after death (neoformation) or in urine post-sampling, owing to the action of bacteria or yeasts on any glucose present (Jones et al., 2000). Failure to find EtG in the blood sample supports the suggestion that the specimen was contaminated during the sampling, transport or preparation for analysis.

Figure 3.7 illustrates the fate of ethanol in the body with the relative amounts eliminated unchanged and metabolized shown.

3.16 Metabolism of Ethanol

Alcohol is an endogenous substance produced in trace amounts by fermentation of carbohydrates in the gut as well as other putative biochemical reactions (Logan and Jones, 2000). Any ethanol generated in the gut must pass with the portal venous blood through the liver before reaching the systemic circulation. Accordingly, trace amounts of ethanol produced by fermentation in the colon are cleared by first pass metabolism in the liver. However, if hepatic ADH is inactivated (e.g., by giving the drug 4-methyl pyrazole), the concentration of endogenous ethanol increased slightly (Sarkola and Eriksson, 2001). The physiological role of ADH at least in part

was to protect the organism from inadvertent intake of ethanol from eating over ripe fruits and fruit juices or any fermented sugars.

A. Alcohol and aldehyde dehydrogenases

The principal enzyme involved in the oxidation of ethanol is the NAD^+-dependent alcohol dehydrogenase (ADH, EC I.I.I.I.), which is located in the cytosol, and aldehyde dehydrogenase (ALDH, EC 1.2.1.3.) located in the mitochondria (Crabb, 1995; Jörnvall and Högg, 1995). These enzymes are not specific for oxidation of ethanol because other aliphatic alcohols such as methanol and isopropanol as well as diols such as ethylene glycol serve as substrates (Eder et al., 1998; Barceloux et al., 2001). It was earlier thought that ethanol was oxidized to some extent also by catalase, which is an enzyme located in the peroxisomes. However, the lack of hydrogen peroxide necessary for this reaction to proceed makes this pathway less likely to play a role for in-vivo metabolism of ethanol (Lieber, 1997a; Lieber, 1999; Bosron et al., 1993).

Human alcohol dehydrogenase exists in multiple molecular forms and these closely related isozymes

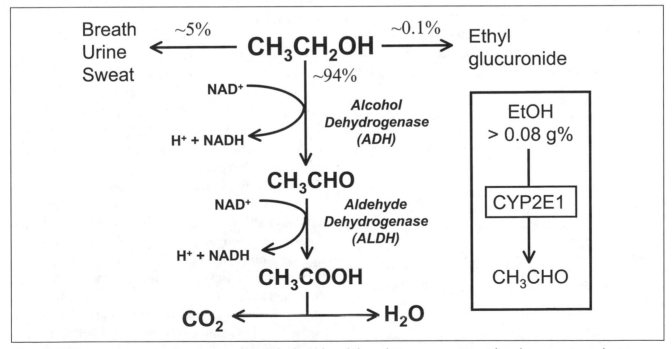

Figure 3.7 Scheme showing the metabolism of ethanol and the relative amounts oxidized (approximately 94 percent) and excreted (approximately 6 percent) and the small fraction (approximately 0.1 percent) that undergoes a phase-II conjugation reaction to produce ethyl glucuronide. Both the alcohol dehydrogenase (ADH) and cytochrome P450 (CYP2E1) pathways are indicated.

have distinct kinetic properties including different V_{max} and k_m and also specificity for different substrates (Crabb et al., 1987). Depending on the particular variants of ADH a person inherits, this can determine the rate of elimination of ethanol from blood and the overall sensitivity to alcohol and alcoholism (Li, 2000; Li et al., 2001; Whitfield and Martin, 1994; Whitfield et al., 2001). The k_m of the most abundant form of human ADH is relatively low (~0.05 g/L), which means that the enzyme quickly becomes saturated after one or two drinks.

The scheme shown in Figure 3.8 compares the oxidative metabolism of ethanol and methanol to produce the respective aldehydes and carboxylic acids along with the various isozymes involved in these reactions (Crabb, 1995; Ramchandani et al., 2001b).

It has long been known that liver ADH is more selective for oxidation of ethanol than methanol so when both these alcohols are present in the blood, the oxidation of methanol into its toxic metabolites formaldehyde and formic acid is prevented (Roe, 1955; Roe, 1982; Barceloux et al., 2002). The first-aid treatment for methanol poisoning entails intravenous administration of ethanol to reach a BAC of ~1 g/L and maintain this level for several hours to divert ADH away from oxidation of methanol to oxidize ethanol instead. The acidosis caused by the formic acid metabolite of methanol can be treated with bi-carbonate and the unchanged methanol is suitably removed from the blood by hemodialysis. An alternative treatment, which is more appropriate for use in children and alcoholics, is to give IV injections of the drug 4-methyl pyrazole, which is a potent competitive inhibitor of class-I ADH (Weintraub and Standish, 1988). This drug is called fomepizole and has been approved by the FDA as an antidote for treatment of methanol and ethylene glycol poisoning (Bekka et al., 2001; Eder et al., 1998).

B. Polymorphism of ADH and ALDH

After moderate drinking when BACs below 0.8 g/L are reached, the principal enzyme involved in the metabolism of ethanol is class-I ADH, which is located in the cytosol fraction of the hepatocyte (Li, 2000). This enzyme is encoded by three kinds of genes denoted ADH*1, ADH*2 and ADH*3 and the latter two are polymorphic giving rise to different molecular forms of the same enzyme each with a slightly different sequence of amino acids (Hittle and Crabbe, 1988; Li et al., 1998; Li, 2000). The rate of ethanol elimination from blood depends on a combination of both genetic and environmental factors that influence activity of the alcohol metabolizing enzymes.

Table 3.3 shows the various class-I ADH and ALDH isozymes in different racial and ethnic groups and one notes a predominance of the β_2 form in Asians and β_3 in African-Americans and γ_3 in Caucasians. (Crabb et al., 1993). The aldehyde dehydrogenase enzyme also shows polymorphism and many people of Asian descent (Japanese, Chinese and Koreans) have a predominance of the ALDH2*2 genotype, which gives them a protection against becoming heavy drinkers, owing to the nausea they experience after drinking ethanol (Higuchi et al., 1995). Among other things, they show visible facial flushing, sometimes very intense, as well as a higher skin-blood flow and unpleasant cardiovascular effects after a single drink (Eriksson, 2001). In essence, they have an inborn aversion to drinking alcohol and the mechanism is similar to the alcohol-disulfiram reaction (Swift, 1999).

The second stage in ethanol degradation involves the conversion of acetaldehyde into acetic acid by the ALDH1 (k_m 30–50 μm) and ALDH2 (k_m

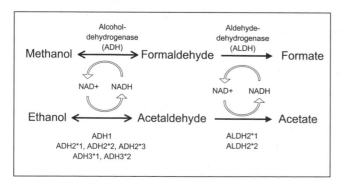

Figure 3.8 *Scheme showing the hepatic metabolism of ethanol and methanol first into their respective aldehydes and then carboxylic acids and the various forms of alcohol (ADH) and aldehyde dehydrogenase (ALDH) that catalyze these reactions. NAD+ and NADH are the oxidized and reduced forms of the coenzyme nicotinamide adenine dinucleotide, respectively*

Table 3.3
Polymorphic Forms of Class I-Enzymes of Alcohol Dehydrogenase (ADH) and Class-II Aldehyde Dehydrogenase (ALDH) Showing Amounts of Isozymes in Different Ethnic Groups
(Hittle and Crabb, 1988)

Gene locus	Subunit type	Populations with high frequency of particiular enzyme
ADH2*1	β_1	Caucasians (90–95 percent), African-Americans (85 percent), Asians (35 percent)
ADH2*2	β_2	Caucasians (< 5 percent), African-Americans (< 5 percent), Asians (65 percent)
ADH2*3	β_3	Caucasians (< 5 percent), African-Americans (15 percent), Asians (< 5 percent)
ADH3*1	γ_1	Caucasians (50–60 percent), African-Americans (85 percent), Asians (95 percent)
ADH3*2	γ_2	Caucasians (40–50 percent), African-Americans (15 percent), Asians (5 percent)
ALDH2*1	High activity	Dominant in Caucasians and African-Americans
ALDH2*2	Low activity	Dominant in East Asians (Chinese and Japanese)

0.1–0.2 µm) enzymes, located in the cytosol and the mitochondria, respectively. Both these enzymes are inhibited by disulfiram (Antabuse) and people treated with this drug become hypersensitive to alcohol owing to an accumulation of acetaldehyde in blood. They experience a drop in blood pressure (hypotension) and an accelerated heart beat (tachycardia) intense flushing and nausea and sometime vomiting (Crabb et al., 1989; Gill et al., 1999). This kind of treatment strategy for alcohol dependence is called aversion therapy because the aim is to scare the patient from continuing to drink because of the various unpleasant effects he or she experiences (Swift, 1999).

The ALDH2 enzyme exhibits polymorphism and the normal allele is denoted ALDH2*1 and the inactive mutant form ALDH2*2 owing to a single change in the amino acid sequence. There is a pronounced deficiency in the low k_m ALDH2*2 variant in many people of Asian descent who are thus afforded a protection from developing alcohol problems, especially those homozygous for ALDH2*2 (Crabb et al., 1993; Wall et al., 1997). The causative agent is acetaldehyde, which is a highly reactive and toxic metabolite of ethanol that can bind to cell membranes and tissues and cause peroxidation of lipids (Panes et al., 1993; Harada et al., 2001; Eriksson, 2001). Indeed, acetaldehyde has been incriminated in many of the untoward effects of too much drinking including liver disease, various forms of cancer as well as addiction and dependence

(Lumeng and Crabb, 1994; McBride et al., 2002; Eriksson, 2001). Asians who are homozygous for ALDH2*2 are extremely sensitive to even the smallest amounts of alcohol (0.1 g/kg) and react by flushing in the face (Enomoto et al., 1991). Those who are heterozygous for ALDH2 drink less alcohol but still develop higher blood concentrations of acetaldehyde compared with those without the inherited deficiency in the ALDH2*2 allele (Wall et al., 1997).

C. Microsomal enzymes cytochrome P450

Enzymes located in a subcellular component of liver cells called smooth endoplasmic reticulum, especially the microsomal fraction, are capable of oxidizing ethanol as well as many other drugs and xenobiotics (Lieber, 1999; Lieber, 1997a). The microsomal enzymes comprise a large family of proteins with broad and overlapping substrate specificity (Nebert and Russell, 2002). The P450s were originally known as mixed function oxidase because of the diverse number of oxidation reactions they catalyzed (e.g., aromatic and aliphatic hydroxylation, N-deamination, O-demethylation and N-demethylation). Cytochrome P450 enzymes are involved in the metabolism of a large number of prescription drugs, which has important consequences for many adverse drug-alcohol and drug-drug interactions. Indeed, some P450s exhibit polymorphism leading to poor, rapid or ultra-rapid metabolizers of some drugs with implications for efficacy and toxicity of drug therapy (Weinshilboum, 2003; Park et al., 1996; Evans and McLeod, 2003).

The form of the P450 enzyme mainly responsible for oxidation of ethanol is denoted CYP2E1 and other low-molecular alcohols are also among potential substrates. This same CYP2E1 enzyme metabolizes various anesthetic gases, volatile hydrocarbons, acetone and certain endogenous substrates. The underlying mechanism of many adverse drug-alcohol interactions (e.g., acetaminophen) can be attributed to competition for or induction of the CYP2E1 enzymes. The CYP2E1 enzyme has a higher k_m for ethanol oxidation compared with class-I ADH, being about 0.6–0.8 g/L, which are concentrations barely reached after social drinking.

Perhaps the most important feature of the CYP2E1 enzyme in the metabolism of ethanol is the fact that this protein is activated (enzyme induction) after continuous exposure to substrate (Song, 1996). The CYP2E1 plays an increasingly important role in ethanol metabolism in heavy drinkers and alcoholics who regularly reach very high BACs during a drinking binge. Moreover, in its induced form there is also a greater potential for drug-alcohol interactions, especially with drugs having toxic metabolites (e.g., acetaminophen). Many organic solvents are substrates for CYP2E1 and some of these produce carcinogenic metabolites, which increases the risk of toxicity in alcohol abusers and others with activated microsomal enzymes. Induction of CYP2E1 after chronic drinking also explains the ability of alcoholics to eliminate alcohol much faster because they have developed a metabolic tolerance (Jones and Sternebring, 1992).

D. Phase-II conjugation of ethanol

A small portion of ethanol (~0.1 percent) undergoes conjugation with glucuronic acid to form a water-soluble product called ethyl glucuronide, which is excreted in the urine (for review see Seidl et al., 2000). The remainder of the ethanol a person ingests becomes excreted unchanged in the breath, urine and sweat (2–5 percent). The amount of alcohol expelled in the breath is proportional to the concentration reaching the pulmonary blood and breath tests for alcohol are widely used in law enforcement (e.g., for testing drunk drivers).

E. Factors influencing the rate of ethanol disappearance from blood

Increasing the rate of ethanol elimination from blood would be a useful strategy in some clinical situations such as treatment of poisoned patients, but this has not been feasible so far. To accelerate the metabolism of ethanol would require speeding up the person's basal metabolism and therefore the rate of conversion of ethanol into its metabolites acetaldehyde and acetic acid.

Well-known species differences exist in the rate of ethanol metabolism and rats and mice oxidize ethanol three to five times faster than dogs or humans (Derr, 1993; Wallgren, 1970). Studies have shown that the rate of ethanol combustion is closely linked with the basal energy requirements of the body including oxygen consumption by the tissues. No effective means has been devised to increase the rate of ethanol metabolism above that found in the well-nourished individual (Bode, 1978). However, in trauma patients suffering from severe burns, the rate of ethanol metabolism was boosted considerably compared with normal values of 0.1–0.2 g/L/h. These patients are in a hypermetabolic state owing to their injuries and under these circumstances all energy processes are boosted including catabolism of glucose and amino acids (Jones et al., 1997b).

A number of alcohol drinking studies have been performed in monzygotic and dizygotic twins to search for a genetic component in the metabolism of ethanol (Martin et al., 1985; Kopun and Propping, 1997). The genetic component was not very strong and the general conclusion was that short-term environmental factors exert more influence on ethanol metabolism particularly during the absorption phase (e.g., determinants of gastric emptying) (Martin et al., 1985). Indeed, the rate of alcohol disappearance from blood seems to vary just as much between as within the same subject from time to time (Wagner and Patel, 1972; Nagoshi and Wilson, 1989; Jones and Jönsson, 1994a). Conducting a controlled drinking experiment to establish a person's ability to metabolize ethanol is therefore rather pointless and one might just as well assume a population average value such as 0.15 g/L/h.

F. Inter- and intra-individual variations

The rate of alcohol disappearance from the blood varies between individuals and also to some extent within individuals depending on the relative importance of genetic and environmental factors that determine activity of alcohol metabolizing enzyme (Passananti et al., 1990; Li et al., 2000). After intake of a moderate dose of ethanol the rate of disappearance of ethanol from blood in the post-absorptive phase might range from 0.1 to 0.2 g/L/h in most moderate drinkers, being slightly faster in women compared with men (Jones, 1993a; Jones and Andersson, 1996a; Piekoszewski and Gubula, 2000; Mishra et al., 1989; Mumenthaler et al., 1999). The total amount of alcohol cleared from the whole body depends on liver weight, which is proportional to body weight and is equivalent to ~0.10 g/kg/h, a rate which is independent of sex.

Figure 3.9 shows the β-slopes found in controlled drinking experiments with healthy men aged twenty to sixty years who consumed 0.68 g/kg ethanol as neat whisky after an overnight fast. The values for the forty-eight men are rank ordered and fall within the range 0.1 and 0.2 g/L/h for the strictly controlled fasting conditions of the experiment (Jones, 1984). Age-related differences in rates of ethanol metabolism were investigated by several research groups, because the activity of CYP450 enzymes decreases with aging (Vestal et al., 1977; Jones and Neri, 1985). However, the kinetic parameter of ethanol that changed the most during aging was the Widmark factor *rho* (volume of distribution), probably because body water decreases in the elderly (Schoeller, 1989; VanLoan, 1996). The rate of alcohol elimination from blood (β-slope) was barely influenced by aging after moderate amounts of alcohol were given when the ADH pathway is mainly responsible for oxidation of ethanol (Lieber, 2000).

G. Sex differences

Attention has also been focused on hormonal influences on ethanol pharmacokinetics, such as the changes occurring during the menstrual cycle and whether use of oral contraceptive steroids affect the rate of ethanol metabolism (Marshall et al., 1983; Jones and Jones, 1984; Mumenthaler et al., 2001).

Support for hormonal influences comes from a study of ethanol metabolism in men who had been castrated owing to testicular cancer (Mezey et al., 1988). The finding of an enhanced elimination rate implicates testosterone as an endogenous factor modulating the activity of alcohol metabolizing enzymes. Although it is fairly well established that alcohol alters behavioral changes including aggression during various stages of the menstrual cycle (Orford et al., 1985; Brick et al., 1986; Jones and Jones, 1976; Gill, 1997) it was more difficult to prove an effect on rate of ethanol metabolism (Haddad et al., 1998). Large numbers of subjects are needed in such studies as well as biochemical analysis of female sex hormones in serum (estrogens, estrone, estradiol, estrol) to unequivocally document the particular phase of the menstrual cycle (follicular, preovulatory, luteal, premenstrual).

H. Physiological range of ethanol elimination rates

Table 3.4 indicates the likely range of values for ethanol elimination rates from blood (β-slopes) that might be found in a properly conducted study in the entire population of drinkers. The conditions under which these rates apply are also listed. Admittedly values beyond these extremes 0.1 and 0.35 g/L/h have occasionally been reported but a detailed analysis of the data shows either flaws in the experimental design or incorrect analysis and interpretation of the results. To calculate the β-slope, the dose of ethanol administered and the number of blood samples taken as well as the sampling time frame must be optimal to allow fitting a straight line to the post-absorptive phase.

Calculating alcohol burn-off rates based on just two blood samples taken sixty minutes apart is not recommended because the phase of alcohol metabolism when sampling occurs cannot be known with certainty. During the post-absorptive state in drunk drivers, taking double blood samples can be used to estimate their alcohol burn-off rate. However, the extreme values are not reliable because some individuals might not have reached their peak BAC at time of sampling and others might be on a BAC plateau. In this population of drinkers, the mean burn-off rate was 0.19 g/L/h (95-percent range 0.09 to

Table 3.4
Expected Rates of Ethanol Disappearance from Blood and
Circumstances under Which Such Values Might Be Observed (Jones, 1993)

Elimination rate from blood	Expected values g/L/h	Experimental conditions/treatment
Slow	0.08–0.1	Malnourished individuals and people eating low-protein diets. Advanced state of liver cirrhosis with portal hypertension. Administration of the ADH inhibitor drug 4-methyl pyrazole (fomepizole).
Moderate	0.1–0.15	Healthy individuals after overnight (10-hour) fast and intake of a moderate dose of ethanol (< 1 g/kg).
Rapid	0.15–0.25	Regular drinkers (e.g., drinking drivers who are not alcoholics and non-fasting). High initial BAC in the fed state. Intravenous administration of the carbohydrate fructose.
Ultra-rapid	0.25–0.35	Alcoholics and binge drinkers during detoxification with very high blood-ethanol levels (> 3.5 g/L). Induction of CYP2E1 enzymes by drugs or ethanol. Genetic predisposition for ultra-rapid metabolism of ethanol. Hypermetabolic state (e.g., induced by drugs or burn trauma).

0.29 g/L/h) and was slightly faster in women (0.22 g/L/h) compared with 0.18 g/L/h for men (Jones and Andersson, 1996a). In another large study in drunk drivers using only those β-values above 0.1 g/L/h to represent the post-absorptive phase, the median rate of ethanol elimination was 0.22 g/L/h (Neuteboom and Jones, 1990). These real-world estimates of alcohol elimination rate from blood are higher than those shown in Figure 3.9 because many drunk drivers are alcoholics and heavy drinkers with an induced capacity to eliminate ethanol (Jones and Andersson, 1996a).

I. Elimination rates in alcoholics during detoxification

Alcohol-dependent people drink daily and often reach very high BAC resulting in a continuous exposure of liver enzymes to alcohol which leads to the development of both cellular and metabolic tolerance to the drug (Kalant, 1996a). Metabolic tolerance means that chronic drinkers have a greater ability to metabolize alcohol and eliminate the drug faster than moderate or first-time drinkers (Lieber,

1997a; Bogusz et al., 1977; Jones and Sternebring, 1992). In studies with alcoholics and binge drinkers admitted to a clinic for detoxification analysis of a series of blood samples taken over twenty-four hours showed that the rate of ethanol elimination could reach 0.35 g/L/h (Bogusz et al., 1977; Jones and Sternebring, 1992). In another study in alcoholics during detoxification and again after they had sobered up for a couple of days the rate of elimination of ethanol had returned to the values expected for nontolerant individuals, namely 0.10 to 0.20 g/L/h (Keiding et al., 1983). The accelerated rate of alcohol elimination in alcoholics is a result of induction of CYP2E1 enzymes by the constant exposure to high concentrations of ethanol (Lieber, 1999; Klotz and Ammon, 1998; Fuhr, 2000). The ability to dispose of ethanol faster is lost when P450 enzymes are no longer engaged in metabolism of ethanol (e.g., during abstinence and withdrawal from the drug) (Gonzalez et al., 1991; Oneta et al., 2002).

Diurnal variations in rate of ethanol metabolism have been investigated (e.g., by serving alcohol (0.75 g/kg) at 9 A.M., 3 P.M., 9 P.M. and 3 A.M. in ran-

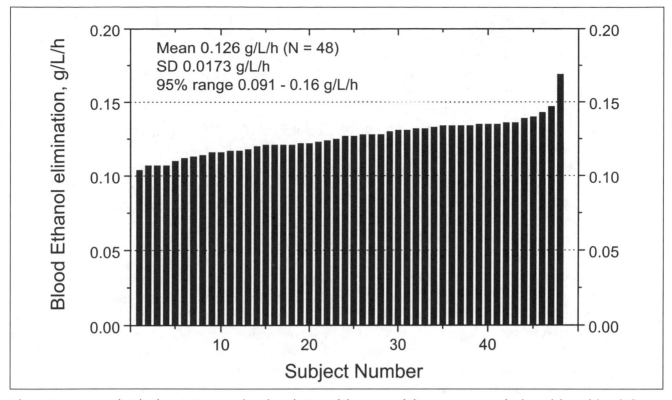

Figure 3.9 *Inter-individual variations and rank ordering of the rates of disappearance of ethanol from blood (β-slopes) in forty-eight healthy men after they drank 0.68 gram per kilogram as neat whisky on an empty stomach (Jones, 1984)*

dom order). Apart from a higher C_{max} in the 9 A.M. drinking session, no differences in pharmacokinetic parameters of ethanol were observed as a function of time of day of the test (Yap et al., 1993). The higher C_{max} at 9 A.M. can probably be explained by a faster gastric emptying secondary to low blood glucose in the morning (Schvarcz et al., 1995; Jones et al., 1999; Lötterle et al., 1989).

J. Liver cirrhosis and ethanol elimination rate
Because the liver is the principal site for oxidative metabolism of ethanol, one might think that in people with liver cirrhosis the rate of ethanol oxidation would be substantially decreased (Hoyumpa and Schenker, 1982; Panes et al., 1989; Jones, 2000b). However, in a controlled study with five patients suffering from liver cirrhosis, the rate of ethanol elimination from blood was 0.1 g/L/h and was not much less than in a control group of healthy individuals (0.13 g/L/h) tested under the same conditions (Jokipii, 1951). In cirrhotic patients suffering from portal hypertension the rate of clearance of

ethanol from blood was decreased below 0.10 g/L/h but the reason was attributed to restriction in hepatic blood flow rather than cirrhosis (Leube and Mallach, 1980). Seemingly, the human liver contains so much ADH that even with advanced necrosis of the tissue the enzyme is sufficient for the combustion of ethanol. Jokipii (1951) also investigated such conditions as obesity, diabetes mellitus, acute hepatitis and hyperthyrosis but failed to find an altered rate of ethanol elimination from blood compared with a control group of healthy subjects.

K. Inhibition and acceleration of ethanol metabolism
Administering the drug 4-methyl pyrazole (fomepizole) would certainly slow the rate of ethanol elimination from blood because this agent competes with ethanol for active sites on the ADH enzyme (Shannon, 1998). Indeed, this drug is currently recommended for treatment of patients poisoned with methanol and ethylene glycol, instead of giving ethanol as the antidote (Brent et al., 2001). People

who are malnourished or restricted to low-protein diets tend to show abnormally low rates of ethanol elimination from blood (Bode, 1978). The underlying mechanism is probably related to lowered activity of ADH enzyme owing to a limited supply of exogenous protein. Some support for this was obtained from animal models and different starvation diets followed by analysis of liver weight, protein and enzyme activity (Bosron et al., 1984; Mezey, 1998). The pharmacokinetics of ethanol was also studied in patients undergoing dialysis because of renal failure but this condition did not decrease the rate of ethanol elimination from the body (Jones and Hahn, 1997). Although the kidneys have some metabolic activity, including presence of ADH enzymes, this represents only a small fraction of the hepatic ADH activity.

Drugs capable of boosting the elimination of ethanol, so called sobering-up agents, have attracted research interest but none seem to be especially effective compared with the oxidative capacity of the liver in healthy, well-nourished individuals (Jones, 1991a; Mascord et al., 1988). The carbohydrates fructose and sucrose have probably attracted most attention as sobering-up agents but in many instances the results are conflicting and depend to a great extent on the experimental conditions, such as the dose, the timing and the route of administration relative to ethanol (Soterakis and Iber, 1975; Goldberg et al., 1979; Crownover et al., 1986; Jones, 1991a). The fructose effect was one of the things covered in the third edition of this book and not much has happened since then, so the topic will not be dealt with further (Baselt, 1996).

L. Blood concentration-time profiles of ethanol

Discussion and debate about forensic aspects of ethanol require a thorough knowledge of the many factors that influence the concentration-time profile of man's favorite drug. Furthermore, there is a need for large-scale human studies in which the volunteers are allowed to consume various drinks and different doses of alcohol. In this connection, it is important to ensure that the blood-sampling schedule is optimal to allow an unequivocal determination of the post-absorptive elimination phase. Without this information it is simply not feasible to arrive at a reliable estimate of the rate of elimination of alcohol from the bloodstream.

1. Fasting versus fed conditions

Figure 3.10 shows the general features of the blood-alcohol concentration time curves after drinking alcohol (0.8 g/kg) on an empty stomach or immediately after breakfast. The relevant pharmacokinetic parameters of ethanol are shown on the plot and the ratio of dose (g/kg)/C_0 gives the Widmark *rho* factor. The plots are average curves (± SD) for N = ten men who drank 95-percent ethanol diluted to 20 percent v/v with orange juice in exactly thirty minutes. In the fed state, the BAC curve runs below the fasted curve for the entire sampling period and this gives the impression that a smaller dose of ethanol was administered. By extrapolating the rectilinear elimination portions back to the time of starting to drink. one obtains the y-intercept (C_0), which represents the BAC expected if absorption and distribution were instantaneous and without any metabolism taking place.

The pharmacokinetic parameters of ethanol with and without food are compared in Table 3.5 based on the curves drawn in Figure 3.10. The C_{max} was lowered by about 0.30 g/L after the subjects had eaten food before drinking and t_{max} occurred considerably later, 120 minutes compared with 45 minutes from start of drinking. The C_0 values for fed and fasting conditions differed by 0.19 g/L (1.16 g/L versus 0.97 g/L) and gives an indication of the size of the absorption deficit. The lower C_0 after food means that Widmark's *rho* factor is abnormally high for men in the fed state (Table 3.5). The extrapolated time to reach zero BAC ($time_0$) was also shorter in the fed state by 102 minutes or 1.7 hours and is roughly the time needed to metabolize completely the absorption deficit of 0.19 g/L. The size of the absorption deficit might differ for different drinking conditions (e.g., fast versus slow absorbers, beer versus liquor, big versus small meal before drinking).

The disappearance rate of ethanol from the bloodstream did not depend on the fed or fasting state of the subjects as verified by comparing the β-slopes (0.14 g/L/h) in Table 3.5. However, when the rate of alcohol elimination per unit body weight was calculated (B_{60}) (e.g., by dividing the dose [g/kg] by

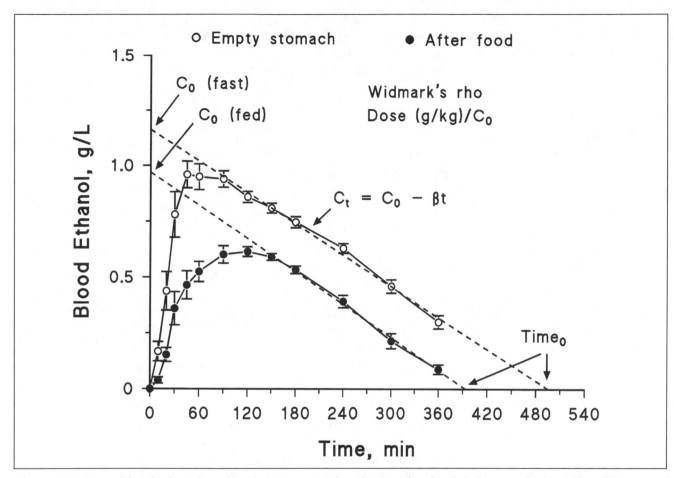

Figure 3.10 *Mean blood-ethanol profiles for N = ten male subjects who drank 0.8 gram of ethanol per kilogram of body weight after an overnight fast or immediately after eating breakfast (Jones and Jönsson, 1994b). The main pharmacokinetic parameters of ethanol are indicated on the curves and one notes a lower C_0 parameter under fed conditions, which indicates an absorption deficit or an apparent loss of ethanol.*

the extrapolated time to zero BAC [min_0]), the overall rate of metabolism was significantly faster after eating the meal. This dichotomy can only be explained if some of the ethanol underwent FPM either in the stomach, the liver or both organs. This ability of food in the stomach to lower the BAC profile was noticed already by Widmark and he referred to it as "loss of alcohol" or absorption deficit but the underlying mechanism at the time was not known (Widmark, 1932).

It is important to realize that if ethanol had been determined in samples of serum or plasma the parameters C_{max}, *rho*, and β-slope would have been slightly different from those derived from whole blood. This follows because the concentrations of ethanol in these biofluids depend on the water content of the specimens as discussed earlier. The slope

in the post-absorptive phase is therefore steeper for plasma giving a higher C_0 value and a correspondingly smaller *rho* factor. However, the extrapolated time to zero BAC (min_0) and the rate of elimination from the whole body dose/min_0 remain the same regardless of whether plasma or whole blood was analyzed.

2. Sex-related differences

Figure 3.11 shows BAC profiles for twenty-two subjects (twelve women and ten men) who drank 0.4 g/kg ethanol in fifteen minutes at two to three hours after they had eaten lunch. The drink was made from ethanol solvent (95 percent v/v) after dilution with a soft drink to 20 percent v/v. Large variation in the shapes of these individual profiles is obvious. The horizontal dotted line represents the theoretical

Table 3.5

Pharmacokinetic Parameters[1] of Ethanol in Healthy men (N = 10) Who Ingested 0.8 Gram Ethanol per Kilogram Body Weight in a Crossover Design Study Either after an Overnight Fast or Immediately after Eating a Standardized Breakfast

(Jones and Jönsson, 1994b)

Conditions	C_{max} g/L	t_{max} min	C_0 g/L	ρ L/kg	min_0 min	β-slope (k_0) g/L/h	B_{60} g/kg/h
Fed	0.62	45	0.97	0.82	393	0.15	0.123
Fasted	0.96	120	1.16	0.69	495	0.14	0.097

[1] The blood-alcohol parameters shown in this table were derived from the mean BAC curves depicted in Figure 3.10 and not from results for individual subjects as described in the article by Jones and Jönsson (1994b).

maximum BAC arising for 100 percent availability of the 0.4 g/kg dose and assuming a distribution volume of 0.7 L/kg for both men and women. Only one male subject exceeded this BAC and evidently he had not eaten any lunch. In all the other subjects, the actual BAC curves were considerably lower than those expected theoretically, which suggests a reduced bioavailability probably being caused by first-pass metabolism or some other mechanism. The average curves (insert top right) agreed well with no marked sex-related differences in patterns of absorption, distribution or elimination.

Statistical summaries of the kinetic parameters for men and women and differences between the sexes are shown in Table 3.6. The rate of disappearance of ethanol from blood (β-slope or k_0) were determined as described by Widmark by fitting a straight line to the concentration-time points on the post-absorptive portions, normally starting ninety minutes after end of drinking. The *rho* factors for both men and women were larger than expected, which probably reflects the fact subjects had not fasted overnight before drinking the alcohol. Also 95 percent ethanol was diluted to ~20 percent v/v with a soft drink instead of consumption of neat spirits as recommended by Widmark (1932). Nevertheless, the mean values for C_0 and *rho* parameters differed significantly between the sexes as expected for sex-related difference in total body water. The β-slope was slightly steeper in women compared with men (p < 0.01) but the overall rate of ethanol elimination

per kilogram body weight (B_{60}) was independent of sex.

3. Time to reach peak blood-ethanol concentration

The peak BAC (C_{max}) and the time of reaching the peak (t_{max}) after drinking depend on the rate of absorption of ethanol, which in turn depends on the speed of gastric emptying. The area under the concentration-time curve (AUC) is another useful parameter and gives an indication of the time of exposure of the body organs and tissue to alcohol for the particular dose administered. The rate of elimination of alcohol from the whole body, sometimes denoted as B_{60}, is the product of β and volume of distribution V_d or can be derived as the ratio of dose/$time_0$.

In a recent survey of the literature dealing with time to reach peak BAC after end of drinking Iffland and Jones (2002) produced the data shown in Table 3.7. The results illustrate the large inter-subject and inter-study differences with peak BAC being reached between zero and thirty minutes as well as more than ninety minutes after end of drinking. It is important to note that the doses of alcohol and duration of drinking in the various studies cited are much smaller than for the typical drunk driver. Nevertheless, the table illustrates that two blood samples taken thirty to sixty minutes apart is not sufficient to allow making an unequivocal statement of whether the person was in the post-peak phase at the time of driving.

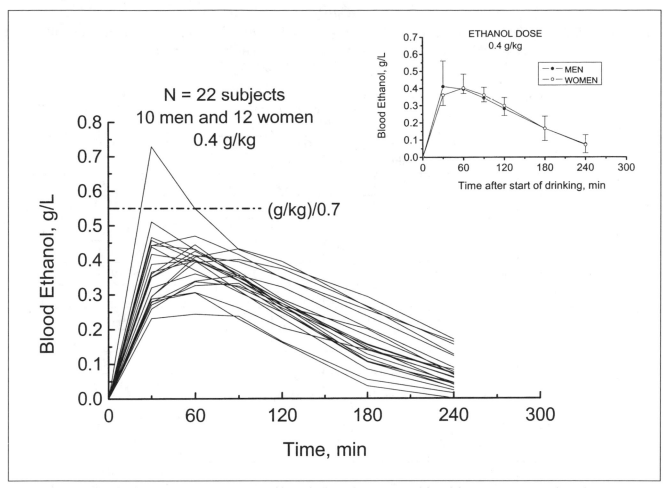

Figure 3.11 *Individual concentration-time profiles of ethanol in venous blood from ten men and twelve women after they consumed 0.4 gram of ethanol per kilogram body weight starting at approximately two hours after their last meal. The mean curves for the two sexes are shown as an insert graph (top right). The dotted horizontal line gives the BAC expected for the dose ingested (0.4 g/kg) and Widmark r factor of 0.7 independent of sex.*

Table 3.6
Pharmacokinetic Parameters of Ethanol in Ten Men and Twelve Women Who Drank 0.4 Gram Ethanol per Kilogram Body Weight in Fifteen Minutes, Two to Three Hours after Eating Lunch. Values Shown Are Mean ± SD
(Jones and Fransson, unpublished data)

Parameter[1]	Men (N = 10)	Women (N = 12)
C_{max} mg/g	0.426 ± 0.136	0.417 ± 0.027
t_{max} min	48.00 ± 15.49	60.00 ± 24.49
C_0 mg/g	0.510 ± 0.064	0.577 ± 0.038[2]
β-slope or k_0 mg/g/h	0.115 ± 0.016	0.138 ± 0.019[2]
V_d or ρ	0.796 ± 0.103	0.696 ± 0.047[2]
AUC mg × h/g	56.82 ± 17.67	58.66 ± 7.56
B_{60} mg/kg/h	0.090 ± 0.016	0.096 ± 0.014

[1] For definitions of parameters see main text.
[2] Statistically significant difference between the sexes (p <0.01).

Table 3.7
Number of Subjects Reaching Their Peak Blood-Alcohol Concentration as a Function of Time after End of Drinking According to a Number of Controlled Experiments
(Iffland and Jones 2002)

Dose g/kg	Drinking time (min)	Time (h) after last meal	N	Number of subjects reaching their peak blood ethanol concentration within				Reference
				0–30 min	31–60 min	61–90 min	> 90 min	
0.3	60	not given	12	12	-	-		Heifer (1976)
0.3	30	> 4	10	9	1	-	-	Kühnholz et al. (1993)
0.34	15	> 8	6	5	1	-	-	Jones et al. (1991)
0.5	5	> 8	20	-	19	1	-	Alha (1951)
0.5	60	not given	12	11	1	-	-	Heifer (1976)
0.5	30	> 4	10	9	1	-	-	Kühnholz et al. (1993)
0.51	15	> 8	16	11	3	1	1	Jones et al. (1991)
0.68	20	> 8	83	33	26	21	3	Jones et al. (1991)
0.75	10	0	23	8	9	5	1	Krauland et al. (1966)
0.75	10	1	15	-	1	6	8	Krauland et al. (1966)
0.75	10	3	30	-	10	14	6	Krauland et al. (1966)
0.75	10	6	55	7	21	13	14	Krauland et al. (1966)
0.8	5	> 8	31	-	20	4	7	Alha (1951)
0.8	60	not given	12	9	2	1	-	Heifer (1976)
0.8	50–55	3	19	2	10	4	3	Gerchow and Steigleder (1961)
0.8	30	> 4	10	6	2	1	1	Kühnholz et al. (1973)
0.8	30	> 8	65	40	19	3	1	Jones (unpublished work)
.85	25	> 8	44	13	24	7	-	Jones et al. (1991)
1.0	5	> 8	41	1	21	13	6	Alha (1951)
1.02	25	> 8	3	-	1	1	1	Jones et al. (1991)
1.2	50–55	3	17	2	5	5	5	Gerchow and Steigleder (1961)
1.25	5	> 8	38	1	14	14	9	Alha (1951)
1.6	50–55	3	19	5	8	6	-	Gerchow and Steigleder (1961)

Zink and Reinhardt (1984) in a classic study showed that during a period of continuous heavy drinking with some of the volunteers reaching BACs of 3–4 g/L, the blood-ethanol concentration increased gradually as drinking proceeded and by the end of drinking the BAC was sometimes very close to its maximum concentration even before the last drink was finished. After continuous heavy drinking much of the alcohol becomes absorbed into the bloodstream and distributed throughout the body compartments during the drinking period so that the amount contained in the last drink is insufficient to raise the BAC further. In reality however much depends on the frequency of drinking and the amount of alcohol contained in the last drink.

4. BAC curves after divided doses of alcohol
Figure 3.12 is a rare example of an experiment in which the alcohol was given in divided doses (Jones, unpublished work). The two male subjects drank a

moderate dose of neat whisky in fifteen minutes after an overnight fast and the same dose of alcohol was ingested again about two hours later. After the first dose the peak BAC was reached fifteen minutes after end of drinking compared with 55–60 minutes after the second dose of whisky was consumed. More studies are needed that involve repetitive drinking, which is closer in keeping with real-world drinking scenarios.

5. Variability in BAC in controlled drinking experiments

Table 3.8 presents the mean and median blood-alcohol concentrations at various sampling times after healthy men drank a moderate amount of alcohol (0.68 g/kg) as neat whisky on an empty stomach (Jones, 1984). Besides mean and median BAC the coefficient of variation and the 95-percent range of BAC are shown for forty-eight male subjects. If the

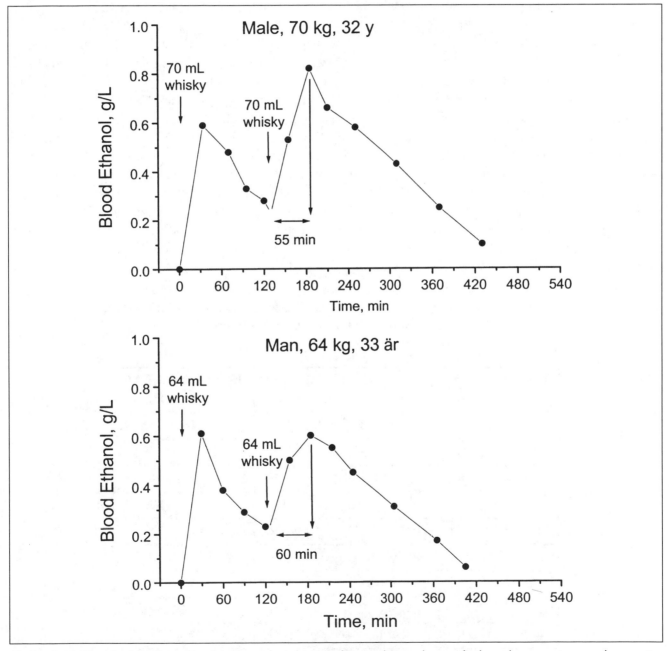

Figure 3.12 *Blood ethanol profiles in two male subjects after moderate doses of ethanol were consumed as neat whisky in divided doses after an overnight fast (Jones, unpublished work)*

coefficient of variation (CV%) is taken as a relative measure of uncertainty in BAC, it is obvious that the errors incurred are greatest early after the end of drinking and also late in the post-absorptive phase six hours later. Least variation (CV = 8%) was found at 100 minutes after end of drinking but even at this time point the BAC might range from 0.59 to 0.83 g/L in ninety-five of 100 subjects. Once again, this example from actual human drinking studies highlights the need to allow for uncertainty when called on to make forward projections of a person's BAC for legal purposes based on Widmark's formulae or some modified version.

6. Effect of age on Widmark factors

In a little-known German study, twenty men over sixty years of age drank ethanol (0.68 g/kg) either as wine or spirits during a time of sixty minutes and the resulting BAC profiles and parameters of ethanol kinetics were compared with literature data for younger men (Hein and Vock, 1989). The absorption of alcohol was slightly slower after drinking the wine compared with the spirits although C_{max} oc-

curred thirty minutes after end of drinking for both beverages. There were no beverage-related differences (spirits versus wine) in β-slope (0.137 ± 0.013 versus 0.138 ± 0.015), C_0 (1.09 ± 0.094 versus 1.06 ± 0.076), and *rho* factor (0.627 ± 0.053 versus 0.645 ± 0.045). These values agree well with those found in younger men aged twenty to sixty years after the same dose of alcohol was taken as neat whisky on an empty stomach (Jones and Neri, 1985).

7. Blood-alcohol profiles after drinking beer

More studies are needed to characterize the shapes of BAC or BrAC profiles after subjects drink various kinds of beer to complement the many bolus dose drinking studies with neat spirits as the alcoholic beverage consumed.

In one such study 500 milliliters of a low-strength beer (2.25 percent v/v) corresponding to 8.8 grams of ethanol was given to eight women (body weight 47–80 kilograms) and four men (body weight 67–100 kilograms). The drink was consumed in fifteen minutes after an overnight fast. The resulting C_{max} and t_{max} showed wide variations with the small-

Table 3.8
Magnitude of Inter-Individual Variability of the Blood-Alcohol Concentration (BAC) Measured at Various Times after Healthy Men (N = 48) Drank Neat Whisky Equivalent to 0.68 Gram of Ethanol per Kilogram Body Weight on an Empty Stomach
(Jones, 1984)

Time, min[1]	Mean blood-alcohol g/L ± SD[2] (median blood alcohol)	CV%[3]	95% range of BAC (± 2 × SD)
10	0.80 ± 0.279 (0.88)	35%	0.24– 1.35
40	0.82 ± 0.141 (0.85)	17%	0.54– 1.1
70	0.77 ± 0.083 (0.78)	11%	0.60– 0.94
100	0.71 ± 0.059 (0.72)	8%	0.59– 0.83
160	0.61 ± 0.062 (0.61)	10%	0.49– 0.73
220	0.50 ± 0.063 (0.54)	13%	0.37– 0.63
280	0.39 ± 0.071 (0.4)	18%	0.25– 0.53
340	0.24 ± 0.074 (0.25)	30%	0.09– 0.39
400	0.10 ± 0.072 (0.08)	72%	0.00– 0.24

[1] Time from the end of drinking, which lasted exactly twenty minutes. [2] Standard deviation. [3] Coefficient of variation.

est woman reaching a peak BAC of 0.28 g/L and the heaviest man reaching 0.09 g/L and the t_{max} occurred between ten and thirty minutes after end of drinking (Magnisdottir and Johannesson, 2000).

The title of an article by Holford (1997), namely "Complex PK/PD models—An alcoholic experience" gives a hint about the complicated nature of ethanol kinetics. He compared the BAC profiles after subjects drank beer containing different concentrations of ethanol, 2.75 percent v/v and 4.0 percent v/v. The low-alcohol beer (2.75 vol %) was compared with a medium brew (4.0 vol %) and each subject drank 2.5 liters of each beer over a two-hour period in a careful double blind study. When results were adjusted for the different amounts of alcohol in the beers, the area under the BAC time curve after drinking the weaker beer was only 52 percent of the AUC for the normal strength beer and C_{max} was halved. The reason for the lower apparent bioavailability of alcohol in the weaker drink was not investigated further but it was felt that differences in absorption rate, first pass metabolism and changes in hepatic blood flow might have contributed (Holford, 1997).

In a study with ten men who drank 0.75 g/kg ethanol as either 4-percent, 8-percent, 20-percent or 44-percent alcohol in water on an empty stomach the BAC profiles were plotted for six hours post-dosing (Springer, 1972). No statistically significant differences in BAC profiles or kinetic parameters were noted although AUC for the 44-percent drink was less than for the weaker ones. It seems that other constituents of the alcoholic beverages (sugar, CO_2 and so on) can probably explain differences noted in some studies (Pfeiffer et al., 1992).

So-called nonalcoholic beers have gained popularity in some quarters, although these drinks often contain between 0.5–1 percent v/v ethanol. In a study with twenty men who drank 3,000 milliliters of low-alcoholic beer over three hours, their blood-ethanol concentration was not measurable after the beverage containing 0.5-percent v/v ethanol and was always less than 0.1 g/L after drinking the 0.9-percent v/v beer (Neuteboom and Vis, 1991). Drinking 3,000 milliliters (100 oz) of 0.9-percent v/v beer correspond to an intake of 21 grams of ethanol, which is almost exactly the amount the liver can metabolize over the three hours drinking time for a 70-kilogram male (0.1 g/kg/h).

In another study with beer, sixteen students (eight men and eight women) drank three pints of larger beer (4.2 percent v/v ethanol) over 30 minutes, which must be considered forced drinking for such a large volume (Ward et al., 1991). The resulting C_{max} was 0.74 ± 0.07 g/L ($\pm$ SD) and t_{max} 60 minutes after end of drinking in the men compared with C_{max} of 1.13 ± 0.17 g/L and t_{max} of 90 minutes in the women. Intake of three pints of low-alcohol beer (1-percent v/v) under the same conditions gave a peak BAC of 0.13 g/L whereas no measurable BAC was evident after drinking three pints of nonalcoholic lager (< 0.05-percent v/v).

In a study with people classified as light (N = 13), moderate (N = 12), heavy (N = 12) and very heavy (N = 14) drinkers depending on a survey of their previous drinking habits, both C_{max} and t_{max} were measured after lager beer (4-percent v/v) was consumed corresponding to an ethanol dose of 0.79 g/kg body weight. This required drinking about two liters of beer (3.5 pints) in a man weighing 80 kilograms and the speed of drinking was staggered over the one hour. The mean C_{max} ranged from 0.39 to 0.44 g/L and the t_{max} from 10 to 25 minutes in the different groups of subjects after end of drinking, which began five hours after the last meal. Even after drinking beer, the overall range of t_{max} was 5–95 minutes after end of drinking (Wright and Cameron, 1998).

3.17 Excretion of Ethanol

The excretion of ethanol takes place through the skin, the lungs and the kidney although in quantitative terms these routes of elimination represent only a small fraction of the total dose administered (Kalant, 1971; Wallgren, 1970). Attempts to enhance the rate of ethanol removal from the body (e.g., by physical exertion to increase lung ventilation, by drinking water to increase production of urine or sauna bathing to increase sweating) will not be effective in speeding up alcohol elimination (Wallgren, 1970; Kalant, 1996b).

A. Ethanol in body fluids

Ethanol is a small neutral molecule, which remains unionized at physiological pH and can therefore easily penetrate cell membranes by diffusion through aqueous channels. Ethanol mixes completely with all the water in the body and is transported to all organs and tissues and enters both extracellular and intracellular fluid compartments as reviewed by Rosenfeld (1996). Ethanol is not bound to plasma proteins and can be used as a marker substance to estimate total body water by noninvasive analysis of end-expired breath (Norberg et al., 2000). Those body fluids and tissues containing most water will contain most ethanol when equilibration has been reached. The time required for equilibration depends on the blood flow to the various organs and tissues. This means that heart, brain, lungs and kidneys with their high minute-blood volume quickly reach equilibrium with the concentration of alcohol in the arterial blood. By contrast the skeletal muscles, where the bulk of the water resides, takes a longer time to reach an equilibrium with arterial blood ethanol because the ratio of blood flow to tissue mass is smaller for the resting muscles (Chiou, 1989).

Plasma, serum, saliva, urine, and cerebrospinal fluid contain more water than whole blood and are therefore expected to also contain more alcohol at equilibrium. However, besides differences in the water content, the time of sampling and the pharmacokinetics of ethanol need to be considered. Indeed, the concentrations of ethanol in arterial (A) and venous (V) blood are the same at only one time point after drinking ends (Martin et al., 1984; Jones et al., 1997a). A-V differences are largest during the time alcohol is being ingested and absorbed a time when the concentration gradient from the gut to the venous return to the heart is greatest. The A-V difference is positive for the first ninety minutes after end of drinking by about 0.2 g/L on average and decreases as time after end of drinking increases. By ninety minutes post-drinking the A-V difference is zero and at all later times the venous blood holds slightly more alcohol than the arterial blood (~0.05 g/L) (see Figure 3.6). What this means is that blood/body fluid distribution ratios of ethanol depend in part on the source of blood taken for analysis and the time after drinking.

Many publications appearing since the 1930s have reported blood/body fluid ratios of alcohol but care is needed when these articles are reviewed and cited. Beside average values for the ratios found the articles sometimes include wide ranges of values that are physiologically just not possible, such as, a plasma/whole blood ratio of less than unity, which implies more water in whole blood than in plasma. Such unusual results depend on errors of some kind in either the sampling or analysis (or both) of ethanol in the blood, the plasma or both media. Concentration ratios of ethanol should not be calculated after drinking very small doses because at the resulting low BAC extreme and unrealistic values are obtained. Small sex-related differences in blood/body fluid ratios might be expected because of the lower hematocrit and slightly more water present in whole blood from females. People with anemia would have more water per unit volume of blood owing to the deficiency in erythrocytes and accordingly different blood/body fluid ratios of ethanol.

B. Breath

Recognizing the smell of alcohol on the breath of a drinker is probably as old as Noah. The first scientific studies reporting quantitative analysis of exhaled ethanol date back to the work of Anstie (1874), who proved convincingly that the amount of ethanol exhaled in breath represented only a small fraction of the total amount ingested. An important early paper by Liljestrand and Linde (1930) established the physiological principles of breath-alcohol testing and also determined the blood/air distribution ratios of ethanol both in-vivo and in-vitro. The blood- and breath-alcohol concentrations were highly correlated and followed a similar time course except that the concentration in the end-expired breath was approximately 2,000 times less than in an equal volume of blood, which suggests a 2,000:1 blood/breath ratio. This study was the starting point for future applications of breath-alcohol analysis in forensic science to provide an indirect way of estimating the concentration of ethanol in blood (Jones, 1996b).

The amount of ethanol excreted from the body in exhaled air can be calculated as follows. Assume a blood-alcohol concentration of 1.0 g/L and a blood-to-breath ratio of 1,800:1 at the alveolar-capillary membrane at a body temperature of 37°C. It follows that one liter of alveolar air will contain 0.55 milligrams of ethanol. The amount of air inspired and expired per minute, known as the respiratory minute volume, is about 6 liters (500 milliliters per breath × 12 breaths per minute). But about 150 mL of each breath does not reach the alveolar regions of the lungs to undergo gas exchange and this volume is known as the dead space air. The alveolar ventilation at a respiratory minute volume of 6 L/min will be only 4.2 L/min or 252 liters per hour so that every hour only 138 mg of ethanol (0.55 × 252) is eliminated from the body via the breath. This corresponds to 1.7–2.3 percent of the total amount eliminated from the body per hour being 6–8 grams per hour. Obviously these values will depend on the underlying blood-ethanol concentration and the actual lung ventilation rate of the subject.

Measuring alcohol in the breath is an excellent screening test to prove that a person has been drinking and this technique has found many applications in research, forensic science and clinical medicine (Jones, 1996b). However, such tests should not be made sooner than fifteen minutes after the last drink to avoid contamination of the breath with high concentrations of residual alcohol in the mucosa membranes of the mouth from the drink consumed. This phenomenon is well recognized and is called the mouth-alcohol effect and can be minimized by washing the mouth with warm water after the end of drinking and before the breath-alcohol test is made. The past fifteen years has witnessed major developments in the methods available for breath-alcohol testing with improved analytical technologies, better routines for sampling end-expired alveolar air and microprocessors and computer technology to monitor and control the entire test sequence. Most countries worldwide now accept breath-alcohol analysis as evidence for prosecuting drunk drivers (Jones, 1998; Jones, 1996b).

Because of much discussion and debate about the value of the blood/breath ratio for an individual subject and variations during the metabolism of alcohol the old practice of translating BrAC into BAC for legal purposes has been abandoned (Emerson et al., 1980; Jones, 1996b; Jones, 2000c). Instead, threshold limits of BrAC are defined by statute in most countries and these operate alongside the equivalent BAC limits (Jones, 2000d; Jones and Andersson, 1996b). However, there is no escaping

the fact that the BrAC limits were derived from the pre-existing BAC limits and an assumed average blood/breath ratio for the population. In this connection, Great Britain and Holland opted for 2,300:1 whereas most other countries in Europe were content to use 2,000:1. In Germany and the Scandinavian countries BAC is reported in units of mg/g or g/kg and a 2,000:1 BAC/BrAC ratio was used to calculate the threshold BrAC limit in mass/volume units (mg/L). In studies when BAC/BrAC ratios of ethanol were determined in actual drinking drivers, median values of 2,400:1 were found with no sex-related differences; males 2,428 ± 261 (± standard deviation N = 369) and females 2,444 ± 232 (N = 39) (Jones and Andersson, 1996b). Clearly this gives a definite advantage to the person who provides breath as opposed to blood when a 2,000:1 or 2,100:1 BAC/BrAC ratio is used to establish the critical threshold value for prosecution.

1. Comparison of venous blood and breath-alcohol profiles

Figure 3.13 compares BAC profiles for venous blood and BrAC profiles in nine men and nine women after they drank moderate amounts of alcohol as wine or whisky under controlled conditions. All the breath-alcohol tests were done with Intoxilyzer 5000S, a quantitative infrared analyzer. The venous blood-alcohol concentration was determined by headspace gas chromatography (Jones and Andersson, 2003). The BAC and BrAC curves agreed well except that BrAC was sometimes higher than BAC for up to ninety minutes post-dosing and thereafter the BAC was always less than BrAC by about 10 percent on the average. This dependence on phase of ethanol metabolism can be explained by arterial-venous differences in ethanol concentration as discussed earlier in this chapter and the fact that pulmonary ethanol is closer to the arterial blood-ethanol concentration. If the blood/breath factor is increased from mg/2 L to mg/2.3 L, this would bring the BAC and BrAC values closer together during the post-absorptive phase but would exaggerate the differences during the rising phase of the alcohol curves. With the critical BrAC defined by statute, interconversion between BAC and BrAC is not necessary because both are equally objective ways to demonstrate over-

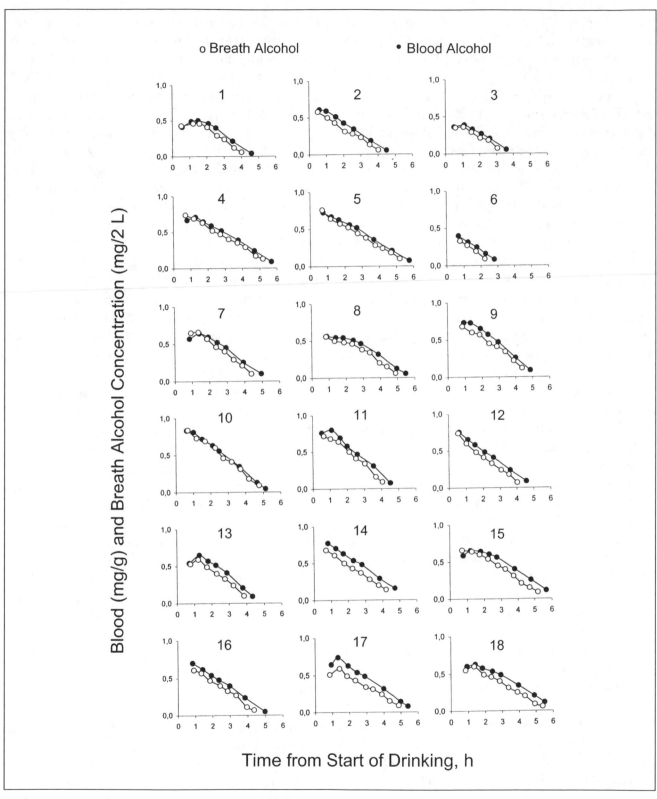

Figure 3.13 *Individual concentration-time profiles of ethanol for nine men and nine women with venous blood alcohol concentration (BAC) determined by gas chromatography and end-expired breath alcohol measured with a quantitative infrared analyzer Intoxilyzer 5000S (Jones and Andersson, 2003). The units of alcohol concentration are those used for legal purposes in Sweden, namely mg/g for blood and mg/L for breath with the latter plotted as mg/2 L for direct comparison with BAC values.*

consumption of alcohol. The differences in the blood and breath curves shown in Figure 3.13 would be the same even if BAC had been reported as g/100 mL and BrAC as g/210 L owing to the density of whole blood being 1.055 on average.

The experiments in Figure 3.13 were done with nine men and nine women and the observed mean (± SD) BAC/BrAC ratios under these test conditions were 2,553 ± 576 and 2,417 ± 494, respectively, and the sex difference was not statistically significant (p > 0.05). The mean rate of ethanol elimination from venous blood was 0.157 mg/g/h, which was very close to the rate of elimination from breath of 0.161 mg/2 L/h (Jones and Andersson, 2003).

2. Factors influencing breath-alcohol concentration

The physiological principles of breath-alcohol analysis and the theory of gas exchange in the lungs have been reviewed elsewhere (Jones, 1990; Hlastala, 1998). Besides equilibration of ethanol between blood and air at the alveolar-capillary membrane of the lungs there is an air-alcohol exchange taking place during a prolonged expiration. Ethanol vapor is highly water soluble and equilibrates with the mucous membranes covering the upper airway, nose and mouth and this equilibrium is sensitive to changes in the subject's breathing pattern. Early proponents of breath-alcohol testing had not appreciated the importance of equilibration of ethanol in the airways and such interactions probably account for much of the variability in blood/breath ratios of ethanol observed in practice (Hlastala, 1998). Hypoventilation elevates the expired BrAC whereas hyperventilation lowers the exhaled BrAC compared with a normal inhalation and exhalation maneuver (Jones, 1982). The BrAC changes are caused in part by disrupting the air-liquid exchanges of ethanol and partly by altered temperature of the equilibrium; hypoventilation raises the temperature and hyperventilation lowers the temperature. The temperature coefficient of alcohol solubility is ± 6.5 percent per degree change in temperature (Jones, 1990).

Diseases of the lungs such as asthma as reflected in inflammation of the airways or chronic obstructive pulmonary disease (COPD) could mean that some individuals might not be able to provide a proper deep-lung sample with modern breath analyzers (Gullberg, 2000). In studies with COPD patients the BAC/BrAC ratios were consistently higher than for an age-matched control group suggesting overall lower concentration of alcohol in the breath (Hahn et al. 1991). Table 3.9 summarizes some of the main factors that might be associated with finding high or low BrAC and a corresponding change in the BAC/BrAC ratio.

C. Saliva

1. General

Saliva, which is commonly referred to nowadays as oral fluid, is being increasingly used as the specimen for analysis of drugs of abuse as well as therapeutic agents during monitoring of patients (Haeckel and Bucklitsch, 1987). Saliva is a watery fluid produced in the mouth by submaxillary, sublingual and parotid glands. Over a twenty-four-hour period, an adult person produces approximately 500–1,500 milliliters of saliva but most of this is swallowed so the alcohol or drugs it might contain are reabsorbed from the gut. Mixed whole saliva is the specimen generally obtained for analysis of ethanol and other drugs and this matrix is mainly composed of water (99 percent) (Lentner, 1981).

The first attempts to compare the concentrations of ethanol in saliva with those in blood can be traced to the 1930s, and a number of early publications testify to this. Perhaps the best early work was done by Linde (1932) from Sweden, who looked at the relationship between ethanol in blood and parotid saliva. He obtained samples of saliva by means of a special silver cannula thus avoiding contamination of the specimen with the mucous secretions from the mouth. The absorption, distribution and elimination stages of ethanol disposition could be monitored by analysis of saliva and the time lag between ethanol entering the blood and appearing in the parotid saliva was negligible. According to this seminal article, the mean saliva/blood ratio of alcohol was 1.21:1 and the concentration-time profile in saliva was on a slightly higher elevation than blood owing to the more water in saliva (Linde, 1932).

The vast majority of studies dealing with ethanol content of blood and saliva have been done with mixed saliva obtained by making tongue and lip

Table 3.9
Factors Influencing Breath Alcohol Concentration (BrAC) and Blood/Breath Ratios of Ethanol

High BrAC and low blood/breath ratios

- long time of exhalation into the breath analyzer
- sampling breath during the absorption stage of ethanol into the bloodstream a time when arterial-venous difference are most pronounced.
- presence of mouth alcohol (sampling too soon after end of drinking)
- rebreathing the first exhalation a number of time before analysis of the final exhalation
- breath-holding (hypoventilation) before sampling breath
- elevated body temperature (hyperthermia)
- nonspecific method of analysis and presence of interfering substance

Low BrAC and high blood/breath ratios

- hyperventilation before breath sampling
- chronic obstructive pulmonary disease (COPD)
- sampling breath too soon after the start of exhalation
- hypothermia
- calculating ratio at low BrAC
- low calibration factor (2,000:1 or 2,100:1 instead of 2,300:1 or 2,400:1)

movements and then spitting the specimen into a small tube. If necessary, the production of saliva can be stimulated by allowing the subject to chew on parafilm or some other inert material or by dropping lemon juice onto the tongue, which also enhances the flow rate. More recently, special saliva-sampling devices called salivetts have been developed for obtaining the required specimen for analysis of drugs of abuse. The subject chews on a cotton wool pad for about one minute and this is later removed from the mouth, placed into a special plastic tube and centrifuged to obtain a clear salivary fluid suitable for analysis of alcohol and other drugs (Haeckel and Peiffer, 1992; Samyn et al., 1999).

Only the free plasma fraction of a drug is available for passage into the saliva, which makes ethanol a good candidate substance because ethanol is not bound to plasma proteins, which explains the strong association found between BAC and SAC (Haeckel, 1993). In an experiment involving forty-eight healthy men who were dosed with 0.68 gram of ethanol per kilogram body weight, the mean saliva/blood ratio of alcohol was 1.08 to 1 and did not depend on the sampling time after the start of drinking (Jones, 1979). In a later study, using the same set of data, the pharmacokinetic profiles of ethanol where compared for serial samples of saliva and capillary whole blood. The results showed that serial samples of saliva were just as valid as blood for use in pharmacokinetic studies and investigations of the disposition and fate of ethanol on the body (Jones, 1993b).

The most recent investigation of saliva/blood ratios of ethanol (Gubala and Zuba, 2002) reported a mean value of 1.02 when mixed saliva was taken for analysis. This was a large study involving thirty-eight subjects (twenty-six men and twelve women) with multiple samples being taken to give a total of 1,152 saliva-blood pairs for statistical evaluation. The saliva-blood values were highly correlated $r = 0.94$ and 50 percent of them were within ± 0.05 g/L of each other. The authors recommend saliva as a useful medium for testing driver sobriety (Gubala and Zuba, 2002) supporting earlier work in hospital casualty patients who had been drinking (McColl et al., 1979).

2. Ethanol-concentration time profiles in saliva

Figure 3.14 shows the mean concentration-time profiles of ethanol in mixed whole saliva (SAC) and capillary blood after three different doses of alcohol (Jones, unpublished work). This clear-cut dose-concentration relationship supports the use of saliva as a body fluid for analysis of ethanol in forensic and biomedical research.

Most of the current interest in the analysis of ethanol in saliva relates to on-site alcohol testing, such as in the workplace or in clinical settings (Dubowski, 2002). Several on-the-spot devices for collection and analysis of saliva are available and these yield either a qualitative response (alcohol present or not) or a semiquantitative response (0.2, 0.3, 0.4 g/L and so forth) (Bates et al., 1993; Biwasaka et al., 2001). The analytical principle involves enzymatic (ADH-NAD$^+$) oxidation with a color endpoint,

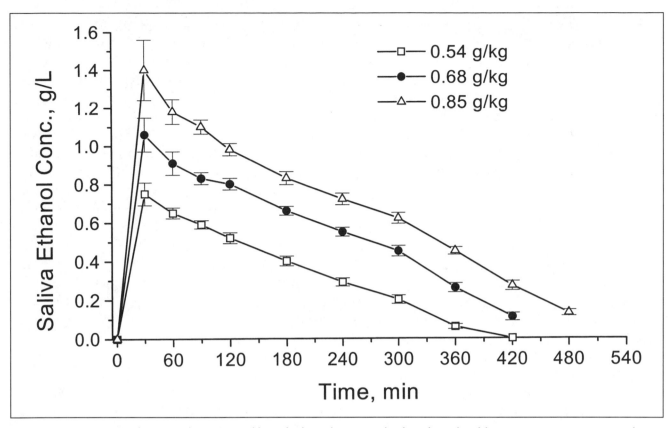

Figure 3.14 Average pharmacokinetic profiles of ethanol in mixed saliva from healthy men (N = sixteen per dose) after they drank 0.54, 0.68 and 0.85 gram per kilogram of body weight as neat whisky (Jones, unpublished work)

which can be read from a linear scale or by a simple photometer device. Several evaluation studies of these on-site saliva kits show their usefulness for the intended purpose. With the QED device, there was a high correlation between and SAC and near simultaneous measurements of venous blood and breath-alcohol concentrations (Jones, 1995; Bates and Martin, 1997). This on-the-spot test for alcohol has found applications in clinical settings such as for monitoring those attending outpatient clinics or emergency medicine departments for alcohol influence (Bendtsen et al., 1999; Biwasaka et al., 2001). Saliva-alcohol testing devices have also been approved for use in the workplace including pre-employment, post-accident and probable-cause situations (Dubowski, 2002).

Saliva specimens are being increasingly used for therapeutic drug monitoring and for many substances good correlations have been found with the levels in plasma (Drobitch and Svensson, 1992; Malamund and Tobak, 1993). The main advantage of saliva is that it can be obtained by noninvasive

methods and has become the preferred specimen for drugs-of-abuse testing at the roadside in impaired drivers (Schramm et al., 1992; Cone, 1993). A disadvantage of saliva is that drugs that are highly bound to plasma proteins (e.g., benzodiazepines) will not pass over into the saliva in sufficient amounts to allow a reliable analysis by conventional methods (Haeckel and Hänecke, 1993; Lentner, 1981).

D. Urine

Urine was the first body fluid used in clinical and forensic science for determination of ethanol probably because it was available in sufficient quantities and without invasion of the body. Ethanol diffuses from the renal artery blood into the glomerular filtrate and the concentration in the primary urine should be the same as that in the water fraction of the arterial blood entering the kidney (Iffland and Jones, 2002). However, the concentration of ethanol in bladder urine depends on many factors including the time after drinking when the bladder was emptied. Any residual alcohol-free urine present before the person started to drink the alcohol tends to dilute the concentration in the freshly produced urine (Jones, 2002). The production rate of urine (diuresis) changes during the time alcohol is being absorbed, distributed and eliminated from the body and the higher the BAC at peak diuresis the higher is the voided UAC. The problem posed by renal failure or use of medication that alters urine flow rate or retention are other confounding factors that have not yet been investigated in controlled studies.

1. Diuresis and ethanol concentration in urine

Figure 3.15 is from a seminal article by Widmark (1914), dealing with the analysis of ethanol in urine and the influence of drinking water on UAC and diuresis. After drinking the alcohol, the rate of urine production increased as shown by the vertical bars, although by ninety minutes post-dosing this increased flow of urine had subsided. After drinking 500 milliliters of water, the production of urine increased again for about forty-five minutes and thereafter returning to a normal rate of 1–2 milliliters per minute. The total amount of ethanol excreted, which is given by the product of volume and concentration, is higher after drinking the water but the concentration of ethanol is unchanged, as shown by the steady decline in UAC despite the increased urinary flow rate. Ethanol enters the ureter urine by passive diffusion from the arterial blood water and the concentration difference determines the UAC. To dilute the concentration of ethanol in urine by drinking water would require diluting the blood-ethanol concentration and this is not feasible under normal conditions of hydration. These early results reported by Widmark were verified in a recent paper by Bendtsen and Jones (1999), who also measured creatinine and osmolality of urine as biochemical markers for highly dilute specimens. Both dilution markers decreased precipitously after drinking ethanol and after drinking 500 milliliters water, but the concentration of ethanol in the successive urine samples collected in the post-absorptive phase were as expected.

A high concentration of ethanol in a person's urine gives evidence to support any clinical signs and symptoms of drunkenness and, indeed, the first drunk-driving laws relied on urine tests to prove under the influence of alcohol. Collecting urine specimens for forensic analysis of ethanol needs to be carefully supervised to avoid any tampering with or attempts at adulterating the specimens (e.g., by dilution with water or other liquids). The first applications of UAC for legal purposes were intended to provide an indirect way to estimate BAC using a population average UAC/BAC ratio of 1.3:1 (Walls and Brownlie, 1985). It is also important that the bottles or tubes used to hold the urine contain a preservative such as 1–2 percent NaF, which will prevent any sugars present being converted to ethanol in-vitro after sampling by fermentation. Urine from diabetics might be loaded with glucose and infections in the urinary tract with *Candida albicans* (yeast) generates ethanol after allowing the specimens to stand at room temperature for at least twenty-four hours (Jones et al., 2000).

A recommended sampling strategy is to obtain two successive voids from DUI suspects about thirty to sixty minutes apart. The aim of the first void is to empty the bladder of old urine produced during an unknown time when the BAC might have changed appreciably (Cooper et al., 1979; Walls and Brownlie, 1985). The concentration of ethanol in the second void provides the important information about the BAC during the sampling interval of about thirty to sixty minutes since the bladder was last emptied. Dividing UAC in the second void by 1.3 gives a good estimate of the BAC at the midpoint of the sampling interval (Cooper et al., 1979). However, the UAC/BAC ratio varies widely both between individuals and also within individuals depending on the stage of ethanol metabolism, the specific gravity of urine and the completeness of emptying the bladder from residual urine.

2. Ratios of ethanol concentration in urine and blood

The UAC/BAC ratios in both first and second voids were recently evaluated for a large number of drinking drivers. An initial void was made soon after arrest before a specimen of venous blood was drawn and this was followed by a second void (Jones, 2002; Jones, 2003). The resulting UAC/BAC ratios for each void are shown in Table 3.10 where it can be seen that the first void is higher than the second void as expected for post-absorptive specimens. The

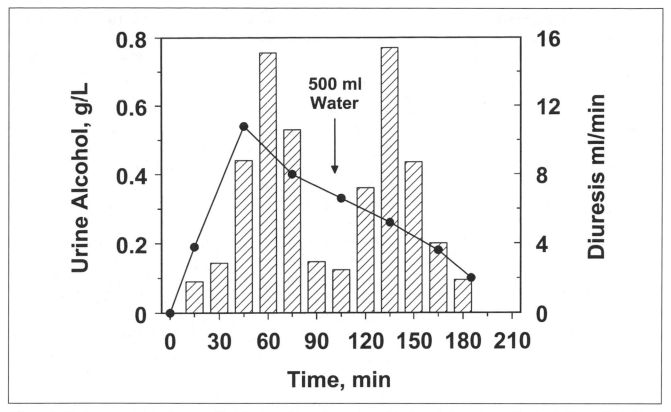

Figure 3.15 *Concentration-time profile of ethanol in urine, ethanol-induced diuresis and lack of effect of drinking water on the concentration of ethanol in successive urine voids (redrawn from Widmark, 1914)*

UAC/BAC ratios are also shown after adjusting sampling of blood and urine to the same time by assuming that all individuals are in the post-absorptive state and are eliminating alcohol at a constant rate of 0.20 g/L/h (Jones and Andersson, 1996a). The time-corrected UAC/BAC values agreed well with a ratio of 1.3:1 and the close agreement between the two voids suggests that even the first random specimen represents fairly fresh urine for this population of drinkers (Jones, 2003).

Urine is voided in batches and during the storage interval in the bladder the BAC might have changed appreciably depending on how much time has elapsed after the drinking ended (Walls and Brownlie, 1985). For a rising BAC curve, some of the urine collected in the bladder was produced at a lower BAC than existed when the urine was actually voided (Biasotti and Valentine, 1985). This leads to an abnormally low UAC/BAC ratio and this is made even lower if there was an alcohol-free pool of urine

Table 3.10
Urine/Blood Ratios of Ethanol in First and Second Voids from Drunk Drivers before and after Adjusting for the Time Differences between Sampling Blood and Urine
(Jones, 2002; Jones, 2003)

Urine sample	Mean (SD) UAC/BAC	95% range	Mean (SD) UAC/BAC[1]	95% range
First void	1.34 (0.192)	0.94– 1.79	1.30 (0.122)	1.11– 1.60
Second void	1.22 (0.119)	0.99– 1.46	1.32 (0.131)	1.10– 1.67

[1] Values adjusted for metabolism of ethanol from blood at a rate of 0.20 g/L/h, between the times of sampling blood and urine.

in the bladder before drinking began. In the post-absorptive phase when the BAC is decreasing at a constant rate of about ~0.15 g/L/h the UAC reflects the BAC existing some time earlier since the previous void. The UAC/BAC ratios might be higher than expected if the bladder had not been emptied for several hours in the post-absorptive period (Biasotti and Valentine, 1985).

As an example of urine retention, consider a person who drinks alcohol during an evening, voids the bladder before bedtime with a BAC of 1.0 g/L. If the person remains in bed for ten hours, the UAC in the first morning void will reflect the BAC prevailing during the night, whereas the BAC in the morning is probably zero owing to complete metabolism of the ethanol during the night. This should not cause any major problem in practice because the first thing people do in the morning is to visit the bathroom, especially if they have been drinking the night before. Accordingly, the UAC/BAC ratio furnishes useful information about the position of the BAC curve when the samples were taken and also the BAC during the collecting interval (UAC/1.3). If the

person was in the absorption phase with the BAC rising, this calculation UAC/1.3 would underestimate the persons BAC because the actual UAC/BAC ratio is less than or close to unit shortly after drinking.

3. Ethanol concentration-time profiles in blood and urine

Figure 3.16 shows mean concentration-time curves of ethanol in blood and urine in thirty subjects who drank 0.68 g/kg ethanol on an empty stomach (Jones, 1990). The bladder was emptied before drinking started so an alcohol-free pool of urine did not exist. The UAC is less than the BAC during the absorption phase, it then crossed the BAC curve and continued to rise above BAC to reach a higher C_{max} and a later t_{max}. After the end of drinking in the post-peak phase the UAC is always above the BAC until all alcohol has been cleared from the bloodstream (Jones, 1992a). The curves also show that obtaining two consecutive urine samples about one hour apart can be used to check when the person last consumed alcohol. If the UAC-1 < UAC-2 this makes it likely that BAC was still rising and the person had prob-

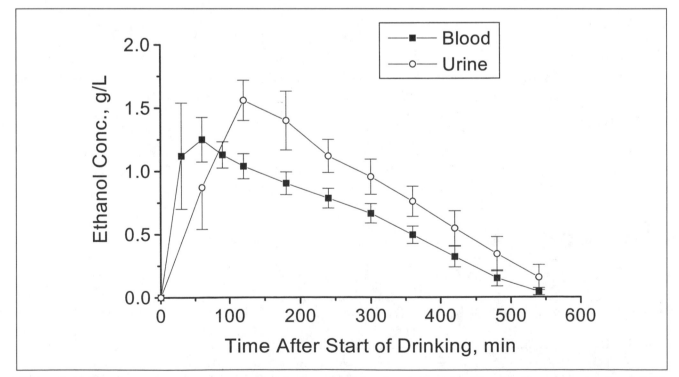

Figure 3.16 Mean concentration-time profile of ethanol in blood and urine for thirty healthy men who drank 0.68 gram of ethanol per kilogram of body weight as neat whisky on an empty stomach. Note that the bladder was emptied before drinking started (Jones, 1992a)

ably just finished drinking. When UAC-1 = UAC-2, the peak BAC was probably just passed and a longer time of one to two hours probably elapsed after the end of drinking. Finally, if UAC-1 > UAC-2 the person with high probability was already in the post-absorptive phase when urine was voided and about two hours or more must have elapsed after the last drink (Jones, 1990; Jones, 2002; Iffland, 1999).

E. Cerebrospinal fluid

1. General

The brain and the spinal cord are surrounded by a watery fluid, which is known as the cerebrospinal fluid (CSF), which fills the ventricles within the brain. CSF is a clear watery fluid (> 99 percent water) secreted by various central nervous system structures and equilibrates between blood and adjacent brain tissue. The biochemical profile of CSF reflects to some extent the chemical reactions taking place within the brain and this has diagnostic potential as an indirect way to monitor brain chemistry in various neurological and psychiatric disorders (Guyton, 1986). The CSF is generally collected from the subarachnoid space (lumbar CSF) and less frequently from the cisterna magna (cisterna CSF). The volume of CSF in adults is about 135 mL and of this 35 mL is found in the ventricles, 25 mL in the subarachnoid space and cisterna and 75 mL in the spinal canal. Because CSF is mostly water and its relative density is very close to 1.0 the ratio of concentrations of ethanol in CSF and whole blood should be 1.2:1 as expected from water-content differences.

In postmortem toxicology CSF is sometimes used for the analysis of ethanol and other drugs but finds most use in clinical medicine, for example whenever patients suffer from skull trauma and bleeding in the brain is suspected. The CSF contains enzymes, proteins and a host of other endogenous substances some of which are useful for clinical diagnosis of various neurological conditions. The CSF has also found applications in neurology for analysis of hemoglobin, lactate, and proteins (e.g., albumin), neuropeptides, as well as catecholamines such as dopamine, norepinephrine, and serotonin.

Alcohol and other drugs that cross the blood-brain-barrier will enter CSF and a few early studies took serial samples of blood and CSF by lumbar puncture from patients who had consumed alcohol. This allowed monitoring the rate of uptake and elimination of ethanol in lumbar CSF samples and the concentration-time course could be compared with blood-ethanol profiles. Although ethanol reaches the brain almost immediately after it is absorbed into the blood, like urine the CSF is produced gradually over a period of time. The concentrations of ethanol appearing in blood and CSF are displaced in time depending on the rates of absorption, distribution and elimination of alcohol in the body. Moreover, an alcohol-free pool of CSF before the person starts to drink will dilute the ethanol content of freshly produced CSF. The combined influences of the time-lag and the dilution means that the concentration-time course of ethanol in CSF and BAC is comparable to that of bladder urine and BAC when voids are collected sequentially over a period of time.

2. Concentration-time profiles

Figure 3.17 compares blood-ethanol with lumbar CSF ethanol in two subjects from an article by Abramson and Linde (1932), who investigated the concentration-time profiles of ethanol in these body fluids. The specimens were lumbar CSF, which were taken at regular intervals after the volunteers had consumed a moderate dose of alcohol. The traces for CSF show a pronounced time lag, which reflects in part the water content difference for CSF (99 percent) and whole blood (80 percent) and also the longer time required for the alcohol to enter the brain and reach the lumbar region. If cisterna CSF had been sampled as is done in autopsy work, this would have shown a higher concentration and earlier occurring C_{max} and less of a time lag (Cooper et al., 1979).

F. Other fluids and tissues

Forensic toxicologists are interested in the analysis of ethanol and other drugs of abuse in a wide variety of biological fluids and matrices (e.g., saliva, tears, hair, sweat, nails and cerebrospinal fluid), in addition to the conventional specimens of blood and urine (see Inoue and Seta, 1992; Pichini et al., 1996 for reviews). There are applications for these alternative specimens in therapeutic drug monitoring, post-

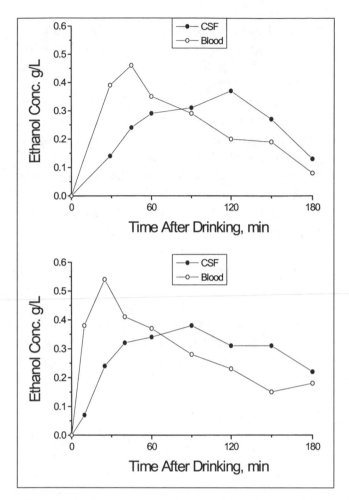

Figure 3.17 Concentration-time profiles of ethanol in blood and cerebrospinal lumbar fluid from experiments in two volunteer subjects (redrawn from Abramson and Linde, 1930)

mortem toxicology, workplace drug testing, and in sports medicine (Rivier, 2000; Cone, 2001).

1. Tears

All body fluids and tissues containing water will take up alcohol. A rather unusual body fluid seldom used for determination of ethanol is tear fluid (Lund, 1984). In one study, the concentrations of ethanol in blood and tears were highly correlated over the absorption, distribution and elimination stages of metabolism. The experiment involved twelve healthy subjects who drank 75 grams of ethanol with food before serial samples of venous blood and tear fluid were taken for analysis of ethanol enzymatically by the ADH method. Several methods were used to enhance the production of tears including direct irrita-

tion of the mucous membranes of the eye with cigarette smoke or chemical irritation of the nose with ammonia vapor or by tickling the nostril with a horse hair. At the appearance of tears in the eyes, the fluid was collected in capillary tubes ready for analysis. The distribution ratio of ethanol between tear fluid and blood was 1.14:1 (SD 0.037) with a range from 1.08 to 1.20. These results were in good agreement with values expected for the difference in water content of tears (100 percent) and whole blood (80 percent) (Lentner, 1981).

2. Sweat

When the skin heats up because of stress, exercise or temperature change, sweat is formed in eccrine glands and its composition is mainly water. Eccrine glands produce sweat to cool the body and if there is ethanol in the blood some will cross the sweat gland epithelium by passive diffusion from the blood supply to the gland. The concentration relationship between ethanol in blood and sweat was first investigated as early as 1936 in a study when healthy men were exposed to steam in a hot-room (Nyman and Palmlöv, 1936). The ethanol concentration in sweat was only 81 percent of the blood-ethanol concentration, and the authors warned about losses of ethanol during the collection of sweat for analysis. More recently using a special device for collecting sweat to avoid losses by evaporation, Buono (1999) found a high correlation between sweat-ethanol and blood-ethanol and the sweat contained about 20 percent more ethanol than an equal volume of whole blood. This difference was explained by the more water in sweat compared with that in whole blood and the recommendation was made that ethanol concentrations should be expressed in terms of the water content of the materials analyzed (e.g., milligrams ethanol per liter water).

Use of sweat as a body fluid for analysis of ethanol has received attention in connection with treatment of alcoholics as a way to verify that they don't drink alcohol (Phillips and McAloon, 1980; Phillips, 1984). A tamper-proof sweat-patch was designed to collect and retain any alcohol that might diffuse through the skin. By periodically removing the patch and analyzing any ethanol it might contain gives evidence to verify or challenge claims of abstinence

(Phillips and McAloon, 1980). Some studies showed the feasibility of monitoring absorption, distribution and elimination stages of ethanol metabolism by serial sampling of sweat using a wearable sensor designed for transdermal diffusion of alcohol (Swift, 2000; Swift et al., 1992). The pharmacokinetics of ethanol were investigated in perspiration although the sampling procedures were not easy to control (Brown, 1985).

3. Mother's milk

Alcohol passes over into the mother's milk and some concern has arisen whether or not infants are being dangerously exposed to ethanol if the mother had been drinking before feeding (Mennela and Beauchamp, 1991). However, experiments have shown that the concentration of ethanol in the milk of lactating women is very close to the concentration in the blood (Olow, 1923). Assuming a baby drinks 300 mL of milk in one feed and if this milk contains one g/L ethanol, this corresponds to an intake of only 0.3 gram ethanol (Jones, 1992b). If this amount of alcohol is distributed into total body water of a 5-kilogram infant with an ethanol distribution volume of 0.85 L/kg, a simple Widmark calculation gives a theoretical BAC of 0.07 g/L. Studies with human fetal livers obtained in connection with legal abortions and from children and adults undergoing abdominal surgery showed the presence of alcohol dehydrogenase activity in all specimens. ADH activity was detectable in two-month-old fetuses, albeit lower than in children and adults, so even at birth babies are capably of metabolizing ethanol (Pikkarainen and Räihä, 1974).

4. Brain and body organs

Knowledge about the concentrations of ethanol in various body organs and tissues has been derived from medical examiner cases and animal studies. The available evidence seems to suggest that the concentrations of ethanol in body tissues bear a close relationship to values expected from the water content of these specimens (Garriott, 1991). However, after death some body organs (e.g., kidney and liver) might retain metabolic activity as the body cools and the concentration of ethanol can decrease by up to 10 percent owing to oxidative metabolism

(Jenkins et al., 1995). The rate of uptake of ethanol depends on blood flow to the various organs and tissue so skeletal muscles take a longer time than brain and kidney to equilibrate with the alcohol in arterial blood. Ethanol is not evenly distributed within the brain and gray matter seems to contain a slightly higher concentration compared with white matter, probably because of regional differences in water content and vascularity (Budd, 1983). The question of distribution of ethanol within different regions of the brain and the best choice of specimen for forensic analysis of ethanol was discussed by Moore et al. (1997).

Some recent studies have monitored the penetration of ethanol into human brain tissue noninvasively by use of spectroscopic and magnetic resonance methods (Fein and Meyerhoff, 2000; Hetherington et al., 1999). Use of a homogenate of whole brain tissue might be the best approach to determine the average concentrations of ethanol present.

5. Vitreous humor

In postmortem toxicology vitreous humor (VH) fluid from the eye is a useful specimen for determination of ethanol. Moreover, the required specimen can be obtained with syringe and needle without the need to perform a complete autopsy (Jones, 2000b). VH is primarily composed of water and the concentration of ethanol in this fluid will therefore be higher than in the whole blood by a factor of approximately 1.2:1. Indeed a mean VH/blood ratio of 1.19:1 with standard deviation 0.285 and a 95 percent range from 0.63 to 1.75 was reported in a recent study by Jones and Holmgren (2001) based on 706 forensic autopsies. The average and range of values agreed well with those reported by other investigators such as Pounder and Kuroda (1994). Although BAC and VH were highly correlated ($r = 0.97$) the large scatter of the data points around the regression line means that there is a large uncertainty if VH is used to estimate BAC in any individual case (Jones and Holmgren, 2001; Pounder and Kuroda, 1994).

The time-lag between ethanol entering the bloodstream and passing into the fluids of the eye is relatively short owing to the rich blood supply to the central nervous system and visual centers. The advantage of VH over other body fluids as specimen for alcohol analysis is that the eyeball is well protected and far removed from the gut, which minimizes the risk of contamination with bacteria that might spread from the gut during autolysis after death (O'Neal and Poklis, 1996). The concentration of ethanol in VH is a useful way to verify the blood-ethanol concentrations whenever postmortem synthesis of ethanol is likely (e.g., in decomposed bodies) (Jones, 2000b). Finding a close agreement between the concentrations of ethanol measured in VH and blood gives confidence to the autopsy toxicology results and speaks against any postmortem synthesis of ethanol by putrefaction processes. VH should always be the specimen of choice for analysis of alcohol when the body has undergone extensive trauma (e.g., in explosions and casualties on the road or air crashes) (Jones, 2000b).

3.18 Concluding Remarks

The basic principles governing absorption, distribution and elimination of ethanol in the human body were established more than seventy years ago (Widmark, 1932; Kalant, 1991). The major conclusions drawn then still remain true today, namely that ethanol distributes into the total body water, that the bulk of the dose ingested (95 percent) is metabolized by enzymes in the liver and that only a small fraction (5 percent) is excreted unchanged in breath, urine and sweat (Wallgren, 1970). The availability of more sensitive and specific methods for determination of ethanol in blood and other body fluids has allowed investigators to refine and enlarge upon many of the fundamental concepts. Research on the disposition and fate of ethanol in the body continues unabated and articles regularly appear in both forensic and biomedical journals.

The blood-alcohol concentration (BAC) reached after drinking alcoholic beverages gives important information about the quantity of ethanol a person has consumed and the degree of influence on performance and behavior (Kalant, 1996a; Jones, 2000c; Wagner et al., 1990). This kind of information obviously has importance in clinical and forensic medicine. The threshold limits of alcohol in blood for driving are 0.08 g%, 0.10 g% or 0.02 g% for novice drivers. However, setting these limits depends more on political forces rather than scientific issues. For

example, in European countries the alcohol and traffic politics are different and 0.05 g% (France, Germany, Spain) and 0.02 g% (Norway, Sweden) are the corresponding threshold values, although a few countries like UK and Ireland still enforce a BAC of 0.08 g% (Jones, 1996b; Jones, 2000c).

The person's BAC can be translated into the amount of alcohol in the body at the time of sampling the blood and if the time of starting to drink is known the total quantity of alcohol consumed can be calculated. These calculations are feasible because unlike other drugs, ethanol mixes with the total body water and does not appear to bind to plasma proteins or other endogenous structures (Kalant, 1996b; Jones, 1996a; Jones et al., 1992). Furthermore, during most of the concentration-time profile, the metabolism of ethanol occurs at a constant rate per unit time (zero-order kinetics) and not at a rate proportional to the prevailing BAC (first-order kinetics), which applies to most other drugs and xenobiotics (Rowland and Tozer, 1980; Gabrielsson and Weiner, 2000).

Ethanol is a central nervous system depressant drug and a quantitative relationship exists between the amount consumed and the BAC reached (Kalant et al., 1971). The degree of alcohol influence on the individual is also a function of BAC although the relationship is complicated by development of acute and chronic tolerance after drinking ethanol (Kalant, 1996a). This means that the clinical signs and symptoms of drunkenness are not always closely correlated with BAC, particularly during the post-absorptive period, a time when the acute impairment effects have subsided (Alha, 1951). The degree of impairment of body functions after drinking alcohol depends on many factors including the person's age, body weight, sex, amount of alcohol consumed, type of beverage and speed of drinking (Alha, 1951). Other important factors are whether alcohol was consumed on an empty stomach or after eating a meal and also the blood sampling site, whether an artery or vein, and the water content of the biological specimen analyzed, whether blood, urine, saliva or breath (Chiou, 1989). Impairment of psychomotor performance and altered behavior are more pronounced on the ascending limb of the concentration-time profile compared with the descending portion of the curve, a phenomenon known as acute tolerance (Alha, 1951; Kalant, 1996a). Many people can seemingly adapt to psychomotor impairment caused by the drug a few hours after reaching the peak BAC provided that no more alcohol is imbibed (Martin and Moss, 1993; Martin and Earleywine, 1990). Although the most obvious acute signs and symptoms of alcohol's effects might have disappeared, this does not make a person a safe driver, especially in critical situations.

Most of the information available about the disposition and fate of ethanol in the body comes from bolus dose drinking studies, which usually entail giving moderate amounts of ethanol (< 1.0 g/kg) after an overnight fast (Wilkinson et al., 1977b). The BACs reached rarely surpass 1.0 g/L to avoid the nausea and other ill effects associated with rapid absorption of ethanol into the blood, which might trigger a vomit reflex. Most controlled drinking experiments reported in the literature are therefore far removed from real-world drinking patterns, which often extend over several hours and includes drinking different beverages (beer, wine, spirits). More studies are needed along the lines described by Kalant et al. (1975) and more recently Ganert and Bowthorpe (2000) and Zink and Reinhardt (1984).

Widmark's equations and other issues important for forensic pharmacokinetics of ethanol deserve to be reanalyzed with larger numbers of subjects and if possible gathering data from use of breath-alcohol instruments (Friel et al., 1995b; Jones and Andersson, 2003). The uncertainty inherent in making theoretical calculations of BAC and the magnitude of first-pass metabolism of ethanol needs to be established under real-world drinking conditions (Baraona et al., 2001). Questions such as the time required to reach the peak BAC (t_{max}) after the end of drinking as well as how much the BAC increased after the last drink needs to be answered by reference to articles appearing in peer-reviewed journals (Gullberg, 1982; Winek et al., 1996). Requests to back extrapolate BAC from time of sampling to time of driving are common in DUI litigation although this is a dubious practice with many variables to consider (Lewis, 1986a; Stowell and Stowell, 1998; Al-Lanqawi et al., 1992). The scientific foundations for making BAC projections are not always well founded and many assumptions are necessary. The main problem is the highly variable absorption of ethanol after the last drink and difficulties in knowing when the maximum BAC was reached (Iffland and Jones, 2002). The situation is not much improved if various kinds of computer software are used to make the BAC calculations and retrograde extrapolations (Rockerbie and Rockerbie, 1995). In many drinking situations the BAC determined at the time of sampling is quite different from the peak BAC, which depends on various time elements and patterns of drinking and estimating t_{max} requires various assumptions and probability theory (Lewis, 1986a; Montgomery and Reasor, 1992; Jackson et al., 1991).

The analysis of ethanol for legal purposes, especially in connection with DUI investigations, is increasingly done with the aid of evidential breath-alcohol instruments (Emerson et al., 1980; Gullberg, 2000). Our current knowledge of the pharmacokinetic parameters of ethanol including values of β and *rho* is based on blood-concentration time profiles of ethanol (Friel et al., 1995b; Jones and Andersson, 2003). It is not satisfactory to convert BrAC to BAC and then plug the numbers into the Widmark equation. Instead, kinetic parameters of ethanol need to be derived from the breath-alcohol profiles.

Calculating β-slopes after drinking small doses of alcohol leading to a relatively low C_{max} and also taking just a few measurements of BAC or BrAC without mapping the entire concentration-time profile is not satisfactory. Such a practice can probably explain some of the bizarre values for alcohol burn-off rate reported in the literature (Winek and Murphy, 1984).

More efforts are needed to investigate the absorption, distribution and elimination of ethanol in various disease states (liver dysfunction, diabetes, hyperthyrosis or other metabolic disturbances) and then compare the values with normal healthy volunteers. One might wonder whether it can be justified to apply knowledge gathered from bolus dose drinking experiments with healthy young student volunteers (mainly men) or physically fit policemen to draw conclusions about disposition and fate of alcohol in the body of the average drinking driver.

References

Abramson, L. and Linde, P. Zum Übergang des Äthyl-lalkohols in die Spinalflüssigkeit beim menschen. *Arch. Intern. Pharmacodynam. Therap.* 39:325–333, 1930.

Alha, A. Blood alcohol and clinical inebriation in Finnish men: A medicolegal study. *Annals Acad. Sci. Fenn. Series A; V Medico-Anthropologica* 26: 1951 pp 1–54.

Al–Lanqawi, Y. et al. Ethanol kinetics: Extent of error in back extrapolation procedures. *Br. J. Clin. Pharmacol.* 34:316–321,1992.

Amir, I. et al. Ranitidine increases the bioavailability of imbibed alcohol by accelerating gastric emptying. *Life Sci.* 58:511–518, 1996.

Ammon, E. et al. Disposition and first-pass metabolism of ethanol in humans: Is it gastric or hepatic and does it depend on gender? *Clin. Pharmacol. Ther.* 59:503–513, 1996.

Andersson, C., Andersson, T. and Molander, M. Ethanol absorption across human skin measured by in vivo microdialysis technique. *Acta. Derm. Venerol.* 71:389–393 1991.

Andréasson, R. and Jones. A.W. The life and work of Erik M.P. Widmark. *Am. J. Forensic. Med. Pathol.* 17:177–190, 1996.

Anstie, F.E. Final experiments on the elimination of alcohol from the body. *Practitioner* 13:15–28, 1874.

Arora, S., Baraona, E. and Lieber, C.S. Alcohol levels are increased in social drinkers receiving ranitidine. *Am. J. Gastroenterol.* 95:208–213, 2000.

Baraona, E. Site and quantitative importance of alcohol first-pass metabolism. *Alcohol. Clin. Exp. Res.* 24: 405–406, 2000.

Baraona, E. et al. Lack of alcohol dehydrogenase isoenzyme activity in the stomachs of Japanese subjects. *Life Sci.* 49:1929–1934, 1991.

Baraona, E., Gentry, R.T. and Lieber, C.S. Bioavailability of alcohol: Role of gastric metabolism and its interaction with other drugs. *Dig. Dis.* 12:351–367,1994.

Baraona, E., et al. Gender differences in pharmacokinetics of alcohol. *Alcohol. Clin. Exp. Res.* 25:502–507, 2001.

Barbour, A.D. Simplified estimation of Widmark "r" values by the method of Forrest. *Sci & Justice* 41:53–54, 2001.

Barceloux, D.G. et al. American academy of clinical toxicology practice guidelines on the treatment of methanol poisoning. *J. Toxicol. Clin. Tox.* 40:415–48, 2001.

Baselt, R.C. (ed.). *Principles and Applications of Medicolegal Alcohol Determinations.* (Translation of Widmark's 1932 monograph). Foster City, CA: Biomedical Publications, 1981.

Baselt, R.C. Disposition of alcohol in man. In: Garriott, J.C. (ed.), *Medicolegal Aspects of Alcohol*, 3rd ed. Tucson: Lawyers & Judges Publishing Company, 1996, pp 65–83.

Bates, M.E., Brick, J. and White, H.R. The correspondence between saliva and breath estimates of blood alcohol concentration: Advantages and limitations of the saliva method. *J. Stud. Alcohol* 54:17–22, 1993.

Bates, M.E. and Martin, C.S. Immediate, quantitative estimation of blood alcohol concentration from saliva. *J. Stud. Alcohol* 58:531–538, 1997.

Batt, R.D. Absorption, distribution and elimination of alcohol. In: Crow, K.E. and Batt, R,D, (eds.), *Human Metabolism of Alcohol*, Vol 1. *Pharmacokinetics, Medicolegal Aspects and General Interest.* Boca Raton: CRC Press, 1989, pp 3–8.

Bekka, R. et al. Treatment of methanol and isopropanol poisoning with intravenous fomepizole. *J. Toxicol. Clin. Tox.* 39:59–67, 2001.

Bendtsen, P. and Jones, A.W. Impact of water-induced diuresis on urine-ethanol profiles, urine-creatinine, and urine-osmolality. *J. Anal. Toxicol.* 23:565–569, 1999.

Bendtsen, P. et al. Monitoring ethanol exposure in a clinical setting by analysis of blood, breath, saliva and urine. *Alcohol. Clin. Exp. Res.* 23:1448–51, 1999.

Benet, L.Z., Mitchell, J.R. and Sheiner, L.B. Pharmacokinetics: The dynamics of drug absorption, distribution and elimination. In: Gilman, A.G. et al. (eds.), *Goodman & Gilman's The Pharmacological Basis of Therapeutics.* Pergamon Press, New York, 1990, pp 3–32.

Berggren, S.M. and Goldberg, L. The absorption of ethyl alcohol from the gastrointestinal tract as a diffusion process. *Acta. Physiol. Scand.* 1:246–270, 1940.

Biasotti, A.A. and Valentine, B.A. Blood alcohol concentration determined from urine samples as a practical equivalent or alternative to blood and breath alcoohl tests. *J. Forensic Sci.* 30:194–207, 1985.

Biwasaka, H. et al. Application of quantitative ethanol detector (QED) test kit to measure ethanol concentrations in blood samples. *Forensic Sci. Intern.* 124:124–129, 2001.

Bode, C. The metabolism of alcohol: Physiological and pathophysiological aspects. *J. Roy. Coll. Phys.* 12:122–135, 1978.

Bogusz, M., Pach, J. and Stasko, W. Comparative studies on the rate of ethanol elimination in acute poisoning and in controlled conditions. *J. Forensic Sci.* 22:446–451, 1977.

Borkan, G.A. and Norris, A.H. Fat redistribution and the changing body dimensions of the adult male. *Hum. Biol.* 49:495–513, 1977.

Bosron, W.F. et al. Effect of fasting on the activity and turnover of rat liver alcohol dehydrogenase. *Alcohol. Clin. Exp. Res.* 8:196–200, 1984.

Bosron, W.F., Ehrig, T. and Li, T.K. Genetic factors in alcohol metabolism and alcoholism. *Semin. Liver Dis.* 13:126–135, 1993.

Breen, M.H. et al. The effect of a "one for the road" drink of hard liquor, beer or wine on peak breath alcohol concentration in a social drinking environment with food consumption. *Med. Sci. Law* 38: 62–69, 1998.

Brent, J. et al. Fomepizole for the treatment of methanol poisoning. *N. Engl. J. Med.* 344:424–429, 2001.

Breslin, F.C. et al. Gender and alcohol dosing: A procedure for producing comparable breath alcohol curves for men and women. *Alcohol. Clin. Exp. Res.* 21:928–930, 1997.

Brick, J. et al. The effect of menstrual cycle on blood alcohol levels and behavior. *J. Stud. Alcohol* 47: 472–477, 1986.

Brown, D.J. The pharmacokinetics of alcohol excreted in human perspiration. *Methods Find. Clin. Pharmacol.* 7:539–544, 1985.

Budd, R.D. Post-mortem brain ethanol levels. *J. Chromatog.* 259:353–355, 1983.

Buono, M.J. Sweat ethanol concentrations are highly correlated with coexisting blood values in humans. *Exp. Physiol.* 84:401–404, 1999.

Bye, A. et al. Effect of ranitidine hydrochloride (150 mg twice daily) on the pharmacokinetics of increasing doses of ethanol (0.15, 0.3, 0.6 g/kg). *Br. J. Clin. Pharmacol.* 41:129–133, 1996.

Caballeria, J. et al. Effects of cimetidine on gastric alcohol dehydrogenase activity and blood ethanol levels. *Gastroenterology* 96:388–392, 1989a.

Caballeria, J. et al. Gastric origin of the first-pass metabolism of ethanol in humans: Effect of gastrectomy. *Gastroenterology* 97:1205–1209, 1989b.

Charlebois, R.C., Corbett, M.R. and Wigmore, J.G. Comparison of ethanol concentrations in blood, serum and blood cells for forensic applications. *J. Anal. Toxicol.* 20:171–178, 1996.

Chiou. W.L. The phenomenon and rationale of marked dependence of drug concentrations on blood sampling site: Implications in pharmacokinetics, pharmacodynamics, toxicology and therapeutics. *Clin. Pharmacokinet.* 17:175–199, 1989.

Clemmesen, J.O., Ott, P. and Sestoft, L. The effect of cimetidine on ethanol concentrations in fasting women and men after two different doses of alcohol. *Scand. J. Gastroenterol.* 32:217–220, 1997.

Cohen, H.M. and Green, J.B. *Apprehending and Prosecuting the Drunk Driver.* NY: Mathew Bender, 1995.

Cone, E.J. Saliva testing for drugs of abuse. *Ann. N. Y. Acad. Sci.* 694:91–127, 1993.

Cone, E.J. Legal, workplace and treatment drug testing with alternate biological matrices on a global scale. *Forensic Sci. Intern.* 121:7–15, 2001.

Cooke, A.R. The stimultaneous emptying and absorption of ethanol from the human stomach. *Am. J. Dig. Dis.* 15:449–454, 1970.

Cooke, A.R. and Birchall, A. Absorption of ethanol from the stomach. *Gastroenterology* 57:269–272, 1969.

Cooper, W.E., Schwär, T.G. and Smith, L.S. *Alcohol, Drugs and Traffic Safety.* Cape Town: Juta & Company Ltd., 1979.

Cortot, A. et al. Gastric emptying and gastrointestinal absorption of alcohol ingested with a meal. *Dig. Dis. Sci.* 31:343–348, 1986.

Cowan, J.M. et al. Determination of volume of distribution for ethanol in male and female subjects. *J. Anal. Toxicol.* 20:287–290, 1996.

Crabb, D.W. Ethanol oxidizing enzymes: Roles in alcohol metabolism and alcoholic liver disease. *Prog. Liver. Dis.* 13:151–172, 1995.

Crabb, D.W. First pass metabolism of ethanol: Gastric or hepatic, mountain or molehill? *Hepatology* 25: 1292–1294, 1997.

Crabb, D.W., Bosron, W.F. and Li, T.K. Ethanol metabolism. *Pharmacol. Ther.* 34:59–73, 1987.

Crabb, D.W. at al.. Genotypes for aldehyde dehydrogenase deficiency and alcohol sensitivity: The inactive ALDH2*2 allele is dominant. *J. Clin. Invest.* 83:314–316, 1989.

Crabb, D.W., Dipple, K.M. and Thomasson, H.R. Alcohol sensitivity, alcohol metabolism, risk of alcoholism, and the role of alcohol and aldehyde dehydrogenase genotypes. *J. Lab. Clin. Med.* 122:234–240, 1993.

Crownover, B.P. et al. Activation of alcohol metabolism in humans by fructose: Importance of experimental design. *J. Pharmacol. Exp. Ther.* 236:574–579, 1986.

Davidson, D., Camara, P. and Swift, R. Behavioral effects and pharmacokinetics of low-dose intravenous alcohol in humans. *Alcohol. Clin. Exp. Res.* 21:1294–1299, 1997.

Davies, B.T. and Bowen, C.K. Total body water and peak alcohol concentration: A comparative study of young, middle-age, and older females. *Alcohol. Clin. Exp. Res.* 23:969–975, 1999.

Dedrick, R.L. and Forrester, D.D. Blood flow limitations in interpreting Michaelis constants for ethanol oxidation in-vivo. *Biochem. Pharmacol.* 22: 1133–1140, 1973.

Derr, R.F. Simulation studies on ethanol metabolism in different human populations with a physiological pharmacokinetic model. *J. Pharm. Sci.* 82:677–682, 1993.

DiPadova, C. et al. Effects of ranitidine on blood alcohol levels after ethanol ingestion: Comparison with other H_2–receptor antagonists. *JAMA* 267: 83–86, 1992.

Drobitch, R.K. and Svensson, C.K. Therapeutic drug monitoring in saliva. *Clin. Pharmacokinet.* 23: 365–379, 1992.

Droenner, P. et al. A kinetic model describing the pharmacokinetics of ethyl glucuronide in humans. *Forensic Sci. Int.* 126:24–29 2002.

Dubowski, K.M. Absorption, distribution and elimination of alcohol: Highway safety aspects. *J Stud. Alcohol Suppl.* 10:98–108, 1985.

Dubowski, K.M. Analysis of ethanol in saliva. In: Jenkins, A.J. and Goldberger, B.A. (eds.), *On–Site Drug Testing.* Humana Press, 2002, pp 77–93.

Edelbroek, M.A. et al. Effects of erythromycin on gastric emptying, alcohol absorption and small intestinal transit in normal subjects. *J. Nucl. Med.* 34: 582–588, 1993.

Edelman, I.S. and Leibman, J. Anatomy of body water and electrolytes. *Am. J. Med.* 27:256–277, 1959.

Eder, A.F. et al. Ethylene glycol poisoning: Toxicokinetic and analytical factors affecting laboratory diagnosis. *Clin. Chem.* 44:168–177, 1998.

Emerson, V.J. et al. The measurement of breath alcohol: The laboratory evaluation of substantive breath test equipment and the report of an operational police trial. *J. Forensic Sci. Soc.* 20:3–70, 1980.

Endres HG, Grüner O. Comparison of D_2O and ethanol dilutions in total body water measurements in humans. *Clin. Investig.* 72: 830–837, 1994.

Enomoto, N. et al. Acetaldehyde metabolism in different aldehyde dehydrogenase-2 genotypes. *Alcohol. Clin. Exp. Res.* 15:141–144, 1991.

Eriksson, C.J.P. The role of acetaldehyde in the actions of alcohol (update 2000). *Alcohol. Clin. Exp. Res.* 25:15S–32S, 2001.

Erwin, R. *Defense of Drunk Driving Cases.* NY: Matthew Bender, 1991.

Evans, W.E. and McLeod, H.L. Pharmacogenomics: Drug disposition, drug targets, and side effects. *N. Engl. J. Med.* 348:538–549, 2003.

Fein, G. and Meyerhoff, D.J. Ethanol in human brain by magnetic resonance spectrometry: Correlation with blood and breath levels, relaxation, and magnetization transfer. *Alcohol. Clin. Exp. Res.* 24: 1227–1235, 2000.

Ferner, R.E. and Norman, E. *Forensic Pharmacology: Medicines, Mayhem, and Malpractice.* Oxford: Oxford University Press, 1996.

Fitzgerald, E.F. *Intoxication Test Evidence*, 2nd ed. St. Paul, MN: West Group (Clark Boardman Callaghan), 2001.

Flegal, K.M. et al. Prevalense and trends in obesity among U.S. adults, 1999–2000. *JAMA* 288:1723–1727, 2002.

Forrest, A.R.W. The estimation of Widmark's factor. *J. Forensic Sci. Soc.* 26:249–252, 1986.

Fraser, A.G. Pharmacokinetic interactions between alcohol and other drugs. *Clin. Pharmacokinet.* 33: 79–90, 1997.

Fraser, A.G. Is there an interaction between H_2-antagonists and alcohol? *Drug Metabol. Drug Interact.* 14:125–45, 1998.

Fraser, A.G at al. Ranitidine, cimetidine and famotidine have no effect on post-prandial absorption of ethanol 0.8 g/kg taken after an evening meal. *Aliment. Pharmacol. Ther.* 6:693–700, 1992.

Fraser, A.G. et al. Inter-individual and intra-individual variability of ethanol concentration-time profiles: Comparison of ethanol ingestion before or after an evening meal. *Br. J. Clin. Pharmacol.* 40:387–392, 1995.

Frezza, M. et al. High blood alcohol levels in women: The role of decreased gastric alcohol dehydrogenase activity and first-pass metabolism. *N. Engl. J. Med.* 322:95–99, 1990.

Friel, P.N., Baer, J.S. and Logan, B.K. Variability of ethanol absorption and breath concentrations during a large-scale alcohol administration study. *Alcohol Clin. Exp. Res.* 19:1055–1060, 1995a.

Friel, P.N., Logan, B.K. and Baer, J. An evaluation of the reliability of Widmark calculations based on breath alcohol measurements. *J. Forensic Sci.* 40: 91–94, 1995b.

Fuhr, U. Induction of drug metabolising enzymes: Pharmacokinetic and toxicological consequences in humans. *Clin. Pharmacokinet.* 38:493–504, 2000.

Gabe, A. Reappraisal of the Watson formulae for BAC calculation. *Sci. & Justice* 37:145–147, 1997.

Gabrielsson, J. and Weiner, D. *Pharmacokinetic and Pharmacidynamic Data Analysis: Concepts and*

Applications, 3rd ed. Stockholm: Swedish Pharmaceutical Press, 2000.

Ganert, P.M. and Bowthorpe, W.D. Evaluation of breath alcohol profiles following a period of social drinking. *Can. Soc. Forensic Sci. J.* 33:137–143, 2000.

Garriott, J.C. Skeletal muscle as an alternative specimen for alcohol and drug analysis. *J. Forensic Sci.* 36:60–69, 1991.

Garriott, J.C. (ed.). *Medicolegal Aspects of Alcohol*, 3rd ed. Lawyers & Judges Publishing Company, Tucson, 1996, pp 1–500.

Gentry, R.T. Effect of food on the pharmacokinetics of alcohol absorption. *Alcohol Clin. Exp. Res.* 24:403–404, 2000a.

Gentry, R.T. Determinants and analysis of blood alcohol concentrations after social drinking. *Alcohol Clin. Exp. Res.* 24:399, 2000b.

Gentry, R.T., Baraona, E. and Lieber, C.S. Agonist: Gastric first pass metabolism of alcohol. *J. Lab. Clin. Med.* 123:21–26, 1994.

Gentry, R.T. et al. Mechanism of the aspirin-induced rise in blood alcohol levels. *Life Sci.* 65:2505–2512, 1999.

Gerchow, J. and Steigleder, E. Zur Frage der Resorptionsgeschwindigkeit und der Rückrechnung bei kurzen Trinkzeiten. *Blutalkohol* 1:43–57, 1961.

Gibbons, D.O. and Lant, A.F. Effects of intravenous and oral propantheline and metoclopramide on ethanol absorption. *Clin. Pharmacol. Therap.* 17:578–584, 1975.

Gill, J. Women, alcohol and the menstrual cycle. *Alc. Alcohol.* 32:435–441, 1997.

Gill, K. et al. An examination of ALDH2 genotype, alcohol metabolism and the flushing response in native Americans. *J. Stud. Alcohol* 60:149–158, 1999.

Goldberg, L., Jones, A.W. and Neri, A. Effects of a sugar mixture on blood-ethanol profiles and on ethanol metabolism in man. *Blutalkohol* 16:421–438, 1979.

Goldstein, D.B. *Pharmacology of Alcohol*. Oxford University Press, Oxford, 1983.

Goldstein, D.B. and Zaechelein, R. Time course of functional tolerance produced in mice by inhalation of ethanol. *J. Pharmacol. Exp. Ther.* 227:150–153, 1983.

Gonzalez, F.J. et al. Microsomal ethanol oxidizing system: Transcriptional and posttranscriptional regulation of cytochrome P450, CYP2E1. *Alc. Alcohol. Suppl.* 1:97–101, 1991.

Goo, R.H. et al. Circadian variations in gastric emptying of meals in humans. *Gastroenterology* 93:15–18, 1987.

Graham, K. et al. Should alcohol consumption measures be adjusted for gender differences? *Addiction* 93:1137–1147, 1998.

Greenblatt, D.J. and Koch-Weser, J. Drug Therapy: Clinical pharmacokinetics, part 1. *N. Engl. J. Med.* 293:702–705, 1975a.

Greenblatt, D.J. and Koch-Weser, J. Drug Therapy: Clinical pharmacokinetics, part 2. *N. Engl. J. Med.* 293:964–970, 1975b.

Gubala, W. and Zuba, D. Comparison of ethanol concentrations in saliva and blood. *Can. Soc. Forensic. Sci. J.* 35:229–235, 2002.

Gullberg, R.G. Variability in blood alcohol concentrations following the last drink. *J. Police Sci. Admin.* 10:289–296, 1982.

Gullberg, R.G. Methodology and quality assurance in forensic breath alcohol analysis. *Forensic Sci. Rev.* 12:50–68, 2000.

Gullberg, R.G. and Jones, A.W. Guidelines for estimating the amount of alcohol consumed from a single measurement of blood alcohol concentration: Reevaluation of Widmark's equation. *Forensic Sci. Int.* 69:119–130, 1994.

Gupta, A.M., Baraona, E. and Lieber, C.S. Significant increase of blood alcohol by cimetidine after repetitive drinking of small alcohol doses. *Alcohol. Clin. Exp. Res.* 19:1083–1097, 1995.

Gustafson, R. and Källmen. H. The blood alcohol curve as a function of time and type of beverage: Methodological considerations. *Drug Alc. Depend.* 21:243–246, 1988.

Guyton, A.C. *Textbook of Medical Physiology*, 7th ed. Philadelphia: W.B. Saunders, 1986.

Haddad, L. et al. Effect of the menstrual cycle in ethanol pharmacokinetics. *J. Appl. Toxicol.* 18:15–18, 1998.

Haeckel, R. Factors influencing the saliva/plasma ratio of drugs. *Ann. N. Y. Acad. Sci.* 694:128–142, 1993.

Haeckel, R. and Bucklitsch, I. The comparability of ethanol concentrations in peripheral blood and saliva: The phenomenon of variation in saliva to blood concentration ratios. *J. Clin. Chem. Clin. Biochem.* 25:199–204, 1987.

Haeckel, R. and Peiffer, U. Comparison of ethanol concentrations in saliva and blood from police controlled persons. *Blutalkohol* 29:342–349, 1992.

Haeckel, R. and Hänecke, P. The application of saliva, sweat and tear fluid for diagnostic purposes. *Ann. Biol. Clin.* 50:903–010, 1993.

Hahn, R.G. et al. Expired breath ethanol measurements in chronic obstructive pulmonary disease: Implications for transurethral surgery. *Acta. Anaesth. Scand.* 35:393–397, 1991.

Hahn, R.G., Jones, A.W. and Norberg, Å. Abnormal blood-ethanol profile associated with stress. *Clin. Chem.* 38:1193–1194, 1992.

Hahn, R.G. et al. Eating a meal increases the clearance of ethanol given by intravenous infusion. *Alc. Alcohol.* 29:673–677, 1994.

Hahn, R.G., Norberg, Ä. and Jones, A.W. Rate of distribution of ethanol into the total body water. *Am. J. Ther.* 2:50–56, 1995.

Hahn, R.G., Norberg, Ä. and Jones, A.W. Overshoot of ethanol in the blood after drinking on an empty stomach. *Alc. Alcohol.* 32:501–505, 1997.

Hak, E.A. et al. Determination of serum alcohol:blood alcohol ratios. *Can. J. Forensic Sci.* 28:123–126, 1995.

Hanson, M. and Lilja, B. Gastric emptying in smokers. *Scand. J. Gastroenterol.* 22:1102–1104, 1987.

Harada, S. et al. Metabolic and ethnic determinants of alcohol drinking habits and vulnerability to alcohol-realted disorders. *Alcohol Clin. Exp. Res.* 25:71S–75S, 2001.

Heifer, U. Untersuchungen zur Rückrechnung der Blutalkoholkonzentration nach "normalem Trinkverlauf." *Blutalkohol* 13:305–313, 1976.

Hein, P.M. and Vock, R. Alkoholtrinkversuche mit über 60 Jahre alten männlichen Personen. *Blutalkohol* 26:98–105, 1989.

Hetherington, H.P. et al. Spectorscopic imaging of the uptake kinetics of human brain ethanol. *Magn. Reson. Med.* 42:1019–1026, 1999.

Higuchi, S. et al. Alcohol and aldehyde dehydrogenase polymorphisms and the risk for alcoholism. *Am. J. Psychiatry* 152:1219–1221, 1995.

Hittle, J.B. and Crabb, D.W. The molecular biology of alcohol dehydrogenase: Implications for the control of alcohol metabolism. *J. Lab. Clin. Med.* 112:7–15, 1988.

Hlastala, M.P. The alcohol breath test: A review. *J. Appl. Physiol.* 84:401–408, 1998.

Holford, N.H.G. Clinical pharmacokinetics of ethanol. *Clin. Pharmacokinet.* 13:273–292, 1987.

Holford, N.H.G. Complex PK/PD models: An alcoholic experience. *Int. J. Clin. Pharm. Therap.* 35:465 468, 1997.

Holt, S. Observations on the relation between alcohol absorption and the rate of gastric emptying. *CMAJ* 124:267–277, 1981.

Holt, S. et al. Alcohol, absorption, gastric emptying and a Breathalyzer. *Br. J. Clin. Pharmacol.* 9:205–208, 1982.

Horowitz, M. et al. Relationships between gastric emptying of solid and caloric liquid meals and alcohol absorption. *Am. J. Physiol.* 257:G291–298, 1989.

Host, U. et al. Haemodynamic effect of eating: The role of meal composition. *Clin. Sci.* 90:269–276, 1996.

Hoyumpa, A.M. and Schenker, S. Major drug interactions: Effect of liver disease, alcohol and malnutrition. *Ann Rev. Med.* 33:113–149, 1982.

Hume, D.N. and Fitzgerald, E.F. Chemical tests for intoxication: What do the numbers really mean? *Anal. Chem.* 57: 876A–882A 1985.

Iffland, R. Nachtrunk und Harnprobe. *Blutalkohol* 36: 99–105, 1999.

Iffland, R. and Jones, A.W. Evaluating alleged drinking after driving: The hip-flask defence, part 1: Double blood samples and urine-to-blood alcohol relationship. *Med. Sci. Law* 42:207–224, 2002.

Iffland, R. and Jones, A.W. Evaluating alleged drinking after driving: The hip-flask defence, part 2: Congener analysis. *Med. Sci. Law* 43:39–68, 2003.

Iffland, R. et al. Zur Zuverlässigkeit der Blutalkoholbestimmung Das Verteilungsverhältnis des Wassers zwischen Serum und Vollblut. *Rechtsmedizin* 9:123–130, 1999.

Iimuro, Y. et al. Glycine prevents alcohol-induced liver injury by decreasing alcohol in the rat stomach. *Gastroenterology* 110:1536–1542, 1996.

Inoue, T. and Seta, S. Analysis of drugs in unconventional samples. *Forensic Sci. Rev.* 4:89–107, 1992.

Jackson, P.R., Tucker, G.T. and Woods, H.F. Backtracking booze with Bayes: The retrospective interpretation of blood alcohol data. *Br. J. Clin. Pharmacol.* 31:55–63, 1991.

Jenkins, A.J., Levine, B.S. and Smialek, J.E. Distribution of ethanol in postmortem liver. *J. Forensic Sci.* 40:611–613, 1995.

Johnson, R.D. et al.. Cigarette smoking and rate of gastric emptying: Effect on alcohol absorption. *Br. Med. J.* 302:20–23, 1991.

Jokipii, S.G. Experimental studies on blood alcohol in healthy subjects and in some diseases. Thesis, University of Helsinki, 1951, pp 1–99.

Jonderko, K. et al. Gastric emptying and hyperthyroidism. *Am. J. Gastroenterol.* 92:835–838, 1997.

Jones, A.W. Inter- and intra-individual variations in the saliva/blood alcohol ratio during ethanol metabolism in man. *Clin. Chem.* 25:1394–1398, 1979.

Jones, A.W. How breathing technique can influence the results of breath-alcohol analysis. *Med. Sci. Law* 22:275–280, 1982.

Jones, A.W. Inter-individual variations in disposition and metabolism of ethanol in healthy men. *Alcohol* 1:385–391, 1984.

Jones, A.W. Physiological aspects of breath–alcohol measurement. *Alc. Drugs Driving*, 6:1–25, 1990.

Jones, A.W. Forensic science aspects of ethanol metabolism. In: Mahley, A. and Williams, R.L. (eds.), *Forensic Science Progress*, vol. 5. Berlin: Springer Verlag, 33–90, 1991a.

Jones, A.W. Top-ten defence challenges among drinking drivers in Sweden. *Med. Sci. Law* 31:229–238, 1991b.

Jones, A.W. Ethanol distribution ratios between urine and capillary blood in controlled experiments and in apprehended drinking drivers. *J. Forensic. Sci.* 37:21–34, 1992a.

Jones, A.W. Alcohol in mother's milk. *N. Engl. J. Med.* 326:766, 1992b.

Jones, A.W. Disappearance rate of ethanol from blood in human subjects: Implications in forensic toxicology. *J. Forensic Sci.* 38:104–118, 1993a.

Jones, A.W. Pharmacokinetics of ethanol in saliva: Comparison with blood and breath ethanol profiles, subjective feelings of intoxication and diminished performance. *Clin. Chem.* 39:1837–1844, 1993b.

Jones, A.W. Measuring ethanol in saliva with QED enzymatic test device: Comparison of results with blood and breath alcohol concentrations. *J. Anal. Toxicol.* 19:169–174, 1995.

Jones, A.W. Biochemistry and physiology of alcohol: Applications to forensic science and toxicology. In: Garriott, J.C. (ed.), *Medicolegal Aspects of Alcohol*, 3rd ed. Tucson: Lawyers & Judges Publishing Company, 1996a, pp 85–136.

Jones, A.W. Measuring alcohol in blood and breath for forensic purposes: A historical review. *Forensic Sci. Rev.* 8:13–44, 1996b.

Jones, A.W. Ethanol metabolism in patients with liver cirrhosis. *J. Clin. Forensic Med.* 7:48–51, 2000b.

Jones, A.W. Alcohol postmortem. In: Siegel, J.A., Saukko, P.J. and Knupfer. G.C. (eds.), *Encyclopedia of Forensic Sciences*. London: Academic Press, 112–126, 2000c.

Jones, A.W. Medicolegal alcohol determinations: Blood- or breath-alcohol concentration? *Forensic Sci. Rev.* 12:23–47, 2000d.

Jones, A.W. Reference limits for urine/blood ratios of ethanol concentration in two successive voids from drinking drivers. *J. Anal. Toxicol.* 26:333–339, 2002.

Jones, A.W. Time-adjusted urine/blood ratios of ethanol in drinking drivers. *J. Anal. Toxicol* 27:167–168, 2003.

Jones, A.W. and Neri, A. Age-related differences in blood-ethanol parameters and subjective feelings of intoxication in healthy men. *Alc. Alcohol.* 20:45–52, 1985.

Jones, A.W. and Neri, A. Evaluation of blood-alcohol profiles after consumption of alcohol together with a large meal. *Can. Soc. Forensic. Sci. J.* 24:165–173, 1991.

Jones, A.W. and Sternebring, B. Kinetics of ethanol and methanol in alcoholics during detoxication. *Alc. Alcohol.* 27:641–647, 1992.

Jones, A.W. and Jönsson, K-Å. Between-subject and within-subject variations in the pharmacokinetics of ethanol. *Brit. J. Clin. Pharmacol.* 37:427–431, 1994a.

Jones, A.W. and Jönsson, K-Å. Food-induced lowering of blood-ethanol profiles and increased rate of elimination immediately after a meal. *J. Forensic. Sci.* 39:1084–1093, 1994b.

Jones, A.W. and Andersson, L. Influence of age, gender, and blood-alcohol concentration on the disappearance rate of alcohol from blood in drinking drivers. *J. Forensic Sci.* 41:922–926, 1996a.

Jones, A.W. and Andersson, L. Variability of the blood/breath alcohol ratio in drinking drivers. *J. Forensic Sci.* 41:916–921, 1996b.

Jones, A.W. and Hahn, R.G. Pharmacokinetics of ethanol in patients with renal failure before and after hemodialysis. *Forensic Sci. Intern.* 90:175–183, 1997.

Jones, A.W. and Rajs, J. Appreciable blood ethanol concentration after washing abraised and lacerated skin with surgical spirits. *J. Anal. Toxicol.* 21:587–588, 1997.

Jones, A.W. and Holmgren, P. Uncertainty in estimating blood-alcohol concentration by analysis of vitreous humor. *J. Clin. Pathol.* 54:699–702, 2001.

Jones, A.W. and Holmgren, P. Comparison of blood-ethanol concentration in deaths attributed to acute alcohol poisoning and chronic alcoholism. *J. Forensic Sci.* 48:874–879, 2003.

Jones, A.W. and Andersson, L. Comparison of ethanol concentrations in venous blood and end-expired breath during a controlled drinking study. *Forensic Sci. Intern.* 132:18–25, 2003.

Jones, A.W., Jönsson, K-Å. and Jorfeldt, L. Differences between capillary and venous blood-alcohol concentrations as a function of time after drinking with emphasis on sampling variations in left vs right arms. *Clin. Chem.* 35:400–404, 1989.

Jones, A.W., Hahn, R.G. and Stalberg, H.P. Distribution of ethanol and water between plasma and whole blood: Inter- and intra-individual variations after administration of ethanol by intravenous infusion. *Scand. J. Clin. Lab. Invest.* 50:775–780, 1990.

Jones, A.W., Jönsson, K-Å. and Neri, A. Peak blood-alcohol concentration and time of its occurrence after rapid drinking on an empty stomach. *J. Forensic Sci.* 36:376–385, 1991.

Jones, A.W., Hahn, R.G. and Stalberg, H.P. Pharmacokinetics of ethanol in plasma and whole blood: Estimation of total body water by the dilution principle. *Eur. J. Clin. Pharmacol.* 42:445–448, 1992.

Jones, A.W., Hahn, R.G. and Norberg, Å. Concentration-time profiles of ethanol in arterial and venous blood and end-expired breath during and after intravenous infusion. *J. Forensic Sci.* 42:1086–1092, 1997a.

Jones, A.W. et al. Accelerated metabolism of ethanol in patients with burn-injury. *Alc. Alcohol.* 32:628–630, 1997b.

Jones, A.W., Jönsson, K-Å. and Kechagias, S. Effect of high-fat, high-protein, and high-carbohydrate meals on the pharmacokinetics of a small dose of alcohol. *Br. J. Clin. Pharmacol.* 44:521–526, 1997c.

Jones, A.W., Eklund, A. and Helander, A. Misleading results of ethanol analysis in urine specimens from rape victims suffering from diabetes. *J. Clin. Forensic Med.* 7:144–146, 2000.

Jones, B.M. and Jones, M.K. Alcohol effects in women during the menstrual cycle. *Ann. N. Y. Acad. Sci.* 273:576–587, 1976.

Jones, K.L. et al. The effect of erythromycin on gastric emptying is modified by physiological changes in the blood glucose concentration. *Am. J. Gastroenterol.* 94:2074–2079, 1999.

Jones, M.K. and Jones, B.M. Ethanol metabolism in women taking oral contraceptives. *Alcohol Clin. Exp. Res.* 8:24–28 1984.

Jönsson, K-Å. et al. Lack of effect of omeprazole, cimetidine, and ranitidine on the pharmacokinetics of ethanol in fasting male volunteers. *Eur. J. Clin. Pharmacol.* 42:209–212, 1992.

Jörnvall, J. and Höög, J.O. Nomenclature of alcohol dehydrogenase. *Alc. Alcohol.* 30:153–161, 1995.

Kalant, H. Absorption, diffusion, distribution, and elimination of ethanol: Effects on biological membranes. In: Kissin, B. and Begleiter, H. (eds.), *The Biochemistry of Alcoholism.* NY: Plenum Press, pp 1–62, 1971.

Kalant, H. Research on alcohol metabolism: A historical perspective. *Keio. J. Med.* 1991:40:113–117, 1991.

Kalant, H. Current state of knowledge about the mechanism of alcohol tolerance. *Add. Biol.* 1:133–141, 1996a.

Kalant, H. Pharmacokinetics of ethanol: Absorption, distribution, and elimination. In: Begleiter, H. and Kissin, B. (eds.), *The Pharmacology of Alcohol and Alcohol Dependence.* New York-Oxford: Oxford University Press, pp 15–58, 1996b.

Kalant, H., Leblanc, A.E. and Gibbins, R.J. Tolerance to and dependence on some on-opiate psychotropic drugs. *Pharmacol. Rev.* 23:135–191, 1971.

Kalant, H. et al. Sensorimotor and physiological effects of various alcoholic beverages. *Can. Med. Assoc. J.* 112:953–958, 1975.

Kechagias, S., Jönsson, K-Å. and Jones, A.W. Impact of gastric emptying on the pharmacokinetics of ethanol as influenced by cisapride. *Br. J. Clin. Pharmacol.* 48:728–732, 1999.

Kechagias, S. et al. Low-dose aspirin decreases blood alcohol concentrations by delaying gastric emptying. *Eur. J. Clin. Pharmacol.* 53:241–246, 1997.

Keiding, S. et al. Ethanol metabolism in heavy drinkers after massive and moderate alcohol intake. *Biochem. Pharmacol.* 32:3097–3102, 1983.

Khanna, J.M., LeBlanc, A.E. and Mayer, J.M. Alcohol pharmacokinetics and forensic issues: A commentary. In: Crow, K.E. and Batt, R.D. (eds.), *Human Metabolism of Alcohol*, vol. 1: *Pharmacokinetics, Medicolegal Aspects and General Interest*. Boca Raton: CRC Press, 1989, pp 59–70.

Klockhoff, H., Näslund, I. and Jones, A.W. Faster absorption of ethanol and higher peak concentration in women after gastric-bypass surgery. *Br. J. Clin. Pharmacol.* 54:587–591, 2002.

Klotz, U. and Ammon, E. Clinical and toxicological consequences of the inductive potential of ethanol. *Eur. J. Clin. Pharmacol.* 54:7–12, 1998.

Kong, M.F. and Horowitz, M. Gastric emptying in diabetes mellitus: relationship to blood-glucose control. *Clin. Geriatr. Med.* 15:321–338, 1999.

Kopun, M. and Propping, P. The kinetics of ethanol absorption and elimination in twins and supplementary repetitive experiments in singleton subjects. *Eur. J. Clin. Pharmacol.* 11:337–344, 1997.

Krauland W., Mallach H. J. and Freudenberg K. Der Gipfelpunkt der Blutalkoholkonzentration nach Belastung mit 0.75 g AlkohoL/kg Körpergewicht. *Blutalkohol* 3:397–404, 1966.

Kruhoffer, P.W. Handling of inspired vaporized ethanol in the airways and lungs: With comments on forensic aspects. *Forensic Sci. Intern.* 21:1–17, 1983.

Kühnholz, B. et al. Zur Dauer der Resorptionszeit bei einer Ethanolbel-astung von 0.3, 0.5 und 0.8 g Alkohol pro kg Körpergewicht in 30 Minuten. *Blutalkohol* 30:158–165, 1993.

Kwo, P.Y. et al. Gender differences in alcohol metabolism: Relationship to liver volume and effect of adjusting for body mass. *Gastroenterology* 115:1552–1557, 1998.

Lammers, S.M., Mainzer, D.E. and Breteler, M.H. Do alcohol pharmacokinetics in women vary due to the menstrual cycle? *Addiction* 90:23–30, 1995.

Lands, W.E. A review of alcohol clearance in humans. *Alcohol* 15:147–160, 1998.

Langford, N.J., Marshall, T. and Ferner, R.E. The lacing defence: Double blind study of thresholds for detecting addition of ethanol to drinks. *Brit. Med. J.* 319:1610, 1999.

Lautt, W.W. and Macedo, M.P. Hepatic circulation and toxicology. *Drug. Metab. Rev.* 29:369–395, 1997.

Lentner, C. Units of measurement, body fluids, composition of the body, nutrition. In: *Ciba-Geigy Scientific Tables*, 8th ed., vol. 1. Basle, Switzerland: Ciba-Geigy, Ltd., 1981.

Lester, D. and Greenberg, L.A. The inhalation of ethyl alcohol by man. *Quart. J. Stud. Alcohol* 12:167–178, 1951.

Leube, G. and Mallach, H.J. Zur Alkoholelimination bei einem Leberkranken mit portocavalen Schunt. *Blutalkohol* 17:15–25, 1980.

Levitt, M.D. Antagonist: The case against first-pass metabolism of ethanol in the stomach. *J. Lab. Clin. Med.* 123:28–31, 1994.

Levitt, M.D. and Levitt, D.G. The critical role of the rate of ethanol absorption in the interpretation of studies purporting to demonstrate gastric metabolism of ethanol. *J. Pharmacol. Exp. Ther.* 269:297–304, 1994.

Levitt, M.D. and Levitt, D.G. Use of a two-compartment model to assess the pharmacokinetics of human ethanol metabolism. *Alcohol Clin. Exp. Res.* 22:1680–1688, 1998.

Levitt, M.D. and Levitt, D.G. Use of a two-compartment model to predict ethanol metabolism. *Alcohol Clin. Exp. Res.* 24:409–410, 2000a.

Levitt, M.D. and Levitt, D.G. Appropriate use and misuse of blood concentration measurements to quantitate first-pass metabolism. *J. Lab. Clin. Med.* 136:275–280, 2000b.

Levitt, M.D. et al. Can the liver account for first-pass metabolism of ethanol in the rat? *Am. J. Physiol.* 267:G452–457, 1994.

Levitt, M.D. et al. Use of measurements of ethanol absorption from stomach and intestine to assess human ethanol metabolism. *Am. J. Physiol.* 273: G951–957, 1997.

Lewis, M.J. A theoretical treatment for the estimation of blood alcohol concentrations arising from inhalation of ethanol vapours. *J. Forensic. Sci. Soc.* 25: 11–22, 1985.

Lewis, M.J. Blood alcohol: The concentration-time curve and retrospective estimation of level. *J. Forensic Sci. Soc.* 26:95–113, 1986a.

Lewis, M.J. The individual and the estimation of his blood alcohol concentration from intake, with particular reference to the "hip-flask" drink. *J. Forensic Sci. Soc.* 26:19–27, 1986b.

Ley, N.J. *Drink Driving Law and Practice*, 2nd ed. London: Sweet and Maxwell, 1997, pp 1–526.

Li, T.K. Pharmacogenetics of response to alcohol and genes that influence alcohol drinking. *J. Stud. Alcohol* 61:5–12, 2000.

Li, T.K. et al. Variation in ethanol pharmacokinetics and perceived gender and ethnic differences in alcohol elimination. *Alcohol Clin. Exp. Res.* 24: 415–416, 2000.

Li, T.K. et al. Genetic and environmental influences on alcohol metabolism in humans. *Alcohol Clin. Exp. Res.* 25:136–144, 2001.

Lieber, C.S. Cytochrome P–4502E1: Its physiological and pathological role. *Physiol. Rev.* 77:517–544, 1997a.

Lieber, C.S. Gastric ethanol metabolism and gastritis: Interactions with other drugs, helicobacter pylori, and antibiotic therapy (1957–1997): A review. *Alcohol Clin. Exp. Res.* 21:1360–1366, 1997b.

Lieber, C.S. Microsomal ethanol-oxidizing system (MEOS): The first 30 years (1968–1998): A review. *Alcohol Clin. Exp. Re.s* 23:991–1007, 1999.

Lieber, C.S. Alcohol: Its metabolism and interaction with nutrients. *Annu. Rev. Nutr.* 20:395–430, 2000.

Liljestrand, G. and Linde, P. Über die Ausscheidung des Alkohols mit der Expirationsluft. *Skand. Arch. Physiol.* 9:273–298, 1930.

Lim, R.T. et al. First-pass metabolism of ethanol is predominantly gastric. *Alcohol Clin. Exp. Res.* 17: 1337–1344, 1993.

Linde, P. Der Überggang des äthylalkohols in den Parotisspeichel beim Menschen. *Arch. Exp. Path. Pharmakol.* 167:285–291, 1932.

Logan, B.K. and Jones, A.W. Endogenous ethanol "autobrewery syndrome" as a drunk driving defense challenge. *Med. Sci. Law* 40:206–215, 2000.

Lötterle, J. et al. Tageszeitliche Unterschiede der Alkoholresorption. *Blutalkohol* 26:369–375, 1989.

Lucey, M.R. et al The influence of age and gender on blood ethanol concentrations in healthy humans. *J. Stud. Alcohol* 60:103–110, 1999.

Lumeng, L. and Crabb, D.W. Genetic aspects and risk factors in alcoholism and alcoholic liver disease. *Gastroenterology* 107:572–578, 1994.

Lund, A. The secretion of alcohol in the tear fluid. *Blutalkohol* 21:51–54, 1984.

Lundquist, F. and Wolthers, H. The kinetics of alcohol elimination in man. *Acta. Pharmacol. Toxicol.* 14: 265–289, 1958.

Magnusdottir, K. and Johannesson, T. Ethanol in blood after ingestion of light alcoholic beverages (maximal 2.23 percent v/v). *Pharmacol. Toxicol.* 87: 297–298, 2000.

Malamund, D. and Tabak, L. (eds.). Saliva as a diagnostic fluid. *Ann. N. Y. Acad. Sci.* 694, 1993.

Marshall, A.W. et al. Ethanol elimination in males and females: relationship to menstrual cycle and body composition. *Hepatology* 3:701–706, 1983.

Martin, C.S. and Moss, H.B. Measurement of acute tolerance to alcohol in human subjects. *Alcohol. Clin. Exp. Res.* 17:211–216, 1993.

Martin, C.S. and Earleywine, M. Ascending and descending rates of change in blood alcohol concentrations and subjective intoxication ratings. *J. Sub. Abuse* 2:345–352, 1990.

Martin, E. et al. The pharmacokinetics of alcohol in human breath, venous and arterial blood after oral ingestion. *Eur. J. Clin. Pharmacol.* 26:619–626, 1984.

Martin, N.G. et al. A twin study of ethanol metabolism. *Behav. Genet.* 15:93–109, 1985.

Mason, J.K. and Blackmore, D.J. Experimental inhalation of ethanol vapour. *Med. Sci. Law.* 12:205–208, 1972.

Mascord, D. et al. Effect of oral glucose on the rate of metabolism of ethanol in humans. *Alc. Alcohol.* 23: 365–370, 1988.

Mather, L.E. Anatomical-physiological approaches in pharmacokinetics and pharmacodynamics. *Clin. Pharmacokinet.* 40:707–722, 2001.

Matsumoto, H. and Fukui, Y. Pharmacokinetics of ethanol: A review of the methodology. *Add. Biol.* 7:5–14, 2002.

McBride, W.J. et al. Involvement of acetaldehyde in alcohol addiction. *Alcohol Clin. Exp. Res.* 26:114–119, 2002.

McColl, K.E.L. et al. Correlation of ethanol concentrations in blood and saliva. *Clin. Sci.* 56:283–286, 1979.

McFarlane, A. et al. How does dietary lipid lower blood alcohol concentrations? *Gut* 27:15–18, 1986.

Mennella, J.A. and Beauchamp, G.K. The transfer of alcohol to human milk: Effect on flavor and the infant's behavior. *N Engl J. Med.* 225:581–585, 1991.

Mezey, E. Stress and ethanol metabolism. *Alc. Alcohol.* 33:310, 1998.

Mezey, E., Oesterling, J.E. and Potter, J.J. Influence of male hormones on ethanol elimination in man. *Hepatology* 8:742–744, 1988.

Mirand, A.L. and Welte, J.W. Total body water adjustment of mean alcohol intakes. *J. Subst. Abuse.* 6: 419–425, 1994.

Mishra, L. et al. More rapid elimination of alcohol in women as compared to their male siblings. *Alcohol Clin. Exp. Res.* 13:752–754, 1989.

Montgomery, M.R. and Reasor, M.J. Retrograde extrapolation of blood alcohol data: An applied approach. *J. Toxicol. Environ. Health* 36:281–292, 1992.

Moore, K.A. et al. A comparison of ethanol concentrations in the occipital lobe and cerebellum. *Forensic Sci. Intern.* 86:127–134, 1997.

Moreno, A. and Pares, X. Purification and characterization of a new alcohol dehydrogenase from human stomach. *J. Biol. Chem.* 266:1128–1133, 1991.

Mumenthaler, M.S. et al. Gender differences in moderate drinking effects. *Alcohol Res. Health* 23:55–64, 1999

Mumenthaler, M.S., Taylor, J.L. and Yesavage, J.A. Ethanol pharmacokinetics in white women: Nonlinear model fitting versus zero-order elimination analyses. *Alcohol Clin. Exp. Res.* 24:1353–1362, 2000.

Mumenthaler, M.S. et al. Influence of the menstrual cycle on flight simulator performance after alcohol ingestion. *J. Stud. Alcohol* 62:422–433, 2001.

Nagoshi, C.T. and Wilson, J.R. Long-term repeatability of human alcohol metabolism, sensitivity and acute tolerance. *J. Stud. Alcohol* 50:162–169, 1989.

Nebert, D.W. and Russell, D.W. Clinical importance of the cytochromes P450. *Lancet* 360:1155–1162, 2002.

Neuteboom, W. and Jones, A.W. Disappearance rate of alcohol from the blood of drunk drivers calculated from two consecutive samples: What do the results really mean? *Forensic Sci. Intern.* 45:107–115, 1990.

Neuteboom, W. and Vis, A.A. The effects of low alcohol beers on the blood alcohol concentration. *Blutalkohol* 28:393–396, 1991.

Norberg, A. et al. Within- and between-subject variations in pharmacokinetic parameters of ethanol by analysis of breath, venous blood and urine. *Br. J. Clin. Pharmacol.* 49:399–408, 2000.

Norberg, A. et al. Role of variability in explaining ethanol pharmacokinetics: Research and forensic applications. *Clin. Pharmacokinet.* 42:1–31, 2003.

Nowak, T.V. et al. Highly variable gastric emptying in patients with insulin dependent diabetes mellitus. *Gut* 37:23–29 1995.

Nyman, E. and Palmlöv, A. The elimination of ethyl alcohol in sweat. *Scand. Arch. Physiol.* 74:155–159, 1936.

O'Connor, S. et al. Clamping breath alcohol concentration reduces experimental variance: Application to the study of acute tolerance to alcohol and alcohol elimination rate. *Alcohol Clin. Exp. Res.* 22:202–210, 1998

Olow, J. Über den übergang des Äthylalkohols in die Milch stillender Frauen. *Biochem. Z.* 134:553–558, 1923.

O'Neal, C.L. and Poklis, A. Postmortem production of ethanol and factors that influence interpretation. *Am. J. Forensic Med. Pathol.* 17:8–20, 1996.

O'Neill, B., Williams, A.F. and Dubowski, K.M. Variability in blood alcohol concentrations. Implications for estimating individual results. *J. Stud. Alcohol.* 44:222–230, 1983.

Oneta, C.M. et al. First pass metabolism of ethanol is strikingly influenced by the speed of gastric emptying. *Gut* 43:612–619, 1998.

Oneta, C.M. et al. Dynamics of cytochrome P4502E1 activity in man: Induction by ethanol and disappearance during withdrawal phase. *J. Hepatol.* 36:47–52, 2002.

Orford, J. and Keddie, A. Gender differences in the functions and effects of moderate and excessive drinking. *Br. J. Clin. Psychol.* 24:265–279, 1985

Österlind, S., Ahlen, M. and Wolff, E. Investigations concerning the constants β and r according to Widmark, especially in women. *Acta. Pathol. Microbiol. Scand.* Supp. 54:489–498, 1944.

Panes, J. et al. Influence of liver disease on hepatic alcohol and aldehyde dehydrogenases. *Gastroenterology* 97:708–714, 1989

Panes, J. et al. Determinants of ethanol and acetaldehyde metabolism in chronic alcoholics. *Alcohol Clin. Exp. Res.* 17:48–53, 1993

Park, B.K. et al. Relevance of induction of human drug-metabolizing enzymes: Pharmacological and toxicological implications. *Br. J. Clin. Pharmacol.* 41:477–491, 1996.

Passananti, G.T., Wolff, C.A. and Vesell, E.S. Reproducibility of individual rates of ethanol metabolism in fasting subjects. *Clin. Pharmacol. Ther.* 47:389–396, 1990.

Pedrosa, M.C. et al. Gastric emptying and first-pass metabolism of ethanol in elderly subjects with and without atrophic gastritis. *Scand. J. Gastroenterol.* 31:671–677, 1996.

Pendlington, R.U. et al. Fate of ethanol topically applied to skin. *Food Chem. Toxicol.* 39:169–174, 2001.

Peng, G.W. and Chiou, W.L. Analysis of drugs and other toxic substances in biological samples for pharmacokinetic studies. *J. Chromatogr.* 531:3–50, 1990.

Pfeiffer, A., Högl, B. and Kaess, H. Effect of ethanol and commonly ingested alcoholic beverages on gastric emptying and gastrointestinal transit. *Clin. Invest.* 70:487–491, 1992.

Phillips, M. Sweat patch testing detects inaccurate self-reports of alcohol consumption. *Alcohol. Clin. Exp. Res.* 3:51–53, 1984.

Phillips, M. and McAloon, M.H. A sweat-patch test for alcohol consumption: Evaluation in continuous episodic drinkers. *Alcohol. Clin. Exp. Res.* 4;391–395, 1980.

Pichini, S. et al. Drug monitoring in nonconventional biological fluids and matrices. *Clin. Pharmacokinet.* 30:211–228, 1996.

Piekoszewski, W. and Gubala, W. Inter- and intra-individual variability of ethanol pharmacokinetics over a long period of time. *Pol. J. Pharmacol.* 52: 389–395, 2000.

Pikkarainen, P.H. and Räiha, N.C.R. Development of alcohol dehydrogenase activity in the human liver. *Pediatr. Res.* 1:165–168, 1967.

Pikaar, N.A., Wedel, M. and Hermus, R.J. Influence of several factors on blood alcohol concentrations after drinking alcohol. *Alc. Alcohol.* 23:289–297, 1988.

Pounder, D.J. and Kuroda, N. Vitreous humor is of limited value in predicting blood alcohol. *Forensic Sci. Intern.* 65:73–80, 1994.

Ramchandani, V.A., Kwo, P.Y. and Li, T.K. Effect of food and food composition on alcohol elimination rates in helathy mern and women. *J. Clin. Pharmacol.* 41:1345–1350, 2001a.

Ramchandani, V.A., Bosron, W.J. and Li, T.K. Research advances in ethanol metabolism. *Pathol. Biol.* 49:676–682, 2001b.

Rangno, R.E., Kreeft, J.H. and Sita,r D.S. Ethanol "dose–dependent" elimination: Michaelis-Menten v classical kinetic analysis. *Br. J. Clin. Pharmacol.* 12:667–673, 1981.

Raufman, J.P. et al. Histamine-2-receptor antagonists do not alter serum ethanol levels in fed, non-alcoholic men. *Ann. Intern. Med.* 118:488–494, 1993.

Rivier, L. Techniques for analytical testing of unconventional samples. *Baillieres Best. Pract. Res. Clin. Endocrinol. Metab.* 14:147–165, 2000.

Roche, A.F., Heymsfield, S.B. and Lohman, T.G. (eds.). *Human Body Composition.* Champaign, IL: Human Kinetics, 1996.

Rogers, J. et al. Differing effects of carbohydrate, fat and protein on the rate of ethanol metabolism. *Alc. Alcohol.* 22:345–353, 1987.

Roine, RP. et al. Aspirin increases blood alcohol concentrations in humans after ingestion of ethanol. *JAMA* 264:2406–2408, 1990.

Roine, R.P. et al. Effect of concentration of ingested ethanol on blood alcohol levels. *Alcohol Clin. Exp. Res.* 15:734–738, 1991.

Roine, R.P. et al. Comparison of blood alcohol concentrations after beer and whiskey. *Alcohol Clin. Exp. Res* 17:709–711, 1993.

Rockerbie, RA. *Alcohol and Drug Intoxication.* Victoria, BC: Trafford, 1999.

Rockerbie, D.W. and Rockerbie, R.A. Computer simulation analysis of blood alcohol. *J. Clin. Forensic Med.* 2:137–141, 1995.

Roe, O. The metabolism and toxicity of methanol. *Pharmacol. Rev.* 7:399–412, 1955.

Roe, O. Species differences in methanol poisoning. *CRC Critical Rev. Toxicol.* 10:275–286, 1982.

Rose, E.F. Factors influencing gastric emptying. *J. Forensic Sci.* 24:200–206, 1979.

Rosenfeld, L.M. Physiology of water. *Clin. Dermatol.* 14:555–561, 1996.

Ross, E.M. Pharmacodynamics: Mechanisms of drug action and the relationship between drug concentration and effect. In: Gillman, A.G. et al. (eds.), *Goodman & Gilman's The Pharmacological Basis of Therapeutics.* NY: Pergamon Press, 1990, pp 33–48.

Rowland, M. and Tozer, T.N. *Clinical Pharmacokinetics: Concepts and Application.* Philadelphia: Lea and Febiger, 1980.

Salmela, K.S. et al. Helicobacter infection and gastric ethanol metabolism. *Alcohol. Clin. Exp. Res.* 18: 1294–1299, 1994.

Samyn, N. et al. Analysis of drugs of abuse in saliva. *Forensic Sci. Rev.* 11:1–19, 1999.

Sarkola, T. and Eriksson, C.J.P. Effect pf 4-methyl pyrazole on endogenous plasma ethanol and methanol levels in humans. *Alcohol Clin. Exp. Res.* 25:513–516, 2001.

Schoeller, D.A. Changes in total body water with age. *Am. J. Clin. Nutr.* 50:1176–1181, 1989.

Schramm, W. et al. Drugs of abuse in saliva: A review. *J. Anal. Toxicol.* 16:1–9, 1992.

Schvarcz, E. et al. Hypoglycemia increases the gastric emptying rate in healthy subjects. *Diabetes Care* 18:674–676, 1995.

Schwartz, J.B. The influence of sex on pharmacokinetics. *Clin. Pharmacokinet.* 42:107–121, 2003.

Sedman, A.J., Wilkinson, P.K. and Wagner, J.G. Concentrations of ethanol in two segments of the vascular system. *J. Forensic Sci.* 21:315–322, 1976a.

Sedman, A.J. et al. Food effects on absorption and metabolism of alcohol. *J. Stud. Alcohol* 37:1197–1214, 1976b.

Seidl, S., Jensen, U. and Alt, A. The calculation of blood ethanol concentrations in males and females. *Int. J. Legal Med.* 114:71–77, 2000.

Seidl, S., Wurst, F.W. and Alt, A. Ethyl glucuronide: A biological marker for recent alcohol consumption. *Add. Biol.* 6:205–212, 2001.

Schmitt, G. et al. Ethyl glucuronide: An unusual ethanol metabolite in humans: Synthesis, analytical data, and determination in serum and urine. *J. Anal. Toxicol.* 19:91–94, 1995.

Schmitt, G. et al. Ethyl glucuronide concentration in serum of human volunteers, teetotalers, and suspected drinking drivers. *J. Forensic Sci.* 42:1099–1102, 1997.

Shannon, M. Toxicology reviews Fomepizole: A new antidote. *Pediat. Emerg. Care* 14:170–172, 1998.

Sharma, R. et al. First-pass metabolism of alcohol: Absence of diurnal variation and its inhibition by cimetidine after evening meal. *Dig. Dis. Sci.* 40: 2091–2097, 1995.

Shultz, J., Weiner, H. and Westcott, J. Retardation of ethanol absorption by food in the stomach. *J. Stud. Alcohol* 41:861–870, 1980.

Simanowski, U.A. et al. Helicobacter pylori infection decreases gastric alcohol dehydrogenase activity and first-pass metabolism of ethanol in man. *Digestion* 59:314–320, 1998.

Singh, B.N. Effects of food on clinical pharmacokinetics. *Clin Pharmacokinet* 37:213–255, 1999.

Smith, G.D. et al. Mathematical modelling of ethanol metabolism in normal subjects and chronic alcohol misusers. *Alc. Alcohol.* 28:25–32, 1993.

Song, B.J. Ethanol-inducible cytochrome P450 (CYP2E1): Biochemistry, molecular biology and clinical relevance: 1996 update. *Alcohol Clin. Exp. Res.* 20: 138A–146A, 1996.

Soterakis, J. and Iber, F.L. Increased rate of alcohol removal from blood with oral fructose and sucrose. *Am. J. Clin. Nutr.* 28:254–257, 1975.

Springer, E. Blutalkoholkurven nach Gabe von wässrigen Aethanollösungen verschiedner Konzentrationen. *Blutalkohol* 9:198–206, 1972.

Stowell, A.R. and Stowell, L.I. Estimation of blood alcohol concentrations after social drinking. *J Forensic Sci* 43: 14–21, 1998.

Swift, R.M. Drug therapy for alcohol dependence. *N. Engl. J. Med.* 340:1482–1490, 1999.

Swift, R.M. Transdermal alcohol measurement for estimation of blood alcohol concentration. *Alcohol Clin. Exp. Res.* 24:422–423, 2000.

Swift, R.M. et al. Studies on a wearable, electronic transdermal alcohol sensor. *Alcohol Clin. Exp. Res.* 16:721–725, 1992.

Tagliaro, F. et al. Chromatographic methods for blood alcohol determination. *J. Chromatogr.* 580:161–190, 1992.

Takala, M., Pihkanen, T.A. and Markkanen, T. *The Effects of Distilled and Brewed Beverages*. Helsinki: Finnish Foundation for Alcohol Studies, vol. 4, 1957, pp 1–195.

Thomasson, H.R. Alcohol elimination: Faster in women? *Alcohol Clin. Exp. Res.* 24:419–420, 2000.

Thomasson, H.R. Gender differences in alcohol metabolism. Physiological responses to ethanol. *Recent Dev. Alcohol* 12:163–179, 1995.

Toon, S. et al. Absence of effect of ranitidne on blood alcohol concentration when taken morning, midday and evening with or without food. *Clin. Pharm. Therap.* 55:385–391, 1994.

VanLoan, M.D. Total body composition: Birth to old age. In: Roche, A.F, Heymsfield, S.B. and Lohman, T.G. (eds.), *Human Body Composition*. Champaign, IL: Human Kinetics, 1996, pp 205–215.

Vantrappen, G. Methods to study gastric emptying. *Dig. Dis. Sci.* 39:91S–94S, 1994.

Vestal, R.E. et al. Aging and ethanol metabolism. *Clin. Pharmacol. Ther.* 21:343–354, 1977.

Wagner, J.G. Lack of first pass metabolism of ethanol in blood concentrations in the social drinking range. *Life Sci.* 39:407–414, 1986.

Wagner, J.G. *Pharmacokinetics for the Pharmaceutical Sciences*. Basel, Switzerland: Technomic Publishing Company, 1993.

Wagner, J.G. and Patel, J.A. Variations in absorption and elimination rates of ethyl alcohol in a single subject. *Res. Commun. Chem. Pathol. Pharmacol.* 4:61–76, 1972.

Wagner, J.G., Wilkinson, P.K. and Ganes, D.A. Parameters Vm and Km for elimination of alcohol in young male subjects following low doses of alcohol. *Alc. Alcohol.* 24:555–564, 1989

Wagner, J.G., Wilkinson, P.K. and Ganes, D.A. Estimation of the amount of alcohol ingested from a single blood alcohol concentration. *Alc. Alcohol.* 25:379–384, 1990.

Wall, T.L. et al. Alcohol elimination in Native American mission Indians: An investigation of inter-individual variation. *Alcohol Clin. Exp. Res.* 20: 1159–1164, 1996.

Wall, T.L. et al. Alcohol metabolism in Asian-American men with genetic polymorphisms of aldehyde dehydrogenase. *Ann. Intern. Med.* 127:376–379, 1997.

Wallgren, H. Absorption, diffusion, distribution and elimination of ethanol: Effect on biological membranes. In: Tremolieres, J. (ed.), *International Encyclopedia of Pharmacology and Therapeutics*, vol. 1: *Alcohols and Derivatives*. Oxford: Pergamon Press, 1970, pp 161–188.

Walls, H.J. and Brownlie, A.R. *Drink, Drugs and Driving*, 2nd ed. London: Sweet and Maxwell, 1985.

Wang, M.Q. et al. Acute alcohol intoxication, body composition, and pharmacokinetics. *Pharmacol. Biochem. Behav.* 43:641–643, 1992.

Ward, R.J. et al The topping-up effect: Differences between low and non-alcoholic lager on blood ethanol. *Alc. Alcohol.* 26:399–402, 1991.

Wartburg, von J-P: Pharmacokinetics of alcohol. In: Crow, K.E. and Batt, R.D. (eds.), *Human Metabolism of Alcohol*, vol. 1, *Pharmacokinetics, Medicolegal Aspects and General Interest*. Boca Raton: CRC Press, 1989, pp 9–22.

Watkins, R.L. and Adler, E.V. The effect of food on alcohol absorption and elimination patterns. *J. Forensic Sci.* 38:285–291, 1993.

Watson, P.E., Watson, I.D. and Batt, R.D. Prediction of blood alcohol concentrations in human subjects: Updating the Widmark equation. *J. Stud. Alcohol* 42:547–556, 1981

Wedel, M. et al. Application of a three-compartment model to a study of the effects of sex, alcohol dose and concentration, exercise and food consumption on the pharmacokinetics of ethanol in healthy volunteers. *Alc. Alcohol* 26:329–336, 1991.

Weinberg, D.S., Burnham, D. and Berlin, J.A. Effect of histamine-2-receptor antagonists on blood alcohol levels. *J. Gen. Intern. Med.* 13:594–599, 1998.

Weinshilbourn, R. Inheritance and drug response. *N. Engl. J. Med.* 348:529–537, 2003.

Weintraub, M. and Standish, R. 4-methyl pyrazole: An antidote for ethylene glycol and methanol intoxication. *Hosp. Formul.* 23:960–969, 1988.

Welling, P.G. et al. Pharmacokinetics of alcohol following single low doses to fasted and nonfasted subjects. *J. Clin. Pharmacol.* 17:199–206, 1977.

Westenbrink, W. Cimetidine and the blood alcohol curve: A case study and review. *Can. Soc. Forensic Sci. J.* 28:165–170, 1995.

Whitfield, J.B. and Martin, N.G. Alcohol consumption and alcohol pharmacokinetics: Interactions within the normal population. *Alcohol. Clin. Exp. Res.* 18:238–243, 1994.

Whitfield, J.B. et al. Variation in alcohol pharmacokinetics as a risk factor for alcohol dependence. *Alcohol. Clin. Exp. Res.* 25:1257–1253, 2001.

Widmark, E.M.P. Om alkoholens övergång i urinen samt om en enkel, kliniskt använbar metod för diagnosticering av alkoholförekomst i kroppen. *Uppsala Läkareförenings Förhandlingar N. F.* 19:241–272, 1914.

Widmark, E.M.P. Eine Mikromethode zur Bestimmung von Äthylalkohol im Blut. *Biochem. Z.* 131:473–484, 1922.

Widmark, E.M.P. *Die theoretischen Grundlagen und die praktische Verwendbarkeit der gerichtlich–medi-zinischen Alkoholbestimmung*. Berlin: Urban & Schwarzenberg, 1932.

Wilkinson, P.K. Pharmacokinetics of ethanol: A review. *Alcohol. Clin. Exp. Res.* 4:6–21, 1980.

Wilkinson, P.K. et al. Blood ethanol concentrations during and following constant-rate intravenous infusion of alcohol. *Clin. Pharmacol. Ther.* 19:213–223, 1976.

Wilkinson, P.K. et al. Pharmacokinetics of ethanol after oral administration in the fasting state. *J. Pharmacokinet. Biopharm.* 5:207–224, 1977a.

Wilkinson, P.K. et al. Fasting and nonfasting blood ethanol concentrations following repeated oral administration of ethanol to one adult male subject. *J. Pharmacokinet. Biopharm.* 5:41–52, 1977b.

Wilkinson, P.K. et al. Nonlinear pharmacokinetics of ethanol: The disproportionate AUC-dose relationship. *Alcohol. Clin. Exp. Res.* 4:384–390, 1980.

Winek, C.L. and Murphy, K.L. The rate and kinetic order of ethanol elimination. *Forensic Sci. Intern.* 25:159–166, 1984.

Winek, C.L. and Carfagna, M. Comparison of plasma, serum and whole blood ethanol concentrations. *J. Anal. Toxicol.* 11:267–268, 1987.

Winek, C.L., Wahba W.W. and Dowdell, J.L. Determination of absorption time of ethanol in social drinkers. *Forensic Sci. Intern.* 77:169–177, 1996.

Wright, N.R. and Cameron, D. The influence of habitual alcohol intake on breath alcohol concentrations following prolonged drinking. *Alc. Alcohol.* 33:495–501, 1998.

Yanovski, S.Z. and Yanovski, J.A. Obesity. *N. Engl J. Med.* 346:591–602, 2002.

Yap, M. et al. Studies on the chronopharmacology of ethanol. *Alc. Alcohol.* 28:17–24, 1993.

Zink, P. and Reinhardt, G. Der Verlauf der Blutalkohol-kurve bei grossen Trinkmengen. *Blutalkohol* 21:422–442, 1984.

Chapter 4

The Biochemistry and Physiology of Alcohol: Applications to Forensic Science and Toxicology

A.W. Jones, Ph.D., D.Sc.

4.1 Introduction

Ethanol[1] has a remarkably simple chemical structure considering its wide spectrum of biochemical, behavioral, and pharmacological effects on the body. Together with other organic solvents such as ether and chloroform as well as anesthetic gases such as aliphatic hydrocarbons and nitrous oxide, ethanol belongs to a class of pharmacological agents known as central nervous system (CNS) depressants (Goldstein, 1994). Because ethanol is much more soluble in water than in lipids (fatty tissue), large quantities must be administered to produce stupor and anesthe-

sia compared with other depressant drugs. Some of the effects of ethanol on brain chemistry, such as the alleviation of anxiety and loss of motor coordination, resemble what happens after taking sedative-hypnotic drugs such as barbiturates and benzodiazepines. Although the exact mechanisms and sites of action of ethanol in the CNS are not fully understood, recent research suggests that some of the cognitive and behavioral changes associated with heavy drinking result from disruption in the normal functioning of membrane receptors for neurotransmitter molecules gamma aminobutyric acid (GABA) and glutamate (Tabakoff and Hoffman, 1993; Korpi, 1994).

The pharmacokinetics and pharmacodynamics of ethanol differ from most other psychotropic drugs used by mankind. First and foremost, the dose of ethanol needed to elicit a pharmacological effect is several orders of magnitude greater than for other drugs of abuse. Secondly, the enzyme systems that clear ethanol from the bloodstream quickly become saturated with substrate and therefore are working at full capacity. To achieve an analgesic effect from opiates such as morphine and codeine, a person has to take ten milligrams and 100 milligrams respectively. This compares with intake of 15,000–20,000 milligrams of ethanol to reach a feeling of mild euphoria ("tipsy"), or the amount contained in 1.5 ounces of spirits (40 percent v/v), one glass (150 milliliters) of wine (12 percent v/v) or one bottle (330 milliliters) of export beer (5 percent v/v). People consume enormous quantities of ethanol compared with other drugs and medication they might use. In 1989 the average per capita annual consumption of alcohol in the U.S. for individuals over fourteen years of age amounted to a staggering 2.43 gallons of absolute (100 percent) ethanol. Because many people are abstainers the amounts consumed by those who actually indulge in drinking alcohol vastly exceeds this average amount (Williams and DeBakey, 1992).

Trace amounts of ethanol are produced naturally in the body in the course of normal metabolic processes, such as during the end-stages of carbohydrate metabolism. Pyruvate and acetaldehyde are considered as likely precursors of endogenous ethanol (EE) (Jacobsen, 1950; Ostrovsky, 1986). Another source of EE is through the microbial fermentation of dietary sugars in the gut. However, because blood from the portal vein must pass through the liver before reaching the systemic circulation the concentrations of EE reaching the peripheral blood are extremely small owing to an effective first-pass metabolism. When reliable and specific analytical methods are used to analyze blood and other body fluids from abstinent subjects, the median concentration of EE is only about 1 mg/L (0.0001 g/dL) with a span from 0.5 to 2 mg/L (0.00005-0.0002 g/dL), depending on genetic (racial), dietary, and environmental factors (Sprung et al., 1981; Jones et al., 1983). Clearly, the concentrations of EE present in body fluids lack any clinical or forensic significance. However, this notion was challenged in two recent papers originating from the same group of investigators (Agapejev et al., 1992a and 1992b). Ethanol was determined in blood and cerebrospinal fluid from ostensibly abstinent subjects, who were patients at a psychiatric hospital. The concentrations of EE showed large inter-subject variations and in some individuals, as much as 40–50 mg/dL were reported. However, an obsolete chemical oxidation method of analysis was used and these abnormally high levels of "apparent" ethanol probably reflect a nonspecific oxidation of other endogenous metabolites in blood and CSF or the kind of medication being prescribed to the patients (Jones, 1994).

For most people ethanol is a harmless socially accepted drug, and moderate intake of wine and beer constitute an important part of the diet and daily life in many countries. Unfortunately, for about 10–15 percent of those who indulge in drinking alcohol, especially among men, chronic consumption leads to profound psychological and physical disturbances with dependence on alcohol and craving as the consequences (Goldstein, 1994). The withdrawal symptoms that develop after ending a prolonged heavy drinking spree include hallucinations, blackouts, seizures, and delirium tremens. If not properly treated, abrupt withdrawal of alcohol might prove fatal.

Alcohol can also be considered a food because it provides easily available energy, actually 7.1 kcal/g (29 kj/g) when oxidized in the body to carbon dioxide and water. This compares with 9 kcal/g from fat and 4 kcal/g from protein and carbohydrate. However, the calories derived from alcohol are usually referred to as "empty" calories because they cannot be stored for later use when needed, for example, as glucose is converted into glycogen (Lieber, 1994a). Furthermore, alcoholic beverages lack the vitamins and minerals present in conventional foodstuffs and a deficiency in certain vitamins (e.g., thiamine, folate, pyridoxine, and vitamin A) represents a common sequel to abuse of alcohol and the development of alcoholism (Lieber 1994b).

Solutions of ethanol (70 percent v/v) are used in clinical medicine as an antiseptic to disinfect the skin before taking blood samples and infusion flasks with 10 percent v/v solutions are always available in the emergency department for the purpose of treating patients poisoned with methanol or ethylene glycol (Jacobsen and McMartin, 1986). Maintaining a moderately high blood-ethanol concentration of about 100 mg/dL blocks the conversion of methanol and ethylene glycol into their toxic metabolites, formic acid and oxalic acid, respectively. These more dangerous alcohols and their metabolites are subsequently removed from the blood by dialysis. This method of treatment works because class-I alcohol dehydrogenase (ADH), the enzyme chiefly responsible for detoxification of alcohols, has a higher affinity for oxidizing ethanol compared with methanol or ethylene glycol (Ehrig et al., 1988; Jones et al., 1990; Haffner et al., 1992). Some recent prospective studies have found that small quantities of alcohol (about 1.5 ounces) taken daily might be effective as a prophylactic treatment for cardiovascular or cerebrovascular disease but this therapeutic approach still remains controversial in some circles (Criiqui and Ringel, 1994; Doll et al., 1994). Red wine (two to three glasses per day) seems to be the most effective alcoholic beverage to reduce mortality according to a recent survey (Grønbaeck et al., 1995).

In this chapter, research dealing with various biochemical and physiological aspects of alcohol metabolism is reviewed and ramifications in forensic science and toxicology are highlighted. The biochemical mechanisms that clear ethanol from the body are discussed, especially the enzymes involved in this process and their distribution in human populations and different racial groups (Agarwal and Goedde, 1990). Moreover, the existence of ADH enzymes in the gastric mucosa is a topic much discussed and debated in connection with the use of alcohol together with drugs such as aspirin and H_2-receptor antagonists[2] cimetidine and ranitidine (Gentry et al., 1994; Levitt, 1994).

Acetaldehyde (AcH), the first product of ethanol oxidation by all known pathways, has long been at the center of biomedical alcohol research (Brien and Loomis, 1983; Von Wartburg and Bühler, 1984). This toxic metabolite of ethanol has been incriminated in many of the untoward effects of heavy drinking including liver cirrhosis, pancreatitis and certain forms of cancer (Lindahl, 1992; Lieber 1994b). The concentrations of AcH in blood and breath after drinking can span a wide range depending on various genetic (racial) and environmental influences such as a person's drinking and smoking habits, the activity of aldehyde dehydrogenase, and whether alcohol-sensitizing drugs are being used (Goedde and Agarwal, 1990). Publications reporting the concentrations of acetaldehyde in the expired air are also reviewed here because this question often arises when breath alcohol analyzers are used in traffic law enforcement to test drinking drivers, namely whether acetaldehyde should be considered an interfering substance (Jones, 1995a).

The magnitude of inter- and intra-individual variations in the pharmacokinetics of ethanol and the factors influencing the peak BAC reached and the time of its occurrence are questions of interest in medicolegal casework. Recent studies of this topic are covered, with emphasis on the influence of food in the stomach before drinking and how this not only lowers the peak BAC but also boosts the rate of me-

tabolism of ethanol (Jones, 1993; Jones and Jönsson, 1994a). The rate of disappearance of ethanol from the bloodstream (β-slope) is important to consider when forward or backward extrapolations of a person's BAC become an issue in drinking and driving litigation. The magnitude of variation in this parameter for a wide variety of drinking conditions is reported here. Finally the impact of various pathological states such as liver cirrhosis on the disposition kinetics of ethanol is reviewed.

4.2 The Fate of Alcohol in the Body

The fate of alcohol in the body is usually illustrated by plotting the blood-alcohol concentration (BAC) as a function of time after volunteer subjects ingest a known amount of alcohol under controlled experimental conditions. Figure 4.1 gives examples of BAC profiles obtained after nine healthy men ingested the same dose of ethanol (0.80 g/kg) as 96 percent v/v ethanol solvent diluted with orange juice to give a cocktail of 15–20 percent v/v. Despite these standardized test conditions, a considerable variability in the pharmacokinetic profiles was evident. The peak BAC, the time required to reach the peak, the area under the curve and the time to reach a zero BAC varied from subject to subject and also within the same subject over time (Jones and Jönsson, 1994b). The shape of the BAC-time course depends on a host of experimental variables including the dose of alcohol taken, the speed of drinking, the kind of beverage consumed (beer, wine, spirits), the fed or fasting state of the subject as well as the individual's age, sex, and body composition (proportion of fat:lean tissue). Furthermore, one should not forget pre-analytical and analytical sources of variations inherent in the methods used to draw the blood samples and determine the concentration of ethanol. The contribution of these analytical factors as sources of variation in the pharmacokinetics of ethanol and other drugs is often overlooked.

The disposition of ethanol in the body after drinking can be subdivided into three stages: (1) uptake from the gut (absorption), (2) transport to all parts of the body by the blood (distribution) and, finally, (3) removal from the body (elimination) both by excretion through the kidneys, the lungs, and the skin and by metabolic degradation. The bulk of the dose of ethanol, actually between 95–98 percent is removed from the body by enzymatic oxidation in a process that occurs mainly in the liver. A very small fraction of the ingested ethanol becomes conjugated to glucuronic acid and this metabolite has been identified in the urine (Schmitt et al., 1995). Although most experimental work on the disposition kinetics of ethanol has been done by sampling and analyzing specimens of whole blood, other body fluids such as breath, urine and saliva are practical but are seldom used for quantitative analysis of ethanol when tracing the time-course of this drug in the body (Jones 1993).

4.3 Enzymes Involved in the Metabolism of Alcohol

Figure 4.2 shows the main metabolic pathway for enzymatic oxidation of ethanol. The first step involves the oxidation of ethanol into acetaldehyde and this reaction is catalyzed by alcohol dehydrogenase, an enzyme located in the cytosol fraction of the hepatocyte (liver cell). The second stage of the metabolism involves oxidation of acetaldehyde into acetate with the help of the enzyme aldehyde dehydrogenase which is mainly located in the mitochondria. Both these biochemical reactions require the presence of a coenzyme, nicotinamide adenine dinucle-

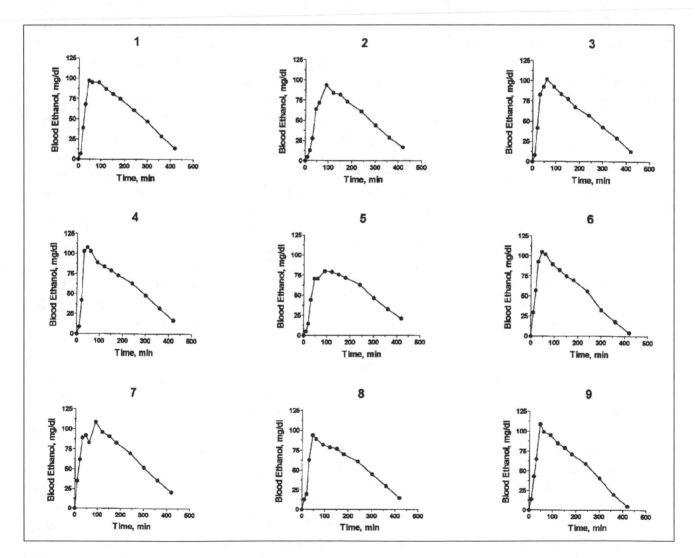

Figure 4.1 *Examples of blood-ethanol profiles in experiments with nine healthy men who drank 0.8 gram of ethanol per kilogram of body weight in thirty minutes after an overnight (ten-hour) fast. The drink was made from ethanol solvent (96% v/v) diluted with orange juice to make a 15–20% v/v cocktail.*

otide (NAD+), which becomes converted into its reduced form (NADH) during the reaction. The acetate produced in the course of ethanol biotransformation enters into normal pathways of metabolism and is converted into acetyl coenzyme A. The end products of ethanol metabolism are carbon dioxide and water. Forensic science aspects of ethanol metabolism were reviewed in detail by Jones (1991).

The increase in the ratio NADH/NAD+ observed during the metabolism of ethanol has important influences on the normal functioning of the liver (Day and Yeaman, 1994). Biochemical processes that involve NAD-dependent redox reactions are perturbed during combustion of ethanol (Lieber 1990; Lieber, 1994a). Accordingly, the redox state of the liver changes towards a more reduced environment, and among other things, the oxidation of fatty acids is hampered, gluconeogenesis (production of glucose) is impaired, and the ratios of lactate to pyruvate, and β-hydroxy-butyrate to acetoacetate increase appreciably. Many of the untoward effects of heavy drinking, including development of fatty liver, lactic acidosis, and gout can be explained by this altered redox state in the hepatocyte (Lieber, 1990).

4.4 Isoenzymes of Alcohol Dehydrogenase

The enzyme mainly responsible for the conversion of ethanol into acetaldehyde is called alcohol dehydrogenase (alcohol; NAD+ oxidoreductase, EC I.I.I.I.), abbreviated simply as ADH. This enzyme is widely distributed in body organs and tissue such as stomach, kidney, and lungs but is predominantly located in the cytosol of the liver cell. Mammalian ADH was first purified from horse liver in the late 1940s by Bonnichsen and Wassén (1948) and its physiological role during evolution was probably to protect the body from alcohols produced endogenously or ingested with overripe fruits or sugar-containing substances such as berries or honey that might have become fermented (Krebs and Perkins, 1970). Few enzymes have been studied so extensively as mammalian ADH and with the tools of molecular biology, the genes encoding these peptides have now been cloned (Hittle and Crabb, 1988).

Mammalian ADH belongs to a family of enzymes organized into six different classes (I to VI) depending on their structure, physicochemical properties including substrate specificity and sensitivity to inhibitors (Jörnvall and Höög, 1995). The ADH

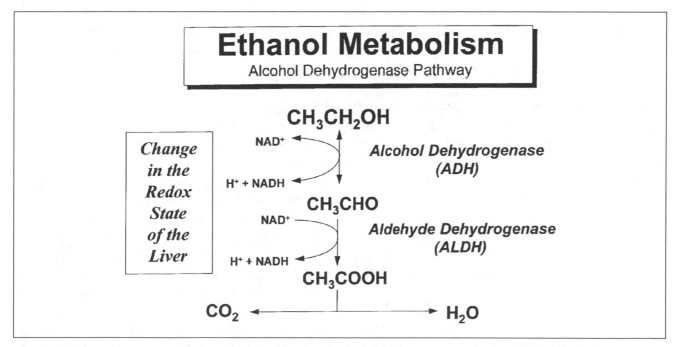

Figure 4.2 *The enzymatic oxidation of ethanol by the alcohol dehydrogenase pathway. ADH = alcohol dehydrogenase, ALDH = Aldehyde dehydrogenase, NAD^+ = oxidized form of the coenzyme nicotinamide adenine dinucleotide, NADH = reduced form of the coenzyme. Note that the first step, the oxidation of ethanol to acetaldehyde, is a reversible reaction.*

molecule is a polypeptide chain consisting of about 375 amino acid residues and has a molecular weight of 40,000 daltons. Each active enzyme is a dimeric molecule comprised of two ADH subunits. Depending on the way that the individual polypeptide subunits combine together, various isozymes are possible (Von Wartburg and Papenberg, 1966). However, individual subunits within the six different enzyme classes do not cross-hybridize to give active dimeric molecules. Each enzyme contains two atoms of zinc and this metal is essential for maintaining catalytic activity (Pettersson, 1987). The class-I ADH is genetically polymorphic and the various allelic forms encode polypeptide chains with tiny differences in the positioning of one or more amino acids. Switching the position of a single amino acid making-up the peptide chains might dramatically influences the catalytic properties of the enzyme. Indeed, the polymorphism of class-I ADH is considered as a likely explanation for the observed differences in rates of ethanol metabolism in different individuals and between racial groups (Crabb et al., 1987; Ehrig et al., 1990; Mizoi et al., 1994).

Table 4.1 gives details of isoenzymes of human class-I ADH which is the main hepatic enzyme involved in the oxidation of ethanol. The three subunits of Class-I ADH are denoted with the Greek letters alpha (α), beta (β), and gamma (γ) and these can associate randomly to produce six possible active enzyme dipeptides. Moreover, the genes ADH1 and ADH2 that encode the beta and gamma peptides are polymorphic which results in the production of alleloenzymes comprising three different β subunits (β_1, β_2, β_3) and two different γ subunits (γ_1, γ_2). These alleloenzymes can also combine in various ways to produce dipeptides and examples of homodimers and heterodimers are shown in Table 4.1 (Crabb et al., 1993). The three β homodimers are interesting because they have widely different catalytic properties and are expressed with different frequencies in different racial groups (Borson and Li, 1986). Studies have shown that European Caucasians have a predominance of the homodimer $\beta_1\beta_1$ isozyme whereas 85 percent of Orientals have $\beta_2\beta_2$ as the dominant form (known previously as atypical ADH). In about 25 percent of African Americans there is an abundance of the $\beta_3\beta_3$ form. Oriental populations

who inherit the β_2-ADH could therefore have both homodimer $\beta_2\beta_2$ and heterodimer $\beta_2\beta_1$ isozymes in liver cells (Harada, 1990; Harada and Okuda, 1993). The $\beta_2\beta_2$ form of the enzyme has a high V_{max} for the oxidation of ethanol and accordingly individuals inheriting this isozyme should be able to eliminate ethanol faster than those with a preponderance of the β_1-ADH which has a lower V_{max} compared with the β_2 isozymes. Despite the well documented differences in ADH isoenzyme in different racial groups the rates of ethanol disposal were surprisingly not much influenced by this (Adachi et al., 1993; Mizoi et al., 1994). This probably stems from large intra-ethnic group variability in the rates of ethanol metabolism owing to dietary and environmental factors. Indeed, in well controlled studies in which the test subjects were carefully matched for age, body composition, use of drugs and their smoking and drinking habits, no statistically significant racial differences in the rate of ethanol disposal have been found (Bennion and Li, 1976; Reed, 1978).

The Class-I ADH enzymes also metabolize secondary alcohols but the oxidation products are ketones instead of aldehydes. Thus 2-propanol and 2-butanol are oxidized into acetone and 2-butanone respectively. Under appropriate conditions (e.g., excess NADH in the hepatocyte) these ketones can also be reduced to the corresponding alcohols (Jones, 1995b).

4.5 The Existence of ADH in the Stomach

Recent studies have shown that ADH (class IV) is widely expressed in the stomach of various species, including man, and this has been confirmed by immuno-histochemical methods that are difficult to fault (Seitz et al., 1993). The class-IV stomach ADH shows differences in catalytic activity depending on a person's age, sex, drinking habits and ethnic group (Danielsson et al., 1994). The existence of gastric ADH has attracted considerable interest among workers in biomedical alcohol research as an explanation for the lower bioavailability of ethanol after oral compared with intravenous administration of the same dose. This work has spin-off effects in forensic toxicology whenever theoretical estimates of BAC are made (e.g., according to Widmark's method). The gastric ADH has a much higher k_m

value for ethanol than liver class-I ADH (Parés et al., 1994), which means that the enzyme is active in an environment with high concentrations of ethanol such as the stomach shortly after drinking. Indeed, some investigators believe that gastric ADH has an important physiological function by starting the metabolism of ethanol already in the stomach. It has been suggested that inter-subject differences in activity of gut-ADH might be one reason for the inherent differences in ethanol-induced organ toxicity and untoward effects of alcohol on the body (Lieber, 1994a and 1994b). In-vitro experiments have demonstrated that gastric ADH is inhibited by various drugs (e.g., aspirin, ranitidine and cimetidine) and it was suggested that these examples of drug-alcohol interaction might have important social-medical consequences (Hernandez-Munoz et al., 1990; Roine et al., 1990). This topic will be discussed in more detail later.

4.6 Aldehyde Dehydrogenase

The second stage in the metabolism of ethanol involves the oxidation of acetaldehyde into its nontoxic metabolite, acetate, and this process occurs through an irreversible reaction (Figure 4.2). This biological oxidation is catalyzed by the enzyme aldehyde dehydrogenase (ALDH; aldehyde: NAD+ oxidoreductase, EC 1.2.1.3) which is a tetrameric enzyme composed of four protein subunits (Goedde and Agarwal 1990). At least two major isoenzymes exist, denoted ALDH-1 and ALDH-2 and these are located in different subcellular compartments. The mitochondrial isoenzyme (ALDH-2) has a low k_m (1 µM or 44 mg/L) which helps to ensure that very low concentrations of AcH circulate in the blood during oxidation of ethanol. The ALDH-1 isozyme has a higher k_m for acetaldehyde (50–100 µM or 2.2–4.4 mg/L) and is mainly located in the cytosol fraction of the hepatocyte. Besides the presence of ALDH in the liver, this enzyme is widely distributed in other body organs and tissue such as kidney, stomach, intestine, lung, brain, muscle and in the erythrocytes (Helander, 1993). The mitochondrial ALDH is encoded for by the ALDH2 gene which exhibits polymorphism. The low-k_m mitochondrial enzyme encoded in 40–50 percent of Japanese and also in other Oriental races (Chinese, Koreans, Vietnamese and Thais) lacks enzymatic activity. Individuals inheriting this mutant form of ALDH are highly sensitive to even small doses of alcohol and this imparts in them a natural protection against heavy drinking and alcoholism (Agarwal and Goedde, 1992; Thacker et al., 1984). The rate of ethanol elimination was slightly slower in Japanese subjects who were deficient in

Table 4.1
Isoenzymes of Human Class-I Alcohol Dehydrogenase

The various isoenzymes and allelozymes have slightly different arrangement of the amino acids, different electrophoretic and kinetic properties, and catalytic activity.

Gene Locus[1]	Allele	Protein Product[2]	Kinetic Constant	Genetic Occurrence
ADH1		α		
ADH2	ADH2*1	β_1	low k_m	90% Whites
	ADH2*2	β_2	high k_m & V_{max}	85% Orientals
	ADH3*3	β_3		25% Blacks
ADH3	ADH3*1	γ_1		
	ADH3*2	γ_2		

[1] The genes encoding ADH enzymes are located on chromosome 4.

[2] Each subunit or protein product (α, β, and γ) contains two atoms of zinc and 90–95% of the amino acid positions in each subunit are identical. The active enzymes are formed by random dimeric association of the three polypeptide subunits and homodimers ($\beta\beta$) and heterodimers ($\alpha\beta$) are possible. The ADH2 and ADH3 genes encoding the β and γ subunits are polymorphic resulting in allelic variants differing in a single amino acid residue (e.g., argine instead of histidine at the forty-seventh position). The subunits combine to form active enzymes and both homodimers, $\beta_1\beta_1$, $\gamma_2\gamma_2$ and heterodimers $\beta_1\beta_2$, $\gamma_1\gamma_2$ are possible.

the low-k_m mitochondrial ALDH (Mizoi et al., 1987). In the normal ALDH subjects, the β-slope was 15.8 mg/dL/h compared with 13.6 mg/dL/h in the alcohol-sensitive ALDH deficient group.

4.7 Microsomal Ethanol Oxidizing System

Besides the alcohol dehydrogenase pathway, enzymes that metabolize ethanol are also located in the microsomal fraction of the liver cell, actually within the smooth endoplasmic reticulum. The discovery of this additional pathway of ethanol disposal, originally called the microsomal ethanol oxidizing system (MEOS), opened up exciting new areas of research such as studies of the mechanism of drug-alcohol interactions (Lieber and DeCarli, 1972). MEOS belongs to the cytochrome P450 family of enzymes that play such a crucial role in the metabolism of many endogenous and exogenous substances (Teschke and Gellert, 1986; Gonzalez 1989). The cytochrome P450 enzymes are a primary defence mechanisms for detoxifying xenobiotics imbibed with the diet or inhaled with the air we breath. Several kinds of cytochrome P450 molecules are present in the liver and these have a broad and overlapping substrate specificity (Koop and Coon, 1986). The cytochrome P450 enzyme involved in the metabolism of ethanol has been designated P450IIE1 and is also responsible for the detoxification of aromatic hydrocarbons such as toluene and benzene as well as chlorinated alkanes (trichloroethylene, chloroform), acetone, 1-butanol, and 2-propanol (Teschke and Gellert, 1986).

The P450IIE1 system has a higher k_m for ethanol, being about 60–80 mg/dL compared with 2–5 mg/dL for class-I ADH (Lieber and DeCarli, 1970). This means that the BAC must exceed the k_m value and therefore be above about 100 mg/dL before the P450 enzyme starts to play a significant role in the disposal of ethanol. More importantly, the microsomal enzymes are inducible, that is, they become more effective in the oxidation of drugs and xenobiotics after repeatedly being exposed to substrate owing to increased synthesis of the enzyme (Mezey, 1972). Accordingly, alcoholics and heavy drinkers acquire an enhanced capacity to metabolize ethanol in the course of their chronic drinking episodes (Mezey and Tobon, 1971). However, this hy-

peractivity is rapidly reversible and after a few days of abstinence the ability of an alcoholic to oxidize ethanol faster than a moderate drinker is lost (Mezey, 1972; Keiding et al., 1983). The enhanced activity of P450IIE1 enzymes is one biological mechanism accounting for metabolic tolerance and the observation that alcoholics sometimes have burn-off rates exceeding 30 mg/dL/h (0.03 g% per hour). A recent study in twenty-two chronic alcoholics reported that the rate of ethanol disappearance from blood (β-slope) ranged from 13 to 36 mg/dL/h with a mean of 22 mg/dL/h (Jones and Sternebring, 1992). Similar rapid rates of ethanol disposal in alcoholics during detoxification have been reported by other investigators (Bogusz et al., 1977; Adachi et al., 1989; Haffner et al., 1991).

Because many other drugs and environmental chemicals serve as substrates for P450 enzymes, the potential for pharmacodynamic drug-alcohol interactions is obvious (Lieber, 1990; Lieber, 1994a). Thus alcoholics might respond differently to a certain dose of drug or medication that proved effective for a patient with moderate drinking habits. Furthermore, the enhanced activity of the P450IIE1 enzymes in alcoholics means they also metabolize a host of environmental chemicals and toxins faster than expected creating a potential danger from highly reactive metabolites of these substances (Lieber 1994a). This renders alcoholics more vulnerable to the toxic and carcinogenic effects of organic solvents such as aromatic hydrocarbons (benzene, toluene), trichloroethylene and carbon tetrachloride. The ethanol-inducible cytochrome P450 is also activated by dietary influences such as prolonged fasting and eating low carbohydrate diets (Sato and Nakajima, 1985; Sato and Nakajima, 1987).

4.8 Biomedical Research on Acetaldehyde

Biomedical research on acetaldehyde began to gather momentum during the early fifties and coincided with the development and testing of tetraethylthiuram disulfide (disulfiram) the prototype alcohol-sensitizing drug. The pharmacology of the interaction between alcohol and disulfiram was studied extensively by researchers in Denmark and their work eventually culminated in the marketing of

Antabuse® now widely used as aversion therapy for the treatment of alcohol dependence (Hald et al., 1948). People who drink alcohol after taking Antabuse experience a multitude of unpleasant effects including throbbing headache, giddiness, accelerated pulse, tachycardia and difficulties in breathing (Asmussen et al., 1948). An intense flushing of the face develops sometimes spreading to the neck and upper arms and hence the expression alcohol-flush reaction. Hald and Jacobsen (1948) discovered that the concentrations of acetaldehyde in blood and breath were appreciably higher during the alcohol-antabuse reaction, compared with the same dose of alcohol taken alone or after a placebo treatment. Abnormally high concentrations of acetaldehyde in the body appear to be responsible for the adverse effects seen during the alcohol-Antabuse interaction (Christensen et al., 1991; Mizoi et al., 1979).

The enzymology and metabolism of acetaldehyde has been studied extensively in Japan where about 40–50 percent of the population normally experience unpleasant effects including facial flushing after drinking small amounts of alcohol. We now know that these alcohol-sensitive Japanese have an inactive mutant form of the low-k_m mitochondrial isoenzyme of aldehyde dehydrogenase (ALDH-2) (Mizoi et al., 1979; Yoshida, 1994). Accordingly, alcohol-sensitive individuals generate considerably higher concentrations of acetaldehyde in blood and breath after drinking alcohol. However, large inter-individual variations in the sensitivity to alcohol exist within the same ethnic group depending on the particular genotypes of ALDH inherited (Johnsen et al., 1992; Takeshita et al., 1993). Those with an inactive or deficient ALDH-2 isozyme (homozygous) are afforded a protection against heavy drinking and alcoholism because of their extreme sensitivity to the effects of acetaldehyde (Yin et al., 1992; Higuchi et al., 1994).

Acetaldehyde research entered the spotlight again in the 1970s when it was found that biogenic amines, such as dopamine and the indolamine serotonin reacted to produce pharmacologically active products (Cohen and Collins, 1970; Davis and Walsh, 1970). Dopamine reacts with acetaldehyde to form salsolinol and serotonin produces a β-carboline (Deitrich and Erwin, 1980). These Picket-Spengler condensation products, known as tetrahydroisoquinolines (TIQs), resemble the structure of intermediate products in the biosynthesis of opium alkaloids. Indeed, some experimental work showed that when TIQs were injected directly into the brain of mice or rats, the animals showed a preference for drinking alcohol in free-choice situations (Myers, 1976). These observations were thought to provide a possible molecular basis for alcohol dependence and addiction. Unfortunately, this research became suspect when it was shown that TIQs could be formed in-vitro during the analytical work-up procedure after blood and tissue were sampled (Eriksson, 1983; Lindros, 1983). Moreover, evidence began to appear suggesting that the concentrations of acetaldehyde reported in blood after drinking were artefactually high, unless special precautions had been taken immediately after sampling the blood (Eriksson and Fukunaga, 1993; Fukunaga et al., 1994).

The concentrations of ethanol in body fluids after drinking moderate amounts of alcohol are about 1,000–10,000 times higher than the concentration of acetaldehyde present. This means that even if minute quantities of ethanol are oxidized in the test tubes after sampling blood, the actual in-vivo concentrations of acetaldehyde are grossly overestimated. Besides a spontaneous formation of AcH from ethanol, it was discovered that a rapid disappearance was also occurring but to a lesser extent, so the overall effect was an abnormally high concentration of blood-acetaldehyde (Eriksson, 1983; Nuutinen et al., 1983; Eriksson and Fukunaga, 1993). Large variability in analytical results seemed to depend on the kind of sample pretreatment used before quantitative analysis. Scores of publications appeared describing various ways to minimize and correct for this artifact formation (e.g., by rapidly (<1 minute) removing erythrocytes, or by precipitation of plasma proteins with perchloric acid or trapping acetaldehyde as its semicarbizone derivative before removal of proteins) (reviewed by Eriksson, 1983). All these methods as well as numerous modifications have been reviewed in detail elsewhere and will not be covered here (Eriksson, 1980; Eriksson, 1983; Lindros, 1983; Stowell, 1989; Eriksson and Fukunaga, 1993). Because of these difficulties, the appearance of an acetaldehyde peak on the gas chromatogram when blood samples from drunk drivers or autopsy blood specimens are analyzed, should not be interpreted as reflecting the in-vivo concentrations of AcH at the time of sampling blood or when death occurred. Reports of high concentrations of blood-acetaldehyde in forensic toxicology casework should be considered with caution.

It was becoming increasingly apparent that another approach was needed for studying the metabolism of acetaldehyde and its role in ethanol-induced organ toxicity and alcohol dependence. Some investigators focused attention on the analysis of acetaldehyde in the expired air as an alternative and indirect way to monitor the concentrations of AcH in pulmonary blood (Stowell 1989; Jones 1995a). Like ethanol, acetaldehyde crosses the alveolar-capillary membrane of the lungs and can be detected in the exhaled air. Breath tests for acetaldehyde were therefore considered a more practical and convenient approach for clinical purposes because of the non-invasive sampling technique (Jones et al., 1988; Fukunaga et al., 1989). The plasma-to-air partition ratio of acetaldehyde at 34°C is about 190:1 compared with 2,100:1 for ethanol (Jones, 1995a). Unfortunately, breath-tests for acetaldehyde are also fraught with difficulties because of the possibility of this compound being formed locally within the upper-airway and the mouth (Jauhonen et al., 1982). The concentrations of acetaldehyde actually present in the pulmonary blood were therefore overestimated by analyzing breath samples (Stowell et al., 1984).

Nevertheless, the analysis of acetaldehyde in the breath provides a fast and non-invasive way to monitor the exposure of the lungs and upper-airway to this toxic volatile metabolite of ethanol. The results of analyzing breath AcH should be reported as the concentration in the specimen analyzed without attempting to translate into the presumed blood or plasma concentration. The concentration of AcH in end-expired breath mirrors the concentration in the pulmonary blood as well as any produced in the lungs and upper airway by bacterial action and microorganisms (Jones, 1995a).

Table 4.2 gives the concentrations of acetaldehyde in human breath for different test conditions. The very low levels of AcH produced endogenously were determined with the aid of a highly sensitive gas chromatographic technique after the breath-AcH content in the specimens was enriched by freeze-trapping (Dannecker et al., 1981; Hesselbrock and Shaskan, 1985). Much higher concentrations of AcH appear in exhaled air during the oxidation of ethanol, especially in individuals with genetically inactive ALDH enzyme such as many Japanese and other Asians (Fukunaga et al., 1989). The highest concentrations of breath AcH were seen after the low-k_m mitochondrial ALDH enzyme was blocked by taking

Table 4.2
Concentrations of Acetaldehyde Measured in Human Expired Air under Different Conditions

Subjects and Test Conditions		Breath Acetaldehyde Concentration (µg/L)
Alcoholics (endogenous level)	Smokers	0.25 ± 0.002
	Non-smokers	0.014 ± 0.003
Non-Alcoholics (endogenous level)	Smokers	0.016 ± 0.003
	Non-smokers	0.004 ± 0.001
Intake of EtOH (0.40 g/kg)	Flushers[1]	10.8 ± 5.5
	Non-flushers	2.1 ± 1.4
Intake of EtOH (0.25 g/kg)	Placebo[2]	range 0.4–1.5[4]
	Calcium carbimide[3]	range 9.2–56[4]

[1] Alcohol-sensitive Japanese subjects with inactive form of ALDH

[2] European Caucasians

[3] Calcium carbimide (50 mg), a potent inhibitor of ALDH, taken one hour before ethanol

[4] N = ten subjects

the drug calcium carbimide before drinking a small dose of ethanol (Jones et al., 1988). However, even under these extreme test conditions, the peak breath AcH only reached 56 μg/L and this concentration was insufficient to give an "apparent ethanol" response when breath samples were analyzed with a single wavelength (3.4 μm) infrared analyzer called Intoxilyzer 4011 (Jones 1986). Accordingly, allegations that elevated concentrations of acetaldehyde, the proximate metabolite of ethanol by all known pathways, is a potential interfering substance when breath-alcohol instruments are used for medicolegal purposes is yet another "red herring" (Jones, 1995a). Moreover those individuals with a very high concentration of acetaldehyde in their breath also had an intense flushing of the face and neck, complained of tachycardia (rapid beating of the heart), difficulties in breathing and feelings of nausea (Jones et al., 1988), providing some physiological evidence of the validity of the analytical findings.

4.9 Aspects of Ethanol Pharmacokinetics

The subject of pharmacokinetics is concerned with the way that drugs and their metabolites are absorbed, distributed, and eliminated from the body (Roland and Tozer, 1980). The elimination process encompasses both biotransformation and excretion of the parent drug unchanged together with its metabolites. The work of Erik M. P. Widmark published during the 1930s is still widely accepted and cited in medicolegal practice when the pharmacokinetics of ethanol are discussed (Widmark, 1932). The Widmark equation and its application in forensic casework have been dealt with in depth in other chapters in this book and will not be repeated here. Instead, results of more recent studies of the pharmacokinetics of ethanol will be highlighted with emphasis on factors that influence the peak BAC reached after drinking and the rate of disappearance of ethanol from the bloodstream (Jones, 1993).

It is important to remember that Widmark's experiments were carried out under the following strictly controlled conditions. First, the volunteer subjects were healthy men (N = 20) and women (N = 10), all of whom were moderate drinkers. Second, they ingested a moderate dose of ethanol (0.50–0.90 g/kg), given in the form of undiluted spirits (30–40

percent v/v) and taken on an empty stomach within about fifteen minutes. Third, samples of capillary (fingertip) blood were drawn at thirty to sixty minute intervals and the concentrations of ethanol were determined by a chemical oxidation method. The analytical results were reported in mass/mass units of concentration actually mg ethanol per gram whole blood (mg/g) because the aliquots taken for analysis were weighed on a torsion balance. If Widmark's experimental conditions are changed, such as by switching beer or wine for spirits or giving alcohol together with or after food instead of an empty stomach, or measuring breath-alcohol instead of blood-alcohol, the resulting pharmacokinetic parameters (β and "r") will not agree with those reported in his monograph (Widmark 1932). The β-slope was defined by Widmark as the rate of disappearance of ethanol from blood per minute although today the rate of elimination per hour is widely used (β_{60}). The average β-slope was slightly steeper for women compared with men, but on the average being 0.0025 mg/g/min or 0.15 mg/g/h (span 0.10–0.24 mg/g/h)[3]. Because the concentration units used to report blood-ethanol in this pioneer work by Widmark were mass/mass, the r factor relating the concentration of alcohol in the body (g/kg) to the concentration in the blood (mg/g) is a dimensionless ratio. The units most commonly used today for r are liters/kilogram because mass/volume units such as (mg/mL, g/dL, g/L) are used when reporting blood-ethanol concentrations. In the terminology used in pharmacokinetics, the Widmark r factor corresponds to the volume of distribution for ethanol which is sometimes abbreviated V_d and its value corresponds well with a person's total body water (Roland and Tozer, 1980; Jones et al., 1992).

Variability in r depends primarily on the person's body composition, especially the amount of water per kilogram of body weight and therefore the proportion of fat to lean tissue in the organism (Watson et al., 1981; Wang et al., 1992). Body water decreases in the elderly and r factors for men 20–29 years, 30–39 years, 40–49 years and 50–59 years were 0.72 ± 0.042, 0.71 ± 0.036, 0.68 ± 0.026, and 0.66 ± 0.041 L/kg (mean ± SD), respectively (Jones and Neri, 1985). Because women have less water per unit body mass compared with men, they can be expected to have a smaller volume of distribution—lower *r* factor (Goist and Sutker, 1985). Widmark reported an average *r* value of 0.68 for men (span 0.51–0.85) and 0.55 for women (span 0.44–0.66). These *r* values for men have been confirmed in several recent controlled studies of the pharmacokinetics of ethanol (Jones, 1984; Joncs and Neri, 1985).

The metabolism and pharmacokinetics of ethanol in women have not been investigated as thoroughly as in men. However, one early study with twenty women found values of *β* and *r* in close agreement with those reported by Widmark (Österlind et al., 1944). Some studies in women have focused on the influence of oral contraceptive steroids and also hormonal changes associated with the menstrual cycle (Jones and Jones 1984; Hobbes et al., 1985; Marshall et al., 1983; Brick et al., 1986). The results of this research are conflicting and definite conclusions cannot be drawn because increases, decreases, and no changes in *β*-slope have been reported in various studies of the interaction between ethanol and contraceptive steroid drugs (Sutker et.

al, 1987). Women tend to have a slightly faster rate of elimination of ethanol from blood compared with men as reflected in a steeper *β*-slope and this observation has been confirmed by numerous investigators (Dubowski, 1976; Marshall et al., 1983; Cole-Harding et al., 1987; Jones, 1989). However a steeper *β*-slope in combination with a smaller volume of distribution in females (lower *r* factor) means that the overall rate of clearance of ethanol from the body expressed as g/kg/h and defined as the product of *β* and *r* was not statistically significant between the sexes (Jones 1989). As a rule of thumb, the rate of body clearance of alcohol is about 0.10 g/kg/h and therefore a person weighing 70 kilograms can eliminate 7 grams of pure ethanol per hour or roughly the amount contained in one bottle of light beer.

Examples of blood-alcohol profiles obtained after intake of alcohol on an empty stomach are shown in Figure 4.1. Certain key features of these curves of particular interest in forensic science are illustrated in Figure 4.3. The time needed to reach the peak BAC after the end of drinking, the increment in the

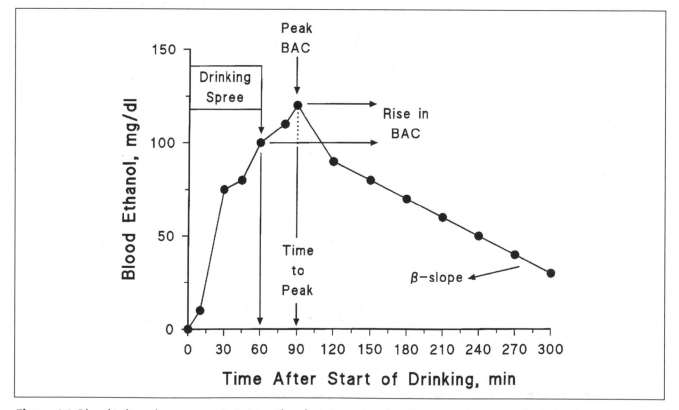

Figure 4.3 *Blood-ethanol concentration-time plot showing some key features of interest in medicolegal casework (e.g., driving under the influence of alcohol (DUI)). Alcohol was ingested over sixty minutes and the peak BAC was reached thirty minutes after the end of drinking.*

BAC before reaching the maximum concentration and the slope of the rectilinear post-peak disappearance phase (β-slope) are indicated. The results of measuring β-slope in a large number of controlled drinking experiments are collected together in Table 4.3 which highlights the considerable inter-individual variability in this pharmacokinetic parameter, spanning from 9 to 36 mg/dL/h. The lowest values were seen in fasted subjects who ingested a bolus dose of ethanol in the morning and the highest values were observed in alcoholics during detoxification. This fourfold difference emphasizes the dangers associated in assuming an average burn-off rate when retrograde extrapolations of a person's BAC from time of sampling to the time of driving are contemplated; such a practice which is sometimes required by law.

Another critical element in any attempt at retrograde extrapolation is the position of the BAC curve at the time of driving and at the time of obtaining the blood sample, that is, whether the blood-alcohol concentration increases, remains unchanged, or decreases after the actual driving incident. Table 4.3 presents the median and range of times necessary to reach peak BAC after the end of drinking for various experimental protocols. Most of these studies involved rapid drinking of a moderate dose of alcohol on an empty stomach and these conditions are not very comparable with real-life situations and drinking practices. Moreover, time to peak as a measure of the rate of absorption of ethanol is always skewed to the right so the median or mode are better statistics to indicate central tendency than the arithmetic mean. Table 4.3 shows that most subjects reached peak BAC within sixty minutes after the end of drinking but some required 120 minutes or more. A more prolonged absorption phase and a later occurring peak was frequently observed when alcohol was taken together with or after a meal compared with drinking on an empty stomach. But even when an exceptionally long time was necessary to reach a maximum BAC much of the alcohol was absorbed by the time drinking ended. Thereafter, the BAC increased further at a variable rate before reaching the maximum level. Sometimes, a very gradual increase was seen or no change at all in BAC for thirty to ninety minutes before the curve started to decrease in the post-peak phase. Occasionally, a flat-topped BAC time-course is seen when the rate of absorption is matched by the rate of elimination and the BAC tends to remain at a constant level. But remember that even during the absorption phase and on a plateau, the molecules of alcohol are still being cleared from the body by enzymatic oxidation in the liver at a rate of about 0.1 g/kg body weight per hour. Although the BAC might be decreasing, which gives

Table 4.3
Rates of Disappearance of Ethanol from Blood (Mean and Range) and the Times of Reaching Peak BAC on Controlled Experiments for Various Drinking Conditions

Conditions	N[1]	Mean β-slope	Time to peak[2]
Straight whisky[3]	150	13.4 (9–18)	30 (5–105)
EtOH[3] + juice	65	14.1 (12–17)	60 (0–120)
Drinks + food	15	16.0 (13–21)	78 (0–230)
Alcohol + food	10	17.4 (14–20	90 (15–90)
Alcohol alone[3]	10	14.2 (12–17)	45 (0–60)
Beer[4] + food	9	12.0 (9–15)	7 (5–25)
Beer alone	9	15.0 (10–18)	16 (5–45)
Alcoholics[5]	20	23.0 (14–36)	##[5]

[1] Number of subjects

[2] After end of drinking, median and range

[3] Alcohol on empty stomach after overnight fast

[4] Two bottles of beer

[5] Tests made during detoxification all were in the post-peak phase

the impression of a post-absorptive phase, absorption from the gut can still be taking place but more slowly than the rate of clearance of ethanol from the bloodstream, being approximately 15 mg/dL/h.

Figure 4.4 shows plots of blood-ethanol concentration against time for two men accustomed to heavy drinking. In this experiment they drank beer or spirits according to choice at regular intervals for about six to ten hours (Zink and Reinhardt, 1984). Blood samples were drawn from an indwelling catheter every fifteen minutes during and after the drinking so the time of reaching the peak BAC was carefully noted. These plots show that with this kind of

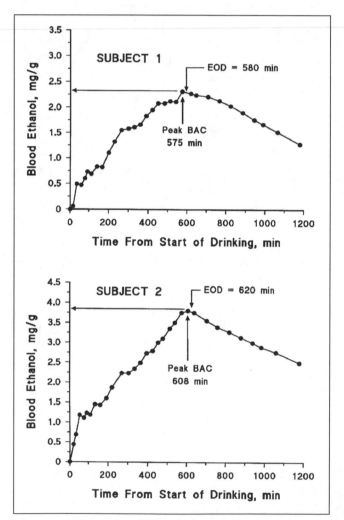

Figure 4.4 *Examples of blood-alcohol concentration profiles in two men during continuous heavy drinking lasting for about ten hours. Blood samples were taken every fifteen minutes from an indwelling catheter. (Figure redrawn from data published by Zink and Reinhardt, Blutalkohol 21;422–442, 1984).*

drinking pattern the highest BAC was sometimes reached even before the end of drinking. During prolonged heavy drinking, it seems that so much alcohol has become equilibrated with body fluids and tissues that the quantity of alcohol contained in the last gulp of alcoholic beverage is insufficient to raise the BAC any further. Obviously, this conclusion depends on how much alcohol was contained in the last drink consumed and this information was not made perfectly clear in the report by Zink and Reinhardt (1984). However, six of the volunteer subjects had reached their maximum BAC before the end of drinking, two subjects at the same time as they finished the drink and six subjects at various times after the last drink was taken.

Another interesting aspect of this same study arose when the peak BAC, which ranged from 2.2–3.8 mg/g (220–380 mg/100 g or 232–400 mg/dL), was compared with the theoretical expected values based on the amount of alcohol consumed, the drinking time frame, and the subject's body weight. The BAC calculated according to Widmark's equation vastly exceeded the actual BAC sometimes by as much as 50 percent or more. The reason for this discrepancy is not fully understood but it seems likely that the rate of ethanol disposal was much faster than expected during the six-to-ten-hour drinking spree. Whether this can be explained by the induction of P450IIE1 enzymes in these regular heavy drinkers or an effective first-pass metabolism remains unsettled. The more effective clearance of ethanol seemed to be occurring during the absorption (drinking) period because in the post-peak phase the rate of disappearance of ethanol from blood was not abnormally high, the β-slopes ranging from 0.11–0.27 mg/g/h (12–28 mg/dL/h).

4.10 Widmark or Michaelis-Menten Pharmacokinetics?

According to Widmark, the decrease in BAC during the post-peak phase occurs at a constant rate per unit time and zero-order elimination kinetics are said to operate. This process can be described mathematically with the simple equation, $C_t = C_o - \beta t$ (Widmark, 1932; Von Wartburg, 1989). However, when the BAC decreases and has reached a concentration below 10 mg/dL (0.01 g%) the straight line changes to a curvilinear disappearance profile. Accordingly, the entire post-peak elimination phase starting at a moderately high BAC and extending down to very low BAC (<0.01 g/dL) takes the shape of a hockey-stick (Wilkinson, 1980). The rectilinear phase and the hockey-stick part of the curve can be fitted to the Michaelis-Menten (M-M) equation. Here the rate of decrease in concentration with time ($-dC/dt$) depends on three parameters: (1) V_{max}, the maximum velocity of the enzymatic reaction, (2) k_m, the Michaelis constant or the concentration of substrate (ethanol) at half the maximum velocity and (3) the underlying initial blood-alcohol concentration (C). The M-M equation is depicted as

$$-dC/dt = [V_{max} \times C]/[k_m + C]$$

and can be converted into two limiting forms depending on the concentration (C) of ethanol in the blood. When C is much greater than the value of k_m (2–5 mg/dL for human class-I ADH), the M-M rate equation simplifies to

$$-dC/dt = V_{max}$$

and the elimination of ethanol occurs at a constant maximum velocity (zero-order kinetics). At very low concentrations much less than the k_m value, the rate of reaction becomes proportional to the prevailing concentration:

$$-dC/dt = [V_{max}/k_m] \times C$$

which is the same as

$$-dC/dt = k_1 \times C$$

corresponding to the equation for first-order kinetics.

The M-M equation has a long established history in biochemistry and a solid theoretical basis for enzymatic reaction processes when a single enzyme is involved. However, because of the existence of multiple forms of ADH (Table 4.1) with different k_m and V_{max} values a series of parallel M-M equations might be more appropriate to describe the elimination kinetics of ethanol. Moreover, a single M-M elimina-tion function takes no account of the participation of P450IIE1 enzymes in the elimination process.

Lundqvist and Wolthers (1958) were the first to investigate the elimination kinetics of ethanol in humans by fitting concentration-time data to the M-M equation. This contribution was continued by specialists in pharmacokinetics who subsequently gave their strong support for the use of this kinetic model for describing the post-peak phase of ethanol elimination in mathematical terms (Wagner et al., 1976; Wilkinson et al., 1977a; Wagner et al., 1989). Many papers have appeared pointing out the advantages and limitations of the M-M equation for describing ethanol kinetics compared with the simple one-compartment model with zero-order elimination first proposed by Widmark (for reviews see Wilkinson 1980; Holford, 1987; Von Wartburg, 1989).

Michaelis-Menten kinetics is sometimes referred to as dose dependent or saturation kinetics because the rate of metabolism approaches a limiting value (V_{max}) as the amount of drug administered increases. The enzyme system becomes progressively saturated with substrate as the concentration of drug reaching the reactive site of the enzyme increases. This pharmacokinetic model has attracted considerable interest not only as a model to describe the elimination kinetics of ethanol (Fujimiya et al., 1989) but also for other drugs such as propranolol, acetylsalicylic acid, and phenytoin.

Table 4.4 compares the rates of elimination of alcohol from blood calculated using the M-M equation starting at different initial BAC values (Forrest, 1986). Results are shown for two individuals with widely different V_{max} and k_m values, one being a fast metabolizer (V_{max} = 22.8 mg/dL/h and k_m = 9.5 mg/dL) and the other a slow metabolizer (V_{max} = 16.0 mg/dL/h and k_m = 6.0 mg/dL). For both individuals, the biggest difference in the rate of disposal of ethanol are evident at relatively low BAC (10–50 mg/dL). At higher blood-ethanol levels (100–300 mg/dL) the rate of elimination was relatively constant because the enzyme (ADH) is now almost fully saturated with substrate. The higher range of BAC has most relevance in forensic work because drunk drivers are heavy drinkers with an average BAC of 150 mg/dL in many countries. One might wonder whether much is gained by using the M-M equation

Table 4.4
Rates of Elimination of Ethanol as a Function of Initial Blood-Alcohol Concentration According to the Michaelis-Menten Equation: $-dC/dt = [V_{max} \times C]/[k_m + C]$

Values are shown for a fast and slow metabolizer of ethanol (data from Forrest 1986).

Blood Alcohol (mg/dL)	Fast Metabolizer[1] $-dC/dt$ (mg/dL/h)	Slow Metabolizer[2] $-dC/dt$ (mg/dL/h)
10	11.6	10.0
20	15.4	12.3
50	19.1	14.2
100	20.8	15.0
150	21.4	15.3
200	21.7	15.5
300	22.1	15.6

compared with the Widmark model with its assumption of a constant value for the β-slope independent of the BAC (Rango et al., 1981; Adachi et al., 1993). However, M-M kinetics should be the model of choice for questions where low BAC are of interest such as after intake of small doses of ethanol (Lewis, 1986).

4.11 The Magnitude of Inter- and Intra-Individual Variations

Human beings show an enormous variation in their response to ethanol as well as other drugs. Besides difference in behavioral response the disposition kinetics show marked variations from person to person and also within the same person from time to time. Jones and Jönsson (1994b) showed that 42 percent of the variance in β-slope was attributable to between subject variation and 58 percent was accounted for by variation within subjects. In the same study, other important pharmacokinetic parameters such as peak BAC, r, C_o, and AUC showed significantly more variation between than within subjects. The notion of conducting an alcohol tolerance test to establish a person's rate of alcohol disposal (β-slope) seems hardly worthwhile considering the large within subject variance component. Instead, a range of elimination rates such as 9 to 25 mg/dL/h can be assumed to apply and in my experience this should encompass actual values for the vast majority of individuals. Indeed, drunken drivers who are also heavy drinkers and often dependent on alcohol, would be more likely to have β-slopes of 20 mg/dL/

h or more rather than 10 mg/dL/h or less. Studies of ethanol metabolism in monozygotic and dizygotic twins have also demonstrated the involvement of both genetic and environmental influences on the pharmacokinetics of ethanol (Martin et al., 1985).

Figure 4.5 gives an indication of the repeatability of estimating the β-slope in controlled drinking experiments (Schonheyder et al., 1942). Three men drank fifty grams of alcohol on ten separate occasions and the post-peak parts of the curves were determined by analyzing a series of blood samples. The β-slope clearly varied as much within the same subject as between subjects. Note that all results fell within the range published by Widmark, namely 11–24 mg/100g/h (mean 15 mg/g/h).

The peak BAC reached after drinking ethanol as a bolus dose also exhibits considerable inter-subject variations and this seems to depend to a great extent on individual variations in the rate of gastric emptying (O'Neill et al., 1983; Jones et al., 1991). Although the absorption of ethanol starts in the stomach immediately after drinking, the rate of absorption is considerably faster from the upper part of the small intestine because of the much larger surface area available. Indeed, after drinking neat spirits on an empty stomach, the rate of absorption of ethanol is sometimes so fast that an overshoot peak is seen. The maximum BAC is higher than expected for the dose ingested because ethanol enters the bloodstream faster than it can be removed and diluted with the other water compartments of the body. An overshooting BAC arises whenever ethanol is given by

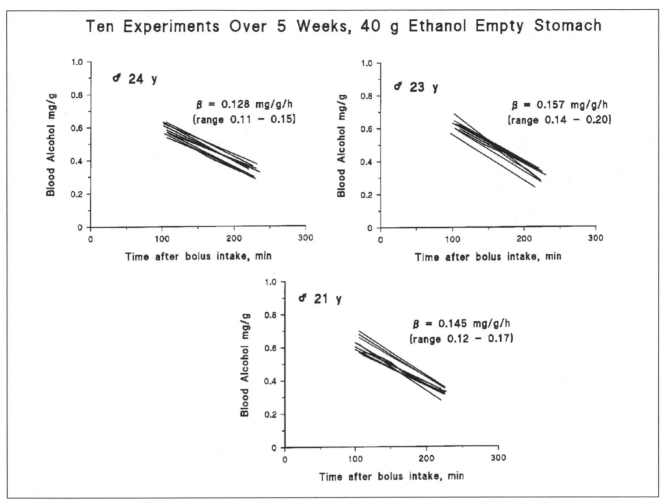

Figure 4.5 *Intra-individual variations in the elimination kinetics of ethanol in three subjects who ingested 0.5 g/kg on ten separate occasions. Data redrawn from paper by Schonheyder et al. (1942).*

rapid intravenous infusion. However, the overshoot is immediately followed by a diffusion plunge and the $t_{1/2}$ of this redistribution phase was recently estimated as 7 minutes (Hahn et al., 1995). Accordingly, 35 minutes ($5 \times t_{1/2}$) are required for ethanol molecules to equilibrate between blood and other body fluids. This new finding regarding the time for equilibration of ethanol after an overshoot peak might be useful to consider in drunk-driving litigation when bolus ingestion of alcohol just before driving is raised as a defence challenge.

4.12 The Zig-Zag or Steepling Effect

The notion of a zig-zag or irregular blood or breath-alcohol time course instead of a smooth post-absorptive elimination phase has attracted unprecedented attention in some quarters because of the obvious implications in forensic science practice (e.g., when

making back-estimation or forward projection of a person's BAC). Figure 4.6 shows blood-ethanol concentration-time data from an experiment described by Teige et al. (1974). Samples of venous blood were taken every one to two minutes through an indwelling catheter and ethanol was determined by gas chromatography. When plotted as a function of time an irregular zig-zag pattern is clearly seen. But this zig-zag trend can be accounted for by a combination of pre-analytical and analytical variations inherent in the methods of sampling blood and determination of alcohol. The insert shows the blood-ethanol time course for samples taken every twenty to thirty minutes. The zig-zag effect is now obliterated which underscores the importance of sampling protocol when studying this curious steepling phenomenon.

Figure 4.7 shows the concentration-time profiles of ethanol determined in our own ongoing experi-

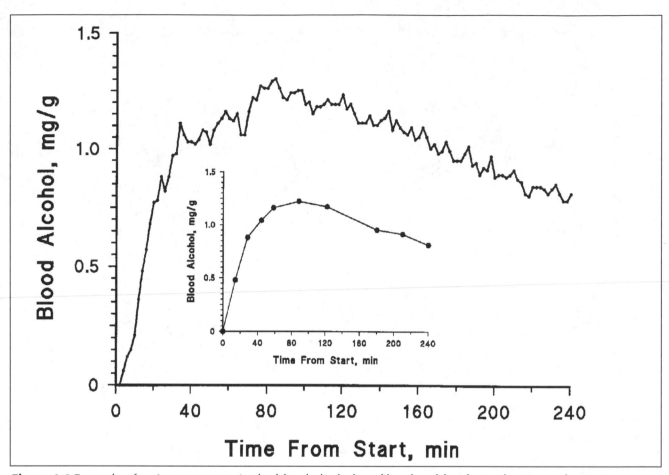

Figure 4.6 Example of a zig-zag pattern in the blood-alcohol profile when blood samples were taken every one to two minutes through an indwelling venous catheter. Ethanol 1.0 g/kg was ingested as wine (data from Teige et al., Blutalkohol 11;29–39, 1974). The small insert is the same data except that results for blood samples taken every thirty to sixty minutes are plotted.

ments concerning the zig-zag effect (unpublished work, 1995). A healthy male subject received the same dose of ethanol (0.4 g/kg) by intravenous infusion on two consecutive days. A long series of blood samples were taken into Vacutainer tube (5 mL each) with the aid of an indwelling venous catheter. Samples were taken every five minutes for four hours and then every ten to fifteen minutes for a further three hours. Note the lack of any marked irregularity or zig-zag pattern in these plots with a five-minute interval between successive samples. The linear decay profile can be seen to change into a hockey-stick shape at low BAC. The values of β-slope and r agreed perfectly on the two successive days for this subject who happened to be a relatively slow metabolizer of ethanol (β-slope 0.096 mg/mL/h or approximately 0.01 g% per hour). Blood samples were analyzed with a well proven gas chro-

matographic method of analysis so that the analytical sources of variation do not contribute to the zig-zag effect. Indeed, zig-zag effects might be expected to be more pronounced when various breath-alcohol analyzers are used to trace the alcohol time-course when very short intervals (one to two minutes) elapse between successive exhalations (Dubowski, 1985). This follows because of the additional physiological sources of variation inherent in methods of breath-alcohol analysis such as variations in body and breath temperature over time, depth of inhalation and exhalation, and the flow rate of breath into the instrument used for analysis and so on. (Jones et al., 1989).

In conclusion, it seems that the zig-zag patterns in blood- and breath-alcohol profiles are mainly a consequence of pre-analytical and analytical variations in the methods used for blood-alcohol analysis

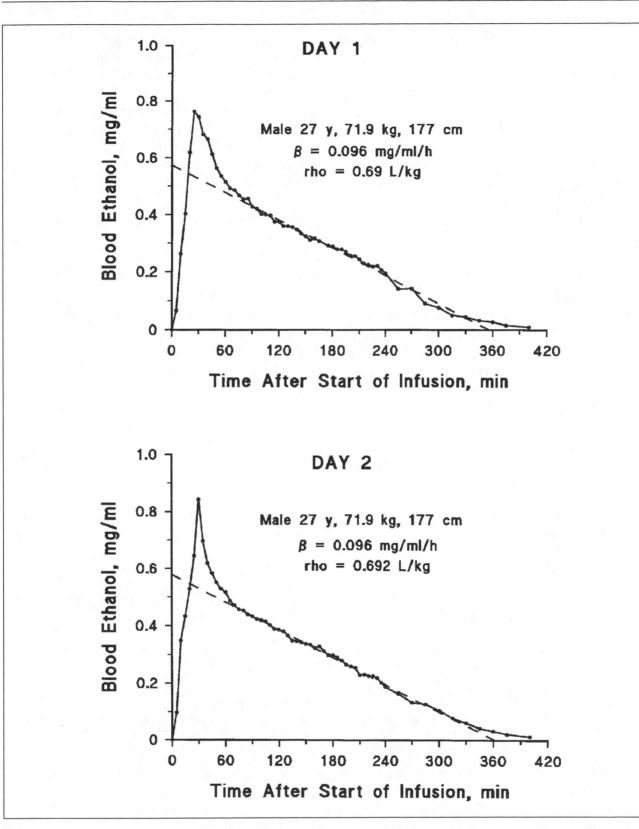

Figure 4.7 *Blood-concentration time profiles of ethanol in the same subject on two consecutive days. The dose of ethanol (0.4 g/kg) was administered by intravenous infusion over thirty minutes. For the first four hours Vacutainer tubes (5 mL) were filled every five minutes and then at fifteen to thirty minute intervals for another three hours. The blood ethanol concentration was determined by headspace gas chromatography.*

or breath sampling parameters when breath-instruments are used and breath-to-breath physiological variations in alcohol concentration. However, during the absorption of ethanol from the stomach an irregular rising phase has often been observed owing to the sudden and unpredictable opening and closing of the pyloric sphincter, a muscle that controls emptying of the stomach contents into the duodenum. This might produce a series of short bursts in absorption of alcohol into the portal blood flowing to the liver resulting in a sudden rise in the peripheral blood-alcohol concentration.

4.13 The Rate of Alcohol Elimination in Pathological Conditions

The bulk of the dose of ethanol administered is metabolized in the liver. Accordingly, liver disease such as hepatitis and cirrhosis might be expected to influence the rate of ethanol metabolism (Bode, 1978). For ethical reasons, conducting drinking experiments with hospitalized patients suffering from cirrhosis are not feasible. However, some older literature on this subject is available and the work of Jokippi (1951) deserves mention. His studies were done with male and female subjects and the patient material was well characterized clinically. They suffered from hepatitis, cirrhosis, diabetes mellitus, hyperthyroidism and dystonia (impaired functioning of the muscles). After an overnight fast, the subjects were challenged with a bolus dose of alcohol (0.5 g/kg as spirits), under the strictly controlled conditions advocated by Widmark (1932). Table 4.5 gives the mean and range of β-slopes for the different patient groups in comparison with a control group of healthy individuals. Test subjects with the various diseases had mean β-slopes within the same range as healthy control subjects except for a few low values in the patients. The lowest β-slope in the patient groups was 7 mg/dL/h or 0.007 g% per hour. The distribution of ethanol in the body as reflected in the value of Widmark's r was about the same for the patient groups and the control group of healthy subjects (Jokippi, 1951).

It seems that subjects suffering from various metabolic diseases and liver cirrhosis still maintain their ability to eliminate alcohol from the bloodstream (Mezey and Tobon, 1971; Lieberman, 1961). Most of the alcohol consumed is oxidized in the liver as demonstrated in experiments with hepatectomized or eviscerated animals (Clark et al., 1941). But even with the liver removed, these animals were capable of metabolizing ethanol: in an hepatectomized dog the elimination rate was 5.5 mg/dL/h compared with 14 mg/dL/h in control animals.

Articles citing an unusually wide range of β-slopes and especially the existence of extremely low

Table 4.5
Influence of Various Metabolic Diseases and Pathological Conditions on the Rate of Disappearance of Ethanol from the Bloodstream (β-slope)

The subjects drank 0.5 gram ethanol per kilogram of body weight as a bolus dose of spirits (30–40% v/v) after an overnight fast.

Subjects and Conditions	Mean values for men and women	
	Number of subjects	Mean β-slope[1] (span)
Healthy subjects	42 (19m, 23w)[2]	13 (10–17)
Dystonia[3]	17 (11m, 6w)	11 (7–15)
Hepatitis	19 (8m, 11w)	11 (7–14)
Cirrhosis	6 (5m, 1w)	11 (9–13)
Hyperthyreosis	15 (3m, 12w)	14 (8–19)
Diabetes mellitus	21 (13m, 8w)	12 (7–19)

[1] β = rate of disappearance of ethanol from blood in mg/dL/h

[2] m = men, w = women

[3] Dystonia is a disordered tonicity of muscles.

rates of alcohol elimination (below 8 mg/dL/h) are obviously not very reliable. These abnormal values are usually the result of making statistical projections from distributions with large standard deviation. This might occur, for example, when the mean and variance are calculated for a non-homogenous experimental group of subjects (e.g., by including moderate drinkers and alcoholics, or β-slopes for men and women, or drinking under fed and fasting conditions). Furthermore, drinking studies with an insufficient number of concentration-time points or an unusually large scatter can easily give unreliable estimates of β-slope. A classic example of this can be found in the paper by Winek and Murphy (1984) where a person with a β-value of 1 mg/dL/h was reported in a peer-review journal without comment. This abnormally low result should have been immediately suspect because in another experiment with the same individual the β-slope was 14 mg/dL/h. Finally the practice of calculating a person's β-slope by taking two blood samples one to two hours apart is not recommended. Although the rate of change in BAC over the sampling interval is obtained, this is not the most reliable indication of the person's rate of ethanol disposal (Neuteboom and Jones, 1990). This follows because the results obtained might be influenced by ongoing absorption and distribution of alcohol during the sampling interval. Reliable information about the phase of alcohol metabolism cannot be ascertained from analyzing just two blood samples.

4.14 First-Pass Metabolism of Ethanol

First-pass metabolism is a term associated with the oral administration of drugs and indicates that a certain amount of the active substance has been eliminated before reaching the systemic circulation (Pond and Tozer, 1994). Accordingly, molecules of the drug undergo pre-systemic metabolism either in the gut (stomach or intestine), or more commonly as the portal blood flows through the liver. First-pass metabolism is associated with a reduced and variable bioavailability and the pharmacological effect of the drug at its site of action is also diminished.

After oral administration, ethanol is absorbed from the stomach and intestine and transported with the portal vein through the liver then on to the heart via the hepatic vein before the systemic arteries distribute ethanol throughout the total body water. Experiments by several research groups have indicated that the area under the BAC time curve is considerably less after oral compared with intravenous administration of the same dose. Figure 4.8 compares blood-ethanol profiles in four subjects who were given 0.3 g/kg in a crossover design experiment either as a bolus dose taken orally (fifteen minutes) or by an intravenous infusion lasting thirty minutes. The smaller areas under the curves (AUCs) after oral compared with IV is one indication of a first-pass metabolism of alcohol occurring either in the stomach or during the time blood passes through the liver.

The existence of gastric ADH was considered as a likely mechanism accounting for pre-systemic metabolism of ethanol and one research group in particular embarked on extensive studies to prove the role of the stomach mucosa as a protective barrier against the toxic effects of ethanol (Caballeria et al., 1991; Dipadova et al., 1987; Gentry et al., 1994). The magnitude of first-pass oxidation of ethanol by gastric ADH seemed to be influenced by a host of variable factors: age, sex, drinking habits (alcoholism), type of beverage (beer or spirits) and the concomitant intake of various drugs (for reviews see Levitt, 1993; Lieber 1993, 1994a, 1994b). If significant presystemic metabolism of ethanol occurred this would have implications in forensic science when making theoretical estimates of a person's BAC for a given drinking scenario. The Widmark equation is widely used for this purpose and rests on the assumption of 100 percent availability of the dose of alcohol. One study suggested that the activity of gastric ADH was appreciably less in women compared with men and was also decreased in alcoholics compared with moderate drinkers (Frezza et al., 1990). Moreover, a large proportion of Japanese seemingly lacked an active gastric ADH enzyme. First-pass metabolism should therefore be small or negligible in these individuals (Baraona et al., 1991).

4.15 Histamine$_2$-Receptor Antagonists and the Pharmacokinetics of Ethanol

Two drugs widely used in the treatment of stomach ailments resulting from too much acidity, namely the prototype H$_2$-receptor antagonists cimetidine and

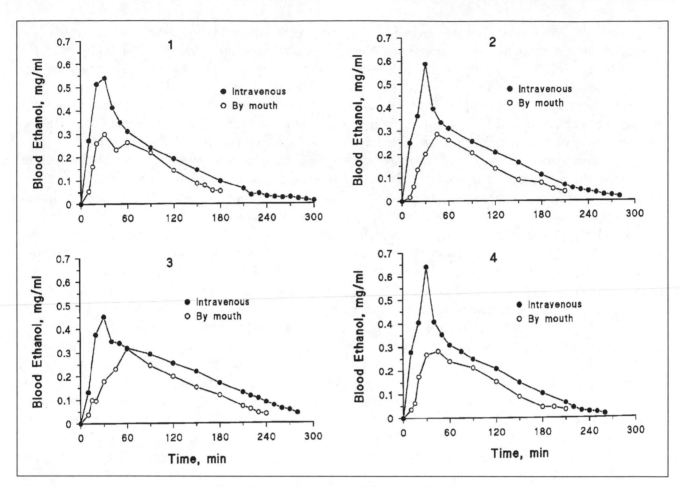

Figure 4.8 *Concentration-time profiles of ethanol in four healthy men after the same small dose of ethanol (0.3 g/kg) was given on two occasions after oral and intravenous administration (Jones et al., unpublished work)*

ranitidine, were shown to inhibit the activity of gastric ADH under in-vitro conditions (Palmer et al., 1991; Caballeria et al., 1991). Figure 4.9 compares the structure of cimetidine with two well-known inhibitors of class-I ADH enzymes namely pyrazole and 4-methyl pyrazole. The existence of a heterocyclic pyrazole-like ring in the cimetidine molecule was thought to account for its inhibitory effect on ADH enzymes. If H_2-receptor antagonists block the action of gastric ADH this might have implications for oral availability of ethanol and the maximum BAC reached after drinking (DiPadova, 1992; Palmer et al., 1991). It was pointed out that people taking these drugs together with alcohol might unknowingly develop higher peak BAC and this might have implications in connection with accidents at work and on the highway (DiPadova et al., 1992). This example of an adverse drug-alcohol interaction received considerable attention in the news media

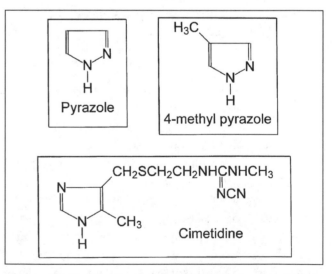

Figure 4.9 *Comparison of the chemical structure of two well known inhibitors of class-I isozymes of alcohol dehydrogenase, namely pyrazole and 4-methyl pyrazole and the prototype H_2-receptor antagonist (cimetidine) used to suppress production of gastric acid*

and even emerged as a defense challenge by some drinking drivers. The suspects or their lawyers maintained that the BAC was above the legal limit because of inadvertent ingestion of alcohol after medication with cimetidine and therefore they were guilty of DUI but without intent. Removing the potential for pre-systemic clearance of ethanol by taking these drugs should theoretically cause a higher blood-alcohol concentration compared with the situation without taking this medication (Levitt, 1994; Gentry et al., 1994). This kind of defense challenge should be vigorously protested because the absorption rate of alcohol and the peak BAC varies widely even within the same individual without any drug treatment. Moreover, drugs such as cimetidine and ranitidine cannot increase the dose of alcohol taken into the body. However, gastric emptying and therefore the rate of absorption into the bloodstream might be influenced by various drugs (Levitt and Levitt, 1994).

The importance of gastric metabolism of ethanol as the mechanism accounting for diminished bioavailability (smaller AUC) was challenged by Levitt (1994) because of the extremely small amount of ADH enzyme in the stomach compared with the abundance of hepatic ADH. He maintained that if a first-pass metabolism occurred it was more likely to take place in the liver rather than the stomach and convincing arguments were developed to support this notion. Moreover, a critical and hitherto unrecognized element in first-pass metabolism of ethanol was the rate of absorption itself (Levitt and Levitt, 1994). The smaller the dose of ethanol and the slower and more prolonged the absorption the greater the likelihood of first-pass metabolism occurring. With a rapid absorption of alcohol, often observed after drinking on an empty stomach, the first-pass metabolism was abolished (Dipadova et al., 1987). Indeed, in the fasting state, total body water can be reliably estimated by the ethanol dilution technique even after oral administration which speaks against first-pass elimination taking place (Jones et al., 1992).

Dr. Charles Lieber and his associates became the main proponents of the importance of gastric ADH in first-pass metabolism of ethanol and still continue to publish on the subject (Ali et al., 1995). However,

in many of their publications, only five to six volunteer subjects were used and human studies were presented together with animal models from rats and baboons (Roine et al., 1990; Caballeria et al., 1991; DiPadova et al., 1992). The results of this research, often published in prestigious scientific journals, gained widespread publicity from the news media, especially regarding sex-related differences in gastric ADH and the potentially greater risk posed to women who indulge in moderate drinking (Frezza et al., 1990; DiPadova et al., 1992). In most of the experimental protocols demonstrating a significant first-pass metabolism very small doses of ethanol were administered (0.15–0.3 g/kg) about one hour after eating a substantial fat-rich breakfast. These are exactly the circumstances known to influence gastric emptying, the absorption rate of alcohol and its systemic availability. Drinking a moderate dose of ethanol (0.6–0.8 g/kg) after an overnight fast abolished the first-pass metabolism of alcohol and H_2-receptor antagonist drugs were ineffective in changing the pharmacokinetics of ethanol (Jönsson et al., 1992; Cook et al., 1994; Daubcey et al., 1993; Fraser et al., 1992; Fraser et al., 1991). Figure 4.10 compares the blood-alcohol profiles in two subjects who ingested 0.8 g/kg ethanol with and without pretreatment with cimetidine for seven days. The pharmacokinetic profiles on the two occasions were remarkably similar which fails to confirm any influence of this kind of drug on the pharmacokinetics of ethanol in the fasting state.

When ethanol was given to subjects with gastrectomy a negligible first-pass metabolism was observed (Caballeria et al., 1989). This finding was thought to support the role of an intact stomach and thus the presence of gastric ADH for pre-systemic metabolism of ethanol. However, as pointed out by Levitt (1993) the rate of absorption of alcohol is also very much faster for individuals with a gastrectomy and this might overwhelm the capacity of the liver ADH to engage in first-pass metabolism. Accordingly, whether first-pass metabolism of ethanol occurs in the stomach or the liver or both remains unresolved.

Because of the widespread use of cimetidine and ranitidine in clinical practice, research groups from several countries embarked on studies to confirm

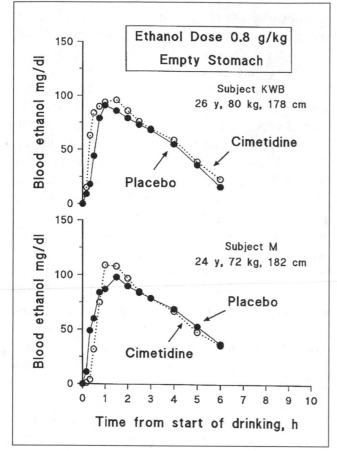

Figure 4.10 *Blood-concentration time profiles of ethanol in two subjects after 0.8 gram of ethanol per kilogram of body weight ingested on an empty stomach both before and after medication with cimetidine (400 mg) daily for seven days*

this adverse drug-alcohol interaction. Despite wide variations in experimental design including the dose of alcohol and use of many more volunteer subjects in the test and control groups, the bioavailability of ethanol was not significantly increased after therapeutic doses of the H_2-receptor antagonists ranitidine and cimetidine (Lewis et al., 1993). This conclusion held when alcohol was ingested by healthy volunteers as well as patients with stomach ulcers (Casini et al., 1994). Ranitidine, a widely prescribed H_2-receptor antagonists, lacked any effect on pharmacokinetics of ethanol when the alcohol was ingested in the morning, at midday, or in the evening and regardless of whether a meal was taken one hour post-drinking (Toon et al., 1994; Raufman et al., 1993; Kendall et al., 1994). All this very extensive experimental work underscores the dangers of drawing conclusions about in-vivo drug-alcohol interac-

tions on the basis of in-vitro experiments (Caballeria et al., 1991).

Summing up the results from extensive studies of this alleged drug-alcohol interaction leads me to conclude that the widely used H_2-receptor antagonists, cimetidine and ranitidine, have no significant influence on the pharmacokinetics and bioavailability of ethanol after small (0.15–0.3 g/kg) or moderate (0.5–0.9 g/kg) doses of ethanol. By contrast, a significant first-pass metabolism of ethanol occurs when small doses (<0.3 g/kg) are taken together with or after a meal. The rate of absorption of ethanol exerts a critical influence on peak BAC and area under the curve (Levitt and Levitt, 1994). Moreover, pronounced variability in the pharmacokinetics of ethanol both between and within individuals means that large numbers of subjects must be investigated to achieve sufficient statistical power to demonstrate effects of a particular drug treatment. With a slow and prolonged absorption of ethanol for whatever reason (food in the stomach or pylorospasm) there seems to be a more effective clearance of ethanol taking place during the absorption phase as the portal vein blood flows through the liver.

4.16 The Effects of Food on the Pharmacokinetics of Ethanol

It has been known since the 1920s that the systemic availability of ethanol is appreciably less if alcohol is ingested together with or after a meal compared with intake under fasting conditions (Widmark 1932). Several mechanisms have been suggested to account for this finding: (1) binding of ethanol molecules to dietary components particularly amino acids, (2) a more effective enzymatic oxidation when alcohol flux through the liver is reduced, (3) formation of ethyl esters in the stomach and intestines, (4) oxidation of ethanol by food components and (5) oxidation in the stomach by gastric alcohol dehydrogenase present in the mucous surfaces (Schmidt and Oehmichen, 1984).

By comparing blood alcohol profiles in the fed and fasting states, Widmark estimated that between 10–12 grams from a moderate dose of 60–70 grams "disappeared" when volunteers drank alcohol after a meal compared with drinking on an empty stomach. He proposed that alcohol became chemically bound to amino acids from the diet such as glycine and was thus prevented from being absorbed into the blood-stream. The effect of food on the bioavailability of ethanol has been confirmed many times since by other investigators (Goldberg, 1943; Sedman et al., 1986; Lin et al., 1976; Jones and Jönsson, 1994a) and in recent years dose-response and time-response studies have been made including variations in the composition of the meal taken, whether in liquid or solid form and the proportions of fat, protein and carbohydrate present (Wilkinson et al., 1977b; Welling, 1977)

The proponents for a biological role of gastric ADH have been quick to suggest that because alcohol is retained in the stomach for a longer time when taken together with food, this gives more opportunity for metabolic breakdown to occur. The areas under the BAC time profiles are appreciably less when the same dose of ethanol is given by oral administration compared with the intravenous route. This was taken to indicate that a significant pre-systemic metabolism was occurring and that gastric ADH was therefore incriminated in this process.

Support for a specific food-induced effect on the rate of ethanol metabolism as opposed to pre-systemic oxidation by gastric ADH was obtained by demonstrating a more rapid rate of disappearance from blood even when the dose of alcohol was given intravenously (Hahn et al., 1994). Furthermore, eating a meal during the post-absorptive phase at about three hours after the end of drinking was also effective in speeding-up the rate of elimination as shown by a steeper β-slope in most subjects (Jones and Jönsson, 1994). Hepatic ADH activity is appreciably less in the fasting state compared with the well nourished organism which might explain the slower rate of disposal of ethanol after an overnight fast (Borson et al., 1980). Protein was especially important in this respect because after feeding a protein-deficient diet to human subjects the rate of ethanol disappearance from blood (β-slope) decreased (Bode, 1978). When a protein-rich meal was reinstated the β-slope recovered and even surpassed the original values after a few days. Furthermore, the liver blood flow is enhanced by feeding and this mechanism may help to facilitate the clearance rate of ethanol from blood

(Svensson et al., 1983; Schmidt and Oehmichen, 1984).

Figure 4.11 gives examples of blood-alcohol profiles obtained in crossover studies designed to investigate the effect of food on ethanol bioavailability. Average curves are shown for two doses of alcohol, 0.3 g/kg and 0.8 g/kg. The major influence of food is seen in a pronounced lowering of peak BAC and diminished area under the curve. After 0.3 g/kg the AUC was lowered by 50 percent and for the higher dose (0.8 g/kg) by 40 percent. The slower absorption and faster rate of metabolism in the fed state means that the BAC profiles return to zero faster than if a person drinks alcohol on an empty stomach.

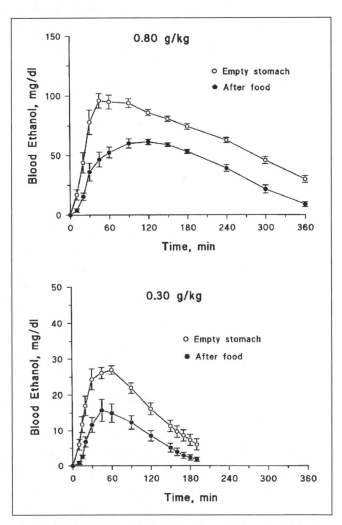

Figure 4.11 *Food-induced lowering of blood-alcohol profiles after volunteer subjects drank either 0.8 g/kg or 0.3 g/kg ethanol in the morning immediately after eating breakfast. Mean curve ± SE are shown for eight subjects after each dose of alcohol.*

Subjective feelings of intoxication were also drastically reduced when alcohol was consumed after a meal.

4.17 Kinetics of Ethanol Metabolites— Acetaldehyde and Acetate

Compared with ethanol itself, there is much less known about the pharmacokinetics of its metabolites acetaldehyde and acetate. These two compounds are normally present in blood and body fluids in extremely small amounts and even after the ingestion of ethanol, the quantitative analysis of blood-acetaldehyde and blood-acetate is more difficult than the determination of blood-ethanol. The acetate produced from ethanol enters the metabolic pool as acetyl coenzyme A and becomes involved in the general pathways for oxidation of fats. The concentrations of acetaldehyde circulating in peripheral blood after drinking ethanol are very low, being about 0.04–0.09 mg/L when reliable methods of analysis are used and when the ALDH enzymes are not inactivated by drugs such as disulfiram or genetic influences on the activity of ALDH (Eriksson and Fukunaga, 1993).

The concentrations of acetaldehyde and acetate generated during the metabolism of ethanol depend in part on the rate of oxidation of ethanol and therefore the reoxidation of NADH which is considered the slowest step in the process. Reoxidation of NADH, which occurs in mitochondria, is dependent on the rate of oxidative phosphorylation (Lundquist et al., 1962). This means that the rate of ethanol disposal is linked to hepatic oxygen consumption within the cell and the person's metabolic rate in general. After drinking ethanol, the concentrations of AcH and acetate in blood rise initially and then remain at a more or less steady-state concentration provided that the alcohol metabolizing enzymes are working at full capacity. Accordingly, swift metabolism of ethanol should lead to a higher steady state concentration of acetate and acetaldehyde compared with slow metabolism of ethanol (Nuutinen et al., 1985). Indeed, subjects having a high steady-state level of blood-acetate during the oxidation of ethanol are usually heavy drinkers with enhanced capacity to oxidize ethanol (Korri et al., 1985). An abnormally high concentration of acetate in blood was

taken as an indication of metabolic tolerance often associated with advanced drinking habits and alcoholism (Roine et al., 1988; Nuutinen et al., 1985).

4.18 Biochemical Markers of Alcohol Abuse and Risk of Alcoholism

Much research effort has been devoted towards developing reliable laboratory tests to identify problem drinkers and individuals at risk for liver disease owing to their continuous exposure to high blood-ethanol (Crabb, 1990). Most of the biochemical screening tests available rely on the analysis of a sample of plasma or serum taken from the individual suspected of dangerously high consumption of alcohol (Rawat, 1992; Rosman and Lieber, 1994). In this context one should distinguish between two kinds of biochemical marker, namely, state markers and trait markers (Salaspuro, 1994; Conigrave et al., 1995; Anton et al., 1994).

Trait markers are genetically transmitted and result in a different biochemical pattern in the individual concerned or a behavioral characteristic making them more susceptible to heavy drinking and alcoholism. One example of a biochemical trait marker is the activity of monoamine oxidase (MAO) an enzyme in the brain involved with catabolism of biogenic amine neurotransmitters, dopamine, norepinephrine, and serotonin. MAO activity can be monitored by analyzing blood platelets and a reduced activity of this enzyme is associated with a greater risk for alcoholism (Gottfries et al., 1975). One goal of a trait marker is to identify those who might be more prone to develop alcoholism before significant exposure to the drug has occurred. Trait markers are therefore one approach to detect individuals with predisposition for becoming dependent on alcohol thus allowing for early prevention and educational programs.

State markers for alcohol abuse on the other hand indicate the development of liver damage as reflected in altered blood chemistry occurring secondary to chronic drinking (Salaspuro, 1994). These diagnostic tests involve laboratory analysis of plasma or serum to detect possible changes in hepatic enzyme systems owing to prolonged heavy drinking. The most widely used biochemical tests for hazardous drinking are various enzymes; aspartate aminotransferase (AST), alanine aminotransferase (ALT), alkaline phosphatase (ALP), gamma glutamyltransferase (GGT), carbohydrate-deficient transferrin (CDT) and a hematological marker called mean corpuscular volume (MCV). The biochemical marker considered to have the best potential for detecting heavy drinkers is CDT because of its >90 percent specificity and reasonably good sensitivity of 65–95 percent in alcoholics and 26–62 percent in heavy drinkers (Jeppsson et al., 1993; Stibler, 1991; Conigrave et al., 1995). However, when alcoholics abstain from drinking for some time, the elevated level (concentration) of a biochemical state marker recovers again to values within the normal range. However, recovery time varies from marker to marker ranging from days (CDT), weeks (GGT) to months (MCV) after stopping drinking. Note that nonalcoholic liver disease and cirrhosis from other causes lead to false positive results with most currently available markers for alcoholism. One forensic application of biochemical state markers is in the rehabilitation of convicted drunk drivers. Frequent monitoring of a person's drinking habits by use of various biochemical tests is often a mandatory requirement before relicensing the driver.

The utility of a biochemical marker or test is often reported in terms of its diagnostic sensitivity and specificity. Sensitivity is the ability of a test to identify correctly individuals who are regular heavy drinkers or alcoholics. Accordingly, a test with a sensitivity of 95 percent would correctly identify ninety-five out of 100 individuals known to be heavy drinkers but the remaining five would go undetected and these are referred to as false negative results. Specificity is the ability of a biochemical test to correctly identify those individuals who are not problem drinkers. The greater the specificity the less likely it is to obtain a positive result when serum from a moderate drinker or abstainer is analyzed. A diagnostic test with 95-percent specificity implies a 5-percent risk of obtaining a false positive result. Obviously, the frequency of false positive tests is an important criteria when choosing a particular state marker for clinical use and combinations of different markers are sometimes advocated. Factors to consider when evaluating false positive results are genetic or environmental factors such as the use of

various drugs or non-alcohol related medical conditions, obesity, exercise or pregnancy.

With most of the diagnostic tests for excessive drinking available today, sensitivity of between 40–60 percent and specificity >90 percent are often reported. The threshold amount of alcohol necessary for an abnormal result is generally reported as 60–70 grams of pure ethanol per day for men and 50–60 grams of ethanol for women. Many alcoholics drink 250 grams alcohol per day or more. When the reliability of biochemical screening tests (specificity and sensitivity) are discussed scant attention seems to have been given to the pattern of alcohol consumption, that is, whether the 60–70 grams is ingested in one hour or in divided doses over the day. (Godsell et al., 1995; Samala et al., 1994). Moreover, results of evaluation studies to ascertain specificity and sensitivity depend on the population being tested, especially the proportion of alcoholics included in the study (Bisson and Milfordward, 1994; Bell et al., 1994).

4.19 Concluding Remarks

Biomedical alcohol research is a good example of an interdisciplinary subject with its roots in biochemistry, physiology, pharmacology, as well as internal medicine. A vast and growing literature has accumulated dealing with all aspects of alcohol and alcoholism. Indeed, several scientific journals specialize in reporting studies on alcohol such as *Alcoholism; Clinical and Experimental Research* (1993 impact factor (IF) = 2.16), *Alcohol and Alcoholism* (IF = 0.95), *Alcohol* (IF = 1.52), *Journal of Studies on Alcohol* (IF = 1.51) and *Drug and Alcohol Dependence* (IF = 1.06). Moreover, papers and reports with information of interest to those working in forensic sciences are sometimes published in the general medical journals such as *JAMA* and *New England Journal of Medicine*. Those who intend to specialize and testify as forensic alcohol experts should develop ways of keeping up-to-date with the biomedical alcohol research literature in addition to reading journals devoted to forensic science and toxicology. An effective way of doing this is by systematically scanning the contents pages of the leading forensic and biomedical periodicals with the use of *Current Contents*, a weekly book now available as a floppy disk.

The information contained in this chapter reflects to a great extent my own alcohol research interests and publications dealing with the metabolism and pharmacokinetics of ethanol. The topics covered here and the associated literature citations will hopefully serve as a review and starting point for those who require more information about specific topics.

References

Adachi, J. et al. Comparative study of ethanol elimination and blood acetaldehyde between alcoholics and control subjects. *Alcoholism, Clin. Exp. Res.* 13:601–604, 1989.

Adachi, J. et al. Is the present standard appropriate to evaluate alcohol elimination rate and degrees of alcohol intoxication in medicolegal examinations. In: Nagata, T. (ed.), *Proc. 30th TIAFT Meeting*, Fukuoka, Japan, 1992, pp 81–84.

Agapejev, S., Vassilieff, I. and Curi, P.R. Alcohol in cerebrospinal fluid (CSF) and alcoholism. *Hum. Exp. Toxicol.* 11:237–239, 1992a.

Agapejev, S., Vassilieff, I. and Curi, P.R. Alcohol levels in cerebrospinal fluid and blood samples from patients under pathological conditions. *Acta Neurol. Scand.* 86:496–500, 1992b.

Agarwal, D.P. and Goedde, H.W. Pharmacogenetics of alcohol dehydrogenase (ADH). *Pharmac. Ther.* 45:69–83, 1990.

Agarwal, D.P. and Goedde, H.W. Medico-biological and genetic studies on alcoholism: Role of metabolic variation and ethnicity on drinking habits, alcohol abuse and alcohol-related mortality. *Clin. Invest.* 70:465–477, 1992.

Ali, S. et al. Metabolism of ethanol in rat gastric cells and its inhibition by cimetidine. *Gastroenterology* 108:737–742, 1995.

Anton, R.F. and Moak, D.H. Carbohydrate-deficient transferrin and gamma-glutamyltransferase as markers of heavy alcohol consumption: Gender differences. *Alcoholism Clin. Exp. Res.* 18:747–754, 1994.

Asmussen, E., Hald, J. and Larsen, V. The pharmacological action of acetaldehyde on the human organism. *Acta Pharmacol.* 4:311–320, 1948.

Baraona, E. et al. Lack of alcohol dehydrogenase isoenzyme activities in the stomach of Japanese subjects. *Life Sci.* 49:1929–1934, 1991.

Bell, H. et al. Carbohydrate deficient transferrin and other markers of high alcohol consumption: A study of 502 patients admitted consecutively to a medical department. *Alcoholism Clin. Exp. Res.* 18:1103–1108, 1994.

Bennion. L.J. and Li, T.K. Alcohol metabolism in American indians and whites: Lack of racial differences in metabolic rate and liver alcohol dehydrogenase. *N. Eng. J. Med.* 294:9–13, 1975.

Bisson, J.I. and Milfordward, A. A comparison of carbohydrate deficient transferrin with other markers of alcohol misuse in male soldiers under the age of 30. *Alc. Alcohol.* 29:315–321, 1994.

Bode, C., Buchwald, B. and Goebell, H. Hemmung des Äthanolabbaues durch Proteinmangel beim Menschen. *Dtsch. Med. Wschr.* 96:1576–1577, 1971.

Bode, C. The metabolism of alcohol: Physiological and pathological aspects. *J. Roy. Coll. Phys.* 12: 122–135, 1978.

Bogusz, M., Puch, J. and Stasko, W. Comparative studies on the rate of ethanol elimination in acute poisoning and in controlled conditions. *J. Forens. Sci.* 22:446–456, 1977.

Bosron, W.F. et al. Effect of fasting on the activity and turnover of rat liver alcohol dehydrogenase. *Alcoholism Clin. Exp. Res.* 8:196–200, 1984.

Bosron, W.F. and Li, T.K. Genetic polymorphism of human liver alcohol and aldehyde dehydrogenases and their relationship to alcohol metabolism and alcoholism. *Hepatology* 6:502–510, 1986.

Brick, J., Nathan, P.E., Westrick, E. et al. The effect of menstrual cycle on blood alcohol levels and behavior. *J. Stud. Alc.* 47:472–477, 1986.

Brien, J.F. and Loomis, C.W. Pharmacology of acetaldehyde. *Can. J. Physiol. Pharmacol.* 61:1–22, 1983.

Bonnischsen, R.K. and Wassén, A. Crystalline alcohol dehydrogemnnase from horse liver. *Arch. Biochem.* 18:361–363, 1948.

Caballeria, J. et al. Gastric origin of the first-pass metabolism of ethanol in humans: Effect of gastrectomy. *Gastroenterol.* 97:1205–1209, 1989.

Caballeria, J. et al. Effects of H_2-receptor antagonists on gastric alcohol dehydrogenase activity. *Dig. Dis. Sci.* 36:1673–1679, 1991.

Casini, A. et al. Prolonged bedtime treatment with H_2-receptor antagonists (Ranitidine and Famotidine) does not affect blood alcohol levels after ethanol ingestion in male patients with duodenal ulcer. *Am. J. Gastroenterol.* 89:745–749, 1994.

Christensen, J.K. et al. Dose-effect relationship of disulfiram in human volunteers, part 1: Clinical studies. *Pharmacol. Toxicol.* 68:163–165, 1991.

Clark, B.B. et al. The role of insulin and the liver in alcohol metabolism. *J. Stud. Alc.* 1:663–683, 1941.

Cohen, G. and Collins, M.A. Alkaloids from catecholamines in adrenal tissue: possible role in alcoholism. *Science* 167:1749–1751, 1970.

Cole-Harding, S. and Wilson, J.R. Ethanol metabolism in men and women. *J. Stud. Alc.* 48:380–387, 1987.

Conigrave, K.M., Saunders, J.B. and Whitfield, J.B. Diagnostic tests for alcohol consumption. *Alc. Alcohol.* 30:15–26, 1995.

Cook, M.D., Cold, J.A. and Strom, J.G. Effect of cimetidine on the pharmacokinetics of alcohol in social and chronic drinkers: A pilot study. *Drug Invest.* 7:84–92, 1994.

Crabb, D.W., Bosron, W.F. and Li, T.K. Ethanol metabolism. *Pharmac. Ther.* 34:59–73, 1987.

Crabb, D.W. Biological markers for increased risk of alcoholism and for quantitation of alcohol consumption. *J. Clin. Invest.* 85:311–315, 1990.

Crabb, D.W., Dipple, K.M. and Thomasson, H.R. Alcohol sensitivity, alcohol metabolism, risk of alcoholism, and the role of alcohol and aldehyde dehydrogenase genotypes. *J. Lab. Clin. Med.* 122:234–240, 1993.

Criqui, M.H. and Ringel, B.L. Does diet or alcohol explain the French paradox? *Lancet* 344:1719–1723, 1994.

Danielsson, O. et al. Fundamental molecular differences between alcohol dehydrogenase classes. *Proc. Natl. Acad. Sci. USA* 91:4980–4984, 1994.

Dannecker, J.R., Shaskan, E.G. and Phillips, M. A new highly sensitive assay for breath acetaldehyde: Detection of endogenous levels in humans. *Anal. Biochem.* 114:1–7, 1981.

Dauncey, H., Chesher, G.B. and Palmer, R.H. Cimetidine and ranitidine: Lack of effect on the pharmacokinetics of an acute ethanol dose. *J. Clin. Gastroenterol.* 17:189–194, 1993.

Davis, V.E. and Walsh, M.J. Alcohol, amines, and alkaloids: A possible biochemical basis for alcoholism. *Science* 167:1005–1006, 1970.

Day, C.P. and Yeaman, S.J. The biochemistry of alcohol-induced fatty liver. *Biochem. Biophys. Acta* 1215:33–48, 1994.

Deitrich, R. and Erwin, V. Biogenic amine-aldehyde condensation products: Tetrahydroisoquinolines and tryptolines (β-carbolines). *Ann. Rev. Pharmacol. Toxicol.* 20:55–80, 1980.

Dipadova, C. et al. Effects of fasting and chronic alcohol consumption on the first-pass metabolism of ethanol. *Gastroenterology* 92:1169–1173, 1987.

DiPadova, C. et al. Effects of ranitidine on blood alcohol levels after ethanol ingestion: Comparison with other H_2-receptor antagonists. *JAMA* 267:83–86, 1992.

Dubowski, K.M. Human pharmacokinetics of ethanol, part 1: Peak blood concentration and elimination in male and female subjects. *Alc. Tech. Rep.* 5:55–63, 1976.

Dubowski, K.M. Absorption, distribution, and elimination of alcohol: Highway safety aspects. *J. Stud. Alc.* Supp 10:98–108, 1985.

Doll, R. et al. Mortality in relation to consumption of alcohol: Thirteen years' observations on male British doctors. *Br. Med. J.* 309:911–918, 1994.

Ehrig, T. et al. Degradation of aliphatic alcohols by human liver alcohol dehydrogenase: Effect of ethanol and pharmacokinetic implications. *Alcoholism Clin. Exp. Res.* 12:789–794, 1988.

Ehrig, T., Bosron, W.F. and Li, T.K. Alcohol and aldehyde dehydrogenase. *Alc. Alcohol.* 25:105–116, 1990.

Eriksson, C.J.P. Human blood acetaldehyde concentration during ethanol oxidation (update 1982). *Pharmacol. Biochem. Behav.* 18:Suppl. 1, 141–150, 1983.

Eriksson, C.J.P. and Fukunaga, T. Human blood acetaldehyde (update 1992). *Alc. Alcohol.* Suppl. 2, 9–25, 1993.

Fraser, A.G. et al. Ranitidine, cimetidine, and famotidine have no effect on post-prandial absorption of ethanol 0.8 g/kg taken after an evening meal. *Aliment. Pharmacol. Therapeut.* 6:693–700, 1992.

Fraser, A.G. et al. The effect of ranitidine, cimetidine or famotidine on low-dose post-prandial alcohol absorption. *Aliment. Pharmacol. Therapeut.* 5: 263–272, 1991.

Frezza, M. et al. High blood alcohol levels in women: The role of decreased gastric alcohol dehydrogenase activity and first-pass metabolism. *N. Eng. J. Med.* 322:95–99, 1990.

Fujimiya, T., Yamaoka, K. and Fukui, Y. Parallel first-order and Michaelis-Menten elimination kinetics of ethanol: Respective role of alcohol dehydrogenase (ADH), non-ADH and first-order pathways. *J. Pharmacol. Exp. Ther.* 249:311–317, 1989.

Fukunaga, T., Sillanaukee, P. and Eriksson, C.J.P. Problems involved in the determination of endogenous acetaldehyde in human blood. *Alc. Alcohol.* 28:535–541, 1993.

Fukunaga, T. et al. Partition ratio of acetaldehyde between blood and breath after ethanol consumption. *Jpn. J. Alcohol & Drug Dependence* 24:405–415, 1989.

Forrest, A.R.W. Non-linear kinetics of ethyl alcohol metabolism. *J. Forens. Sci. Soc.* 26:121–123, 1986.

Gentry, R.T., Baraona, E. and Lieber, C.S. Gastric first pass metabolism of alcohol. *J. Lab. Clin. Med.* 123:21–26, 1994.

Godsell, P.A. et al. Carbohydrate deficient transferrin levels in hazardous alcohol consumption. *Alc. Alcohol.* 30:61–66, 1995.

Goedde, H.W. and Agarwal, D.P. Pharmacogenetics of aldehyde dehydrogenase (ALDH). *Pharmac. Ther.* 45:345–371, 1990.

Goist, K.C. and Sutker, P.B. Acute alcohol intoxication and body composition in women and men. *Pharmacol. Biochem. Behav.* 22:811–814, 1985.

Goldberg, L. Quantitative studies on alcohol tolerance in man. *Acta Physiol. Scand.* 5:1–128, supp. 16, 1943.

Goldstein, A. *Addiction, from Biology to Drug Policy.* NY: W.H. Freeman and Co., 1994.

Gonzalez, F.J. The molecular biology of cytochrome P450s. *Pharmacol. Rev.* 40:243–288, 1989.

Gottfries, C.G. et al. Lowered monoamine oxidase activity in brains from alcoholic suicides. *J. Neurochem.* 25:667–673, 1975.

Grønbaek, M. et al. Mortality associated with moderate intakes of wine, beer, or spirits. *Br. Med. J.* 310:1165–1169, 1995.

Haffner, H.T. et al. Die Äthanol-Eliminationsgeschwindigkeit bei Alkoholikern unter besonderer Berücksichtigung der Maximalwertvariante der forensischen BAK-Rück-rechnung. *Blutalkohol* 28: 46–54, 1991.

Haffner, H.T. et al. The elimination kinetics of methanol and the influence of ethanol. *Int. J. Leg. Med.* 105:111–114, 1992.

Hald, J., Jacobsen, E. and Larsen, V. The sensitizing effect of tetraethylthiuram disulphide (Antabuse) to ethyl alcohol. *Acta Pharamcol.* 4:285–296, 1948.

Hald, J. and Jacobsen, E. The formation of acetaldehyde in the organism after ingestion of Antabuse (tetraethylthiuram disulphide). *Acta Pharamcol.* 4:305–310, 1948.

Hahn, R. et al. Eating a meal increases the rate of alcohol clearance after intravenous infusion. *Alc. Alcohol.* 29:673–677, 1994.

Hahn, R., Norberg, Å. and Jones, A.W. Rate of distribution of ethanol into the total body water. *Am. J. Therap.* 2:50–56, 1995.

Harada, S. Genetic polymorphism of aldehyde dehydrogenase and its physiological significance to alcohol metabolism. *Isozymes* 344:289–294, 1990.

Harada, S. and Okubo, T. Investigation of alcohol dehydrogenase isozymes of biopsy gastric mucosa in Japanese. *Alc. Alcohol.* 28:59–62, 1993.

Helander, A. Aldehyde dehydrogenase in blood: Distribution characteristics and possible use as marker of alcohol abuse. *Alc. Alcohol.* 28:135–145, 1993.

Hernandez-Munoz, R. et al. Human gastric alcohol dehydrogenase: Its inhibition by H_2-receptor antagonists, and its effect on the bioavailability of ethanol. *Alcoholism, Clin. Exp. Res.* 14:946–959, 1990.

Hesselbrock, V.M. and Shaskan, E.G. Endogenous breath acetaldehyde levels among alcoholic and non-alcoholic probands: Effect of alcohol and smoking. *Prog. Neuro-Psychopharmacol. Biol. Psychiat.* 9:259–265, 1985.

Higuchi, S. et al. Aldehyde dehydrogenase genotypes in Japanese alcoholics. *Lancet* 343:741–742, 1994.

Hittle, J.B. and Crabb, D.W. The molecular biology of alcohol dehydrogenase: Implications for the control of alcohol metabolism. *J. Lab. Clin. Med.* 112:7–15, 1988.

Hobbes, J., Boutagy, J. and Shenfield, G.M. Interactions between ethanol and oral contraceptive steroids. *Clin. Pharmacol. Therap.* 38:371–380, 1985.

Holford, N.H.G. Clinical pharmacokinetics of ethanol. *Clin. Pharmacokin.* 13:273–292, 1987.

Jacobsen, E. Is acetaldehyde an intermediary product in normal metabolism? *Biochim. Biophys. Acta* 4:330–334, 1950.

Jacobsen, D. and McMartin, K.E. Methanol and ethylene glycol poisoning: Mechanism of toxicity, clinical course, diagnosis and treatment. *Med. Toxicol.* 1:309–334, 1986.

Jauhonen, P. et al. Origin of breath acetaldehyde during ethanol oxidation: Effect of long-term cigarette smoking. *J. Lab. Clin. Med.* 100:908–916, 1982.

Jeppsson, J.O., Kristensson, H. and Fimiani, C. Carbohydrate deficient transferrin quantified by HPLC to determine heavy consumption of alcohol. *Clin. Chem.* 39:2115–2120, 1993.

Johnsen, J., Stowell, A. and Morland, J. Clinical responses in relation to blood acetaldehyde levels. *Pharmacol. Toxicol.* 70:41–45, 1992.

Jokipii, S.G. Experimental studies on blood alcohol in healthy subjects and in some diseases, Thesis, University of Helsinki, Helsinki, 1951.

Jones, A.W. Inter-individual variations in disposition and metabolism of ethanol in healthy men. *Alcohol* 1:393–396, 1984.

Jones, A.W. Drug-alcohol flush reaction and breath acetaldehyde concentration: No interference with an infrared breath alcohol analyzer. *J. Anal. Toxicol.* 10:98–101, 1986.

Jones, A.W. Metabolism of ethanol in healthy men and women and comparison of Widmark parameters and blood/breath ratios of ethanol between the sexes. In: Valverius, M. (ed.), *Women, Alcohol, Drugs and Traffic.* Stockholm: DALCTRAF, 1989, pp 169–175.

Jones, A.W. Forensic science aspects of ethanol metabolism. In: Maehly, A. and Williams, R.L. (eds.), *Forensic Science Progress*, vol. 5. Berlin: Springer-Verlag, 1991, pp 31–89.

Jones, A.W. Pharmacokinetics of ethanol in saliva: Comparison with blood and breath alcohol profiles, subjective feelings of intoxication, and diminished performance. *Clin. Chem.* 39:1837–1844, 1993.

Jones, A.W. Disappearance rate of ethanol from blood of human subjects: Implications in forensic toxicology. *J. Forens. Sci.* 38:104–118, 1993.

Jones, A.W. Concentration of endogenous ethanol in blood and CSF. *Acta Neurol. Scand.* 89:149–150, 1994.

Jones, A.W. Measuring and reporting the concentration of acetaldehyde in human breath. *Alc. Alcohol.* 30:271–285, 1995a.

Jones, A.W. Biotransformation of acetone to isopropanol observed in a motorist involved in a sobriety control. *J. Forens. Sci.* 40:674–675, 1995b.

Jones, A.W., Mårdh, G. and Änggård, E. Determination of endogenous ethanol in blood and breath by gas chromatography-mass spectrometry. *Pharmacol. Biochem. Behav.* 18:suppl. 1 267–272, 1983.

Jones, A.W. and Neri, A. Age-related differences in blood-ethanol parameters and subjective feelings of intoxication in healthy men. *Alc. Alcohol.* 20:45–52, 1985.

Jones, A.W., Neiman, J. and Hillbom, M. Concentration-time profiles of ethanol and acetaldehyde in human volunteers treated with alcohol sensitizing drug calcium carbimide. *Br. J. Clin. Pharmacol.* 25:213–221, 1988.

Jones, A.W. et al. Physiological variations in blood-alcohol measurements during the post-absorptive state. *J. Forens. Sci. Soc.* 30:273–283, 1990.

Jones, A.W. et al. Metabolic interaction between endogenous methanol and exogenous ethanol studied in human volunteers by analysis of breath. *Pharmacol. Toxicol.* 66:62–65, 1990.

Jones, A.W., Jönsson, K-Å. and Neri, A. Peak blood alcohol concentration and the time of its occurrence after rapid drinking on an empty stomach. *J. Forens. Sci.* 36:376–385, 1991.

Jones, A.W., Hahn, R. and Stalberg, H.P. Pharmacokinetics of ethanol in plasma and whole blood: Estimation of total body water by the dilution principle. *Eur. J. Clin. Pharmacol.* 42:445–448, 1992.

Jones, A.W. and Sternebring, B. Kinetics of ethanol and methanol in alcoholics during detoxification. *Alc. Alcohol.* 27:641–647, 1992.

Jones, A.W. and Jönsson, K-Å. Food-induced lowering of blood-ethanol profiles and increased rate of elimination immediately after a meal. *J. Forens. Sci.* 39:1084–1093, 1994a.

Jones, A.W. and Jönsson, K-Å. Between-subject and within-subject variations in the pharmacokinetics of ethanol. *Br. J. Clin. Pharmacol.* 37:427–431, 1994b.

Jones, M.K. and Jones, B.M. Ethanol metabolism in women taking oral contraceptives. *Alcoholism Clin. Exp. Res.* 8:24–28, 1984.

Jönsson, K-Å. et al. Lack of effect of omeprazole, cimetidine, and ranitidine on the pharmacokinetics of ethanol in fasting male volunteers. *Eur. J. Clin. Pharmacol.* 42:209–212, 1992.

Jörnvall, H. and Högg, J.O. Nomenclature of alcohol dehydrogenase. *Alc. Alcohol.* 30:153–161, 1995.

Keiding, S. et al. Ethanol metabolism in heavy drinkers after massive and moderate alcohol intake. *Biochem. Pharmacol.* 32:3097–3102, 1983.

Kendall, M.J. et al. Lack of effect of H_2-receptor antagonists on the pharmacokinetics of alcohol consumed after food at lunch-time. *Br. J. Clin. Pharmacol.* 37:371–374, 1994.

Korpi, E.R. Role of GABAA receptors in the actions of alcohol and in alcoholism: Recent advances. *Alc. Alcohol.* 29:115–129, 1994.

Koop, D.R. and Coon, M.J. Ethanol oxidation and toxicity: Role of alcohol P450 oxygenase. *Alcoholism Clin. Exp. Res.* 10:Suppl. 6, 44–49, 1986.

Korri, U.M., Nuutinen, H. and Salaspuro, M. Increased blood acetate: A new laboratory marker of alcoholism and heavy drinking. *Alcoholism Clin. Exp. Res.* 9:468–471, 1985.

Krebs, H.A. and Perkins, J.R. The physiological role of liver alcohol dehydrogenase. *Biochem. J.* 118: 635–644, 1970.

Levitt, M.D. Review article: Lack of clinical significance of the interaction between H_2-receptor antagonists and ethanol. *Aliment. Pharmacol. Therapeut.* 7:131–138, 1993.

Levitt, M.D. The case against first-pass metabolism of ethanol in the stomach. *J. Lab. Clin. Med.* 123:28–31, 1994.

Levitt, M.D. and Levitt, D.G. The critical role of the rate of ethanol absorption in the interpretation of studies purporting to demonstrate gastric metabolism of ethanol. *J. Pharmacol. Exp. Ther.* 269:297–304, 1994.

Lewis, M.J. Blood alcohol: The concentration-time curve and retrospective estimation of level. *J. Forens. Sci.* Soc. 26:95–113, 1986.

Lewis, J.H. and McIsaac, R.L. H_2 antagonists and blood alcohol levels. *Dig. Dis. Sci.* 38:569–572, 1993.

Lieber, C.S. Mechanism of ethanol induced hepatic injury. *Pharmac. Ther.* 46:1–41, 1990.

Lieber, C.S. Mechanisms of ethanol-drug-nutrition interactions. *J. Toxicol-Clin. Toxicol.* 32:631–681, 1994a.

Lieber, C.S. Alcohol and the liver: 1994 update. *Gastroenterology* 106:1085–1105, 1994b.

Lieber, C.S. and DeCarli, L.M. Hepatic microsomal ethanol oxidizing system: In-vitro characteristics and adaptive properties in vivo. *J. Biol. Chem.* 245:2505–2512, 1970.

Lieber, C.S. and DeCarli, L.M. The role of the hepatic microsomal ethanol oxidizing system (MEOS) for ethanol metabolism in vivo. *J. Pharmacol. Exp. Ther.* 181:279–287, 1972.

Lieberman, F.L. The effect of liver disease on the rate of ethanol metabolism in man. *Gastroenterol.* 44:261–266, 1961.

Lin, Y.J. et al. Effects of solid food on blood levels of alcohol in man. *Res. Commun. Chem. Pathol. Pharmacol.* 13:713–722, 1976.

Lindahl, R. Aldehyde dehydrogenases and their role in carcinogenesis. *Crit. Rev. Biochem Molec. Biol.* 27:283–335, 1992.

Lindros, K.O. Human blood acetaldehyde levels: With improved methods, a clearer picture emerges. *Alcoholism Clin. Exp. Res.* 7:70–75, 1983.

Lundquist, F. and Wolthers, H. The kinetics of alcohol elimination in man. *Acta Pharmacol. Toxicol.* 14:265–289, 1958.

Lundquist, F. et al. Ethanol metabolism and production of free acetate in the human liver. *J. Clin. Invest.* 41:955–961, 1962.

Marshall, A.W. et al. Ethanol elimination in males and females; Relationship to menstrual cycle and body composition. *Hepatology* 3:701–706, 1983.

Martin, N.G. et al. A twin study of ethanol metabolism. *Behav. Gen.* 15:93–109, 1985.

Mezey, E. Duration of the enhanced activity of the microsomal ethanol-oxidizing enzyme system and rate of ethanol degradation in ethanol-fed rats after withdrawal. *Biochem. Pharmacol.* 21:137–142, 1972.

Mezey, E. and Tobon, F. Rates of ethanol clearance and activities of the ethanol-oxidizing enzymes in chronic alcoholic patients. *Gastroenterol.* 61:707-715, 1971.

Mezey, E., Hamilton, B. and Potter, J.J. Effect of testosterone administration on rates of ethanol elimination in hypogonadal patients. *Alcohol* 6:331–333, 1989.

Mizoi, Y. et al. Relationship between facial flushing and blood acetaldehyde level after intake. *Pharmacol. Biochem. Behav.* 10:305–311, 1979.

Mizoi, Y. et al. Individual and ethnic differences in ethanol elimination. *Alc. Alcohol.* Suppl. 1:389–394, 1987.

Mizoi, Y. et al. Involvement of genetic polymorphism of alcohol and aldehyde dehydrogenases in individual variation of alcohol metabolism. *Alc. Alcohol.* 29:707–714, 1994.

Myers, R.D. Tetrahydroisoquinolines in the brain: The basis of an animal model of alcoholism. *Alcoholism Clin. Exp. Res.* 3:364–367, 1979.

Nuutinen, H. et al. Elevated blood acetate as indicator of fast ethanol elimination in chronic alcoholics. *Alcohol* 2:623–626, 1985.

Nuutinen, H., Lindros, K. and Salaspuro, M. Determinants of blood acetaldehyde level during ethanol oxidation in chronic alcoholics. *Alcoholism Clin. Exp. Res.* 7:163–168, 1983.

Nuutinen, H. et al. Blood acetaldehyde concentration gradients between hepatic and antecubital venous blood in ethanol intoxicated alcoholics and controls. *Eur. J. Clin. Invest.* 14:306–311, 1984.

Nuutinen, H. et al. Elevated blood acetate as indicator of fast ethanol elimination in chronic alcoholics. *Alcohol* 2:623–626, 1985.

Neuteboom, W. and Jones, A.W. Disappearance rate of ethanol from the blood of drunk drivers calculated from two consecutive samples: What do the results really mean? *Forens. Sci. Int.* 45:107–115, 1990.

O'Neill, B., Williams, A.F. and Dubowski, K.M. Variability in blood alcohol concentrations: Implications for estimating individual results. *J. Stud. Alc.* 44:222–230, 1983.

Ostrovsky, Y.M. Endogenous ethanol: Its metabolic, behavioral and biomedical significance. *Alcohol* 3:239–247, 1986.

Österlind, S., Åhlén, M. and Wolff, E. Investigations concerning the constants β and r according to Wid-

mark, especially in women. *Acta Pathol. Microbiol. Scand.* Supp 54:489–498, 1944.

Palmer, R.H. et al. Effects of various concomitant medications on gastric alcohol dehydrogenase and the first-pass metabolism of ethanol. *Am. J. Gastroenterol.* 86:1749–1755, 1991.

Parés, X. et al. Mammalian class IV alcohol dehydrogenase (stomach alcohol dehydrogenase): Structure, origin, and correlation with enzymology. *Proc. Natl. Acad Sci.* (USA) 91:1893–1897, 1994.

Pettersson, G. Liver alcohol dehydrogenase. *CRC Crit. Rev. Biochem.* 21:349–389, 1987.

Pond, S.M. and Tozer, T.N. First-pass elimination: Basic concepts and clinical consequences. *Clin. Pharmacokin.* 9:1–25, 1984.

Rango, R.E., Kreeft, J.H. and Sitar, D.S. Ethanol "dose-dependent" elimination: Michaelis-Menten vs. classical kinetic analysis. *Br. J. Clin. Pharmacol.* 12:667–673, 1981.

Raufman, J.P. et al. Histamine-2 receptor antagonists do not alter serum ethanol levels in fed, nonalcoholic men. *Ann. Intern. Med.* 118:488–494, 1993.

Rawat, A.K. Role of biochemical markers in the diagnosis of alcoholism. *Res. Commun. Substance Abuse* 13:219–230, 1992.

Reed, T.E. Racial comparisons of alcohol metabolism: Background, problems and results. *Alcoholism Clin. Exp. Res.* 2:83–87, 1978.

Roine, R.P. et al. Aspirin increases blood alcohol concentrations in humans after ingestion of ethanol. *JAMA* 264:2406–2408, 1990.

Roine, R.P. et al. Increased serum acetate as a marker of problem drinking among drunken drivers. *Alc. Alcohol.* 23:123–126, 1988.

Roland, M. and Tozer, T.N. *Clinical Pharmacokinetics: Concepts and Applications.* Philadelphia: Lea & Febiger, 1980.

Rosman, A.S. and Lieber, C.S. Diagnostic utility of laboratory tests in alcoholic liver disease. *Clin. Chem.* 40:1641–1651, 1994.

Salmela, K.S. et al. Carbohydrate-deficient transferrin during three weeks' heavy alcohol consumption. *Alcoholism Clin. Exp. Res.* 18:228–230, 1994.

Salaspuro, M. Biological state markers of alcohol abuse. *Alc. Health. Res. World* 18:131–135, 1994.

Sato, A. and Nakajima, T. Enhanced metabolism of volatile hydrocarbons in rat liver following food deprivation, restricted carbohydrate intake and administration of ethanol, phenobarbital, polychlorinated biphenyl and 3-methyl-cholantrene. *Xenobiotica* 15:67–75, 1985.

Sato, A. and Nakajima, T. Pharmacokinetics of organic solvent vapors in relation to their toxicity. *Scand. J. Environ. Health* 13:81–93, 1987.

Schmidt, V. and Oehmichen, M. Alkoholkinetik und Nahrungszufuhr. *Blutalkohol* 21:403–421, 1984.

Schmitt, G. et al. Ethyl glucuronide: An unusual ethanol metabolite in humans: Analytical data, and determination in serum and urine. *J. Analyt. Tox.* 19:91–94, 1995.

Schonheyder, F. et al. On the variation of the alcoholemic curve. *Acta Med. Scand.* CIX:460–470, 1942.

Sedman A.J. et al. Food effects on absorption and metabolism of alcohol. *J. Stud. Alc.* 37:1197–1214, 1976.

Seitz, H.K. et al. Human gastric alcohol dehydrogenase activity: Effect of age, sex, and alcoholism. *GUT* 34:1433–1437, 1993.

Sprung, R. et al. Zum Problem des endogenen Alkohols. *Blutalkohol* 18:65–70, 1981.

Stibler, H. Carbohydrate-deficient transferrin in serum: A new marker of potentially harmful alcohol consumption reviewed. *Clin. Chem.* 37:2029–2037, 1991.

Stowell, A.R. et al. A reinvestigation of the usefulness of breath analysis in the determination of blood acetaldehyde concentration. *Alcoholism Clin. Exp. Res.* 8:442–447, 1984.

Stowell, A.R., Measurement of acetaldehyde and ethanol in blood, breath, and other biological material for experimental purposes. In: Crow, K.E. and Batt, R.D. (eds.), *Human Metabolism of Alcohol*, vol. 2. Boca Raton: CRC Press, 1989, pp 163–176.

Sutker, P.B., Goist, K.C. and King, A.R. Acute alcohol intoxications in women: Relationsship to dose and menstrual cycle phase. *Alcoholism Clin. Exp. Res.* 11:74–79, 1987.

Svensson, C.K. et al. Effect of food on hepatic blood flow: Implications in the "food effect" phenomenon. *Clin. Pharmacol. Ther.* 34:316–323, 1983.

Tabakoff, B. and Hoffman, P.L. The neurochemistry of alcohol. *Curr. Opin. Psychiat.* 6:388–394, 1993.

Takeshita, T. et al. Phenotypic differences in low k_m aldehyde dehydsrogenase in Japanese workers. *Lancet* 341:837–838, 1993.

Teschke, R. and Gellert, J. Hepatic microsomal ethanol-oxidizing system (MEOS): Metabolic aspects and clinical implications. *Alcoholism Clin. Exp. Res.* 10:20S–32S, 1986.

Thacker, S.B. et al. Genetic and biochemical factors relevant to alcoholism. *Alcoholism Clin. Exp. Res.* 8:375–383, 1984.

Tiege, K. et al. Unterschiede der Blutalkoholkonzentration bei gleichzeitiger, quasikontinuierlicher Blutabinahime aus den korrespon-dierenden Venen des rechten und des linken Armes. *Blutalkohol* 11:29–39, 1974.

Toon, S. et al. Absence of effect of ranitidine on blood alcohol concentrations when taken morning, midday, or evening with or without food. *Clin. Pharmacol. Ther.* 55:385–391, 1994.

Von Wartburg, J.P. Pharmacokinetics of alcohol. In: Crow, K.E. and Batt, R.D. (eds.), *Human Metabolism of Alcohol*, vol. 1. Boca Raton: CRC Press, 1989, pp. 9–22.

Von Wartburg, J.P. and Papenberg, J. Alcohol dehydrogenase in ethanol metabolism. *Psychosomatic Med.* 28:405–413, 1966.

Von Wartburg, J.P. and Bühler, R. Biology of disease: Alcoholism and aldehydydism: New biomedical concepts. *Lab. Invest.* 50:5–15, 1984.

Wagner, J.G. et al. Elimination of alcohol from human blood. *J. Pharm. Sci.* 65:152–154, 1976.

Wagner, J.G., Wilkinson, P.K. and Ganes, D.A. Parameters V_m and K_m for elimination of alcohol in young male subejcts following low doses of alcohol. *Alc. Alcohol.* 24:555–564, 1989.

Wang, M.Q. et al. Acute alcohol intoxication, body composition, and pharmacokinetics. *Pharmacol. Biochem. Behav.* 43:641–643, 1992.

Watson, P.E., Watson, I.D. and Batt, R.D. Prediction of blood alcohol concentration in human subjects: Updating the Widmark equation. *J. Stud. Alc.* 42: 547–556, 1981.

Welling, P.G. et al. Pharmacokinetics of alcohol following single low doses to fasted and nonfasted subjects. *J. Clin. Pharmacol.* 17:199–206, 1977.

Widmark, E.M.P. *Die theoretischen Grundlagen und die praktische Verwend-barkeit der gerichtlich-medizinischen Alkoholbestimmung.* Berlin: Urban and Schwarzenberg, 1932.

Wilkinson, P.K. Pharmacokinetics of ethanol: A review. *Alcoholism Clin. Exp. Res.* 4:6–21, 1980.

Wilkinson P.K. et al. Pharmacokinetics of ethanol after oral administration in the fasting state. *J. Pharmacokin. Biopharm.* 5:207–224, 1977a.

Wilkinson P.K. et al. Fasting and non-fasting blood ethanol concentrations following repeated oral administration of ethanol to one adult male subject. *J. Pharmacokin. Biopharm.* 5:41–52, 1977b.

Williams, G.D. and DeBakey, S.E. Changes in levels of alcohol consumption: United States 1983–1988. *Brit. J. Addict.* 87:643–648, 1992.

Winek, C.L. and Murphy, K.L. The rate and kinetic order of ethanol elimination. *Forens. Sci. Int.* 25: 159–166, 1984.

Yin, S.J. et al. Genetic polymorphism and activities of human lung alcohol and aldehyde dehydrogenases: Implications for ethanol metabolism and cytotoxicity. *Biochem Genet.* 30:203–215, 1992.

Yoshida, A. Genetic polymorphisms of alcohol metabolizing enzymes related to alcohol sensitivity and alcoholic diseases. *Alc. Alcohol.* 29: 693–696, 1994.

Zink, P. and Reinhardt, G. Der Verlauf der Blutalkoholkurve bei großen Trinkmengen. *Blutalkohol* 21, 422–442, 1984.

Endnotes

1. The words ethanol and alcohol are used interchangeably in this chapter.

2. An antagonist drug produces the opposite effect or blocks the action of a naturally occurring chemical substance such as a neurotransmitter or hormone.

3. One milliliter of whole blood weighs 1.055 grams so the β-factor reported by Widmark should be increased by 5.5 percent and the *rho* value lowered by 5.5 percent to compare with BAC in units of mass/volume (mg/dL).

Chapter 5

Blood, Urine and Other Fluid and Tissue Specimens for Alcohol Analyses

Yale H. Caplan, Ph.D. and Bruce A. Goldberger, Ph.D.

5.1 Blood

A. General considerations

The determination of alcohol is undoubtedly the most widely requested analysis in analytical toxicology. Tests may be required of a living subject, where knowledge of the role of alcohol in a particular situation is needed, or on a deceased person, where alcohol may have contributed to that person's death or to the death of another. In either scenario, a decision as to the type of specimen to be analyzed is important to facilitate proper interpretation of the impact of alcohol in a particular case. Since alcohol affects the brain, a specimen that is reflective of the alcohol content of the brain is most useful. Because the blood compartment is in equilibrium with the brain, the blood alcohol concentration is expected to best reflect the effects of alcohol on the brain. In view of the fact that the majority of tests will be conducted on living subjects, blood or a component of blood is most commonly used. In postmortem cases, the brain itself, among other specimens, becomes available; however, blood is still principally used since comparison to antemortem situations is often required. Blood, available with equal ease from living or deceased persons, becomes the most practical

specimen; hence, the first step in the alcohol analysis is to obtain the proper blood specimens.

Approximately five liters of blood is contained in the average person constituting about 8 percent of the total body weight. There are two principal components of blood: the plasma and the cells. The plasma is the liquid portion and contains the lipids, proteins, ions, vitamins, and other constituents. There are two principal types of blood cells; the red blood cells and the white blood cells. Red blood cells, or erythrocytes, contain hemoglobin which binds oxygen and facilities oxygen transport throughout the body. White blood cells, or leukocytes, are responsible for the cell-mediated immune responses to foreign organisms. There are approximately 500 times more erythrocytes than leukocytes. The ratio that indicates the relative volumes of the plasma and cells is the hematocrit (Hct), which is defined as the volume of red cells divided by the total blood volume. An average Hct is between 40 percent and 50 percent. A low Hct would imply a greater water content of the blood. Alcohol distributes in the body's total water; therefore, its concentration would vary according to whether whole blood or a component of the blood is selected for testing.

Although Chapter 11 deals in more detail with the question of storage and stability of alcohol in blood, a few words must be included here. Ordinarily, days or even weeks may pass between the sampling and analysis of a blood specimen. Since the interest of the analyst is in the blood alcohol concentration at the time that the specimen was drawn, it is important that the integrity of the specimen remain intact over this time period. Specifically, the degradation of the blood by normal biological events and changes in the original ethanol concentration must be avoided. Many reports in the literature have shown that there may be decreases as well as increases in ethanol concentration with time. Improperly sealed containers, microorganism oxidation of ethanol, and temperature-dependent conversion of ethanol to acetaldehyde have resulted in decreases in ethanol concentration (Brown et al., 1973; Smalldon and Brown, 1973; Chang et al., 1984) while increases in ethanol concentration have been attributed to microbial conversion of glucose to alcohol. To prevent these changes, blood specimens should be well sealed and stored at low temperatures. Anticoagulants such as oxalate salts, citrate salts, or heparin should be added to prevent clotting. Microorganism growth can be inhibited by adding fluoride salts, mercuric salts, or azide salts. Postmortem blood specimens are ordinarily obtained without using sterile technique; therefore, they have an increased likelihood of bacterial contamination and may require a greater amount of fluoride to prevent *in vitro* ethanol formation. A combination of potassium oxalate at a concentration of 5 mg/mL of blood, and sodium fluoride at 1 mg/mL of blood is frequently used, along with storage of the blood at 4°C or –20°C.

It is important that the blood specimen, once drawn, be properly handled until it reaches the laboratory for analysis. Specimens should be labeled with the subject's name, the date and time obtained, the location (site) from which the specimen was drawn, and the name of the person who withdrew the blood. The time of blood draw is especially important in living subjects because the blood alcohol concentration determined may be used in the estimation of the blood concentration at an earlier time. The tube should be sealed by the person drawing the blood and chain of custody must be established from the time of draw until the time of analysis. When specimens are mailed in from an outside source, the U.S. Postal Service has been determined by the courts to be an acceptable link in the chain. More recent experiences include overnight couriers as well.

Several studies (Heise, 1959; Dubowski, 1977; Kaye, 1980) using living subjects have demonstrated that externally applied alcohol can produce false-positive results. Although one study suggests that this is not a problem when isopropanol-containing antiseptics are used (Goldfinger and Schaber, 1982), it seems reasonable to use a nonalcohol-containing antiseptic during the venipuncture procedure. For postmortem cases, such antiseptics are not used; however, care must still be exercised in obtaining the specimen. The specimen should be drawn from an exposed area to ensure that the specimen is, in fact, blood. For instance, in trauma cases, it is possible for the blood to be mixed with the stomach contents and if alcohol were present in the stomach contents, an artificially elevated blood alcohol concentration could result.

B. Sources of blood specimens

The location from which the blood specimen is obtained in the body is important. For the most part, alcohol is absorbed from the gastrointestinal (GI) tract and enters the portal circulation; during the early absorption process, the portal blood contains the highest concentration of alcohol. This suggests that portal blood would not be a good blood specimen to obtain in postmortem cases. Past the liver, the portal blood passes into the heart. At this point, the alcohol concentration is diluted by blood from other sources. From the heart, the alcohol is distributed to the rest of the tissues.

During the absorption phase, alcohol concentrations in blood from different parts of the body may vary (Haggard et al., 1940). Numerous studies have reported on the length of time required for alcohol to equilibrate throughout the body (Harger et al., 1956; McCallum and Scroggie, 1960; Forney et al., 1964; Dundee et al., 1971; Sedman et al., 1976). For instance, in one study (Forney et al., 1964) five subjects were administered a fixed dose per weight of alcohol and at subsequent time intervals, blood specimens from the cubital vein and the fingertip were drawn for alcohol analysis. Blood from the fingertip represented capillary blood, which was assumed to be equivalent to arterial blood. At the end of the drinking period, the alcohol concentration in the fingertip blood exceeded that in the cubital vein in each case, ranging from a 12 percent to 40 percent difference. At 30 minutes, differences were still observed, but for the remainder of the two-hour period, no further differences between the two blood sites were noted. Blood from the foot vein had a much lower alcohol concentration than that of the cubital vein.

Another report (Sedman et al., 1976) indicated that it may take somewhat longer for the equilibrium between capillary blood and venous blood to occur. Following equilibrium, a point is reached where the venous blood slightly exceeds the capillary blood concentration. Ideally, arterial blood should be used because arterial blood alcohol concentrations correlate best with central nervous system (CNS) impairment (Mason and Dubowski, 1974). However, the analysis of arterial blood requires arterial puncture, which is more painful, presents greater medical risk, and requires specially trained personnel to draw the blood. Therefore, the more easily and safely obtained venous blood is regularly used. The proper interpretation of the results may require knowledge as to whether or not the blood was drawn in the postabsorptive period, when it can be established that the venous blood alcohol concentration is approximately equal to the arterial blood concentration.

In postmortem cases, the medical examiner or coroner is able to obtain a blood specimen directly from the heart. As mentioned previously, it is important that the blood specimen not be mixed with other bodily fluids, for this may increase or decrease the alcohol concentration. It is also recommended that a second blood specimen from an alternate site, such as the femoral vein or other peripheral site, be obtained at autopsy. The two blood specimens can provide some information as to whether the subject was in the postabsorptive state. More importantly, in those cases where the heart blood may have been contaminated, the alternative specimen can be used to provide an interpretable blood alcohol concentration. Postmortem blood alcohol results should be compared to vitreous humor and urine concentrations to ensure validity.

In a study of 100 cases, Prouty and Anderson (1987) evaluated alcohol distribution data for pairs of heart and femoral blood specimens. The mean heart/femoral blood alcohol ratio was 0.98, with a mean difference between heart blood and femoral blood specimens of 0.019 g/dL. In cases exhibiting differences greater than 0.02 g/dL, the specimens were "suspect" because of their physical appearance, trauma to the decedent in the area of specimen collection, gross differences in hematocrit, or large volume differences in the two specimens. It was concluded that heart blood was a reliable specimen for postmortem alcohol determinations.

In many instances, including death from severe trauma and exsanguination, blood from central and peripheral sites is not readily available during autopsy. However, blood from the chest, thorax or pleural cavity may be available and submitted to the laboratory for alcohol analysis. In an evaluation conducted by Budd (1988), it was determined that chest cavity blood is representative of heart blood when precautions were taken to minimize postmortem diffusion and when there was no perforation of the stomach walls and diaphragm.

Marraccini et al. (1990) assessed the affects of agonal events on postmortem alcohol concentrations. The events studied included aspiration of ethanol-laden vomitus; intravenous fluid therapy; freshwater drowning; and hanging in a vertical position. The investigators concluded that the interpretation of alcohol measurements must take into consideration the possible entry of ethanol into the pulmonary-venous circulation via the respiratory system.

Briglia et al. (1992) studied multiple specimens obtained during autopsy in sixty-one cases. Statistical analysis of the cases revealed no significant differences among the various blood sites (right and left heart, femoral and pericardial) tested. Larger variances occurred in those instances where the stomach alcohol concentration was greater than 0.5 percent. The study further emphasizes the need for multiple blood specimens to be tested, along with vitreous humor and urine in postmortem cases.

5.2 Serum and Plasma

In clinical laboratories, analyses for alcohol are commonly performed on serum or plasma, rather than on the whole blood. Serum and plasma are essentially equivalent. Serum is obtained by allowing the blood to clot, while plasma is prepared by collecting blood in a tube with an anticoagulant. The only difference is that fibrinogen and certain other substances are precipitated or destroyed in the clotting process. For alcohol determinations, the concentration in both serum and plasma are the same. It is important to understand the relationship between blood alcohol and serum or plasma alcohol concentrations. Since alcohol distributes according to the water content of the tissue or fluid and since there is about 12 percent to 18 percent more water in a volume of serum or plasma than in a corresponding volume of whole blood, one would expect that serum or plasma would have a higher alcohol concentration than the corresponding whole blood. Further, by using the Hct of the blood specimen, one can calculate the expected serum/plasma-blood ratio of alcohol concentrations. Several reports (Grumer, 1957; Illchmann-Christ, 1959; Dotzauer et al., 1952) have determined experimentally serum-blood and plasma-blood ratios. Serum-blood ratios vary from 1.12 to 1.17 whereas plasma-blood ratios ranged from 1.10 to 1.35, with an average of about 1.18 (Payne et al., 1968). Thus, there appears to be no significant difference between plasma-blood and serum-blood ratios.

5.3 Urine

In addition to breath and blood, a widely used specimen for determining alcohol has been urine. Urine is the end product of the physiology involving the kidney, which is responsible for the removal of waste products from the body. Each minute, the kidneys receive 1,200 mL of blood, which is approximately one-fourth of the cardiac output. This renal blood flow corresponds to a renal plasma flow of 650 mL per minute. About one fifth, or 130 mL per minute, is filtered by the glomeruli. This means that 180 liters of protein-free filtrate is generated each day. However, only about 1.5 liters is excreted as urine. The remainder is reabsorbed by the renal tubules. Unionized chemicals are more likely to be absorbed while more polar, or water-soluble, compounds remain in the filtrate.

Intrinsically, urine has some advantages over blood. Since urine can be obtained without invading the body, it does not require specialized personnel or equipment. Because of this, many studies have been undertaken to correlate urine alcohol concentrations with blood alcohol concentrations. The majority of these studies suggest that the average urine-blood ratio is about 1.3. However, there is tremendous variation in the ratios determined. For example, in one study (Payne et al., 1967), blood and urine specimens of thirty-five drivers suspected of drunk driving were analyzed; urine-blood ratios were found to vary from 1.10 to 2.44. In postmortem specimens, Kaye and Cardona (1969) obtained blood and urine specimens for alcohol analysis in 148 autopsied cases and found that the urine-blood ratio averaged 1.28, but ranged from 0.21 to 2.66. Using the average ratio, they calculated a blood alcohol concentration from the urine alcohol concentration and compared it to the actual blood concentration. In 21.5 percent of the cases, the calculated blood alcohol concentration exceeded the actual value while in 34.5 percent of the cases, the calculated value underestimated the actual blood alcohol concentration. Another study (Backer et al., 1980) found urine-blood alcohol ratios ranging from 0.53 to 2.17 in postmortem specimens.

Jones (1980) studied twenty-one healthy males by collecting blood and urine specimens at different time intervals for seven hours after drinking. It was determined that the urine-blood alcohol ratio could be divided into two phases: an absorptive phase when the ratio is less than 1.0 and a post absorptive phase when the ratio is greater than 1.3 and may even exceed 2.0. This suggests that although urine alcohol concentrations by themselves are not useful in determining blood alcohol concentrations, when they are used in conjunction with blood alcohol concentrations, some information can be inferred regarding the time frame of the individual's drinking. A low urine-blood alcohol ratio suggests that little time has passed between drinking and sampling such that absorption is still occurring. A higher ratio implies absorption has been completed and the individual is in the elimination phase.

A similar approach to assessing the status of alcohol absorption was used by Levine and Smialek (1990). In a study of 129 decedents (drivers), the urine-blood alcohol ratios were sorted into three ranges corresponding to absorptive (<1.0), plateau (1.0–1.2), and postabsorptive (>1.2) phases of alcohol absorption. Based on this approach, less than 10 percent of the decedents were in the absorptive phase at the time of their death, whereas greater than 90 percent of the decedents were in the plateau or postabsorptive phases at the time of their death.

Kuroda et al. (1995) performed a retrospective study of 435 fatalities in order to assess the statistical relationship between blood and urine alcohol concentrations. The evaluation produced wide prediction intervals that would not be useful in assessing an individual decedent. The investigators concluded that it is not valid to derive a blood alcohol concentration based on a conversion factor applied to a urine alcohol concentration.

In addition to pharmacokinetic considerations, there are other explanations for such a wide variation in urine-blood alcohol ratios. Alcohol has a diuretic effect, resulting from inhibition of the release of antidiuretic hormone (ADH). However, there are great individual differences in sensitivity to this effect. An individual producing more dilute urine would be expected to have a lower urine-blood ratio than one producing a more concentrated urine. A related factor is the frequency of urination between alcohol ingestion and urine collection. To diminish these problems, the following procedure has been used: The bladder is emptied and the urine is discarded. After a twenty-to-thirty-minute wait, a second urine specimen is obtained and this is used for the analysis. The alcohol concentration in the second urine specimen reflects more accurately the blood alcohol concentration at that time.

5.4 Bile

Bile is often collected during postmortem examination for alcohol and drug analysis. Bile is stored in the gall bladder and generally remains intact and free from contamination. Winek et al. (1983) evaluated the relationship between blood and bile alcohol concentrations. The mean blood-bile alcohol ratio was 1.03, with a range of 0.32–2.91. Further studies evaluated the effect of surface tension, specific gravity, viscosity and lipid content on the bile alcohol content. These studies demonstrated no correlation between the blood-bile alcohol ratio and the aforementioned physical properties.

5.5 Saliva

Although blood and urine are the two most popular fluids for alcohol analysis, saliva has been used as an alternate specimen. It has the advantage of urine of being obtainable by noninvasive techniques, but it also has the limitation of urine in that it is a somewhat variable specimen. Saliva is composed of secretions from three major salivary gland sources: the parotid, the submaxillary, and the sublingual glands. The degree to which each gland contributes to the makeup of the saliva depends on numerous factors: type, duration, intensity of stimulation, time of day, diet, age, sex, and disease state (Danhof and Breimer, 1978). Furthermore, the pH of saliva shows greater inter- and intra-individual variation (Mucklow, 1982). Fortunately, this is not a problem with alcohol since, unlike other drugs, alcohol distributes according to the water content and is independent of pH. There are a number of techniques that can be used to collect saliva (e.g., direct collection, stimulation, swabs), with each method producing saliva of variable composition. As a result, the combined saliva exudates in the mouth more recently have been named oral fluid.

In spite of these pitfalls, numerous investigators have attempted to use saliva alcohol concentrations as an estimate of blood alcohol concentrations. Coldwell and Smith (1959) found a good correlation between blood and saliva alcohol concentrations. The saliva-blood alcohol ratio was 1.12. In a study of forty-eight subjects with 336 data pairs conducted by Jones (1979a), saliva and blood values were highly correlated, with a mean saliva-blood alcohol ratio of 1.082. The ratio of saliva to blood was independent of the sampling time (phases of ethanol metabolism) and the blood alcohol concentration. Jones (1979b) additionally reported a ratio of 1.079 for the same subjects. Further studies by Jones (1980) found that after thirty minutes of alcohol ingestion, the saliva-blood alcohol ratio remained constant at 1.10 throughout a seven-hour period.

The saliva to blood ratio is theoretically 1.17, with saliva and whole blood containing 994 and 850 grams of water per kilogram, respectively. However, generally lower ratios have been found in the postabsorptive phase. Saliva alcohol concentrations more closely parallel the blood concentration in the elimination phase thus relating more to capillary rather than venous blood (Cone, 1993; Haeckel and Bucklitsch, 1987).

5.6 Brain and Cerebrospinal Fluid

In postmortem cases, a greater variety of specimens are available for alcohol analysis. It could be assumed that since brain is available, it would be the specimen of choice. However, brain-blood alcohol concentration ratios have also shown a great variability, ranging from 0.31 to 8.0 (Hine, 1951; Freireich, 1960; Budd, 1983). This is not surprising in view of the heterogeneous makeup of the brain. Different parts of the brain have different water contents (gray matter versus white matter) and differential blood flow, and what is generally reported is an average of all of these parts. Regional distribution of alcohol in the brain is rarely reported and extrapolation of blood alcohol values based on brain alcohol values is discouraged unless the brain specimen is representative of the whole brain (Garriott, 2003).

Cerebrospinal fluid (CSF) is another specimen that can be used for alcohol analysis. Intuitively, the CSF might be expected to more closely correlate with the ethanol concentration in the CNS. Gettler and Freireich (1931) reported an average ratio of 1.08 for fifteen subjects. Harger et al. (1937) found a lumbar CSF-blood alcohol ratio of 1.14 in forty-six specimens. Hebold (1959) reported a range of 0.93 to 1.40 in twenty-two subjects. Although no concentrations were published, Marcellini (1961) administered alcohol orally to ten fasting nonalcoholic patients and obtained blood and CSF every half-hour for six hours after drinking. The maximum blood alcohol concentration was reached within ninety minutes in eight of the ten patients, but the maximum CSF concentration was not reached until three hours after drinking in nine of the ten subjects. Moreover, during the elimination phase, the concentration in the CSF exceeded that in the blood. In more recent studies, average ratios of 1.1 and 0.9 were reported in two sets of postmortem cases (Backer et al., 1980; Budd, 1982). The apparent delay in distribution equilibrium, coupled with the difficulty in properly obtaining an uncontaminated specimen, has limited the use of CSF.

5.7 Vitreous Humor

Vitreous humor is a relatively easy specimen for the medical examiner to obtain and is a relatively stable postmortem. Since the vitreous humor is located in a peripheral body compartment, there is a delay in alcohol uptake and removal in vitreous humor compared to blood. Sturner and Coumbis (1966) were the first to show a close correlation between vitreous humor and blood alcohol concentrations in postmortem specimens with an average reported vitreous humor-blood ratio of 1.10. Coe and Sherman (1970) studied 174 cases; the average vitreous humor-blood alcohol ratio was 1.12. Other studies (Backer et al., 1980; Leahy et al., 1968; Felby and Olsen, 1969; Scott et al., 1974; Budd, 1982) have produced average ratios of between 0.90 and 1.38 (See also Chapter 6 for blood-vitreous humor relationships).

Scott et al. (1974) illustrated the potential of using vitreous humor to determine alcohol involvement in those cases where the body has been embalmed. In eight cases in which the blood was positive for alcohol, pre-embalmed and post-embalmed vitreous specimens were obtained and analyzed. The average pre-embalmed vitreous-blood alcohol ratio was 0.91, while the post-embalmed ratio was 0.81. This indicates that vitreous humor can be a useful specimen to analyze for alcohol in embalmed cases. Furthermore, Zumwalt et al. (1982) studied vitreous humor in relation to bacterial infiltration in decomposed bodies after assessing the degree of putrefaction based on eight physical changes. They found that even in moderately decomposed bodies, few bacteria were detected in the vitreous humor, suggesting that postmortem formation of alcohol in vitreous humor would be negligible under these circumstances. Therefore, any alcohol found in the vitreous humor could be presumed to be of exogenous origin.

The interpretation of alcohol concentrations in decomposed specimens without vitreous humor can be a difficult process since concentrations can increase or decrease in biological fluids with time and other factors. Realizing that this information is needed in many cases, it is suggested that a negative alcohol result probably indicates that no alcohol was present at death while a very high blood alcohol concentration was probably not caused by alcohol neoformation alone. Blood alcohol concentrations exceeding 0.1 g/dL in postmortem cases are likely the result of true alcohol ingestion when the analysis is conducted by gas chromatography.

This relationship was confirmed in a more recent study (Caplan and Levine, 1990). Blood ethanol concentrations less than 0.03 g/dL are frequently associated with negative vitreous humor ethanol concentrations, implying that postmortem fermentation may have occurred. A blood ethanol concentration of 0.05 g/dL has an 87 percent chance of being associated with a positive vitreous humor ethanol concentration. A blood ethanol concentration greater than 0.05 g/dL has a 99 percent chance of being associated with a positive vitreous humor ethanol concentration.

5.8 Other Specimens

Very little has been published regarding the distribution of alcohol into the central body compartments, such as liver and kidney. This is surprising because liver is a frequently analyzed specimen for most other drugs. Presumably, since these organs have a rich blood supply, these tissues reach equilibrium with the blood quite rapidly after absorption. This has been confirmed in animal studies. Harger et al. (1937), in dog studies, found no change in liver-blood ratio from five minutes to twelve hours, with a ratio of 0.78. Christopoulos et al. (1973) conducted distribution studies of alcohol in various body tissues and fluids obtained from three postmortem cases involving a violent death with a positive blood alcohol concentration. Liver-blood ratios averaged 0.63 ± 0.1 with a range of 0.51 to 0.83. In ten cases of acute alcohol intoxication (> 0.49 percent) the average liver-blood ratio was 0.6 ± 0.056 with a range of 0.54 to 0.72; the average kidney-blood ratio was 0.66 ± 0.058 with a range of 0.57 to 0.76. In a larger study, Jenkins et al. (1995) reported liver to heart-blood ratios for seventy-one cases in which the heart-blood alcohol concentration was equal to or greater than 0.04 g/dL. The average ratio was 0.56 (SD = 0.3). Seventy-six percent of the cases showed ratios between 0.26 and 0.86. In six cases where the cause of death was acute alcohol intoxication, the average liver to heart-blood ratio was 0.65 (range 0.47–0.85).

In addition to the analysis of the more common toxicologic specimens for alcohol, attempts have been made to correlate blood alcohol concentrations with alcohol concentrations in unusual specimens.

Isokoski et al. (1968) analyzed blood and femur bone marrow for alcohol in twelve postmortem cases. These specimens were analyzed using both the Widmark and ADH methods. The marrow-blood ratios ranged from 0.21 to 0.67 in ten of the cases with an average ratio of 0.34 ± 0.14. Of the remaining two cases, one had a ratio of 1.75, whereas the other had a negative blood and a positive marrow alcohol. The authors concluded that due to the great individual variations in the ratios, it was impossible to determine the exact blood alcohol concentration from a given marrow alcohol concentration.

Winek and Jones (1980) performed similar studies, but instead of using femur marrow, they used rib marrow, and found an average marrow-blood ratio of 0.47 ± 0.066, ranging from 0.34 to 0.61. They postulated that this wide range may be due to differences in the lipid content of the marrow, and in a subsequent study from their laboratory (Winek and Esposito, 1981), an attempt was made to correct for the differences in lipid content in the bone marrow. A weighed amount of marrow was extracted with ether and after centrifugation and separation, the ether layer was evaporated to dryness. The resulting residue was weighed and it was assumed that this fraction of the total weight was the lipid fraction while the remaining weight was the aqueous fraction. This "corrected" marrow concentration was equal to the observed marrow concentration divided by the aqueous fraction. Without the correction, the average marrow-blood ratio was 0.53 with a range of 0.31 to 0.77; with the correction, the average ratio was 0.79 with a range of 0.6 to 1.03.

Skeletal muscle is another unusual specimen studied. Based on water content, the theoretical muscle-blood ratio would be 0.86 (Harger, 1937). Felby and Olsen (1969) determined leg muscle-blood and arm muscle-blood alcohol ratios from fifteen postmortem cases; the average ratios were 0.89 and 0.9, respectively. This was in agreement with the ratio later found by Krauland et al. (1980) of 0.91.

Further studies of medical examiner cases by Garriott (1991) indicated a uniform distribution of alcohol into two groups. In the group with blood alcohol concentrations greater than 0.1 g/dL, the muscle-blood ratio was 1.0 or less with an average of 0.94. In the group with blood alcohol concentrations less than 0.1 g/dL, the muscle-blood ratio was 1.0 or greater with an average of 1.48. These data indicate a muscle-blood ratio that is dependent upon the time course of absorption and distribution, as seen with vitreous humor, but with more rapid equilibration.

Synovial fluid, another unusual specimen, is a viscous, straw-colored fluid found within the joints, bursae, and tendon sheaths. The mean water content of synovial fluid is 96 percent. Winek et al. (1993) and Ohshima et al. (1997) conducted postmortem distribution studies of alcohol in blood and synovial fluid from the bursa sac (knee joint). In the Winek et al. study, the mean synovial fluid-blood alcohol ratio was 1.01 with a range of 0.58 to 2.41. In the Ohshima et al. study, the mean synovial fluid-blood alcohol ratio was 1.31 with a range of 1.07 to 1.67.

Finally, sequestered subdural, epidural and intracerebral hematomas may provide valuable information regarding the concentration of alcohol in the blood at the time of an injury. Analysis of the alcohol content of sequestered hematomas is particularly useful when the injury does not result in immediate death. Although the alcohol content of the sequestered hematomas is not metabolized to any significant degree, changes in alcohol content may occur as a result of intermittent or continual bleeding, perfusion, dehydration, or reabsorption. In addition, since the formation of sequestered hematomas is generally not instantaneous, the concentration of ethanol in the sequestered hematoma may lack uniformity and not correlate well to levels of alcohol in the blood (Hirsch and Adelson, 1973; Smialek at al, 1980; Eisele et al., 1984; and Buchsbaum et al., 1989).

All ratios of the various specimens to blood alcohol concentrations in human studies are summarized in Table 5.1.

Table 5.1
Summary of Ratios of Specimens to Blood Alcohol Concentrations in Human Studies

Specimen	Study	Number	Average	Range
Serum or plasma	Grumer, 1957		1.16	1.13–1.17
	Illchmann-Christ, 1959		1.17 ± 0.06	
	Dotzauer et al., 1952		1.12 ± 0.006	
	Payne et al., 1968		1.18	
Urine	Jetter, 1938	372	1.23	1.0–2.3
	Bavis, 1940	66	1.17	0.81–1.65
	Mozes and Katonak, 1941	100	1.16	0.63–1.65
	Ellenbrook and Van Gaazbeek, 1943	76	1.26	0.69–1.71
	Prag, 1953	75	1.31	1.0–1.64
	Coldwell and Smith, 1959	91	1.24 ± 0.08	
	Lundquist, 1961	55	1.35	1.12–1.51
	Morgan, 1965	518	1.38	0.9–2.4
	Heise, 1967	20	1.4 ± 0.84	1.29–1.58
	Payne et al., 1967	35	1.44	1.1–2.44
	Kaye and Cardona, 1969	148	1.28	0.21–2.66
	Christopoulos et al., 1973	9	1.01 ± 0.15	0.79–1.16
	Backer et al., 1980	92	1.16	0.53–2.17
	Budd, 1982	109	1.5	
	Stone and Rooney, 1984	88	1.29	
Saliva	Friedeman et al., 1938	13	1.1	0.97–1.31
	Elbel, 1949			0.97–1.25
	Prag, 1953	6	1.2 ± 0.13	1.1–1.4
	Coldwell and Smith, 1959	244	1.12	
	DiGregorio et al., 1978		1.04	0.95–1.13
	Jones, 1979a	336	1.082	
	Jones, 1979b	336	1.077	1.065–1.088
	Jones, 1980	21	1.1	
	Haeckel and Bucklitcsh, 1987		1.032	
	Kiesow et al., 1993	56	1.14	
CSF	Gettler and Freireich, 1931	15	1.08	0.42–12.5
	Harger et al., 1937	46	1.18 ± 0.09	
	Christopoulos et al., 1973	7	0.92 ± 0.058	0.84–1.01
	Backer et al., 1980	54	1.14	0.79–1.64
	Budd	5	0.09 ± 0.4	

continued on next page

Table 5.1
Summary of Ratios of Specimens to Blood Alcohol Concentrations in Human Studies (cont'd)

Specimen	Study	Number	Average	Range
Vitreous humor	Sturner and Coumbis, 1966	38	0.99 ± 0.22	0.46–1.4
	Leanhy et al., 1968	20	1.08 ± 0.078	0.89–1.23
	Felby and Olsen, 1969	27	1.34 ± 0.29	0.52–1.82
	Coe and Sherman, 1970	174	1.12	
	Scott et al., 1974	8	0.91 ± 0.17	0.67–1.13
	Backer et al., 1980	110	1.05	0.48–1.72
	Budd, 1982	15	1.3 ± 0.6	
	Stone and Rooney, 1984		1.34	
Brain	Gettler and Freireich, 1931	12	0.96	0.63–1.47
	Ellenbrook and Van Gaasbeek, 1943	19	0.92	0.76–1.13
	Van Hecke et al., 1957	47	0.69	0.37–1.35
	Hine, 1951	100	0.65	0.31–2.0
	Freireich et al., 1960	82	0.94	0.69–1.47
	Herold and Prokop, 1960	35	0.69	0.38–1.3
	Christopoulos et al., 1973	10	0.62 (acute alcohol death)	0.51–0.76
	Backer et al., 1980	33	0.86	0.64–1.2
	Budd, 1982	51	1.24	0.31–8.0
	Moore et al., 1997	18 / 18	0.9 (occipital) / 0.6 (cerebellar)	0.0–1.8 / 0.0–1.2
Liver	Christopoulos et al., 1973		0.63 ± 0.1 (violent death) / 0.6 ± 0.056 (acute alcohol death)	0.51–0.83 / 0.54–0.72
	Jenkins et al., 1995	71	0.56 ± 0.3	0–1.4
Kidney	Christopoulos et al., 1973		0.66 ± 0.058 (acute alcohol death)	0.57–0.76
Bone marrow	Isokoski et al., 1968	10	0.34 ± 0.14	0.21–0.67
	Winek and Jones, 1980	18	0.47 ± 0.066	0.34–0.61
	Winek and Esposito, 1981	36	0.53 (actual) / 0.79 (corrected)	0.31–0.77 / 0.6–1.03

References

Backer, R.C., Pisano, R.V. and Sopher, I.M. The comparison of alcohol concentrations in postmortem fluids and tissues. *J. Forensic Sci.* 25:327–331, 1980.

Bavis, D.F. 145 drunken drivers: A blood alcohol study. *J. Lab. Clin. Med.* 25:2223–273, 1940.

Briglia, E.J., Bidanset, J.H. and Dal Cortivo, L.A. The distribution of ethanol in postmortem blood specimens. *J. Forensic Sci.* 37:991–998, 1992.

Brown, G.A. et al. The stability of ethanol in stored blood, I: Important variables and interpretation of results. *Anal. Chim. Acta* 66:271–283, 1973.

Buchsbaum, R.M., Adelson, L. and Sunshine, I. A comparison of post-mortem ethanol levels obtained from blood and subdural specimens. *Forensic Sci. Int.* 41:237–243, 1989.

Budd, R.D. Ethanol levels in postmortem body fluids. *J. Chromatogr.* 252:315–318, 1982.

Budd, R.D. Postmortem brain alcohol levels. *J. Chromatogr.* 259:353–355, 1983.

Budd, R.D. Validity of postmortem chest cavity blood ethanol determinations. *J. Chromatogr.* 449:337–340, 1988.

Caplan, Y.H. and Levine, B. Vitreous humor in the evaluation of postmortem blood ethanol concentrations. *J. Anal. Toxicol.* 14:305–307, 1990.

Chang, R.B. et al. The stability of ethyl alcohol in forensic blood specimens. *J. Anal. Toxicol.* 8:66–67, 1984.

Christopoulos, G., Kirch, E.R. and Gearrien, J.E. Determination of ethanol in fresh and putrefied post mortem tissues. *J. Chromatogr.* 87:454–472, 1973.

Coe, J.I. and Sherman, R.E. Comparative study of postmortem vitreous humor and blood alcohol. *J. Forensic Sci.* 15:185–190, 1970.

Coldwell, B.D. and Smith, H.W. Alcohol levels in body fluids after ingestion of distilled spirits. *Can. J. Biochem. Physiol.* 37:43–52, 1959.

Cone, E.J. Saliva testing for drugs of abuse. *Ann. N.Y. Acad Sci.* 694:91–127, 1993.

Danhof, M. and Breimer, D.D. Therapeutic drug monitoring in saliva. *Clin. Pharmacokinet.* 3:39–57, 1978.

DiGregorio, G.J., Piraino, A.J. and Ruch, E. Correlations of parotid saliva and blood ethanol concentrations. *Drug Alcohol Depend.* 3: 43–50, 1978.

Dotzauer, G. et al. Eprobung einer spezifischer Ferment-methode zur Mikrobestimmung von Äthylalkohol. *Dtsch. Z. Ges. Gerichtl. Med.* 41:15, 1952.

Dubowski, J. *Manual for Analysis of Ethanol in Biological Liquids.* U.S. Dept. of Transportation Report No. DOT-TSC-NHTSA0-76-4, 1977, pp. 5–7.

Dundee, J.W., Isaac, M. and Taggart, J. Blood ethanol levels following rapid intravenous infusion. *Q. J. Stud. Alcohol* 32:741–747, 1971.

Eisele, J.W., Reay, D.T. and Bonnell, H.J. Ethanol in sequestered hematomas: Quantitative evaluation. *Am. J. Clin. Pathol.* 81:352–355, 1984.

Elbel, H. *Dtsch. Z. Gesamte Gerichtl. Med.* 39:538, 1949.

Ellenbrook, L.D. and Van Gaasbeek, C.B. The reliability of chemical tests for alcoholic intoxication. *JAMA* 122:996–1002, 1943.

Felby, S. and Olsen, J. Comparative studies of postmortem ethyl alcohol in vitreous humor, blood, and muscle. *J. Forensic Sci.* 14:93–101, 1969.

Forney, R.B. et al. Alcohol distribution in the vascular system: Concentration of orally administered alcohol in blood from various parts in the vascular system and in rebreathed air during absorption. *Q. J. Stud. Alcohol* 25:205–217, 1964.

Freireich, A.W., Landau, D.P. and Lukash, L. A comparison of alcohol levels in brain, heart blood, and peripheral blood. Read to the Second Intentional Meeting on Forensic Pathology and Medicine, New York University Medical Center, New York, 1960, abstract 10-1, p. 49.

Friedemann, T.E., Motel, W.G. and Necheles, H. The excretion of ingested alcohol in saliva. *J. Lab. Clin. Med.* 23:1007–1014, 1938.

Garriott, J.C. Skeletal muscle as an alternative specimen for alcohol and drug analysis. *J. Forens. Sci.* 36:60–69, 1991.

Garriott, J.C. Analysis for alcohol in postmortem specimens. In: Garriott, J.C. (ed.), *Medical-Legal Aspects of Alcohol*, 4th ed. Tucson, AZ: Lawyers & Judges Publishing Co., 2003. pp 163–176.

Gettler, A.O. and Freireich, A.W. Determination of alcoholic intoxication during life by spinal fluid analysis. *J. Biol. Chem.* 92:199–209, 1931.

Goldfinger, T.M. and Schaber, D.A comparison of blood alcohol concentration using non-alcohol and alcohol-containing skin antiseptics. *Ann. Emerg. Med.* 11:665–667, 1982.

Grumer, O. The distribution of alcohol in the blood. *Dtsch. Z. Ges. Gerichtl. Med.* 46:10, 1957.

Haeckel, R. and Bucklitsch, I. The comparability of ethanol concentrations in peripheral blood and saliva. The phenomenon of variation in saliva to blood concentration ratios. *J. Clin. Chem. Clin. Biochem.* 25:199–204, 1987.

Haggard, H.W., Greenberg, L.A. and Rakietin, N. Studies on the absorption, distribution, and elimination of alcohol, part 6: The principles governing the concentration of alcohol in the blood and the concentration causing respiratory failure. *J. Pharmacol. Exp. Ther.* 69:252–265, 1940.

Harger, R.N., Forney, R.B. and Baker, R.S. Estimation of the level of blood alcohol from analysis of breath, part 2: Use a rebreathed air. *Q. J. Stud. Alcohol* 17:1–18, 1956.

Harger, R.N., Hulpieu, H.R. and Lamb, E.B. The speed with which various parts of the body reach equilibrium in the storage of ethyl alcohol. *J. Biol. Chem.* 120:689–704, 1937.

Hebold, G. Evaluation of alcohol findings in the CSF: Studies on 68 cadavers. *Dtsch. Z. Ges. Gerichtl. Med.* 48:257, 1959.

Heise, H.A. How extraneous alcohol affects the blood test for alcohol. *Am. J. Clin. Pathol.* 32:160–170, 1959.

Herold, K. and Prokop, O. Postmortem alcohol distribution differences in brain. *Dtsch. Z. Ges. Gerichtl. Med.* 50:1, 1960.

Hine, C.H. Blood/brain distribution in 100 postmortem cases. *Proc. Am. Acad. Forensic Sci.* 1:161, 1951.

Hirsch, C.S. and Adelson, L. Ethanol in sequestered hematomas. *Am. J. Clin. Pathol.* 59:429–433, 1973.

Illchmann-Christ, A. Research on the relation of blood clot-total blood (serum) alcohol values with a contribution to the conversion of serum alcohol to total blood concentrations. *Dtsch. Z. Ges. Gerichtl. Med.* 49:113, 1959.

Isokoski, M., Alha, A. and Laiho, K. Bone marrow alcohol content in cadavers. *J. Forensic Med.* 15:9–11, 1968.

Jenkins, A.J., Levine, B.S. and Smialek, J.E. Distribution of ethanol in postmortem liver. *J. Forensic Sci.* 40:611–613, 1995.

Jetter, W.W. Studies in alcohol: I. The diagnosis of acute alcoholic intoxication by a correlation of clinical and chemical findings. *Am. J. Med. Sci.* 196:475–487, 1938.

Jones, A.W. Distribution of ethanol between saliva and blood in man. *Clin. Exp. Pharmacol. Physiol.* 6:53–59, 1979a.

Jones, A.W. Inter- and intra-individual variations in the saliva/blood alcohol ratio during ethanol metabolism in man. *Clin. Chem.* 25:1394–1398, 1979b.

Jones, A.W. Quantitative relationships among ethanol concentrations in blood, breath, saliva, and urine during ethanol metabolism in man. *Proceedings of the Eighth International conference on Alcohol, Drugs, and Traffic Safety*, Stockholm, Sweden, June 15–19, 1980, pp. 550–569.

Kaye, S. The collection and handling of the blood alcohol specimen. *Am. J. Clin. Pathol.* 74:743–746, 1980.

Kaye, S. and Cardona, E. Errors of converting a urine alcohol value into a blood alcohol level. *Am. J. Clin. Pathol.* 52:577–584, 1969.

Kiesow, L.A., Simons, C.T. and Long, W.B. Quantitative determination and comparison of ethanol in saliva samples of unknown volumes with blood ethanol levels in human test subjects following ethanol ingestion. *Ann. N.Y. Acad. Sci.* 694:293–295, 1993.

Krauland, W., Klug, E. and Toffel, P. Determination of alcohol concentrations in organs of human corpses. *Blutalkohol* 17:198–206, 1980.

Kuroda, N., Williams, K. and Pounder, D.J. Estimating blood alcohol from urinary alcohol at autopsy. *Am. J. Forensic Med. Pathol.* 16:219–222, 1995.

Leahy, M.S., Farber, E.R. and Meadows, T.R. Quantitation of ethyl alcohol in the postmortem vitreous humor. *J. Forensic Sci.* 13:498–502, 1968.

Levine, B. and Smialek, J.E. Status of alcohol absorption in drinking drivers killed in traffic accidents. *J. Forensic Sci.* 45:3–6, 2000.

Lundquist, F. The urinary excretion of ethanol by man. *Acta Pharmacol. Toxicol.* 18:231–238, 1961.

Marcellini, D. Blood alcohol and spinal fluid alcohol. *Q. J. Stud. Alcohol* 22:145–146, 1961.

Mason, M.F. and Dubowski, K.M. Alcohol, traffic, and chemical testing in the United States: A resume and some remaining problems. *Clin. Chem.* 20:126–140, 1974.

Marraccini, J.V. et al. Differences between multisite postmortem ethanol concentrations as related to agonal events. *J. Forensic Sci.* 35:1360–1366, 1990.

McCallum, N.E.W. and Scroggie, J.G. Some aspects of alcohol in body fluids, part 3: Study of alcohol in different parts of the body. *Med. J. Aust.* 2:1031, 1960.

Moore, K.A. et al. A comparison of ethanol concentrations in the occipital lobe and cerebellum. *Forensic Sci. Int.* 86:127–134, 1997.

Morgan, W.H.D. Concentrations of alcohol in samples of blood and urine taken at the same time. *J. Forensic Sci. Soc.* 5:15–21, 1965.

Mozes, E.B. and Katonak, L.J. One hundred drunken drivers. *Ohio State Med. J.* 37:21–24, 1941.

Mucklow, J.C. The use of saliva in therapeutic drug monitoring. *Ther. Drug Monit.* 4:229–247, 1982.

Ohshima, T. et al. Postmortem alcohol analysis of the synovial fluid and its availability in medico-legal practices. *Forensic Sci. Int.* 90:131–138, 1997.

Payne, J.P. et al. Observations on interpretation of blood alcohol levels derived from analysis of urine. *Br. Med. J.* 3:819–923, 1967.

Payne, J.P., Hill, D.W. and Wood, D.G.L. Distribution of ethanol between plasma and erythrocytes in whole blood. *Nature* 217:963–964, 1968.

Prag, J.J. The chemical and the clinical diagnosis of driving under the influence of alcohol and the use of chemical tests in traffic law enforcement. *S. Afr. J. Clin. Sci.* 4:289–325, 1953.

Prouty, R.W. and Anderson, W.H. A comparison of postmortem heart blood and femoral blood ethyl alcohol concentrations. *J. Anal. Toxicol.* 11:191–197, 1987.

Scott, W., Root, I. and Sanborn, B. The use of vitreous humor for determination of ethyl alcohol in previously embalmed bodies. *J. Forensic Sci.* 19:913–916, 1974.

Sedman, A.J., Wilkinson, P.K. and Wagner, I.G. Concentrations of ethanol in two segments of the vascular system. *J. Forensic Sci.* 21:315–322, 1976.

Smalldon, K.W. and Brown, G.A. The stability of ethanol in stored blood, II: The mechanism of ethanol oxidation. *Anal. Chim. Acta* 66:285–290, 1973.

Smialek, J.E., Spitz, W.U. and Wolfe, J.A. Ethanol in intracerebral clot: Report of two homicidal cases with prolonged survival after injury. *Am. J. Forensic Med. Pathol.* 1:149–150, 1980.

Stone, R.E. and Rooney, P.A. A study using body fluids to determine blood alcohol. *J. Anal. Toxicol.* 8:95–96, 1984.

Sturner, W.Q. and Coumbis, R.J. The quantitation of ethyl alcohol in vitreous humor and blood by gas chromatography. *Am. J. Clin. Pathol.* 46:349–351, 1966.

Van Hecke, W., Handovsy, H. and Thomas, F. Analyse statistique de 597 dosages d'alcool éthylique practiques dans le sanq, les humeurs et les organes d'un total de 93 cadavres: Signification physiologique et intérèt médico-légal. *Ann. Med. Legale* 31:291–1957.

Winek, C.L. and Jones, T. Blood versus bone marrow ethanol concentrations in rabbits and humans. *Forensic Sci. Int.* 16:101–109, 1980.

Winek, C.L. and Esposito, F.M. Comparative study of ethanol levels in blood versus bone marrow, vitreous humor, bile and urine. *Forensic Sci. Int.* 17:27–36, 1981.

Winek, C.L., Henry, D. and Kirkpatrick, L. The influence of physical properties and lipid content of bile on the human blood/bile ethanol ratio. *Forensic Sci. Int.* 22:171–178, 1983.

Winek, C.L. et al. Blood versus synovial fluid ethanol concentrations in humans. *J. Anal. Toxicol.* 17:233–235, 1993.

Zumwalt, R.E., Bost, R.O. and Sunshine, I. Evaluation of ethanol concentrations in decomposed bodies. *J. Forensic Sci.* 27:549–554, 1982.

Chapter 6

Analysis for Alcohol in Postmortem Specimens

James C. Garriott, Ph.D.

Analysis for ethyl alcohol is the most frequent determination required of laboratories performing toxicology for medical examiners and coroners. Studies have shown that alcohol is the most common drug found in persons dying of all causes, but with highest incidences in deaths from injuries and violence (Norton et al., 1982; Baselt and Cravey, 1980; Garriott, 1993; Smith et al., 1999).

Ethyl alcohol is also one of the leading causes of death by poisoning, ranking with carbon monoxide and heroin (Garriott et al., 1982; Taylor and Hudson, 1977; Caplan, 1985). Over 1,300 Americans are estimated to die annually because of alcohol overdose or when alcohol is a contributing cause of death (Yoon et al., 2002). It is therefore of great importance in forensic autopsy investigations to perform accurate analyses for alcohol using the optimal specimens for this purpose, and to know the significance (and limitations) of alcohol findings in these specimens. The specimen choices, interpretations and implications of alcohol findings in postmortem cases are discussed in this chapter.

6.1 Analytical Considerations

The blood or other fluids or tissues taken at a postmortem examination for alcohol analysis are more likely to be contaminated with volatile substances that could potentially interfere with alcohol analysis as compared with specimens from living subjects. These interfering substances include methanol and formaldehyde from embalming processes; low boiling decomposition products, such as other alcohols; and abnormal metabolic products, such as acetone (e.g., as is formed in deaths resulting from malnutrition or starvation, or in diabetic ketoacidosis). Alcoholics may ingest liquids that contain rubbing alcohol (isopropanol), wood alcohol (methanol), antifreeze (ethylene glycol) or various other volatile solvents.

Therefore it is essential when analyzing postmortem samples for alcohol to utilize specific techniques. Volatile organic components would interfere most with the nonspecific oxidation techniques and least with gas chromatographic procedures, which are designed to separate all low-boiling compounds eluting in the same range as ethyl alcohol (see Chapter 9 for discussion of methods for alcohol analysis). An advantage in analysis of postmortem cases is that a greater choice of specimens is available than in living persons. It is always desirable to analyze more than one specimen for optimum interpretation of alcohol in postmortem cases.

6.2 Distribution of Alcohol in the Body

Body fluid and tissue distribution of alcohol is discussed in Chapter 5 (see Table 5.1). The following discussion will consider special circumstances relating to postmortem specimens.

A. Blood

Blood is the most important of autopsy specimens to analyze for alcohol, and other specimens are usually related to and compared with blood concentrations. The blood itself is subject to some variation, depending on site of sampling, collection technique, and other factors to be discussed. In living subjects, venous blood is sampled, usually from the anterior cubital vein of the arm. After death, peripheral blood is more difficult to obtain, and sampling is usually from the heart or major vessels. Arterial blood is up to 40 percent higher in alcohol concentration than venous blood in the absorptive phase, whereas there is little difference between the two specimens in the postabsorptive phase (see Chapter 3 for a more detailed discussion of arterial-venous differences).

Thus blood from the heart or other large blood vessels may differ from venous blood in alcohol concentration at death due to incomplete distribution (Forney et al., 1950; Martin et al., 1984). This difference was demonstrated by comparing heart blood with femoral blood in fifty-one cases, thirty-five of which had higher cardiac blood alcohol concentrations, the greatest difference observed being 0.09 g/dL (Turkel and Gifford, 1957). Prouty and Anderson (1987) analyzed heart and femoral blood in 100 autopsy cases, however, and found the heart/femoral blood ratio to be near unity (0.98). Of seventeen cases with differences between the two specimens greater than 20 percent, only six had heart/femoral blood greater than unity. These six cases were either in early stages of absorption, or the femoral blood was artificially low due to low specimen volume in the sample tube. According to the study of Prouty and Anderson, in the great majority of autopsy cases there is little difference in vascular distribution of alcohol. This is not to say that differences cannot occur, however, especially in cases of recent ingestion when the deceased had been in the absorption phase and distribution equilibrium had not been established. Circulatory equilibrium of alcohol occurs rapidly, however, so that significant differences in blood sources in autopsy cases are rare.

B. Antemortem dilution

An injured subject receiving transfusions of blood or fluids may have a diluted blood sample, leading to false low alcohol concentrations. The actual dilution of the blood alcohol concentration can be estimated if the volume transfused is known. Alcohol is distributed in total body water, rather than in blood. Therefore, if two liters of fluid are given to a 150-pound male, with a volume of distribution (V_d) of 0.66 (see Chapters 3 and 4 for discussion of V_d), the body water, and consequently the blood alcohol, has been diluted by 4.4 pounds in 100-pound of body water, so the dilution is only 4.4 percent (Field, 1993). This dilution factor is sometimes magnified, however, when cardiovascular failure occurs and the fluids are not circulated or equilibrated in the body water, resulting in substantial dilutions in heart or other systemic vasculature blood. Vitreous fluid and peripheral blood will present more valid specimens for alcohol analysis when diluting fluids have been administered shortly prior to death.

Table 6.1 shows some case examples of effects of fluid dilution on postmortem and antemortem samples in autopsies of trauma victims. In cases 1 and 2, the antemortem samples are obviously artificially low in alcohol concentration due to fluids administered during treatment for traumatic injury, and the postmortem samples reflect the more accurate blood concentrations as evidenced by the comparative values in vitreous humor. Cases 3 and 4 show an opposite effect, with fluid dilution affecting the postmortem samples. This could result from fluid infusion near the time of death, diluting the heart blood. Case 5 reflects a more normal degradation during a 1.5-hour survival, with no fluids given.

C. Other body tissues

Alcohol is distributed primarily in the body water. Consequently, the alcohol concentration in various organs or body fluids is dependent on the water content of that specimen. Harger et al. (1937), after administering alcohol to dogs, reported that when equilibrium is reached (after two to three hours), the brain, liver, muscle, stomach tissue, upper intestine, and lower intestine store practically the same amount of alcohol per gram of water. Their calculated distribution ratios after equilibrium, based on

Table 6.1
Alcohol Concentrations in Traumatic Deaths After Hospital Treatment

Case No.	BAC (AM)	BAC (PM)	VAC	Treatment
	g/dL			
1	0.018	0.073	0.093	5.5 liters fluid; survived 1.75 hours
2	0.120	0.230	0.210	1.7 liters fluid; survived 0.75 hour
3	0.234	0.071	0.104	1 liter fluid; survived 2.5 hours
4	0.141	0.019	NA	2 liters fluid; survived 4.25 hours
5	0.12 serum −0.16	0.091	0.148	no fluids given; survived 1.5 hours

BAC (VAC) = Blood (vitreous humor) alcohol concentration; AM = antemortem; PM = postmortem

brain as 1.0, were: blood 1.18 ± 0.08; liver 0.94 ± 0.04; muscle 1.01 ± 0.04; stomach contents 1.13 ± 0.08; stomach tissue 0.93 ± 0.06; upper intestine 0.97 ± 0.03, and lower intestine: 0.99 ± 0.05. Since blood is today the most commonly utilized specimen for alcohol analysis (both living and postmortem) the values of Harger et al. as tissue- or fluid-to blood ratios would be: brain, 0.847; liver, 0.797; muscle, 0.856; stomach contents, 0.958; stomach tissue, 0.788; upper and lower intestine, 0.788 and 0.876, respectively; spinal fluid-blood ratios in forty-six human subjects averaged 1.18 ± 0.09 (see also Chapter 5, Table 5.1).

A study of ethanol distribution in human liver at autopsy (Jenkins et al., 1995) yielded an average liver:heart blood ratio of 0.53 ± 0.3 (range 0–1.40) in seventy-one cases with a BAC greater than or equal to 0.04 g/dL. Six cases diagnosed as deaths from acute ethanol intoxication had an average liver:heart blood ratio of 0.65 (range 0.47–0.85), likely reflecting death before complete distribution. The authors also considered the possibility of liver degradation of alcohol or other loss as an explanation for their lower ratios than those of Harger, since their specimens were stored up to one month prior to analysis.

D. Skeletal muscle

A study conducted on rats reported the skeletal muscle-blood ratio of alcohol concentrations to be 0.97 two hours after alcohol dosing, using femoral muscle (Nanikawa et al., 1982). Harger et al. (1937), studying dogs, stated that muscle lagged behind the other tissues during the first hour in reaching equilibrium, but that this was established within three

hours and the femoral muscle-blood ratio was 0.856. The reason for the difference in the ratios reported for the two species is not apparent, and equilibrium times are not known for humans. In the studies of Harger et al., all tissues were in equilibrium at three hours, at which time only 1 percent of the alcohol dose remained unabsorbed in the stomach. At thirty minutes the unabsorbed alcohol was dependent on the dose; 6.2 percent and 49.1 percent, respectively, remained after 0.5- and 6.0-g/kg doses. Garriott (1991), comparing psoas muscle and blood from human autopsies, found a blood/muscle ratio of 0.94 ± 0.086 in cases when the blood alcohol concentration was greater than 0.1 g/dL, and a ratio averaging 1.48 ± 0.13 in cases with BACs less than 0.1 g/dL. The ratios mirrored very closely those found in vitreous humor, and were thought to reflect the state of alcohol absorption. The majority of those with BACs greater than 0.1 g/dL would have been at maximum distribution equilibrium, while those with less than 0.1 g/dL were believed to be far into the postabsorptive phase, and the higher muscle concentrations reflected the lag time for alcohol equilibration as seen in vitreous humor.

Luvoni and Marozzi (1968) studied tissue distribution of alcohol in fifty-nine human autopsies, and found that they could be divided into two groups: those with tissue concentrations of alcohol lower than those in the blood, and those with tissue concentrations higher than those in the blood. Those with lower tissue concentrations were presumed to have been in the preabsorptive phase after alcohol ingestion, while those with higher concentrations were in the postabsorptive phase. They concluded that only when the individual was in the postabsorptive phase at death, could the blood alcohol concentrations be predicted from concentrations of the tissues.

E. Brain

Brain alcohol concentrations appear to be subject to regional differences. Meyer (1959) reported the following brain-blood distribution ratios after administering a 3-g/kg dose to rats and permitting equilibrium to be established: telencephalon 0.689; diencephalon and mesencephalon 0.546; cerebellum 0.55; and medulla oblongata 0.426. He suggested that brain distribution depends more on blood supply than on water content. These ratios are considerably lower than those reported by some other authors, however. In a study of human autopsy tissue, brain-blood ethanol ratios varied from 0.29 to 8.0, with 82 percent of the values between 0.8 and 1.50 (Budd, 1983). The mean ratio was 1.24, with a standard deviation of 1.01. If one eliminates the single 8.00 observation (occurring with a blood alcohol of only 0.01 percent) the range of ratios would be 0.29 to 2.0. From these observations, it would seem unwise to attempt to extrapolate brain alcohol concentrations to those of blood unless one were careful to analyze a sample representative of the whole brain. The study of Harger et al. (1937) used the whole brain.

In general, the organ-blood ratios are relatively consistent, provided the subject was in the postabsorption phase of alcohol distribution. The postabsorptive phase occurs after that point in time when most ingested alcohol has been absorbed from the gastrointestinal (GI) tract, and the maximum BAC has been reached. Harger et al. (1937) found that three hours after a single dose of alcohol given to dogs, virtually all had been absorbed. Observations in human subjects have shown that alcohol is absorbed rapidly during normal drinking circumstances, and that the peak BAC is reached in less than sixty minutes in the majority of subjects (Jones, 1990; Moore, 1991). Prior to one hour, alcohol is present in irregular proportions in various organs, and valid extrapolation to blood concentrations cannot be made.

In order to determine if a deceased subject had been in the postabsorptive phase at the time of death, it has been suggested that an analysis for ethyl alcohol be performed on the gastric contents (Backer et al., 1980). If the gastric concentration is greater than 0.5 g/dL, the subject has most likely ingested alcohol recently, and is in the preabsorptive state, whereas if the level is less than 0.5 g/dL, the individual can be considered to be in the postabsorptive phase. In a study of sixty autopsy cases using these criteria, Backer et al. obtained good agreement between the theoretical ratios and the actual ratios for brain, bile, spinal fluid, and urine in thirty-seven autopsy cases with stomach alcohol concentrations less than 0.5 g/dL. They found that the bile-blood ratio was the least variable and that bile could be used more reliably than other tissues to predict the blood alcohol concentration both in the preabsorptive and the postabsorptive phases. Average tissue-blood ratios obtained from thirty-seven human autopsy cases with stomach alcohols less than 0.5 g/dL were: bile, 0.99; brain, 0.91; spinal fluid, 1.16; vitreous humor, 1.19; and urine, 1.32.

F. Intracerebral blood clots

Under certain unique circumstances, it may be desirable to analyze blood clots for alcohol. Head injuries are a common result of violence, and may lead to subdural, epidural, or intracerebral hematomas. This hematoma would be protected from the general circulation, and, if alcohol were present in the blood at the time the injury occurred, it would theoretically be present in this specimen, even if death were delayed for some hours, and the blood were negative due to metabolism during this interval. This phenomenon was first noted by Freireich et al. (1975), who reported on four cases with negative or very low peripheral blood alcohol, and intracranial clot alcohol concentrations of 0.15, 0.09, 0.18, and 0.08 g/dL. In another reported case, a man died twenty-one hours after suffering head injury from a beating. The blood was negative for alcohol, while the intracerebral blood clot contained 0.04 g/dL. In another similar case, the postmortem blood had an alcohol concentration of 0.04 g/dL, while the clot yielded 0.11 g/dL at death after nine hours in the hospital (Smialek et al., 1980). Buchsbaum et al. (1989) reviewed seventy-five autopsy cases with subdural clots and heart blood analyzed for alcohol. They determined that no information could be gained from the clot when the posttraumatic time interval (PTTI) had been short (less than nine hours). In contrast, in twelve of the sixteen cases with PTTI greater than nine hours, subdural levels were positive in the face of negative blood levels. Two of the twelve had subdural levels in excess of 0.1 g/dL, whereas only four of the sixteen with long PTTIs had positive blood levels. The authors conclude that subdural alcohol testing can provide forensically pertinent information, particularly when the post trauma interval is relatively long.

G. Urine

Urine is usually sampled at autopsy for toxicology purposes, and should be analyzed for alcohol when available. However, it must be recognized that, under some conditions, high concentrations of alcohol can be produced postmortem in urine. Saady et al. (1993) permitted urine samples with varying amounts of glucose to sit at room temperature, without preservatives, for up to twenty days, analyzing for ethanol when initially sampled and at intervals. Alcohol was produced in five of the fourteen urines, in concentrations of 0.036 to 0.326 in four of the five, and in one, 2.383 g/dL was formed. All of the five samples contained both glucose and yeast. Alcohol did not form in less than twelve hours, and samples were maintained at room temperature. Conventional refrigeration would be expected to greatly retard or prevent alcohol formation in urine. It must also be recognized that the urine alcohol concentration is higher than that of the blood at equilibrium, and may be either higher or lower, depending on the status of absorption. See Chapter 5 for urine-blood relationships.

H. Vitreous humor

The vitreous humor of the eye has been used extensively for toxicological analyses in recent years, and is now recognized as an extremely useful specimen for postmortem alcohol determinations (Backer, 1980; Caplan and Levine, 1990; Pounder and Kuroda, 1994). The advantages of its use are that it is readily available and easily collected, there is less

chance of bacterial contamination than in blood and other organs, and alcohol enters the vitreous and establishes equilibrium about as fast or faster than in other body compartments. Approximately 2.0 milliliters of vitreous fluid can be collected from each eye, which is sufficient for alcohol analysis and often for other toxicology procedures.

The ratio of alcohol concentrations in the blood and vitreous humor is dependent upon the time after ingestion, as is that of other body organs and fluids. The time required for the establishment of equilibrium between the two specimens is thought to be about two hours. In experiments reported by Hentsch and Müller (1965), and Garriott (1976), alcohol was given orally to rabbits in a single dose, after which the animals were sacrificed periodically, and vitreous alcohol concentrations were measured. Prior to one hour, the alcohol concentrations were higher in the blood by about 0.05 g/dL but at one to two hours, the two specimens equilibrated, and the concentrations were approximately the same for a short period. After this period, the vitreous humor concentration reached a higher value than blood, and remained so until complete disappearance (Figure 6.1). Olsen (1971) injected a high dose of 3 g/kg of alcohol to a single rabbit, and followed concentrations in vitreous humor and in arterial blood for five hours. His curve is similar to Figure 6.1, but the equilibrium state was not reached until 210 minutes. This suggests that after ingestion of high doses of alcohol in a short period of time, equilibrium may not be reached for three or more hours. Since the average water contents of blood and vitreous humor are 78 percent and 99 percent, respectively, the average vitreous-blood ratio should be about 1.27, when distribution is complete.

A number of investigators have performed blood and vitreous humor analyses for alcohol in human autopsy specimens. In 174 cases, Coe and Sherman (1970) found an average vitreous-blood ratio of 1.12. Felby and Olsen (1969) found an average ratio of 1.37 in thirty-one cadavers. They pointed out that hemoconcentration could account for a higher ratio, and that those dying before diffusion equilibrium is reached (with vitreous-blood ratio of less than 1.0) will have lower ratios.

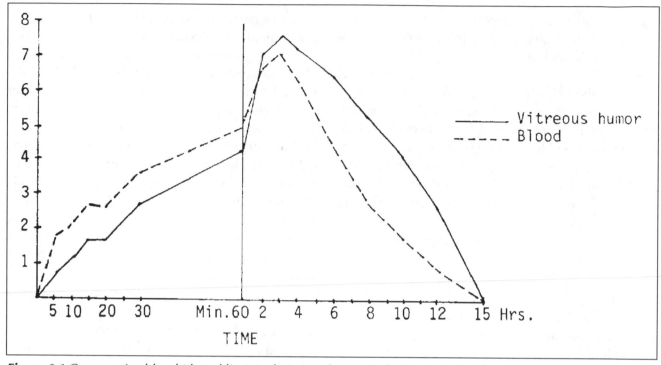

Figure 6.1 *Comparative blood (dotted line) and vitreous humor (solid line) alcohol concentrations after oral dosing in rabbits (reproduced with permission from Hentsch and Muller, 1965)*

Backer et al. (1980) reported an average vitreous humor:blood ratio of 1.19 (range 0.86–1.72) in thirty-seven cases with stomach alcohol concentrations less than 0.5 g/dL. When the stomach concentrations were greater than 0.5 g/dL, indicating recent ingestion, the average ratio was 0.89 (range 0.48–2.0). Sturner and Coumbis (1966) found an average ratio of 1.12 in thirty-eight cases, the ratios varying from 0.46 to 5.4. They reported a wider range between the two specimens in cases with higher blood alcohol levels. Of course, the comparison of blood and vitreous humor alcohol concentrations in postmortem cases depends on the time between ingestion and death. In postmortem cases this is rarely established, so a wide variation can be expected. For this reason, one can not accurately "predict" a BAC from a vitreous alcohol concentration, although reasonable estimates can be made in postmortem cases, the majority of which are in the post absorptive phase. Pounder and Kuroda (1994) provide the regression equation, BAC = 3.03 + 0.852 vitreous humor alcohol concentration (VHAC), with 95-percent prediction interval ± 0.019, and 99 percent prediction interval ± 0.025. They conclude that the prediction interval is too wide to be of real practical use,

and that BAC estimates from VHAC should not be made for evidential purposes without giving 95 percent prediction intervals.

Using the general relationship between the vitreous humor and blood alcohol after a single-dose ingestion shown in Figure 6.1, one could estimate the blood alcohol concentration from the vitreous humor reasonably accurately if it could be assumed that death occurred at least two hours after ingestion of any alcohol. If based on the water contents of the two fluids as exists antemortem, the ratio for conversion would be 1.27, as stated above. This estimate could in fact be more accurate than actual blood analysis, due to the more variable water content of postmortem blood. Audrlicky and Pribilla (1971) reported water contents varying from 68.2 percent to 90.1 percent in twenty postmortem blood samples taken from the subclavian or femoral vein. The postmortem pooling of blood could therefore lead to artificially high or low values for blood alcohol. These aberrations are probably due to variations in the hematocrit values (cell volume) resulting from pooling of the blood, but are probably not significant in most cases since the fluctuation should be within the difference between the alcohol concentration in whole blood (1.0) and that in plasma (1.18) (Mason and Dubowski, 1974; Payne et al., 1968). However, the nearer the bottom of the "pool" from which one takes the sample, the lower the alcohol concentration would be expected to be, due to the increased cell volume and thus the decreased water content. These variations can usually be avoided by taking as nearly a homogeneous blood sample as possible for analysis or by analyzing more than one sample.

6.3 Postmortem Effects on Blood Alcohol Concentrations

A. Diffusion

One of the factors potentially affecting postmortem alcohol determinations is contamination of the specimen by diffusion from another body organ. If one should die shortly after drinking alcoholic beverages, so that the stomach or upper intestine has a high concentration of alcohol, this would continue to diffuse after death into surrounding organs and blood, causing falsely high alcohol concentrations.

It was shown that alcohol present in the stomach at death may diffuse into the pericardial sac and pleural cavity after death. In twenty autopsies in which 500 milliliters of 10 percent ethyl alcohol was instilled into the stomach, false readings greater than 0.15 g/dL were found in the pericardial sacs in six cases. However, blood samples taken from the intact heart chambers or the femoral blood vessels showed no contamination (Plueckhahn and Ballard, 1967; Plueckhahn, 1968). Samples of autopsy blood taken from pooled blood in the pericardial sac or pleural cavities are most liable to contamination by diffusion of stomach alcohol, when present. Pounder and Yonemitsu (1991) demonstrated that alcohol which may enter the trachea due to agonal aspiration of gastric contents can result in falsely elevated concentrations in aortic and pulmonary vessel blood samples. Alcohol and drug slurries were introduced into the tracheas of cadavers, after which blood from the aorta, pulmonary vessels, vena cava, right and left heart was sampled. Highest alcohol concentrations were found in the pulmonary vessels, but contamination by alcohol occurred in aortal, heart, and vena caval blood as well. The authors recommended analysis of femoral blood to avoid the possibility of misinterpretation of alcohol concentrations due to contamination of blood samples by aspiration. Briglia et al. (1991) also found that significant differences can occur in different blood compartments, primarily in cases with stomach alcohol greater than 0.5 g/dL. Four out of sixty-one autopsy cases had differences in alcohol concentrations greater than 50 percent between one or more samples of femoral blood, right atrium blood, and blood from the root of the aorta. Their results are consistent with those of Backer et al. (1980) showing that alcohol present in the gastrointestinal tract at the time of death can result in elevations of some postmortem blood alcohol concentrations.

It has been observed, however, that the stomach is unlikely to contain much alcohol at the time of death. After analysis of numerous autopsies for alcohol distribution, Sunshine (1957) stated that "—people simply do not die with a bellyful of strong liquor." He also concluded that heart blood is not liable to contamination from stomach alcohol. Backer et al. (1980), in a study of thirty-seven autopsy cases with stomach concentrations less than 0.5 g/dL and twenty-three cases greater than 0.5 g/dL, did not report actual concentrations of stomach alcohols, but observed that "In actual cases only a few stomach alcohol levels exceed 5 g/100 mL—". They concluded that the alcohol is absorbed very rapidly from the stomach.

Although alcohol is absorbed from the stomach rapidly, a larger quantity is absorbed from the small intestine. Thus postmortem diffusion into the abdominal cavity could contaminate any abdominal cavity fluid, and surrounding organs. In general, any cavity fluid or blood should be avoided. A combination of heart, femoral, or subclavian blood, vitreous humor and urine, if available, should be used for alcohol analysis, to aid in the interpretation of the state of absorption and in evaluation of the actual blood concentration.

B. Sampling considerations

Falsely elevated blood alcohol concentrations in autopsy samples can arise from contamination of the sample with alcohol present in the gastrointestinal tract. Although this may be a rare occurrence as previously discussed, it is especially of concern in autopsies involving trauma to the gastrointestinal tract, when the heart blood sample is obtained by transthoracic puncture. Winek et al., (1995) found eight cases out of 6,000 in which blood alcohol concentrations were falsely elevated due to laceration or transection of the gastrointestinal tract. This problem can be avoided by taking blood from the intact heart chamber, as well as additional samples for comparison, such as vitreous humor and peripheral blood.

C. Postmortem decomposition

It is well known that decomposing tissues in the body can produce alcohol. The mechanisms and details of this phenomenon are discussed in Chapter 11. A major problem in forensic alcohol analysis lies in attempting to determine if the alcohol found was from antemortem ingestion or if all or a portion of the alcohol was produced postmortem. The object is to determine if the subject was intoxicated at the time of his death and, if so, what blood alcohol concentration had been present. Ethyl alcohol formed by postmortem decomposition is the same ethyl alcohol that is ingested in alcoholic beverages. Therefore one cannot analytically distinguish ingested alcohol from alcohol that may have been formed after death.

Many factors have to be considered in making this interpretation. One of the most important considerations is the distribution of alcohol in the body at postmortem. One can generally utilize the distribution ratios determined in antemortem studies to interpret postmortem values. The vitreous humor and urine are of utmost value in this determination since glucose (the major substrate for alcohol formation) is usually of very low concentration in these specimens. In advanced decomposition, neither these fluids nor blood are usually available. However, in most postmortem cases, vitreous humor is present. Urine is less reliably available due simply to the normal periodic (or agonal) emptying of the bladder. In a study of 130 decomposing bodies, vitreous humor was obtained in 70 percent of cases, while urine was available in only 35 percent. Vitreous humor was reported to be present until advanced decomposition (Zumwalt et al., 1982).

In the mild to moderately decomposed body, the eye chamber is intact, and sufficient vitreous humor

can be obtained for alcohol analysis for comparison with blood or urine. If the vitreous humor contains no alcohol, any alcohol found in blood or other body specimens can be assumed to have been formed postmortem. Vitreous humor is generally protected from bacterial contamination and has not been reported to produce ethanol endogenously.

In the intact, decomposing body, ethyl alcohol is usually not formed rapidly, and rarely reaches high levels in postmortem blood. In the study by Zumwalt et al. (1982), twenty-nine (97 percent) of thirty mildly decomposing bodies contained no ethanol that could have been formed postmortem. Of thirty-three mild to moderately decomposed bodies, eighteen (55 percent) contained no ethanol. Endogenous production was presumed in nine (27 percent) of the thirty-three cases. Endogenous ethanol was present in eight (19 percent) of forty-two moderately decomposed bodies, while no ethanol was found in twelve (29 percent). In 23 severely decomposed bodies, three (13 percent) exhibited endogenously formed alcohol; no alcohol was found in three (13 percent), while exogenous alcohol was found in seven (30 percent). No determination could be reached in the remaining ten cases. Twenty-three (17 percent) of the 130 cases studied had presumed production of alcohol postmortem. Of the twenty-three cases in which presumed endogenous alcohol was found in blood, nineteen (83 percent) had levels of 0.07 mg/dL or less while four cases had 0.11, 0.12, 0.13, and 0.22 mg/dL, respectively. The vitreous humor and urine were used as the criteria for determining the presence of endogenously formed alcohol (Zumwalt et al., 1982).

Gilliland and Bost (1993) evaluated 286 autopsy cases with some degree of decomposition. They concluded alcohol had been formed postmortem in fifty-five of the cases, and was present due to antemortem ingestion in 130 cases. The highest blood alcohol concentration from endogenous production was 0.07 g/dL. The criterion used for determining endogenous production of alcohol, with alcohol presence in blood and bile, was absence of alcohol in vitreous humor and urine. Mayes et al. (1992) measured alcohol in forty-seven victims of a Naval ship explosion, which were autopsied between forty-eight and ninety-two hours after death. Of forty-two blood samples analyzed twenty-three had alcohol detected. Two of these were greater than 0.1 g/dL (0.11 and 0.19 g/dL), and the remainder of the positive cases ranged from 0.01 to 0.09 g/dL.

In the "fresh" body, refrigerated within four hours of death, no endogenous alcohol was found, even in the presence of bacterial contamination (Clark and Jones, 1982).

In the more severely decomposed body, when no vitreous humor, urine, or even blood may be available, the interpretation of alcohol levels is much more difficult. All body tissues can form alcohol, and the amounts formed in organs are usually greater than those in blood. A good indication of putrefactive processes in tissue is the presence of other alcohols and putrefactive products. N-propanol production was found to agree closely with ethyl alcohol production in muscle and blood of rat corpses. The n-propanol concentrations were generally greater than 10 percent of the ethyl alcohol concentration in muscle, and greater than 5 percent of the alcohol concentration in blood. The postmortem production of ethanol was always greater in blood than in muscle. The authors suggest that a concomitant determination of n-propanol in blood or tissues can distinguish between cases in which alcohol was formed postmortem, and those in which it was present antemortem (Nanikawa et al., 1982). In a similar study with dog corpses, stored up to fourteen days, n-propanol was reported to be present in all cases, and in concentrations up to 32 percent of those of ethanol. Traces of amyl alcohol also were present in some cases (Mebs et al., 1978). In badly decomposed bodies, muscle tissue is likely the optimal specimen for alcohol analysis due to its low liability for postmortem production of alcohol in comparison with other body organs.

Another approach for evaluating postmortem alcohol production involves measurement of two serotonin metabolites, 5-hydroxyindoleacetic acid (5-HIAA) and 5-hydroxytryptophol (5-HTOL) in urine. In the absence of alcohol ingestion, the normal ratio of 5-HTOL/5-HIAA is below 0.01. After alcohol ingestion, this ratio becomes increased. Therefore, when alcohol is found in the presence of a normal ratio, postmortem production is implied (Helander et al., 1992). These observations are pre-liminary, however, and the practical application in forensic cases remains to be seen.

There is currently no proven method for determining how much of the alcohol might have been formed postmortem, and how much was present antemortem in cases with advanced putrefaction, but further research on other putrefaction products, such as n-propanol, or butanol, might lead to at least a partial answer to this question.

D. Effects of embalming

The embalmed body has had much of the blood replaced by embalming fluid. Embalming fluids generally contain formalin as the major active component, but also may contain methanol, other alcohols, various odorants, salts and so on. Table 6.2 shows some typical mixtures of embalming fluids (Rendon, 1971).

The most universal contaminants in embalming fluids are formaldehyde and methanol. Although ethanol may be present in some cavity fluids, it is not a standard component of embalming fluids, and would not be expected to contaminate the vitreous humor. Usually in the embalmed body, vitreous humor will contain a low concentration of methyl alcohol, formaldehyde or both. Any ethyl alcohol present in the vitreous humor in fresh or embalmed bodies, other than trace amounts, can be assumed to be the result of antemortem ingestion.

6.4 Acute Ethyl Alcohol Fatalities

Acute alcohol poisoning or death from overdose of alcohol is a frequent phenomenon. In one ten-year study of a major metropolitan area (Dallas, Texas), ninety-one cases of acute alcohol overdose were diagnosed, which amounted to 0.3 percent of all deaths seen, and 8 percent of all deaths resulting from drugs or toxic agents. These alcohol-induced deaths were more frequent than those from any other agent excepting carbon monoxide and narcotics (Garriott et al., 1982). In another comparable survey in Maryland, 157 acute alcohol deaths occurred over a six-year period (Caplan et al., 1985). These amounted to 9.1 percent of all deaths due to drugs or other toxic agents. This compared with 13.4 percent of the cases resulting from acute narcotics overdose. The Medical Examiner's Office of North Carolina

Table 6.2
General Formulations of Embalming Preparations

Ingredient	Composition
Type I (nonformaldehyde)	
EDTA	3.0%
Monosodium phosphate	1.0%
Sodium citrate	1.0%
Sorbitol	10.0%
Methanol	10.0%
Water	74.0%
Nonionic surfactant	1.0%
Type II (primary fluid)	
Borax	4.2%
Boric acid	2.5%
Glycerin	16.8%
Water	47.0%
Methanol	17.5%
Formalin	11.0%
Anionic or nonionic surfactant	0.6%
Reodorant and coloring agents	as desired (0.4%)
Type III (arterial fluid)	
Glutaraldehyde	8%–12%
Formalin	8%–25%
Water	27%–42%
Glycerin	6%–12%
Borax	2%–6%
Methanol	15%–26%
Tetrahydrofurfuryl alcohol	5%–10%
Alkyl aryl sodium sulfonate	0.5%–1.0%
Reodorant and coloring agents	as desired
Type IV (arterial fluid)	
Glycerin	20 lb
Polyarcylic acid (Carbopol 934)	4 lb
Sulfonated naphthenic mineral oil (Atlantic Soluble Oil No. 1)	25 lb
Formaldehyde (46% solution in methanol)	516 lb
P-dichlorobenzene	20 lb
O-dichlorobenzene	42 lb
Pine oil	20 lb
Rhodamine B (2% aqueous solution)	2,000 ml
Bismarck Brown (3% aqueous solution)	2,500 ml
Sodium hydroxide (crystals)	38 oz
Water	528 lb
Methanol	53 lb
Type V (arterial fluid; diluted to 1 pt. (473 ml with water)	
Trimethylolnitromethane	200 g
Potassium carbonate	5 g
Anionic surfactant (a phosphated, higher alcohol)	5 g
Sulfanilimide	1 g
Eosin dye and perfume	as desired
Type VI (cavity fluid)	
Formalin	70.0%
Alcohol (methanol, ethanol, or isopropyl alcohol)	29.5%
Wetting agent (Triton X-100 or equivalent)	0.5%

Reproduced with permission from Rendon (1971).

determined that 2.5 percent of all deaths certified in North Carolina over a twenty-four-month period were due to acute alcohol overdose (Taylor and Hudson, 1977). Yoon et al. (2002) estimates the overall death rate from alcohol poisoning in the U.S. at 0.49 per 100,000 population.

The diagnosis of death from acute ethanol poisoning is usually made on the basis of a high blood ethanol level, combined with circumstances consistent with overdose of alcohol. The usually accepted minimum lethal concentration for alcohol in blood is 0.4 g/dL. Lower concentrations are not necessarily inconsistent with death from alcohol overdose, however. Stress from pre-existent disease, reduced individual tolerance to alcohol, and many other factors may result in lower lethal blood alcohol concentrations at death.

While ethanol levels in excess of 0.3 g/dL indicate severe alcohol intoxication with concomitant respiratory depression, there have been numerous observations of individuals driving a motor vehicle with blood alcohol concentrations greater than 0.3 and occasionally greater than 0.4 g/dL, indicating the wide variation in individual tolerance (Garriott et al., 1977; Taylor and Hudson, 1977; Cimbura et al., 1982).

The acute alcohol fatality usually will have blood ethanol greater than 0.3 g/dL with a vitreous humor level considerably higher, although the ratio will depend on survival time after ingestion of the alcohol dose. When death occurs rapidly after consumption of a large dose of alcohol in a short time period, the blood concentration will be higher than that of the vitreous humor. In 213 cases of acute ethanol deaths examined by Taylor and Hudson (1977), 62 percent of the cases had blood levels greater than 0.40 g/dL, while the remaining 38 percent had levels between 0.3 and 0.4 g/dL.

Of thirty-nine ethanol fatalities in another study, a mean postmortem blood alcohol of 0.416 g/dL was found. Levels ranged from 0.237 to 0.592 g/dL (Garriott et al., 1982; Garriott, unpublished data, 1986). Six of the cases had blood levels less than 0.3 g/dL. In these cases, the subject was assumed to have had a "lethal" blood alcohol concentration some hours before death, and that death was from the resultant brain damage, even though the subject survived to

metabolize a significant proportion of the alcohol. In such cases, urine and vitreous humor are of great value in supporting the previously higher alcohol levels. Blood and vitreous alcohol concentrations in representative ethanol fatalities are compared in Table 6.3.

Table 6.3
Alcohol Concentration in Acute Fatalities (g/dL)

Age/Race/Sex	Blood (Bl)	Vitreous Humor (V)	V/Bl Ratio
30 W/M	0.59	0.47	0.79
60 W/M	0.41	0.43	1.05
45 B/M	0.35	0.48	1.39
43 B/M	0.24	0.38	1.58
31 W/M	0.24	0.37	1.57
48 W/M	0.52	0.54	1.04
30 W/M	0.33	0.46	1.39
45 W/F	0.39	0.45	1.15
51 W/M	0.50	0.59	1.18
54 W/F	0.35	0.46	1.31
20 B/M	0.53	0.48	0.91
40 B/M	0.56	0.59	1.05
24 W/M	0.59	0.66	1.12
43 W/F	0.36	0.46	1.28
65 W/F	0.54	0.31	0.57
41 W/M	0.38	0.47	1.23
48 W/M	0.37	0.42	1.14
37 W/M	0.40	0.51	1.20
49 W/M	0.45	0.53	1.18
37 W/M	0.64	0.77	1.20
17 W/M	0.35	0.39	1.12

References

Audrlicky, I. and Pribilla, O. Vergleichende Untersuchung der Alkoholkon-zentration im Blut, der Glaskörperflüssigkeit, der Synovialflüssigkeit und im Harn. *Blutalkohol* 8:116–121, 1971.

Backer, R.C., Pisano, R.V. and Sopher, I.M. The comparison of alcohol concentrations in postmortem fluids and tissues. *J. Forensic Sci.* 25:327–331, 1980.

Baselt, R.C. and Cravey, R.H. Forensic toxicology. In: Doull, J., Klassen, C. and Amdur, M. (eds.), *Toxicology, the Basic Science of Poisons*, 2nd ed. NY: MacMillan, 1980, p. 663.

Briglia, E.J., Bidanset, J.H. and Dal Cortivo, L.A. The distribution of ethanol in postmortem blood specimens. *J. Forensic Sci.* 37:991–998, 1992.

Budd, R.D. Postmortem brain alcohol levels. *J. Chromatogr.* 259:353–355, 1983.

Buchsbaum, R.M., Adelson, L. and Sunshine, I. A comparison of post-mortem ethanol levels obtained from blood and subdural specimens. *Forens. Sci. Internat.* 41:237–243, 1989.

Caplan, Y.H. et al. Drug and chemical related deaths: Incidences in the state of Maryland, 1975–1980. *J. Forensic Sci.* 30:1012–1021, 1985.

Caplan, Y.H. and Levine, B. Vitreous humor in the evaluation of postmortem blood ethanol concentrations. *J. Anal. Tox.* 14:305–307, 1990.

Cimbura, G. et al. Incidence and toxicological aspects of drugs detected in 489 fatally injured drivers and pedestrians in Ontario. *J. Forensic Sci.* 27:855–867, 1982.

Clark, M.A. and Jones, W.D. Studies on putrefactive ethanol production, part 1: Lack of spontaneous ethanol production in intact human bodies. *J. Forensic Sci.* 27:366–371, 1982.

Coe, J.L. and Sherman, R.E. Comparative study of postmortem vitreous humor and blood alcohol. *J. Forensic Sci.* 15:185–190, 1970.

Felby, S. and Olsen, J. Comparative studies of postmortem ethyl alcohol in vitreous humor, blood, and muscle. *J. Forensic Sci.* 14:93–101, 1969.

Field, P.H. The expert witness. In: Garriott, J.C. (ed.), *Medicolegal Aspects of Alcohol Determination in Biological Specimens.* Tucson, AZ: Lawyers & Judges Publishing Co., 1993, p.290.

Forney, R.B., Hulpieu, H.R. and Harger, R.N. The levels of alcohol in brain, peripheral blood and heart blood ten minutes after oral administration. *J. Pharmacol. Exp. Ther.* 98:8–9, 1950.

Freireich, A.W., Bidanset, J.H. and Lukash, L. Alcohol levels in intracranial blood clots. *J. Forensic Sci.* 20:83–85, 1975.

Garriott, J.C. Relationship of vitreous humor and blood alcohol concentrations in rabbits. *Forensic Sci. Gaz.* 7:4–5, 1976.

Garriott, J.C., Di Maio, V.J.M. and Petty, C.S. Death by poisoning: A ten-year survey of Dallas County. *J. Forensic Sci.* 27:868–879, 1982.

Garriott, J.C. et al. Incidence of drugs and alcohol in fatally injured motor vehicle drivers. *J. Forensic Sci.* 22:383–389, 1977.

Garriott, J.C. Skeletal muscle as an alternative specimen for alcohol and drug analysis. *J. Forensic Sci.* 36:60–69, 1991.

Garriott, J.C. Drug use among homicide victims. *Am. J. Forensic Med. Pathol.* 14:51–53, 1993.

Gilliland, M.G.F. and Bost, R.O. Alcohol in decomposed bodies: Postmortem synthesis and distribution. *J. Forensic Sci.* 38:1266–1274, 1993.

Harger, R.N., Hulpieu, R.H. and Lamb, E.B. The speed with which various parts of the body reach equilibrium in the storage of ethyl alcohol. *J. Biol. Chem.* 120:689–704, 1937.

Helander, A., Beck, O. and Jones, A.W. Urinary 5HTOL/5HIAA as biochemical marker of postmortem ethanol synthesis. *Lancet* 340:1159, 1992.

Hentsch, R. and Müller, H.P. Tierexperimentelle Untersuchungen über die Konzentration von peroral zugeführtem Äthanol in Blut und Glaskörper. *Albrecht Von Graefes Arch. Klin. Exp. Ophthalmol.* 168:330–334, 1965.

Jenkins, A.J., Levine, B.S. and Smialek, J.E. Distribution of ethanol in postmortem liver. *J. Forensic Sci.* 40:611–613, 1995.

Jones, A.W. Status of alcohol absorption among drinking drivers. *J. Anal. Tox.* 14:198–199, 1990.

Luvoni, R. and Marozzi, E. Ethyl alcohol distribution in the various organs and fluids of cadavers. *J. Forensic Med.* 15:67, 1968.

Martin, E. et al. The pharmacokinetics of alcohol in human breath, venous and arterial blood after oral ingestions. *Eur. J. Clin. Pharmacol.* 26:619–626, 1984.

Mason, M.F. and Dubowski, K.M. Alcohol, traffic, and chemical testing in the United States: A resume and some remaining problems. *Clin. Chem.* 20:126–170, 1974.

Mayes, R. et al. Toxicologic findings in the USS Iowa disaster. *J. Forensic Sci.* 37:1352–1357, 1992.

Mebs, D., Schmidt, K. and Gerchow, J. Experimental studies on postmortem alcohol formation. *Blutalkohol* 15:145–150, 1978.

Meyer, K.H. Experimentelle Untersuchung über das Verhältnis des Blutalkohols zum Alkoholgehalt des Gehirns, abstracted from dissertation. *Q. J. Stud. Alcohol* 20:785, 1959.

Moore, R. Concerning breath alcohol measurements during absorption and elimination (letter). *J. Anal. Tox.* 15:346–347, 1991.

Nanikawa R. et al. Medico-legal studies on alcohol detected in dead bodies: Alcohol levels in skeletal muscle. *Forensic Sci. Int.* 20:133–140, 1982.

Norton, L.E., Garriott J.C. and Di Maio, V.J.M. Drug detection at autopsy: A prospective study of 247 cases. *J. Forensic Sci.* 27:66–71, 1982.

Olsen, J.E. Penetration rate of alcohol into the vitreous humor studied with a new in vivo technique. *Acta Ophthalmologica* 49:585–588, 1971.

Payne, J.P., Hill, D.W. and Wood, D.G.L. Distribution of ethanol between plasma and erythrocytes in whole blood. *Nature* 217:963–964, 1968.

Plueckhahn, V.D. The evaluation of autopsy blood alcohol levels. *Med. Sci. Law* 8:168–176, 1968.

Plueckhahn, V.D. and Ballard, B. Diffusion of stomach alcohol and heart blood alcohol concentration at autopsy. *J. Forensic Sci.* 12:463–470, 1967.

Pounder, D.J. and Yonemitsu, K. Postmortem absorption of drugs and ethanol from aspirated vomitus: An experimental model. *Forensic Sci. Int.* 51:189–195, 1991.

Pounder, D.J. and Kuroda, N. Vitreous alcohol is of limited value in predicting blood alcohol. *Forensic Sci. Int.* 65:73–80, 1994.

Prouty, R.W. and Anderson, W.H. A comparison of postmortem heart blood and femoral blood ethyl alcohol concentrations. *J. Anal. Tox.* 11:191–197, 1987.

Rendon, L. Embalming chemicals. In: Snell, F.D. and Ettre, L.S. (eds.) *Encyclopedia of Industrial Chemical Analysis.* NY: Interscience Publishers, 1971, pp. 162–164.

Saady, J.J., Poklis, A. and Dalton, H.P. Production of urinary ethanol after sample collection. *J. Forensic Sci.* 38:1467–1471, 1993.

Smialek, J.E., Spitz, W.U. and Wolfe, J.A. Ethanol in intracerebral clot. *Am. J. Forensic Med. Pathol.* 1:149–150, 1980.

Smith, G.S., Branas, C.C. and Miller, T.R. Fatal non-traffic injuries involving alcohol: A meta-analysis. *Ann. Emerg. Med.* 33:659–668, 1999.

Sturner, W.Q. and Coumbis, M.S. The quantitation of ethyl alcohol in vitreous humor and blood by gas chromatography. *Am. J. Clin. Pathol.* 46:349–351, 1966.

Sunshine, I. *Postmortem Distribution of Ethyl Alcohol.* Presented at the American Academy of Forensic Sciences, Chicago, Feb. 1957.

Taylor, H.L. and Hudson, R.P. Acute ethanol poisoning: A two-year study of deaths in North Carolina. *J. Forensic Sci.* 22:639–653, 1977.

Turkel, H.W. and Gifford, H. Erroneous blood alcohol findings at autopsy, avoidance by proper sampling technique. *JAMA* 164:1077–1079, 1957.

Winek, C.L., Winek, C.L. and Wahba, W.W. The role of trauma in postmortem blood alcohol determination. *Forensic Sci. Int.* 71:1–8, 1995.

Yoon, Y.H., Yi, H. and Dufour, M.C. *Accidental Alcohol Mortality from Poisoning, 1996–1998,* Alcoholism, Clinical and Experimental Res. Suppl. 2, vol. 26 May 2002, Presented at the annual meeting of the Research Society on Alcoholism, San Francisco, CA, June 28–July 3, 2002.

Zumwalt, R.E., Bost, R.O. and Sunshine, I. Evaluation of ethanol concentrations in decomposed bodies. *J. Forensic Sci.* 27:549–554, 1982.

Chapter 7

Breath as a Specimen for Analysis for Ethanol and Other Low-Molecular-Weight Alcohols

Morton F. Mason, Ph.D. and Kurt M. Dubowski, Ph.D.

7.1 Introduction

The use of breath analysis for alcohol[1] in traffic law enforcement arose in order to avoid the involvement of a physician or a nurse in the process of arrest, charge, and trial of a subject suspected of DWI (driving while intoxicated). Their participation was required because to obtain blood as a specimen the body must be entered. Although urine could be collected by police officers it was generally recognized that, for a number of reasons, its concentration of ethanol might vary widely from that in the blood at the time of arrest. The need to use medical personnel often lengthened the time between apprehension and actual drawing of blood and, in addition, the final report on its analysis might be excluded from trial if the physician or nurse were not present to testify, or if there were defects in the record of the chain of custody of the specimen. Further, the specimen, in most instances, was venous blood and thus, except after absorption and distribution had been completed, did not reflect, precisely, the concentration of ethanol in the blood supply of the brain, whereas the ethanol in alveolar (deep lung) air is in equilibrium with that of arterial blood plasma which is the concentration to which the brain is exposed.

To shorten maximally the interval between apprehension and procuring of a specimen of breath requires the use of an instrument or device suitable for being carried in patrol vehicles. Some of the larger instruments (e.g., the Breathalyzer) are stationed at police headquarters or substations so that the interval may be variably prolonged, depending upon distance and traffic density, in which to reach the test site.

For many years the concentration of ethanol found in breath was converted by *calculation* to a presumed blood concentration which was the quantity reported and upon which any charge of violation of law was based. Not only was the calculation difficult for a jury to understand, but "in actual law enforcement practice, when a breath sample is analyzed for alcohol, the quantity found cannot be used to calculate the simultaneously existing actual blood concentration without making assumptions having uncertain validities in any given case because they have not been assessed" (Mason and Dubowski, 1974; Mason and Dubowski, 1976). This view was supported and documented by the unacceptable lack of agreement of found and calculated concentrations in numerous blood-breath correlation studies and in the discordant values reported for the blood-breath concentration ratio for alcohol, which varied considerably from the value of 2,100:1 which, essentially arbitrarily, was employed for many years (Mason and Dubowski, 1974; Borkenstein et al., 1972).

In the United States these matters have been, it is hoped, recently resolved by acceptance of recommendations of the Committee on Alcohol and Other Drugs of the National Safety Council (National Safety Council, 1979) and by the action of the National Committee on Uniform Traffic Laws and Ordinances (1979) to amend section 11-902.1a of the Uniform Vehicle Code (UVC) (1980) to read that "Alcohol concentration shall mean either grams of alcohol per 100 milliliters of blood or grams of alcohol per 210 liters of breath."

Thus the offense of DWI is defined, not only in respect to concentration of alcohol in the blood, but also in terms of exceeding a specified concentration of alcohol, *analytically determined*, in a specimen of breath. It should be noted that alveolar air is not required. Inasmuch as in an otherwise correctly performed breath test, failure to obtain air *only* of alveolar composition gives a nearly proportionately lower result and is without prejudice to the defendant, the question of the specimen being entirely alveolar in origin need not arise.

7.2 The History of Breath Alcohol Analysis

Reports of detection of alcohol in breath and subsequent development of methods for breath analysis considerably preceded forensic applications (e.g., the demonstration of alcohol in human breath after consumption of wine in 1847 and analyses for alcohol in rabbit breath [Bouchardat and Sandras, 1847; Subbotin, 1891]). The earliest English language publication is that of Anstie in 1874 (Anstie, 1874). Since then many methods and instruments have been described and references to them may be found in several sources; (Harger et al., 1950; American Medical Association, 1959; Dubowski, 1973; Forrester, 1960; American Medical Association, 1970; Dubowski, 1970; Mason and Dubowski, 1974; Mason and Dubowski, 1976).

Although presently most breath alcohol analyses are for forensic purposes related to traffic law enforcement, some are done for diagnostic purposes and in evaluation of subjects upon admission to a hospital to determine whether observed symptoms, signs or other immediate causes for need for medical help are alcohol-related. Examples include unexplained coma, signs of cirrhosis of the liver, trauma from unexpected workplace accidents, and, especially, injuries caused by violence such as gunshot, stabbing, blunt weapon trauma or vehicular accidents. Any of these occurrences can lead to later civil litigation or criminal prosecution. Other applications of breath analysis than for alcohol have considerably expanded as technologies for vapor-phase analysis have further developed. Thus, by 1974, 135 compounds had been identified in breath and two to three times as many had been separated (i.e., detected) (Ellin et al., 1973; Ellin et al., 1974; Pauling et al.,

1971, 1976). Dubowski (1974) listed applications that might be encountered in a clinical chemistry laboratory. The list included nine methods or devices for determination of ethanol, four for diagnosis, seven for physiologic and metabolic studies, three for therapeutic monitoring, two for occupational health monitoring, and only two primarily for other forensic purposes. Since that time the number of other clinical applications has greatly increased (Manolis, 1983). For the years 1976 to 1978 a National Library of Medicine literature search revealed forty-nine clinical applications (including several which involved industrial monitoring and could have forensic uses) and only eight with clear-cut relevance to the forensic purposes of breath analysis. The scope of the expanded clinical applications is revealed by (Perman et al., 1978; Schneider et al., 1978; Haines et al., 1977; Schoeller et al., 1977; Lauterburg, 1978).

During the 1920s there were rapid increases in the number of vehicles and miles driven, and irregular increases in traffic density along with increases in vehicular speeds and accelerations attainable. There was an accompanying rise in death and injury from accidents involving drivers, passengers, and pedestrians. After repeal of Prohibition in 1933, a sharp rise in alcohol-related deaths and injuries became apparent, resulting in a demand for statutory control of alcohol in relation to traffic.

A number of states passed legislation requiring a driver "to have command of the normal use of his mental and physical faculties in order to legally operate a motor vehicle." It soon appeared that statutory definition of "normal use" in terms of concentration of alcohol in the blood was desirable, but this required guidelines for specification of the relation between blood alcohol concentration (BAC) and degree of impairment. On the basis of scanty experimental evidence available at the time, the Committee on Tests for Intoxication (now the Committee on Alcohol and Other Drugs) of the National Safety Council (1938) and a committee report approved by the House of Delegates of the American Medical Association in 1939 presented such guidelines which provided the basis for statutory law in a number of states, Indiana in 1939 being the first. These guidelines were to the effect that any individual having a blood alcohol concentration in excess of 0.15 percent wt/vol (1.5 g/L or 150 mg/dL) was to be considered under the influence of alcohol and that if values between 0.05 percent wt/vol and 0.15 percent wt/vol were found he might or might not be under the influence, with the decision to rest upon other evidence. If the concentration found was less than 0.05 percent wt/vol, he was not to be prosecuted for driving while under the influence of alcohol (American Medical Association, 1939). As experimental information on these matters accumulated, these guidelines were modified over the next three decades (Mason and Dubowski, 1976).

The significant changes which took place during this period in the utilization of breath alcohol analysis have been reviewed in detail (Mason and Dubowski, 1974; Mason and Dubowski, 1976). It was soon recognized that estimating the volume of alveolar air in a breath specimen on the basis of the weight of carbon dioxide present was fraught with error and abandonment of this practice was urged by the Committee on Alcohol and Drugs of the National Safety Council, followed by extensive documentation of its position (National Safety Council, 1967, 1968; Dubowski, 1975).

In 1960, the National Safety Council Committee on Alcohol and Drugs recommended that the presumptive definition of alcoholic impairment of drivers be lowered to 0.1 percent wt/vol (National Safety Council, 1979). Although this was not uniformly accepted by the various states in statutory law and enforcement, it resulted in more vigorous scrutiny of breath test results in courts, and with this, airing of such matters as the magnitude of discrepancies in the results of blood-breath studies. Further, there was lack of agreement on the value of the blood-breath ratio for alcohol which was used to convert a breath concentration finding to a presumed blood concentration. At the same time, there was general recognition of the evidence relating driving impairment to BAC and that about 40 percent of vehicular injuries and deaths were alcohol-related. In one notable study of vehicular deaths where driver responsibility could be certainly fixed, 73 percent were alcohol-related (McCarroll and Haddon, 1962).

Federal intervention into traffic matters followed to assure uniformity of traffic laws and procedures,

including the reliability of the latter. In 1966, Congress established the Department of Transportation with one of its units being the National Highway Safety Agency—later designated the National Highway Safety Bureau (NHSB) and, in 1970, as the National Highway Traffic Safety Administration (NHTSA)—charged to study motorized vehicle traffic and to develop program standards for the states to reduce its hazards.

In anticipation of what in 1968 became volume eight of the Highway Safety Program Manual *Alcohol in Relation to Highway Safety* and its "Appendix A, Highway Safety Program Standard 4.4.8," the Committee on Alcohol and Drugs of the National Safety Council had prepared the document, *A Model Program for the Control of Alcohol for Traffic Safety* (National Safety Council, 1967). Most of its elements were incorporated into the program manual presented in 1968, including limiting breath testing instruments to those designed to collect only "substantially alveolar air" and specific requirements for training of breath test operators, administration of tests with use of necessary scientific safeguards, and periodic inspection of instruments (National Highway Safety Bureau, 1968).

A number of breath alcohol analyses of uncertain capability appeared briefly. Following a recommendation by the Committee on Alcohol and Drugs of the National Safety Council, the NHTSA required quantitative evidential breath testers purchased with federal funds to meet federal performance standards developed in cooperation with the National Bureau of Standards (National Safety Council, 1971; *Federal Register*, 1973). Comments and recommendations on these were made by the National Safety Council and were accepted (National Safety Council, 1974). A qualified products list for devices found to meet these standards first appeared in *Federal Register* in 1974. The list was amended in 1979 and again in 1980 and (*Federal Register*, 1979, 1980, 1986). The last list includes seventeen instruments meeting all then existing performance requirements for mobile evidential breath testers, and four devices meeting all existing requirements excluding those for mobile evidential breath testers (i.e., the devices are suitable for evidential testing only at fixed test sites). For analysis of alcohol in remotely collected specimens of breath, nonspecialized gas chromatographs can be used (Dubowski and Essary, 1982). The several remote sampling devices have not as yet had performance standards specified.

7.3 Sampling

The physiologic and physiochemical considerations involved in the relationship between the alcohol in substantially alveolar air and in pulmonary arterial blood have been summarized by Dubowski (1970, 1974, 1975). The practical application of these by a breath test operator include procedural matters common to all types of instrumentation.

The prime objective in sampling is to procure a specimen of substantially alveolar air, free from contamination proximal to the larynx which could contribute to the amount of alcohol subsequently found by analysis, and which is protected from loss of alcohol by condensation before reaching the final measuring device (e.g., an oxidizing solution, an optical path or a gas chromatographic detector).

While not presently (1986) a statutory requirement, the collected air should have a temperature of "close" (± 0.5°C) to 34.5°C. Hyperthermia will increase the partial pressure of alcohol in the vapor phase from blood and hypothermia will have the opposite effect. It seems likely that instrumental measurement of the delivered breath temperature from which a sample is taken for analysis will be a required feature of evidential breath testers in the future.

Contamination of a delivered breath specimen can result from residual alcoholic beverage in the mouth, by the presence of residual vomitus containing alcohol in the mouth, by the regurgitation of stomach contents, or by eructation of gas having a significant component of alcohol. These can be avoided by careful and constant observation of the subject for fifteen minutes to assure that nothing enters his mouth prior to sampling (Dubowski, 1970; National Safety Council, 1968; *Federal Register*, 1979). Salivary flow, reflex swallowing, and absorption into mucous membranes remove the alcohol rapidly and completely from residual beverage and other contaminating materials. Alternatively, and perhaps advisably in the case of denture wearers, the mouth can be rinsed with water at body temperature;

but in order to have the residual water come to equilibrium with alcohol in the salivary and mucous membrane secretions, breath sampling must be delayed for at least six minutes during which the subject must be closely observed (Dubowski, 1960; Dubowski, 1970; Dubowski, 1975; Smith et al., 1969). Immediate sampling would give a falsely low result.

Losses by condensation are prevented by performing the test in a room (or closed squad car) with the air and instrument parts leading to the volume-measuring device or light path presenting a minimal surface at an initial temperature of not less than 35°C. Under these circumstances significant loss by condensation, if any, is restricted to the initial portion of the breath which is discarded (see below).

Delivery of the breath can be made from the sitting or standing position into an inlet equipped with a mouthpiece or saliva trap to prevent aqueous droplets from entering whatever volume or optical path-measuring device is employed, which in turn depends upon which instrument is being used. In any event, at least the first two-thirds of the delivered breath should be discarded before taking the actual "last phase" expiratory portion to be analyzed which has now reached an alveolar plateau, that is, it is now "substantially expired alveolar air" (Dubowski, 1975).

Difficulty in obtaining a suitable breath specimen is occasionally encountered in intoxicated subjects or subjects who have severe bronchopulmonary disorders. In most instances, a sufficient amount of less than substantially alveolar air can be obtained in which it is likely that an alcohol concentration in excess of the statutory threshold will be found if the subject is indeed intoxicated.

The concentration of alcohol appearing in alveolar air at a given concentration in the pulmonary blood is independent of the barometric pressure, provided a measured volume of the air is at existing ambient pressure (Mason, 1974). Following remote sampling, differences in barometric pressure at the time of collection and analysis may be ignored as long as the collected specimen is not reconverted to a volume.

Other suggested safeguards related to sampling include the analysis of at least two breath specimens from a subject (i.e., duplicate, but separate, analyses) even though this may not be a statutory requirement. The results should agree within the limits of 0.02 g/210 L, with the lower or the mean value to the second decimal place being reported. Thus values of 0.13 and 0.139 gram per 210 liters would average 0.1345 g/210 L and would be reported as 0.13 g/210 L. Values of 0.175 g/210 L and 0.17 g/210 L would average 0.1725 g/210 L and would be reported as 0.17 g/210 L and so on.

For vapor from aqueous reference standards or controls of 0.1 to 0.2 g/210 L, duplicate analyses should agree within the range of 0.02 g/210 L. For standards or controls with concentration in excess of 0.2 g/210 L, agreement within 10 percent of the putative values is considered acceptable. Records of all blank analyses, control analyses, and subject breath analyses with the times and dates and location thereof should be a part of each final completed case report. Details of analysis of controls, blank analyses, and analysis of the sample taken from a subject differ according to the instruments employed and the corresponding directions for use of each should be rigorously followed. Presently, there is no valid procedure known for preservation of Breathalyzer reagent ampules and their contents after initial use (Dubowski, 1986). This issue was infrequently raised in some jurisdictions as a result of appellate court decisions arising from the notorious Hitch case (*People v. Hitch*, 1974).

Collection of a breath specimen or its content of alcohol with subsequent analysis at a different place and time is known as "remote sampling" and several procedures have been described. These include adsorption on anhydrous magnesium perchlorate, first used in the original Portable Intoximeter (Jetter et al., 1941) and later in the DPC Intoximeter (Forrester, 1964); on anhydrous calcium chloride with the Breathalyzer Remote Sampling Unit (Dubowski, 1970); indium tube encapsulation of breath for subsequent analysis by the GC-Intoximeter (Penton and Forrester, 1969); collection of breath in a glass tube (Hine et al., 1968), or in an evacuated metal container (Principe, 1974) and several other devices and procedures. A number of early remote sampling devices no longer in general use were described by Harger et al. (1956). Adsorbed alcohol is usually re-

covered by aqueous elution or by distillation with subsequent analysis of the eluate following dilution with distilled water to a known volume.

References

American Medical Association. Report of the Committee to Study Problems of Motor Vehicle Accidents. *JAMA* 108:2137, 1937; 112:2164–2166, 1939.

American Medical Association Committee on Medicolegal Problems. *Chemical Tests for Intoxication*, American Medical Association, Chicago, 1959. [See especially Friedemann, T.E. and Dubowski, K.M. Chemical testing procedures for the determination of ethyl alcohol, pp. 20–44; Appendix B. Procedures for analysis of breath for ethyl alcohol, pp. 45–56.]

American Medical Association. *Alcohol and the Impaired Driver. A Manual on the Medicolegal Aspects of Chemical Tests for Intoxication with Supplement on Breath Alcohol Tests.* Chicago: American Medical Association, 1970, 1972. Reprinted by National Safety Council, Chicago, 1976 [see especially pp. 94–100].

Anstie, E.F. Final experiments on elimination of alcohol from the body. *Practitioner* 13:15–28, 1874.

Borkenstein, R. et al. Statement, Ad Hoc Committee on the Blood/Breath Alcohol Relationship. Indianapolis: Indiana University Law School, Jan 1972.

Bouchardat, M.M. and Sandras. De la digestion des boissons alcooliques et de leur role dans la nutrition physique. *Ann. Chem. Physique. Ser.* 21:448–457, 1847.

Dubowski, K.M. Necessary scientific safeguards in breath alcohol analysis. *J. Forensic Sci.* 5:422–433, 1960.

Dubowski, K.M. Measurement of ethyl alcohol in breath. In: Sunderman, F.W. Jr. (ed.), *Laboratory Diagnosis of Diseases Caused by Toxic Agents*. St. Louis: Warren H. Green, 1970, pp. 316–342.

Dubowski, K.M. *Selected References on Chemical Tests for Alcoholic Influence,* 10th ed. Oklahoma City: University of Oklahoma, 1973.

Dubowski, K.M. Breath analysis as a technique in clinical chemistry. *Clin. Chem.* 20: 966–972, 1974.

Dubowski, K.M. Studies in breath-alcohol analysis: Biological factors. *Z. Rechtsmed.* 76:96–117, 1975.

Dubowski, K.M. Letter to the editor, National Safety Council Committee on Alcohol and Drugs. *Am. J. Forensic Med. Pathol.* 7:266, 1986.

Dubowski, K.M. and Essary, N.A. Alcohol analysis of stored whole–breath samples by automated gas chromatography. *J. Anal. Toxicol.* 6:217–221, 1982.

Ellin, R.l., Farrand, R.L., Oberst, F.W. et al. *Collection, Detection, Identification and Quantitation of Human Effluents,* Edgewood Arsenal Technical Report EB–TR–73007, EATR 4779. Edgewood Arsenal, Aberdeen Proving Ground, MD: Dept. of the Army, Oct 1973.

Ellin, R.I. et al. An apparatus for the detection and quantitation of volatile human effluents. *J. Chromatogr.* 100:137–152, 1974.

Federal Register. 38 (Nov. 5):30459–30463, 1973 [Erratum: Section 5.4.4., line 7, should read: "BAC's are within the range 0.4–0.10 per . . .".].

Federal Register. 39 (Nov. 21): 41,399, 1974.

Federal Register. 44 (July 7): 3,261, 1979.

Federal Register. 45 (Sept. 11): 60,103, 1980.

Federal Register. 51 (April 9): 12,257, 1986.

Forrester, G . *Chemical Tests for Alcohol in Traffic Law Enforcement.* Springfield, IL: Charles C Thomas, 1964.

Forrester, G.C. *Manual for the DPC Intoximeter.* St. Louis: Intoximeters-Midwestern, 1964.

Haines, A. et al. Breath-methane in patients with cancer of the large bowel. *Lancet* 2:481–483, 1977.

Harger, R.N., Forney, R.B. and Baker, R.S. Estimation of the level of blood alcohol from analysis of breath, part 3: Use of re-breathed air. *Q. J. Stud. Alcohol* 17:1–18, 1956.

Harger, R.N., Forney, R.B. and Barnes, H.B. Estimation of the level of blood alcohol from analysis of breath. *J. Lab. Clin. Med.* 36: 306, 1950.

Hine, C.H., Aitchison, J.P. and Parker, K.D. *The Accutube: A New Method for Determination of Alcohol in Breath.* San Francisco: Hine Laboratories, 1968.

Jetter, W.W., Moore, M. and Forrester, G.C. Studies in alcohol. IV. A new method for determination of breath-alcohol. *Am. J. Clin. Pathol.* 5:75–89, 1941.

Lauterburg, B.H., Newcomer, A.D. and Hofmann, A.F. Clinical value of the bile acid breath test: Evaluation of the Mayo Clinic experience. *Mayo Cli. Proc.* 53:227–239, 1978.

McCarroll, J.R. and Haddon Jr., W. A controlled study of fatal Automobile accidents in New York City. *J. Chron. Dis.*15:811–826, 1962.

Manolis, A. The diagnostic potential of breath analysis. *Clin. Chem.* 29:5–15, 1983.

Mason, M.F. A note upon barometric pressure and breath-alcohol analysis. *J. Forensic Sci.* 19:325–326, 1974.

Mason, M.F. and Dubowski, K.M. Alcohol, traffic, and chemical testing in the United States: A resume and some remaining problems. *Clin. Chem.* 20: 126–140, 1974.

Mason, M.F. and Dubowski, K.M. Breath-alcohol analysis: Uses, methods and some forensic problems: Review and opinion. *J. Forensic Sci.* 21:9–41, 1976.

National Committee on Uniform Traffic Laws and Ordinances. Aug. 15–17, Washington, DC, 1979.

National Committee on Uniform Traffic Laws and Ordinances. Uniform Vehicle Code and Model Traffic Ordinance, rev. ed. 1980; Section 11-902.1(a), Michie Company, Charlottesville, VA. [This publication may be obtained from the National Committee on Uniform Traffic Laws and Ordinances, 525 School St., S.W., Washington, DC 20024].

National Highway Safety Bureau. *Highway Safety Program Manual*, vol. 8, *Alcohol in Relation to Highway Safety*. U.S. Dept. of Transportation publication, 1968.

National Safety Council Committee on Tests for Intoxication. *Report: Chemical Test for Intoxication*. Chicago: National Safety Council, 1938.

National Safety Council Committee on Alcohol and Drugs. *A Model Program for the Control of Alcohol for Traffic Safety*. Chicago: National Safety Council, 1967.

National Safety Council Committee on Alcohol and Drugs. *Recommendations of the Ad Hoc Committee on Testing and Training*. Chicago: National Safety Council, 1968. [See Appendix A for sixty-six relevant references to CO_2 in breath.]

National Safety Council Committee on Alcohol and Drugs. *Recommendations of the Ad Hoc Committee on Quantitative Breath Alcohol Instrumentation*. Chicago: National Safety Council, 1971.

National Safety Council Ad Hoc Committee of Committee on Alcohol and Drugs. *Comments on Standards for Devices to Measure Breath Alcohol*. Chicago: National Safety Council, 1974.

National Safety Council. *Minutes of the Executive Board of the Committee on Alcohol and Drugs*, Chicago: Feb. 1975.

National Safety Council. *Recommendations of the Committee on Alcohol and Drugs, 1936–1977*. Chicago: National Safety Council, 1979, p. 15. [The Uniform Vehicle Code was amended to meet this recommendation in 1962.]

Pauling, L. et al. Quantitative analysis of urine vapor and breath by gas-liquid partition chromatography. *Proc. Natl. Acad. Sci.* U.S.A. 68:2374–2376, 1971.

Penton, J.R. and Forrester, M.R. A gas chromatographic breath analysis system with provisions for storage and delayed analysis of samples. In *Proceedings of the Fifth International Conference on Alcohol and Traffic Safety*. Schulz Verlag, Freiburg, West Germany, 1969, pp II-79–86.

People v. Hitch, 527 P2d 372 (Cal. Sup. Ct., 1974).

Perman, J.A., Barr, R.C. and Watkins, J.B. Sucrose malabsorption in children: Non-invasive diagnosis by interval breath hydrogen determination. *J. Pediatr.* 93:17–22, 1978.

Principe, A.H. The Vacu-Sampler: A new device for the encapsulation of breath and other gaseous samples. *J. Police Sci. Admin.* 2:404–413, 1974.

Schneider, J.F. et al. Validation of $^{13}CO_2$ breath analysis as a measurement of demethylation of stable isotope-labeled aminopyrine in man. *Clin. Chem. Acta.* 84:152–162, 1978.

Schoeller, D.A. et al. Clinical diagnosis with the stable isotope ^{13}C in CO_2 breath tests; Methodology and fundamental considerations. *J. Lab. Clin. Med.* 90:412–421, 1977.

Smith, W.C. et al. Breathalyzer experiences under operational conditions recommended by the California Association of Criminalists. *J. Forensic Sci. Soc.* 9:58–64, 1969.

Subbotin, V. Ueber die physiologische Bedeutung des Alkohols für den thierischen Organismus. *Z. Biol.* 7:361–369, 1891.

Endnote

1. Unless otherwise specified, the term "alcohol" will refer to ethanol. For convenience the terms will often be used interchangeably.

Chapter 8

Methods for Breath Analysis

Patrick Harding, B.S.

8.1 Introduction

The analysis of breath as a practical means to clinically assess alcohol intoxication was proposed in this country in 1927 (Bogen, 1927). Breath alcohol analysis has since become widely employed as a primary means of determining alcohol involvement in motor vehicle violations. Breath alcohol analysis is also used in conjunction with the enforcement of juvenile drinking, impaired boating, snowmobiling and off-road vehicle laws. Breath alcohol analysis has found increasing use in hospitals and drug abuse treatment centers for clinical screening of alcohol use and abuse, at worksites for screening employees, and as a means to ensure compliance with probation orders of alcohol abstinence. Breath alcohol analyzers can also be integrated into a vehicle's ignition system to prevent alcohol-impaired drivers from operating it.

The technology of breath alcohol analysis has evolved from the collection of breath in balloons and analysis by cumbersome wet chemical methods to automated, portable, microprocessor-controlled instruments providing immediate results. These instruments are capable of providing reliable results when operated in a non-laboratory environment by individuals with little or no scientific background or training.

8.2 Sampling Breath for Alcohol Analysis

Breath analysis provides a rapid, noninvasive means of determining alcohol concentration that requires minimal subject cooperation. That alcohol is both infinitely soluble in water and significantly volatile at physiological temperatures influences the methodology necessary to measure alcohol in breath.

There are several key aspects of breath sampling for alcohol analysis that relate to instrumental and procedural design.

A. End-expiratory breath is the desired specimen

It is well established that the terminal portion of a prolonged breath expiration provides a sample that reflects the alcohol concentration of arterial blood to which the brain is exposed. (American Medical Association, 1976). In order to obtain the desired specimen, subjects are generally instructed to take a deep breath and provide a steady exhalation into a sampling tube or hose for as long as they are able. During the course of the exhalation, the breath alcohol[1] concentration will increase rapidly until a concentration "plateau" is reached (Figure 8.1, normal breath). Analysis of any portion of the breath sample prior to attaining this plateau will result in a lower breath alcohol concentration reading. It is therefore standard breath sampling practice to provide a continuous exhalation against moderate pressure and to discard at least the initial two-thirds of the sample (Dubowski, 1974).

B. Residual mouth alcohol

Alcohol in the oral cavity arising from recent alcohol ingestion, regurgitation of stomach contents containing alcohol or by eructation of gas containing significant amounts of alcohol can contaminate the breath sample and cause falsely elevated results. During the course of exhalation, breath samples contaminated with residual mouth alcohol are characterized by an initial rapid alcohol concentration rise followed by a rapid decline of the concentration to zero or to the baseline breath alcohol concentration (Dubowski, 1992) (Figure 8.1, mouth alcohol). It is well established that a pretest alcohol deprivation period of at least fifteen minutes provides sufficient time to dissipate residual mouth alcohol.

C. Condensation losses, carryover

If breath is subjected to a reduction in temperature during or after sampling its water vapor component will condense and alcohol will be removed from the sample because of its high affinity for water. Alcohol in the condensate could contribute to a subsequent test if not removed. Potential condensation loss or carryover is more of an issue for screening devices or evidential instruments in mobile service (Conde et al., 2002). This potential loss or carryover is easily

avoided by maintaining the instrument's sample chamber (and any significant length of sampling tubing) at a constant temperature, typically between 45° and 50°C

D. Additional steps

Additional steps are taken in instrument design to prevent evaporative losses of alcohol during sampling and analysis.

8.3 Breath Alcohol Testing Instrumentation
A. Testing instruments

Breath alcohol testing instruments can be classified into four categories of use.

1. Passive alcohol sensor (PAS)

The PAS is designed to easily and rapidly detect the presence of alcohol. It is typically used by law enforcement officers to screen drivers at roadside sobriety checkpoints. The PAS is a handheld, battery-operated unit which is often housed in a modified police service flashlight (Dubowski, 1992). In operation it is held in proximity to the subject's mouth while an internal fan draws expired breath or air from the vehicle interior into the unit for analysis. No subject cooperation is necessary (thus the term "passive"). If alcohol is detected, its presence, and sometimes an approximate amount, will be displayed.

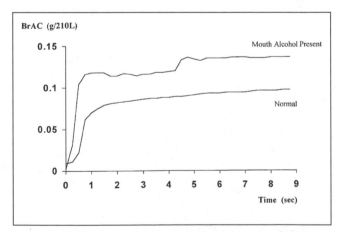

Figure 8.1 *Breath alcohol profiles showing patterns of normal exhalation and mouth alcohol. Data from a BAC DataMaster during exhalation from an alcohol-dosed subject (Rod Gullberg, Washington State Police)*

2. Screening device

Screening devices (also known as preliminary or pre-arrest breath testers) are relatively inexpensive, handheld, portable units which are designed to provide a rapid approximation of alcohol concentration. They are commonly employed by police officers at the scene of traffic offenses where they are incorporated as an adjunct to field sobriety testing to establish probable cause for an arrest. These instruments are also used in hospitals (Falkensson et al., 1989) and are extensively used for workplace testing. Lighted panels display a numerical result or an indication as to whether or not a preset alcohol concentration has been exceeded (if the instrument has a "pass/fail" or "pass/warn/fail" display). In many jurisdictions screening device results are considered unreliable and are not admissible evidence in anything but a probable cause hearing. Even though many of these devices were not originally designed for evidential use, most are capable of producing accurate and reliable results when proper scientific safeguards are applied.

3. Ignition interlock device

A breath alcohol ignition interlock device (BAIID) is an adaptation of screening device technology, which prevents a driver from starting a BAIID-equipped vehicle if a preset alcohol concentration has been exceeded. The devices are installed as a court-ordered sanction with the intent of altering the drinking and driving habits of habitual offenders. The cost of installation and servicing BAIIDs is typically borne by the offender. Various sampling schemes are employed to deter attempts at substituting breath samples from someone other than the driver or altering the breath sample in a way that removes alcohol. Some of these procedures require subject training, such as humming while providing a sample, or blowing in a predetermined pattern of varied pressure. In addition, random, rolling retest requirements are used to prevent an alcohol-free driver from starting the vehicle and leaving it running while alcohol is consumed later. Failure to pass a rolling retest may result in the vehicle's lights flashing or horn blowing. BAIIDs are equipped with an electronic data logger that records the date and time of all breath alcohol results, power interrup-

tions, and all attempts at ignition and breath sampling. The data is periodically downloaded and printed to verify compliance with the terms for use of the BAIID-equipped vehicle.

4. Evidential breath tester

An evidential breath tester (EBT) is designed to provide accurate, precise, quantitative alcohol results. Results obtained from these devices are generally admissible in court proceedings. Although these devices are most often situated at fixed sites such as police stations, the instruments may also be designed for use as mobile units employing batteries or a vehicle's electrical system to obtain power. Mobile units have the advantage of providing the capability to measure an alcohol concentration nearly coincident to the time of a traffic violation and can be used in isolated areas such as waterways, snowmobile trails, and other locations where a significant time delay from apprehension to testing might otherwise result.

B. Calibrating units

An important adjunct to breath alcohol testing instruments are the devices used to calibrate them and verify their accuracy. The most commonly used devices for this purpose are breath alcohol simulators. These devices produce a predictable, known vapor alcohol concentration by passing air through a heated aqueous solution of known alcohol concentration. Any vapor alcohol concentration of practical interest can be produced by varying the alcohol concentration of the aqueous solution. The simulator must be designed to evenly heat the solution and its headspace. The temperature must be carefully regulated to ensure reproducible results and should be accurately verified (Dubowski, 1979). Laboratory and field studies using current generation breath alcohol simulators indicate that these devices perform adequately for both the calibration and verification of calibration of breath alcohol testing instruments (Dubowski and Essary, 1991, 1992). Figure 8.2 is a diagram of one of the commercially available breath alcohol simulators that meets these criteria.

In addition to breath alcohol simulators, alcohol mixtures in inert gas stored in pressurized cylinders or cans have found increased use for calibration and control testing. Care must be taken in the manufacture of these mixtures to ensure that the gas cylinders are chemically inert and that no moisture is present in the mixture gas, hence the oft-used term "dry gas standard." Since gaseous alcohol standards follow the *ideal gas law*, the measured results are dependant on atmospheric pressure at the test site. Atmospheric pressure decreases as altitude increases, therefore dry gas standard results must be corrected for changes in altitude above sea level. Most EBTs capable of using dry gas standards are equipped with pressure transducers and software to automatically make any necessary correction. Absent the above, correction tables are provided to covert the nominal concentration given at standard temperature and pressure (STP) to the ambient pressure. Dry gas standards have been found to compare favorably to breath alcohol simulators for breath alcohol testing applications (Dubowski and Essary, 1996).

Both gaseous standards and breath alcohol simulator solutions should be standardized against reference materials traceable to National Institute of Standards and Technology (NIST) standard reference material (SRM) (Dubowski, 1992). NIST's SRM 1828a, or its successors, provides ethyl alcohol solutions expressly for this purpose.

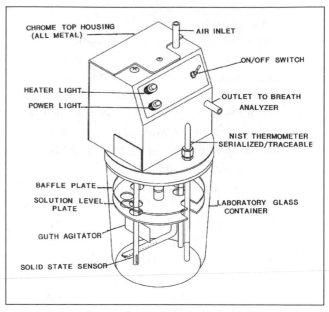

Figure 8.2 Guth Model 34 C breath alcohol simulator (Guth Laboratories)

8.4 Requirements for Evidential Breath Testing

A. General

The adoption of per se laws has made the achievement of a specified alcohol concentration illegal, resulting in increased judicial scrutiny of the breath testing instruments and sampling procedures. Reliable results can be obtained from evidential breath testing instruments under properly controlled conditions that include proper training of operators, proper maintenance of equipment and rigorously following appropriate testing protocols. Many of the factors in such protocols are codified in the statutes or administrative rules and regulations that govern the jurisdiction in which the testing is performed. These may vary widely from one jurisdiction to another. A combination of testing protocols and instrument features is necessary to ensure that a scientifically valid and forensically acceptable alcohol result is obtained.

There are several generally recognized aspects of breath testing which should be part of testing protocols:

- At least a fifteen-minute pretest alcohol deprivation period. During this period the subject must be observed to ensure that no ingestion of alcohol-containing material, regurgitation or emesis occurs.
- Blank analysis prior to any subject or control test. Analysis of a room air sample establishes the absence of environmental contamination and serves to purge the instrument so that there is no contamination from prior samples.
- Analysis of control specimens. Analyzing gaseous alcohol specimens of known concentration establishes the proper functioning of the sampling system and demonstrates proper calibration and maintenance of the instrument (Dubowski, 1986).
- Documentation that all steps of a prescribed testing protocol were conducted. This may be accomplished by printouts from automated instruments or the use of manual checklists.
- Documentation and certification of instrument maintenance and calibration. Compliance with all applicable rules and regulations, routine

maintenance, problems and action taken to solve them should all be documented.

There are additional recommended, but not always required, practices:

- Reporting results as breath alcohol instead of blood alcohol concentration. In the United States breath alcohol results should be expressed in units of grams of alcohol per 210 liters of breath (g/210 L) (Mason and Dubowski, 1976, National Safety Council, 1992, International Association for Chemical Testing, 1993).
- Analysis of at least two separate breath samples. Two sequentially analyzed samples taken two to ten minutes apart will help demonstrate the absence of mouth alcohol contamination and rule out contributions from instrument artifacts such as radio frequency interference or spurious results. In order to be effective the results of such analyses must agree within a prescribed amount of each other, typically 0.02 g/210 L (Dubowski and Essary, 1987, National Safety Council, 1992).

B. Maintaining reliability

To safeguard the testing process and validate the breath alcohol results, evidential breath alcohol testing requires adherence to a comprehensive quality assurance program. This program should monitor and control not only the testing process, but also all applicable rules and regulations, equipment, test sites, personnel, performance and proficiency testing, records and reports, and inspections, reviews and evaluations (Dubowski, 1994). Each of these elements must be reviewed and updated on a regular basis. Inadequacy in any of these areas jeopardizes the reliability of the testing result. Recommended practices for breath alcohol testing have been compiled by the National Safety Council, Committee on Alcohol and Other Drugs (National Safety Council, 1992) and the Canadian Society of Forensic Science (Canadian Society of Forensic Science, 1995).

C. Federal specifications

In the United States, the Department of Transportation, National Highway Traffic Safety Administration (NHTSA) assists states and manufacturers by implementing uniform performance standards and certifying breath alcohol testing instruments and calibrating units that meet those standards. At first, only equipment that complied with these standards could be purchased with federal funds. The mandatory standards were later changed to model specifications (U.S. Department of Transportation, 1984a, 1984b). Manufacturers submit equipment to NHTSA for evaluation of compliance with these specifications. Lists of products conforming to the applicable specifications are periodically published (U.S. Department of Transportation, 1997, 2002). These conforming product lists (CPLs) define qualifying equipment for use under the Omnibus Transportation Employee Testing Act and are used as the primary criteria for choosing evidential equipment in some jurisdictions. The specifications are occasionally amended, as was the case when evaluation of instruments at lower alcohol concentrations was instituted (U.S. Department of Transportation, 1993). In addition to evidential breath alcohol testing instrumentation and calibrating units, NHTSA has also published model specifications and CPLs for breath alcohol ignition interlock devices and screening devices for measuring both breath and saliva (U.S. Department of Transportation, 1992, 1994, 2001).

In Canada instrument standards and approval procedures are recommended by the Alcohol Test Committee of the Canadian Society of Forensic Science (Canadian Society of Forensic Science, 1995). Similar arrangements exist in other countries. International standards for breath testing instruments have been formulated by the International Organization of Legal Metrology (OIML). Adoption of the OIML International Recommendation IR 126, Ethanol Breath Analyzers, will influence the design of instruments intended for sale in OIML member nations.

8.5 Challenges to the Validity of Breath Alcohol Results

The results of breath alcohol testing instruments are often the object of judicial scrutiny. Following are some of the more frequently heard challenges to the validity of breath alcohol results which are related the instrument and its operation.

A. Rules, regulations and documentation

Many successful challenges to the validity of breath alcohol results have resulted from the simple failure to follow the established testing and reporting protocols. It is of the utmost importance that breath alcohol testing be conducted in conformance to all applicable rules and regulations. Adherence to all steps of the proscribed testing protocol must be documented. Documentation must exist showing that the testing instruments have been properly calibrated, maintained and operated by qualified personnel.

B. Specificity

It is often alleged that a breath alcohol result was caused wholly or in part due to compounds other than ethyl alcohol in the subject's breath, thus causing a falsely elevated result. The specificity of an instrument can be defined as its ability to respond exclusively to the compound of interest (in this case ethyl alcohol). Compounds that are indistinguishable from ethyl alcohol to the instrument can potentially interfere with the test. In order to significantly affect a subject's breath alcohol result a potential interferant must

- be a volatile organic compound capable of appearing in the breath of a living, conscious human being;
- be present in sufficiently high concentration to be measured by the instrument after a fifteen-minute pretest observation period; and
- be able to both produce a response and not be recognized as an interferant by the instrument.

Acetone is the only endogenous compound present in breath that can reasonably be considered to be a potential interferant. It may be present in elevated concentrations in the breath of diabetics and fasting dieters. Numerous studies have conclusively shown that endogenous acetone will not have a deleterious effect on breath alcohol results (Dubowski and Essary, 1983, 1984; Flores and Frank, 1985; Jones, 1986, 1988; Oliver and Garriott, 1979). The possible contribution of exogenous compounds to a breath alcohol result is mostly theoretical as it is limited by the physiological restrictions of the potential interferant and the characteristics of the employed detection technology (National Safety Council, 1999). Most potential exogenous interferants are too short-lived in breath, too toxic, or will not cause a significant response on the instrument's detector. The specificity characteristics of various detectors used in breath alcohol testing instruments are discussed later in this chapter.

C. Residual mouth alcohol

The theory of residual mouth alcohol challenges to breath alcohol results is that alcohol remaining in the mouth harmfully contributes to the reading. Most mouth alcohol-based challenges can be successfully avoided by strictly adhering to a pretest observation and alcohol deprivation period and having agreement between duplicate breath tests. Prior to the start of the pretest period the mouth should be visually inspected to ensure that it does not contain any foreign substance, such as chewing tobacco, which may contain or retain alcohol. Many mouthsprays, inhalers and mouthwashes contain alcohol (Westenbrink and Sauve, 1991; Modell et al., 1993; Gomez et al., 1995; Logan et al., 1998). Use of these products during the pretest observation period must be strictly avoided (Denny and Williams, 1987). Additional potential sources of mouth alcohol have been studied, including food and beverages (Logan and Distefano, 1998), breath freshening tablets (Williams, 1996) and gastroesophageal reflux disease (Kechageas et al., 1999, Gullberg, 2001). These sources either have been found to have no effect or if they could, adhering to established safeguards will eliminate the potential challenge.

Some challenges to breath alcohol results are based on factors which allegedly prolong the time period in which alcohol remains in the mouth beyond the usual fifteen minutes, such as alcohol trapped by dentures. Dentures and dental adhesives have not been found to influence mouth alcohol clearance rates (Harding et al., 1992) and need not be treated as foreign objects in the mouth. Similarly, oral jewelry (Logan and Gullberg, 1998) and blood in the mouth (Wigmore and Wilkie., 2001) have been found to have no effect on breath alcohol results.

D. Radio frequency interference

Radio frequency interference (RFI) or electromagnetic interference can arise when radio signals transmitted in proximity to a breath testing instrument are amplified in a way indistinguishable from electronic signals generated by the instrument during an analysis. Most instruments are shielded from such interference, have RFI detectors that prevent testing if significant potential RFI sources are present or both. Breath testing protocols typically prohibit the use of handheld transmitters in the proximity of the instrument while it is being operated (National Safety Council, 1992). Subject testing protocols that include the analysis of air blanks, known alcohol samples and agreement of duplicate subject test results can be used to demonstrate the lack of RFI.

E. Instrument variability

Breath alcohol analysis instruments, like all measuring devices, are subject to random variability. Case law abounds with references to "margin of error." In breath alcohol analysis the variability associated with an instrument's ability to measure the alcohol in a given breath sample is relatively small (Gullberg, 1992). Instruments appearing on NHTSA CPLs meet minimum specifications for accuracy, precision and linearity. Tables 8.1 and 8.2 illustrate the in-vitro accuracy and precision of several instruments as determined in a multi-state study. Listed in the tables are the instrument model, number of individual instruments tested, total number of tests performed for each model, mean value, standard deviation (SD), coefficient of variation (CV), lowest value and highest value obtained.

8.6 Breath Alcohol Testing Instruments

Detection technology. Breath alcohol instruments generally use one of five types of analytical technology. These detection principles and examples of some instruments in which they are employed are listed in Table 8.3.

Numerous breath alcohol-testing instruments have been designed and marketed over the years. Many instruments that are no longer manufactured remain in use in some jurisdictions. New instruments are continually developed and older instruments evolve. Advances in electronic components allow for microprocessor-control of customized test sequences and instrument functions, even in instruments designed to be handheld. Data acquisition software allows for downloading subject results, along with diagnostic and subject demographic information, to an attached or remote computer. Electronic panels and printers display results and other information.

No attempt is made here to cover all breath alcohol testing instruments currently in use. Instead, each of the five analytical technologies commonly used will be described along with representative instruments that incorporate these detection methods. All of the instruments described in this section appear on NHTSA conforming product lists for evidential breath testers.

A. Infrared spectroscopy

Instruments utilizing infrared spectroscopy technology are the most common type of EBT currently in use. They typically feature a high degree of automation and the ability to customize testing and data handling protocols. The underlying analytical principle of these instruments is that all chemicals absorb infrared radiation at specific wavelengths corresponding to various atomic and molecular structural characteristics. Ethyl alcohol absorbs strongly in the infrared energy wavelength range of 3.3 to 3.5 microns utilized by many infrared breath alcohol testing instruments. An additional, more specific absorption band existing around 9.5 microns may also be used. Infrared instruments quantitate the amount of alcohol in the sample by measuring the energy at specific wavelengths entering and emerging from the sample chamber. The amount of infrared energy lost due to absorption by ethyl alcohol molecules is proportional to the alcohol concentration.

The potential for chemical interference is a consideration in infrared-based breath alcohol testing instruments because literally thousands of compounds will absorb infrared radiation in the 3.3–3.5 micron wavelength range that is typically used. The use of two or more analytical wavelengths is commonly employed to increase the specificity of cur-

Table 8.1
Accuracy and Precision of Several Breath Alcohol Analyzers at a Target Value of 0.05 g/210 L[**]

Instrument (number tested)	Number of Replicates	Mean	SD	CV	Range
Intoxilyzer 4011A (15)	150	0.048	0.0017	3.5%	0.044–0.055
Intoxilyzer 5000 (12)	140	0.05	0.0016	3.2%	0.046–0.053
Intoxilyzer 1400 (8)	100	0.05	0.0012	2.4%	0.043–0.053
BAC DataMaster (10)	110	0.05	0.0014	3.8%	0.046–0.054
AlcoMonitor (8)	100	0.051	0.0017	3.3%	0.048–0.054
AlcoSensor IV (8)	30	0.047	0.0011	2.3%	0.043–0.049

* Number of individual instruments of this model tested.
** Data from International Association for Chemical Testing Breath Alcohol Research Project. Unpublished.

Table 8.2
Accuracy and Precision of Several Breath Alcohol Analyzers at a Target Value of 0.1 g/210 L[**]

Instrument (number tested)	Number of Replicates	Mean	SD	CV	Range
Intoxilyzer 4011A (15)	150	0.1	0.0016	1.6%	0.089–0.106
Intoxilyzer 5000 (12)	140	0.1	0.0016	1.6%	0.096–0.103
Intoxilyzer 1400 (8)	100	0.099	0.0024	2.4%	0.089–0.104
BAC DataMaster (10)	110	0.1	0.0018	1.8%	0.095–0.103
AlcoMonitor (8)	100	0.103	0.0025	2.5%	0.096–0.108
AlcoSensor IV (8)	30	0.095	0.0009	0.9%	0.091–0.098

* Number of individual instruments of this model tested.
** Data from International Association for Chemical Testing Breath Alcohol Research Project. Unpublished.

Table 8.3
Detection Technology Employed in Breath Alcohol Testing Instruments

Primary Detection Principle	Instrument
Infrared spectrometry	BAC DataMaster BAC DataMaster cdm Intoxilyzer 1400 Intoxilyzer 5000, 5000 EN Intoxilyzer 8000 Intoxilyzer 4011A*, Intoxilyzer 4011AS-A*
Electrochemical oxidation/fuel cell	Alco-Sensor III, IV Alcolmeter CC Alcotest 7410 A.L.E.R.T. J4X Intoxilyzer S-D2, S-D5 Intox EC/IR LifeLoc FC 10, FC 20 RBT IV, RBT IV XL Breath Alcohol Ignition Interlock Devices (BAIIDs)
Dual detector (infrared/fuel cell)	Alcotest 7110 MKIII-C
Taguchi gas sensor	A.L.E.R.T. J4 Breath Alcohol Ignition Interlock Devices (BAIIDs)
Chemical oxidation/photometry	Breathalyzer models 900*/900A*
Gas chromatography	Alco-Analyzer 2100*

* indicates instruments which are no longer manufactured

rent infrared breath alcohol testing instruments. Deviations from the expected relative response of the detector to ethyl alcohol at the employed wavelengths allow the instrument to notify the operator of the presence of potential interferants. Such systems are typically optimized for detecting acetone and eliminating its contribution from the final result. Most endogenous or exogenous compounds that are otherwise potential interferants do not respond to the more ethyl alcohol-specific 9.5-micron band. Regardless of the wavelengths used, only those compounds capable of appearing in significant concentrations in human breath need be considered potential interferants.

Infrared analyzers are able to continuously measure alcohol in a breath sample during the course of exhalation. This allows for employing "slope detection" to assure the achievement of a near-alveolar sample by monitoring the rate of change of the alcohol concentration and accepting a sample as valid only after consecutive measurements fall within a predetermined minimum rate of change. Slope detection is also used to detect the presence of residual mouth alcohol by recognizing the altered pattern typical of such samples. The absence of mouth alcohol detection by an instrument equipped with slope detection circuitry should not be used as the sole means to ensure that a valid sample has been obtained (Harding et al., 1992; Wigmore and Leslie, 2001). Since the breath sample is not destroyed or altered, infrared instruments may be equipped with a means for the alcohol in the actual analyzed sample to be retained ("trapped") for subsequent retesting.

1. BAC DataMaster

The BAC DataMaster (Figure 8.3) is also available in a smaller configuration as the BAC DataMaster cdm.

Manufacturer. National Patent Analytical Systems, Mansfield, OH.

Analytical characteristics. Dedicated greybody Kanthal infrared source lamp, cooled detector, 1.1-meters optical pathlength (0.87 meter in the cdm), two narrow bandwidth filters: 3.44 microns used for alcohol quantitation, 3.37 microns used for acetone correction and detection of other interfer-

ants. A diagram of the BAC DataMaster optical bench is given in Figure 8.4.

Display, printer. Twenty-four character liquid crystal display, integral printer using multicopy test cards.

Automation. Complete automation of programmed test sequences, microprocessor control of instrument functions. Automated single point calibration procedure. Test sequences can be changed through password-protected keyboard commands. Remote operation from a host computer possible with communication interface option.

Breath sampling. External, heated breath tube with disposable mouthpieces. Sample chamber is fifty milliliters (39.5 mL in the cdm). A thermistor in the breath sample pathway monitors breath flow. Slope detection, flow rate and time are used to determine adequate breath sample.

Calibration or control tests. External wet bath simulator with simulator vapor recirculation used for control tests and calibration. Single alcohol concentration calibration protocol. Dry gas standard may be used for control tests. Dry gas standard results are automatically corrected for pressure. A quartz plate of known absorbance is used as an internal calibration check.

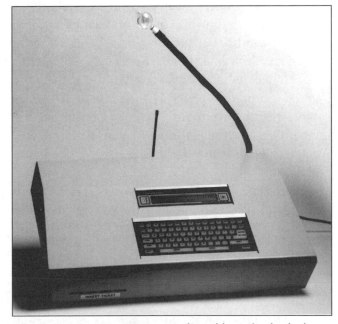

Figure 8.3 *BAC DataMaster infrared breath alcohol analyzer (National Patent Analytical Systems)*

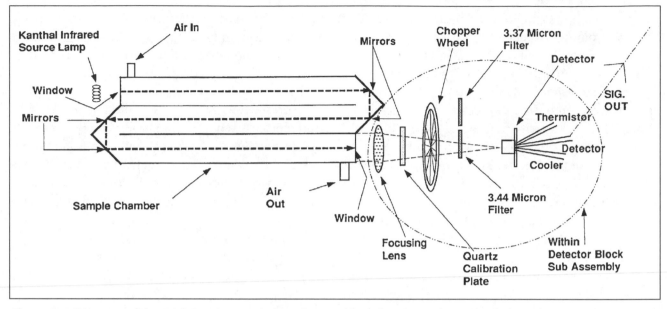

Figure 8.4 Diagram of the BAC DataMaster infrared optical bench (National Patent Analytical Systems)

Data acquisition. Test data and demographic information stored in large capacity memory can be downloaded to computer directly or via modem.

Operation. Depressing the Run key initiates the programmed test sequence. The electronic display panel and audible signals prompt the operator throughout the testing procedure and also indicate any instrument or operational problems or errors.

Each test sequence begins with a system purge with ambient air drawn in by an internal pump. This sample is used to set the analytical baseline and is also checked for interferants. Successful completion of this test is indicated by a 0.000 result display. An internal calibration check is then conducted. Each subject breath or control test is preceded and followed by a system purge and room air blank test. Adequate breath flow is indicated by a steady audible tone.

Both versions of the DataMaster have an available "Delta" filter option that employs an additional 3.5-micron narrow bandwidth filter for enhanced interferant detection.

2. Intoxilyzer 5000, Intoxilyzer 5000 EN

The Intoxilyzer 5000 family of instruments (Figure 8.5) are presently the most widely employed evidential breath alcohol testing instruments. The Intoxilyzer 5000 was first manufactured in 1984 and has undergone continuous revision since that time.

For purposes of this description the original Intoxilyzer 5000 is referred to as the 64/66 series, with major revisions referred to as the 568 series, 768 series and EN. The currently manufactured version is the Intoxilyzer 5000 EN.

Manufacturer. CMI, Inc., Owensboro, KY.

Analytical characteristics. Quartz-iodide IR source, three filters in rotating chopper wheel (64/66, 568 Series). The 568, 768 and EN have a cooled detector. 768 Series and EN instruments are equipped with two additional filters (for added interferant detection). A 3.8-micron filter is used as a ref-

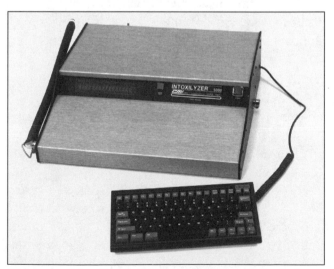

Figure 8.5 Intoxilyzer 5000 infrared breath alcohol analyzer (CMI, Inc.)

erence wavelength, 3.48 (3.47 for 768 and EN) for alcohol quantitation, and 3.39 (3.38 for 768 and EN) for detection of interferants and correction for acetone. The two filters used for enhanced interferant detection capability in the 768 and EN are 3.36 and 3.52 microns (Figure 8.6).

Display, printer. Lighted sixteen-character vacuum fluorescent display, integral printer using multicopy test cards or paper roll. Optional external printer.

Automation. Complete automation of preprogrammed test sequences, microprocessor control of instrument functions. Test sequences changed through switches in locked access panel or through keyboard commands for 768 and EN.

Breath sampling. External, heated breath tube with disposable mouthpieces. Standard sample chamber has a volume of 81.4 mL. Slope detection, time, pressure and volume (EN) are used to determine adequate breath sample.

Calibration or control testing. External wet bath simulator used for control tests and calibration. Simulator vapor recirculation is available as an option. Dry gas standard may be used for control tests (568, 768 and EN). The 568, 768 and EN instruments measure barometric pressure and apply any necessary correction to the dry gas result. An internal electronic calibration check is also available. Remote diagnostic testing possible if equipped with a modem.

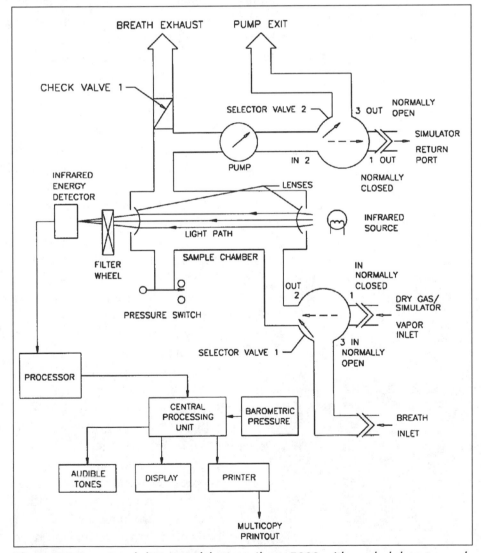

Figure 8.6 *Functional diagram of the Intoxilyzer 5000 with cooled detector and vapor recirculation (CMI, Inc.)*

Data acquisition. Test data and demographic information stored in memory can be downloaded to a host computer via cable or modem.

Operation. Pressing the Start Test button initiates the programmed test sequence. The electronic display panel and audible signals prompt the operator throughout the testing procedure and also indicate any instrument or operational problems or errors.

The sequence begins with an internal check of electronic parameters, printer function and sample chamber temperature. Failure of any portion of the internal check will be indicated and the test will be aborted. Each subject breath or control test is preceded and followed by a system purge and setting of analytical baseline with room air drawn in by an internal pump. Adequate breath pressure is indicated by a steady audible tone. Keyboard commands can also be used to initiate any of the preprogrammed test sequences.

3. Intoxilyzer 8000

The Intoxilyzer 8000 (Figure 8.7) is designed as a compact, mobile or stationary infrared EBT. It is designed to operate from an external 12-volt DC supply, or can use the internal power supply to convert 110 or 220 volts AC to the required 12 volts DC. The instrument is also available with a 12-volt rechargeable battery pack.

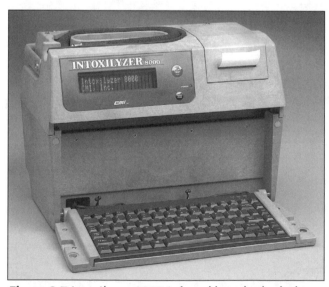

Figure 8.7 *Intoxilyzer 8000 infrared breath alcohol analyzer (CMI, Inc.)*

Manufacturer. CMI, Inc., Owensboro, KY.

Analytical characteristics. Dual pyroelectric detectors. Pulsed infrared source, eliminating the need for chopper wheel. Equipped with two filters (3.4 and 9.4 micron).

Printer, display. Integral thermal or impact printer with paper roll, lighted two line by twenty character vacuum fluorescent display. Able to use external printer.

Automation. Microprocessor control of instrument functions, diagnostic functions and test sequences. Custom programming achieved through keyboard commands.

Breath sampling. Heated breath tube with disposable mouthpieces.
Adequate breath sample determined by slope detection, minimum flow rate, pressure and volume.

Calibration or control tests. Wet bath simulator vapor, with integral simulator vapor recirculation, or dry gas standards may be used for calibration and control tests. Single or multiple concentration automated calibration protocol.

Data acquisition. Integral keyboard used to input subject demographic data, initiate test sequences and program instrument functions. Password protection limits functional access to authorized personnel. Data can be downloaded to computer via internal modem or external cable.

Operation. Test sequences may be started by pressing the Start Test button or through keyboard commands. Test sequences can be user-programmed in any combination of subject and control tests. Air blanks precede and follow each subject or control analysis. The operator is prompted through the display panel and audio signals for each step in a sequence.

B. Electrochemical oxidation or fuel cell

A fuel cell is a device designed to continually convert fuel and an oxidant into direct current. As used for breath testing, alcohol is used as the fuel and oxygen from the atmosphere as the oxidant (Dubowski, 1992). Alcohol is converted in the fuel cell to acetic acid, producing two electrons for each alcohol molecule. These electrons produce an electrical current that serves to quantitate the amount of alcohol. Acetic acid further reacts at a much slower rate to form oxygen, carbon dioxide and water (Figure 8.8). Acetic acid can build up on the fuel cell after several consecutive positive tests, prolonging the time necessary to return to a zero baseline. Fuel cells change in sensitivity as they age, which may require more frequent recalibration than some other types of detectors, depending on how the signal is analyzed. Fuel cells are relatively specific for ethyl alcohol. Fuel cells can potentially respond to other alcohols such as methyl-, isopropyl-, and *n*-propyl alcohol, and to acetaldehyde. All of these compounds appear endogenously in insignificant breath concentrations and are far more intoxicating than ethyl alcohol when ingested.

The size and power requirements of fuel cells allow for small, portable, battery-operated instruments which lend themselves well to screening devices and on-site testing use. When first introduced in the 1970s, fuel-cell instruments were not considered to be sufficiently reliable for use as evidential units.

More recently, fuel cell detector and breath sampling improvements coupled with solid state circuitry and microprocessor technology have led to instrument designs which meet NHTSA model specifications for EBTs and are able to incorporate sophisticated control of instrument functions and data transfer capabilities. Several former screening instruments were reclassified as EBTs and now appear on NHTSA CPLs.

Fuel cell instruments include:

1. Intox EC/IR
The Intox EC/IR (Figure 8.9) is an EBT that uses a fuel cell as the primary analytical technology for alcohol quantitation, coupled with an infrared detector to monitor breath sample quality.

Manufacturer. Intoximeters, Inc., St. Louis, MO.

Analytical characteristics. Rapid recovery fuel cell for alcohol quantitation. Infrared detector used

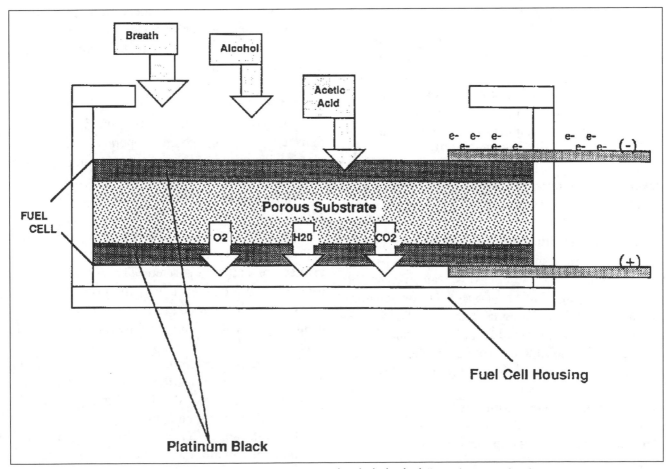

Figure 8.8 *Diagram of a fuel cell showing its reaction with ethyl alcohol (Intoximeters, Inc.)*

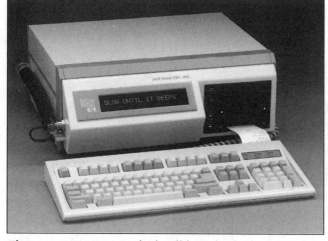

Figure 8.9 *Intox EC/IR fuel cell breath alcohol analyzer (Intoximeters, Inc.)*

to monitor breath sample quality and detect mouth alcohol. Coiled nichrome wire infrared source, three-channel detector measures infrared radiation from two narrow bandpath filters of 3.45 microns and one of 4.26 microns. The 3.45 micron wavelength is used for alcohol detection and the 4.26 micron wavelength for carbon dioxide.

Printer, display. Internal high-speed thermal printer with graphics capability using paper rolls. Two-line, twenty characters each, vacuum fluorescent display. Optional external printer capability.

Automation. Dual microprocessors, one controlling all analytical functions and one for user interfacing. Keyboard command, software-driven test sequences, diagnostics and calibration. Diagnostic testing may be remotely conducted from host computer. Automated features can be customized for the user.

Breath sampling. Heated external breath sampling tube using disposable mouthpieces. A thermistor is used to measure flow rate. Acceptable samples are determined by slope detection and minimum volume. The timing of detection of carbon dioxide in breath compared to that of alcohol by the infrared unit is used to determine whether mouth alcohol is present. If alcohol is detected prior to carbon dioxide the instrument indicates the presence of mouth alcohol. Other algorithms that utilize the data from the IR and flow detectors can also be used to determine acceptable sample and mouth alcohol.

Calibration or control tests. Wet bath simulators or dry gas standards may be used for control tests and single concentration calibration protocol. A pressure transducer is used to correct the dry gas standard result for altitude. Wet bath simulator vapor is introduced by the operator through the breath tube, with an optional simulator vapor port and simulator air input pump available.

Data acquisition. Demographic data may be entered via an attached keyboard and through an optional magnetic card reader. Test results, diagnostic and demographic data may be downloaded to a host computer via serial cable or the instrument's modem. Report and data collection formats can be customized.

Operation. Keyboard commands initiate a preprogrammed test sequence. The fuel cell is electronically zeroed and an ambient air sample is analyzed prior to subject testing. The instrument display prompts the operator throughout the testing procedure. During breath sampling the instrument provides a visual display to indicate that an adequate sample is being delivered. An audible tone alerts the operator when minimum breath sample requirements have been met.

2. RBT IV

The RBT IV (Figure 8.10) combines an Alco-Sensor IV handheld, battery-operated fuel cell detector with a microprocessor and printer. The two units are connected by cable.

Manufacturer. Intoximeters, Inc., St. Louis, MO.

Analytical characteristics. Rapid recovery fuel cell detector (Figure 8.11). Both detector unit and printer are battery operated. The Alco-Sensor IV uses a 9-volt alkaline battery; the printer unit uses 12-volt rechargeable batteries or an optional AC adapter. The detector unit is equipped with an RFI detector.

Printer, display. Impact printer using paper roll. The detector unit has a four-character LCD panel; the printer unit has two-line, lighted LCD with twenty characters for each line.

Automation. Microprocessor in printer unit monitors the detector unit and prompts operator during preprogrammed test sequence.

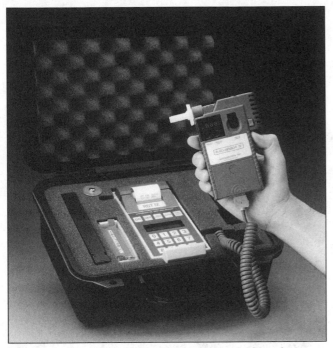

Figure 8.10 *RBT IV fuel cell breath alcohol analyzer (Intoximeters, Inc.)*

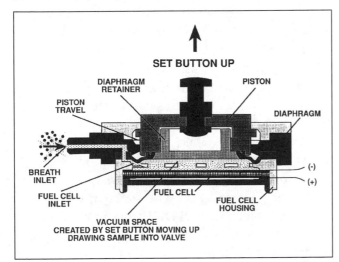

Figure 8.11 *Diagram of RBT IV fuel cell and sampling system (Intoximeters, Inc.)*

Breath sampling. Disposable one-way mouthpieces attach directly to detector unit. Mouthpieces are removed after sampling by depressing an eject button. A flow thermistor monitors flow rate and volume to assure an adequate sample. The thermistor system can be overridden by pressing the Manual button. An electrically operated piston sample pump delivers a one-milliliter sample.

Calibration or control tests. Wet bath simulator or dry gas standards may be used for control tests and the single concentration calibration protocol.

Data acquisition. Test data stored in the RBT IV microprocessor memory can be downloaded via optional cable connection and software to a PC-compatible computer. The RBT IV has sufficient memory to store up to 1,000 tests.

Operation. Pressing the Start button on the printer unit initiates a preprogrammed test sequence. Both the printer and detector unit displays guide the operator through the procedure. The operator must insert a mouthpiece into the detector and depress the Set button when prompted. The detector automatically samples and analyzes a room air blank. After successful completion of the blank analysis the Set button is again pressed and a subject or standard sample is taken. Each subject or standard test in a sequence is preceded by a blank analysis and followed by pressing the Set button.

When the subject blows into the mouthpiece a "+" symbol on the detector unit display panel indicates sufficient flow rate during sampling. A "++" is displayed when a minimum breath volume of approximately 1.2 liters has been delivered. A breath sample is automatically taken when the thermistor senses a decrease in flow after this time. Simulator vapor and dry gas standards are sampled by depressing the Manual button on the detector unit. Test results are printed when a sequence is completed. Additional copies of the just-completed test may be printed. Testing may be aborted or stopped if the subject refuses testing by depressing appropriate keys on the printer unit.

3. Intoxilyzer S-D5

The Intoxilyzer S-D5 (Figure 8.12) is a small, lightweight, battery-operated, handheld device primarily used for screening tests. Designed for use by right or left hand.

Manufacturer. CMI, Inc., Owensboro, KY.

Analytical characteristics. Fuel cell detector, battery-operated.

Printer, display. Three-character LED panel. No printer.

Automation. Instrument prompts operator through automated test sequence.

Breath sampling. Uses disposable breath tube attached directly to instrument. Tube has restriction on one end and small hole in center, which attaches

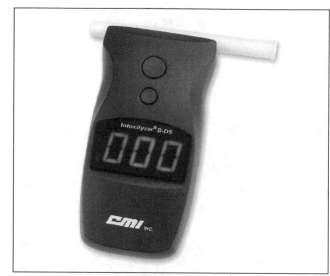

Figure 8.12 *Intoxilyzer S-D5 handheld fuel cell breath alcohol analyzer (CMI, Inc.)*

to instrument. Subject provides sample in unrestricted end. Pressure and time used to calculate minimum acceptable breath volume. A spring-loaded piston draws a sample into the fuel cell once minimum volume achieved and pressure decreases. Sample can be taken manually also. If inadequate sample delivered, "vol" displayed and test aborted.

Calibration or control tests. Wet bath simulator or dry gas standard used for control tests and single concentration automated calibration protocol.

Operation. Pressing the On button initiates test sequence. The instrument first analyzes an ambient air sample. The test is aborted if the air blank shows alcohol present. After air blank, "blo" displayed, with flashing red light to indicate ready for breath sample. Instrument displays "flo" as well as audio tone to indicate adequate breath flow. Result is displayed on LED panel when reaction is complete. Instrument memory retains last test result for display until a new test is conducted.

4. Alcotest 7410

The Alcotest (also Breathalyzer) 7410 (Figure 8.13) is a handheld, portable, battery-operated fuel cell instrument. In addition to using rechargeable batteries, it may be operated with an AC adapter.

Manufacturer. Draeger Safety Inc.—Breathalyzer Division, Durango, CO.

Analytical characteristics. Rapid recovery fuel cell.

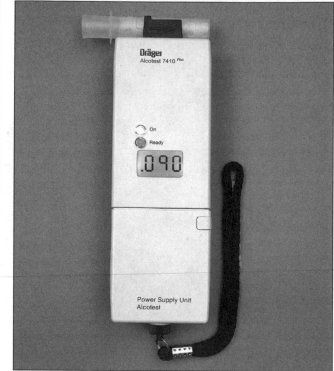

Figure 8.13 *Alcotest 7410 fuel cell breath alcohol analyzer (Draeger Safety—Breathalyzer Division)*

Display, printer. Lighted LCD panel, optional external dot matrix printer using paper roll and opto-electric data transmission from analyzer unit. Three records are printed for each test.

Automation. Manual operation of each test in test sequence. Test mode is indicated on the LCD. Microprocessor controls instrument functions and diagnostics. The instrument is offered in a configuration programmed to meet DOT workplace testing requirements. Software customization of display and printer output is available if the instrument is to be used for other than workplace testing.

Breath sampling. Disposable mouthpieces attach directly to instrument, no breath tube. Time and pressure are used to determine adequate breath sample. An audible tone and ready light indicate acceptable sample. Sample size is one milliliter. An internal pump is used to draw in room air for blank analysis.

Calibration or control tests. External wet bath simulator for control tests and single concentration calibration protocol. Dry gas standard may be used for control tests. Simulator or dry gas must be manually introduced.

Data acquisition. Test data stored in memory can be downloaded to computer directly via interface cable.

Operation. Depressing the single button in various manners determines the test mode (and type of sample to be obtained). The LCD panel, ready light and audible signals prompt the operator throughout the testing procedure and also indicate any instrument or operational problems or errors.

C. Dual detector: Infrared/fuel cell

Alcotest 7110 MKIII-C. The Alcotest 7110 MKIII-C (Figures 8.14 and 8.15) employs both an infrared and fuel cell detector. The instrument can be programmed to utilize any combination of detector results. As one example, the IR detector could be used as the primary means to detect alcohol, with the fuel cell detector used to independently verify the IR result. Any significant discrepancy between the two results would invalidate the test. The instrument is also capable of measuring breath temperature and adjusting the BrAC result to what it would be at 34°C. The instrument is contained in a metal carrying case that is suitable for both permanent and mo-

bile installation. The instrument can operate without modification at 12 volts DC or 80–260 volts AC.

Manufacturer. Draeger Safety Inc.—Breathalyzer Division, Durango, CO.

Analytical characteristics. Dual detector: 9.5 micron infrared and rapid recovery fuel cell (Figure 8.16)

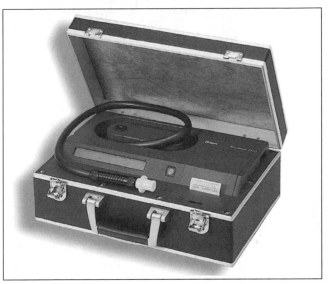

Figure 8.14 *Alcotest 7110 MKIII-C dual detector breath alcohol analyzer (Draeger Safety—Breathalyzer Division)*

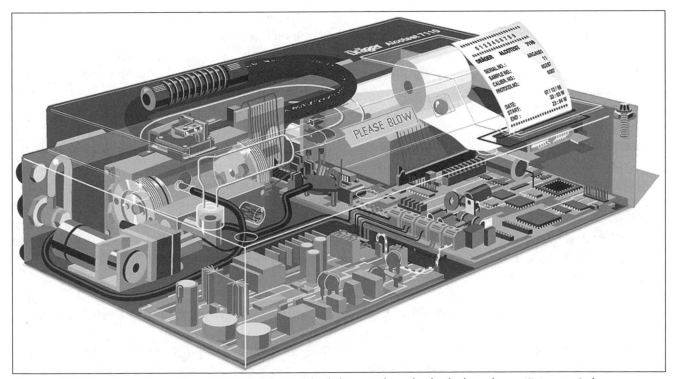

Figure 8.15 *Cut-away view, Alcotest 7110 MKIII-C dual detector breath alcohol analyzer (Draeger Safety—Breathalyzer Division)*

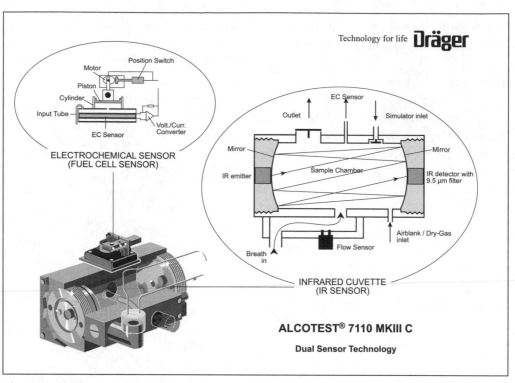

Figure 8.16 *Diagram of Alcotest 7110 MKIII-C sample chamber, infrared and fuel cell detectors (Draeger Safety—Breathalyzer Division)*

Display, printer. Forty-character backlit LCD panel, optional external printer. Internal dot-matrix, ink-ribbon printer using paper roll. Capable of using external printer.

Automation. Complete automation of preprogrammed test sequences, microprocessor control of instrument functions. Programming through keyboard commands.

Breath sampling. External, heated breath tube with disposable mouthpieces. Flow rate monitored by pressure transducer and thermistor. Flow rate, time, volume, and IR slope detection are all used to determine adequate breath sample. Breath temperature is measured at the end of the mouthpiece via dual thermistors attached to the breath tube.

Calibration or control tests. External wet bath simulator or dry gas standards can be used for both calibration and control tests. One point calibration procedure allows both detectors to be calibrated with a single sample. Internal pressure transducer used to correct dry gas result to ambient pressure.

Data acquisition. Subject and operator data input via keyboard, magnetic card reader and barcode reader. Test data and subject-operator data stored in internal memory, up to approximately 1,200 tests. Data can be downloaded to external computer via cable, internal modem or Ethernet connection.

Operation. Test sequence is initiated through button on instrument or via keyboard command. The LCD panel and audible signals are used to prompt the operator throughout the testing procedure and also indicate any instrument problems or errors. Test sequences are customized for the user. Any combination of from the two detectors can be used to obtain a reported value. Air blank analysis is performed before and after each subject or control test. Air blank analysis is conducted strictly using the fuel cell detector, which samples the air in the IR chamber. The measured breath temperature reading may be used to automatically apply a correction factor to the BrAC result for temperatures that deviate from 34°C.

D. Solid-state semiconductor (Taguchi) gas sensor

Breath alcohol testing instruments incorporating solid state semiconductor sensing detectors typically employ Taguchi gas sensors (Dubowski, 1992). Because Taguchi cells are small, inexpensive and have low power requirements they lend themselves well to handheld screening devices. They are also commonly used in breath alcohol ignition interlock devices.

The active element in a Taguchi gas sensor is an N-type semiconductor that consists of a heated, porous, stannic oxide bead mounted in a ceramic cylinder. Gases adsorbed onto the bead will cause the electrical conductivity to rise in proportion to the concentration of the adsorbed gas. Taguchi cells respond to virtually all combustible gases, including ethyl alcohol. A certain degree of specificity can be obtained by modifying the stannous oxide with catalytic elements and optimizing the working temperature of the sensor for the gas to be measured (Watson and Yates, 1985). Taguchi detectors are highly sensitive but are not inherently stable, so breath alcohol testing instruments employing this technology must be frequently recalibrated. Although primarily used as screening devices, some breath testing instruments based on the Taguchi gas sensor have been approved for evidential use by NHTSA.

A.L.E.R.T. Model J4. A small, lightweight, battery-operated, handheld device primarily used for screening tests.

Manufacturer. Alcohol Countermeasure Systems, Inc., Mississauga, Ontario.

Analytical characteristics. Taguchi Gas Sensor detector, heated to approximately 350°C. Operates on three AA rechargeable batteries, AC adapter for recharging is supplied.

Printer, display. Four character LED panel. No printer.

Automation. Microprocessor-controlled. Audible tones and visual display guides operator through sequence and provides indication of instrument status and any errors.

Breath sampling. Uses disposable mouthpiece attached directly to instrument. Minimum acceptable breath sample is obtained by monitoring pressure and time. During exhalation a small portion of the breath is directed to the detector by use of a split flow system.

Calibration or control tests. Wet bath simulator standard is recommended for control tests and the single alcohol concentration calibration protocol.

Operation. Pressing the rocker switch initiates a diagnostic check and conditioning step during which any contaminant gases are purged from the detector. An intermittent audible signal and visual display of "blo" indicates when a subject or control sample should be provided. The three decimal place alcohol result will be displayed for thirty seconds after a successfully delivered sample has been analyzed. Failure to provide an adequate sample will cause a display of "On A" indicating that the test was aborted and the detector is being purged in preparation for another attempt. After three aborted attempts to provide an adequate sample the instruments indicates an error code and powers down.

E. Chemical oxidation and photometry

Chemical oxidation coupled with photometry is the analytical technique that brought breath alcohol testing into widespread law enforcement use. With this method, a breath sample is introduced into a vial or ampoule containing an oxidizing mixture of chemicals. Reaction of the oxidizing compounds with alcohol causes a decrease in the amount of ultraviolet light absorbed by the mixture, which is measured by the photometer.

Breathalyzer Model 900A. The prototype Breathalyzer was invented by Dr. Robert Borkenstein in 1954 and quickly became the predominant instrument used in traffic law enforcement. Breathalyzers using this technology continue to be used with only minor modifications from the original design. The Breathalyzer 900A (Figure 8.17) shares the same oxidation-reduction analytical principle as the Breathalyzer Models 900 and 1000.

Manufacturer. Draeger Safety Inc.—Breathalyzer Division, Durango, CO. Will continue to offer parts and supplies as long as they are available. The instrument is no longer manufactured.

Analytical characteristics (Figure 8.18). The Breathalyzer 900A is a filter photometer that measures the change in transmittance of a potassium dichromate solution through which a fixed volume of breath has been passed. The light source for the photometer is a twelve-volt bulb, which is mounted

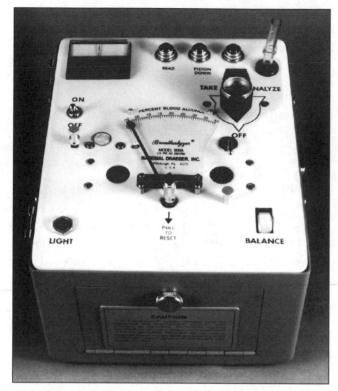

Figure 8.17 *Breathalyzer Model 900A breath alcohol analyzer (Draeger Safety—Breathalyzer Division)*

on a carriage. On either side of the light carriage are sample wells, which hold reagent ampoules. One ampoule is unopened and serves as a reference; the other is the sample ampoule. Light from the source passes through the ampoules, then through 440-millimicron filters and onto photocells. Each ampoule contains three milliliters of 0.025 percent potassium dichromate in 50-percent sulfuric acid with silver nitrate added as a catalyst. In the sample ampoule alcohol is oxidized and potassium dichromate reduced, causing less ultraviolet light to be absorbed (therefore more light is transmitted). The logarithmic change in transmittance is mechanically converted to a linear alcohol result scale.

The analytical system does not depend on constant conditions. Line voltage and light intensity affect each ampoule and photocell the same, so changes in either make no difference. Similarly, the initial potassium dichromate concentration is not important since only the amount used to conduct a test is measured. It is only necessary for the solution to have sufficient initial concentration to conduct all necessary testing. Reagent volume is important, since greater or lesser volume will affect the degree

of color change proportionally (Borkenstein et al., 1962).

Printer, display: Individual test cards for each air blank, subject and control test results are printed by the operator striking a plastic shield covering a pointer, causing an inked marker to strike the test card. One test card is required for each result in a test sequence. Analog display consists of a result scale and movable pointer.

Automation. The instrument is operated manually.

Breath sampling. Retractable breath sampling hose and disposable mouthpieces. Heated sample chamber has 56.5-mL volume. The pressure caused by the breath forces a free-floating piston to the top of the chamber where vent holes allow excess breath to escape. When the subject stops blowing, the piston drops and covers the vent holes, capturing the sample. The captured sample is equivalent to 52.5 mL of expired air at 34°C. The operator must determine that a deep lung breath sample has been delivered.

Calibration or control tests. Wet bath simulator vapor introduced by operator for control tests and calibration. Single concentration calibration protocol.

Operation. To conduct a test, the instrument operator must manipulate the pointer needle and control valve in a prescribed manner. An operator checklist is typically used to document that all steps in the testing procedure are completed. The reagent and reference ampoules must first be checked for proper reagent volume by using a special gauge. Before each analysis, the analytical system is balanced by depressing the Light button to activate the photometer analytical system and moving the light carriage until an equal signal is generated by each photocell, as indicated by a nullmeter. The pointer is then disengaged from the carriage and manually set to zero. After ethanol is introduced into the sample ampoule and allowed to react, the photometer system is brought back into electrical balance. Testing protocols require the analysis of a room air blank as well as flushing the sample chamber with room air between breath samples.

Operation of the 900A consists of three phases:

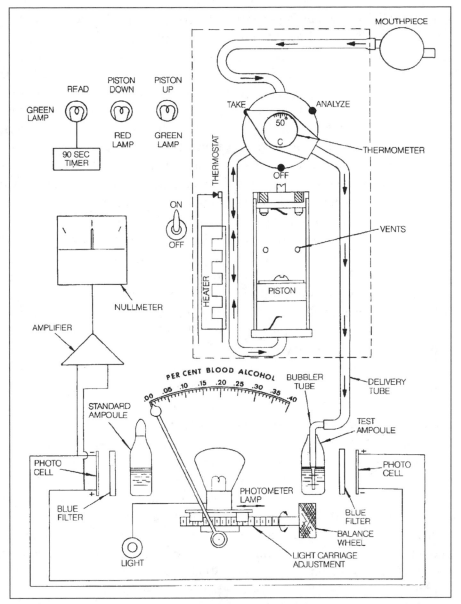

Figure 8.18 *Functional diagram, Breathalyzer Model 900A (Draeger Safety—Breathalyzer Division)*

- collection of a breath sample,
- reaction of alcohol in the reagent ampoule, and
- measurement of the change in potassium dichromate concentration.

Breath sampling. The operator must turn the control valve to the Take position. The Piston Down light indicates that the sample chamber is empty. The subject is required to blow through a disposable mouthpiece into a plastic breath tube. The Piston Up light indicates that the subject is blowing with sufficient pressure.

Chemical reaction of alcohol. Once a sample has been collected, the operator turns the control valve to the Analyze position. This allows the piston to drop, forcing the sample from the cylinder. The breath is routed through a delivery tube and glass bubbler tube into the sample ampoule. Ninety seconds are allowed for this phase of the analysis. A time delay circuit prevents activation of the photometric system during this period.

Measurement. At the end of ninety seconds the timer circuit causes the Read light to illuminate. The operator presses the Light button and rebalances the nullmeter by rotating the balance wheel. When this has been accomplished, the plastic screen is pressed against the inked pointer and a record of the reading is made.

Challenges to Breathalyzer results. Because of the degree of manipulation required to conduct an analysis on the Breathalyzer, operator error and integrity are issues that are often raised in legal proceedings. Results can be "fudged" by the operator simply by moving the pointer more or less than is necessary to bring the electrical system into balance. Some challenges involve the test ampoule and its chemical composition. Variations in the volume and concentration of its components have been shown to influence, at least to some degree, the final analytical results (Coldwell et al., 1963). Proper examination of the ampoule and good quality assurance procedures in the manufacturing of the ampoules and their contents, as well as strict adherence to the prescribed, appropriate breath test protocol will successfully avoid these issues. Challenges to specificity are limited, as the ninety-second optimum reaction time for ethyl alcohol excludes contributions from most other compounds capable of appearing in breath. Those potential interferants that react within the same time period are readily detected by their characteristic odor. (Dubowski, 1964; Coldwell et al., 1963).

It has been occasionally contended that the subject test ampoule may be preserved in such a way that the chemical composition could be determined and the original test result reconstructed. These contentions were studied and found to be lacking in scientific merit by the National Safety Council, Committee on Alcohol and Other Drugs (National Safety Council, 1992).

In a field study of police-operated Breathalyzer 900/900A instruments no evidence was found of operator tampering, RFI or interferants causing falsely elevated results (Harding et al., 1987).

F. Gas chromatography

Gas chromatography is widely used in analytical laboratories to separate and quantitate compounds of interest in mixtures. The technology involves vaporizing a small sample of the mixture and using an inert gas (called the carrier gas) to pass the sample through a length of heated tubing, called the column.

The column is packed with liquid-coated granules or consists of liquid-coated capillary tubing. The coating for this stationary phase is chosen for its ability to reproducibly and predictably interact with the compounds of interest. As the vaporized sample progresses through the column the various components of the mixture are separated from each other in time, depending on their relative affinity for the stationary phase. A detector at the end of the column produces an electrical signal as a function of time, which can be converted, to a quantitative result. Near complete specificity for a given analyte can be achieved by optimizing the analytical conditions. These conditions include temperature, carrier gas flow rate, column packing material, column length and type of detector.

No gas chromatographs designed for breath alcohol analysis are currently manufactured.

Alco-Analyzer 2100 (Figure 8.19).

Manufacturer. Formerly manufactured by U.S. Alcohol Testing of America, Inc., Rancho Cucamonga, CA.

Analytical characteristics. Gas chromatograph. Helium carrier gas, 0.125-inch O.D. × 54 inches (3.2-mm × 1.4-m) stainless steel column, Poropak S packing material, thermal conductivity detector. Analysis time is 2–2.5 minutes.

The instrument is equipped with an RFI detector.

Display, printer. Video color monitor, external 80-character dot-matrix printer using tractor-fed paper.

Automation. An IBM-compatible microprocessor controls all instrument functions. Instrument setup, test sequence protocols and calibration are all initiated through password-protected keyboard commands. Menu driven software can be custom-programmed.

Breath sampling. A short, disposable length of 0.375-inch (9.5-mm) O.D. plastic tubing is affixed to a breath sample port. Minimum time (six seconds) and pressure determine minimum acceptable sample. Breath pressure triggers an internal pump, which draws breath into the sample loop. Sample size is ten milliliters. Figures 8.20a and 8.20b illustrate the instrument's sampling and operational characteristics.

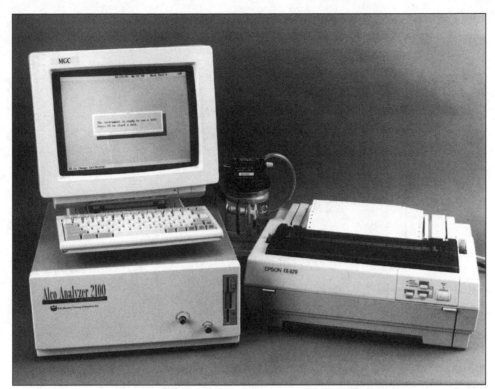

Figure 8.19 *Alco-Analyzer 2100 gas chromatograph breath alcohol analyzer (U.S. Alcohol Testing of America, Inc.)*

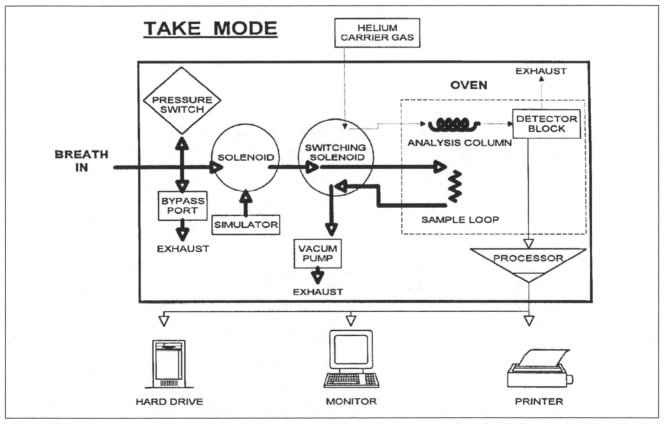

Figure 8.20A *Functional diagram of the Alco-Analyzer 2100 gas chromatograph in the "Take" mode (U.S. Alcohol Testing of America, Inc.)*

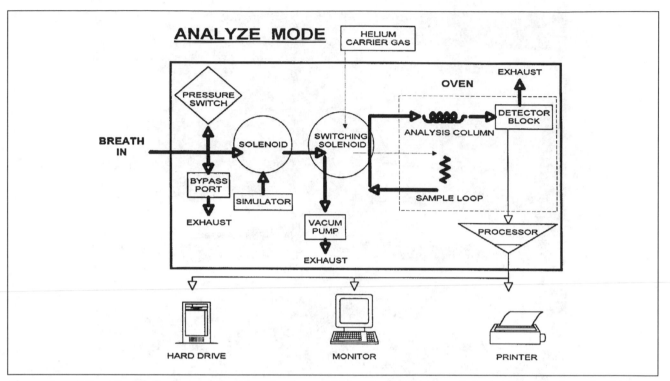

Figure 8.20B *Functional diagram of the Alco-Analyzer 2100 gas chromatograph in the "Analyze" mode (U.S. Alcohol Testing of America, Inc.)*

Calibration or control tests. External wet bath simulator with vapor recirculation is used for control tests and automated single concentration calibration protocol. Dry gas standards may also be used for control tests.

Data acquisition. Test data and associated information is stored in integral computer. Optional software allows use of the internal modem so data can be uploaded to a host computer or transferred via a network service.

Operation. Tests are initiated via keyboard commands with operator access controlled through the use of passwords. The video monitor displays prompts to guide the operator through the programmed test sequence. The monitor graphically displays the detector output over the analysis time and the alcohol concentration.

References

American Medical Association. *Alcohol and the Impaired Driver. A Manual on the Medicolegal Aspects of Chemical Tests for Intoxication with Supplement on Breath Alcohol Tests*, 1970, 1972.

Reprinted by National Safety Council, Chicago, 1976 [see especially pp. 94–100].

Bogen, E.M.H. Drunkeness; A quantitative study of acute alcoholic intoxication. *JAMA* 89:1508–1511, 1927.

Borkenstein, R.F. and Smith, H.W. The Breathalyzer and its applications. *Med. Sci. Law* 2:13–22, 1962.

Canadian Society of Forensic Science. Recommended standards and procedures of the Canadian Society of Forensic Science alcohol test committee. *Can. Soc. Forensic Sci. J.* 28:1–25, 1995.

Coldwell, B.B. and Grant, G.L. A study of some factors affecting the accuracy of the Breathalyzer. *J. Forensic Sci.* 8:149–162, 1963.

Conde, E. Special testing for possible carry over effects using the Intoximeters, Inc. Alco-Sensor IV at 10 degrees celsius. DOT HS 809-424, March. 2002.

Denny, R.C. and Williams, L.C. Mouth alcohol: Some theoretical and practical considerations. In:

Noordiz, P.C. and Roszbach, R. (eds.), *Alcohol, Drugs and Traffic Safety—T86*. Proceedings of the Tenth International Conference on Alcohol, Drugs and Traffic Safety. Amsterdam: Elsevier Science Publishers B.V., 1987, 355–358.

Dubowski, K.M. Specificity of breath-alcohol analyses. *JAMA* 189:1039, 1964.

Dubowski, K.M. Biological aspects of breath-alcohol analysis. *Clin. Chem.* 20:294–299, 1974.

Dubowski, K.M. Breath-alcohol simulators: Scientific basis and actual performance. *J. Anal. Toxicol.* 3:177–182, 1979.

Dubowski, K.M. Recent developments in alcohol analysis. *Alcohol, Drugs, and Driving. Abstracts and Reviews* 2:13–46, 1986.

Dubowski, K.M. *The Technology of Breath-Alcohol Analysis*. Public Health Service, U.S. Department of Health and Human Services, DHSS Publication No. (ADM)92-1728, 1992.

Dubowski, K.M. Quality assurance in breath-alcohol analysis. *J. Anal. Toxicol.* 18:306–311, 1994.

Dubowski, K.M. and Essary, N.A. Response of breath-alcohol analyzers to acetone. *J. Anal. Toxicol.* 7:231–234, 1983.

Dubowski, K.M. and Essary, N.A. Response of breath-alcohol analyzers to acetone: Further studies. *J. Anal. Toxicol.* 8:205–208, 1984.

Dubowski, K.M. and Essary, N.A. Breath-alcohol analysis on duplicate samples. In: Noordiz, P.C. and Roszbach, R. (eds.), *Alcohol, Drugs and Traffic Safety—T86*. Proceedings of the Tenth International Conference on Alcohol, Drugs and Traffic Safety. Amsterdam: Elsevier Science Publishers B.V., 1987, 373–377.

Dubowski, K.M. and Essary, N.A. Evaluation of commercial breath-alcohol simulators: Further studies. *J. Anal. Toxicol.* 15:272–275, 1991.

Dubowski, K.M. and Essary, N.A. Field performance of current generation breath-alcohol simulators. *J. Anal. Toxicol.* 16:325–327, 1992.

Dubowski, K.M. and Essary, N.A. Vapor-alcohol control tests with compressed ethanol-gas mixtures: scientific basis and actual performance. *J. Anal. Toxicol.* 20:484–491, 1996.

Falkensson, M., Jones, W. and Sorbo, B. Bedside diagnosis of alcohol intoxication with a pocket-size breath-alcohol device: Sampling from unconscious subjects and specificity for ethanol. *Clin. Chem.* 35:918–921, 1989.

Flores, A.L. and Frank, J.F. The likelihood of acetone interference in breath alcohol measurement. U.S. Department of Transportation Technical Report HS 806–922, 1985.

Gomez, H. et al. Elevation of breath ethanol measurements by metered-dose inhalers. *Ann. Emerg. Med.* 25:608–611, 1995.

Gullberg, R.G. Letter to the editor, identifying components of variability in breath alcohol analysis. *J. Anal. Toxicol.* 16:208–209, 1992.

Gullberg, R.G. Breath alcohol analysis in one subject with gastroesophageal reflux disease. *J. Forensic Sci.* 46:1498–1503, 2001.

Harding, P.M. and Field, P.H. Breathalyzer accuracy in actual law enforcement practice: A comparison of blood- and breath-alcohol results in Wisconsin drivers. *J. Forensic Sci.* 32:1235–1240, 1987.

Harding, P.M. et al. The effect of dentures and denture adhesives on mouth alcohol retention. *J. Forensic Sci.* 37:999–1007, 1992.

International Association for Chemical Testing Legislative Committee. Reporting of blood and breath test results. Adopted March 26, 1993.

Jones, A.W. Breath acetone concentrations in healthy men: Response of infrared breath-alcohol analyzers. *J. Anal. Toxicol.* 10:98–101, 1986.

Jones, A.W. Breath acetone concentrations in fasting male volunteers: Further studies and effect of alcohol administration. *J. Anal. Toxicol.* 12:75–79, 1988.

Kechagias, S. et al. Reliability of breath-alcohol analysis in individuals with gastroesophageal reflux disease. *J. Forensic Sci.* 44:814–818, 1999.

Logan, B., Distefano, S. and Case, G. Evaluation of the effect of asthma inhalers and nasal decongestant sprays on a breath alcohol test. *J. Forensic Sci.* 43:197–199, 1998

Logan, B. and Distefano, S. Ethanol content of various foods and soft drinks and their potential for interference with a breath-alcohol test. *J. Anal. Toxicol.* 22:181–183, 1998.

Logan, B. and Gullberg, R. Lack of effect of tongue piercing on an evidential breath alcohol test. *J. Forensic Sci.* 43:239–240, 1998b.

Mason, M.F. and Dubowski, K.M. Breath-alcohol analysis: Uses, methods and some forensic problems: Review and opinion. *J. Forensic Sci.* 21:9–41, 1976.

Modell, J.G., Taylor, J.P. and Lee, J.Y. Breath alcohol values following mouthwash use. *JAMA* 270:2955–2956, 1993.

National Safety Council Committee on Alcohol and Other Drugs. Recommendations. *Committee Handbook. Committee on Alcohol and Other Drugs.* Chicago: National Safety Council, 1992.

National Safety Council Committee on Alcohol and Other Drugs. Report on the Specificity of Breath Alcohol Analyzers. *Minutes of the Committee on Alcohol and Other Drugs.* Chicago: National Safety Council, February 1999.

Oliver, R.D. and Garriott, J.C. The effects of acetone and toluene on Breathalyzer results. *J. Anal. Toxicol.* 3:99–101, 1979.

U.S. Department of Transportation, National Highway Traffic Safety Administration. Highway safety programs: Model specifications for evidential breath testing devices. *Federal Register* 49:48,855–48,865, 1984a.

U.S. Department of Transportation, National Highway Traffic Safety Administration. Highway safety programs: Model specifications for calibrating units for breath alcohol testers. *Federal Register* 49:48865–4,872, 1984b.

U.S. Department of Transportation, National Highway Traffic Safety Administration. Model specifications for breath alcohol ignition interlocks (BAIIDs). *Federal Register* 57:11772–11787, 1992.

U.S. Department of Transportation, National Highway Traffic Safety Administration. Highway safety programs: Model specifications for devices to measure breath alcohol. *Federal Register* 58:48,705–48710, 1993.

U.S. Department of Transportation, National Highway Traffic Safety Administration. Highway safety programs: Model specifications for screening devices to measure alcohol in bodily fluids. *Federal Register* 59:39382–39390, 1994.

U.S. Department of Transportation, National Highway Traffic Safety Administration. Highway safety programs: Model specifications for calibrating units for breath alcohol testers; conforming products list of calibrating units. *Federal Register* 62:43416–43425, 1997.

U.S. Department of Transportation, National Highway Traffic Safety Administration. Highway safety programs: Conforming products list of screening devices to measure alcohol in bodily fluids. *Federal Register* 66:22639–22640, 2001.

U.S. Department of Transportation, National Highway Traffic Safety Administration. Highway safety programs: Model specifications for devices to measure breath alcohol. *Federal Register* 67:62091–62094, 2002.

Watson, J. and Yates, R.A. A solid-state gas sensor. *Elec. Eng.* 57:47–57, 1985.

Westenbrink, W. and Sauve, L.T. The effect of asthma inhalers on the A.L.E.R.T. J3A, Breathalyzer 900A and Mark IV G.C. Intoximeter. *Can. Soc. Forensic Sci. J.* 24: 23–25, 1991.

Wigmore, J. and Leslie, G. The effect of swallowing or rinsing alcohol solution on the mouth alcohol effect and slope detection of the Intoxilyzer 5000. *J. Anal. Toxicol.* 35:112–114, 2001.

Wigmore, J. and Wilkie, M. A simulation of the effect of blood in the mouth on breath alcohol concentrations of drinking subjects. *Can. Soc. Forensic Sci. J.* 35:9–16, 2002.

Williams, R. The effect of ethanol in Ice Drops on breath alcohol concentration. *J. Anal. Toxicol.* 20: 271, 1996.

Endnote

1. The unmodified term "alcohol" in this chapter refers to ethyl alcohol unless otherwise specified.

Chapter 9

Methods for Fluid Analysis

Richard F. Shaw, B.S.

Methods for the measurement of alcohol in fluids of biological nature such as blood, cerebral spinal fluid, urine, bile, vitreous humor, and infrequently saliva appeared in the scientific literature as early as 1860 (Jain and Cravey, 1972a; Smith, 1965). Bechamp (1865) is credited with the first method using potassium dichromate and sulfuric acid for the quantitative determination of ethyl alcohol. Since then, numerous analytical approaches have been suggested leading to literally hundreds of published or modifications of published methodologies. Generally, the methods have been classified as (1) chemical, (2) biochemical and (3) instrumental. Comprehensive reviews on the subject have been reported by Jain and Cravey (1972a,b); Cravey and Jain (1974); the American Medical Association Committee on Medicolegal Problems (1973); Dubowski (1977); Caplan (1982); and Tagliaro et al. (1992). A number of these methods require separation and isolation of alcohol from the biological matrix by procedures involving diffusion, aeration, distillation, or headspace production, while others require protein precipitation, or direct mixing of biological fluids with a dilutent just prior to measurement of alcohol.

9.1 Chemical Methods

Alcohol, due to its volatility, is conveniently separated from biological samples by various techniques and, after separation, can be quantitatively measured by means of reaction with oxidizing agents such as dichromate, permanganate, or osmic acid. In the reaction with potassium dichromate and alcohol in strong sulfuric acid solution, the yellow-orange dichromate ion is reduced to the blue-green chromic ion while alcohol is oxidized to acetaldehyde, acetic acid, or carbon dioxide and water, depending on the condition of the reaction.

One of the earliest methods involving diffusion was that of Widmark (1922) utilizing a specially constructed spoon for suspending the biological sample over a known quantity of potassium dichromate solution in a stoppered flask. The flask was heated allowing for the simultaneous distillation and oxidation reactions to be completed. The cooled dichromate was then titrated with standard sodium thiosulfate using potassium iodide and starch as an indicator. Since 1922, a number of very suitable dichromate methods for determining ethyl alcohol in body fluids have been described (Harger, 1935; Cavett, 1938; Kozelka and Hine, 1941; Shupe and Dubowski, 1952; Sunshine and Nenad, 1953; Bradford, 1958; Kirk et al., 1958), involving distillation or desiccation coupled with conventional distillation apparatus, modified Erlenmeyer reaction flasks, or Conway diffusion cells.

One of the most reliable diffusion methods is that reported by Smith (1951). He used a 50-mL glass-stoppered Erlenmeyer flask with an attached glass cup, similar to that of the Widmark flask. The glass stem is fused to the center of the cup and a strip

213

of filter paper is rolled around the stem and fitted into the cup. A known amount of blood or urine is added to the cup which is suspended over the dichromate solution of known concentration. The flask and its contents are heated in an oven for an hour or allowed to remain overnight at room temperature. The liquid specimen diffuses onto the filter paper and a highly exposed surface area provides for rapid evaporation. Any vaporized alcohol combines with the dichromate solution. Any residual dichromate is then determined either colorimetrically or by titration. Blystone and Collins (1984) described a procedure to measure the dichromate concentration directly at 444 nm with a microcomputer-controlled spectrophotometer. The spectrophotometer interfaced with an HP-85 desktop computer provided additional capability to average and store data.

9.2 Biochemical Methods

Alcohol dehydrogenase (ADH), an enzyme, is used in the measurement of alcohol in biological specimens. In the reaction, alcohol is oxidized to acetaldehyde by ADH in the presence of a coenzyme, nicotinamide adenine dinucleotide (NAD), which is further reduced to NADH. This reduced form can be measured spectrophotometrically at 340 nm. In a secondary reaction the NADH can be coupled to a diaphorase-chromogen system producing a red-colored formazan colloidal suspension that may be read spectrophotometrically at 500 nm. This procedure can be automated with microprocessor control and printout providing rapid turnaround time. The enzyme does not react with methyl alcohol or acetone and only reacts to a lesser degree with isopropyl alcohol and butyl alcohol. Bonnichsen and Theorell (1951) described the first use of ADH for the analysis of ethyl alcohol.

Redetzki and Dees (1976) compared results obtained with four commercially available kits for enzymatic determination of ethyl alcohol in blood. Each of the kits yielded reliable results with acceptable reproducibility. Blood samples containing ethyl alcohol (0.045 g/dL) plus varying concentrations of methyl alcohol (0.05 and 0.15 g/dL) and isopropyl alcohol (0.05 and 0.15 g/dL) were analyzed to evaluate the specificity of the assays. As suspected, high concentrations of methyl alcohol increased apparent ethyl alcohol levels only insignificantly, and isopropyl alcohol in low concentrations interfered in all kits.

Vasiliades et al. (1978) reported a case of ethyl alcohol and isopropyl alcohol ingestion that resulted in coma. Erroneous analytical results were obtained using the enzyme method because of the nonselectivity of ADH. In this case, ethyl alcohol was overestimated and the significance of isopropyl alcohol was underestimated. Jung and Ferard (1978) described an automated enzymatic method for ethyl alcohol determination with a centrifugal analyzer by measuring the rate of the reaction catalyzed by ADH and coupled to aldehyde dehydrogenase. This new method has several advantages over an automated ADH method utilizing semicarbazides. Results show an improved linearity and sensitivity, in addition to the method being more rapid due to a shorter equilibrium time.

A rapid electrochemical measurement of ethyl alcohol in blood was proposed by Cheng and Christian (1978). In their method, ethyl alcohol is oxidized by NA+ in the presence of alcohol dehydrogenase, and the NADH produced is aerobically oxidized by horseradish peroxidase. The rate of depletion of buffer-carried oxygen, which is directly proportional to the alcohol in the sample, is amperometrically monitored with a membrane oxygen-sensing electrode. Only 5 mL of blood is required, with no deproteinization, incubation, or dilution needed. Results, obtained in less than one minute, correlate well with those obtained by gas chromatographic and spectrophotometric methods.

Poklis and Mackell (1982) evaluated a new ADH enzymatic assay (ADH-glycine, Sigma Chemical Co.) for ethyl alcohol in blood. The assay differs from Sigma's previous assay (ADH-pyrophosphate) in that glycine replaced pyrophosphate as the buffer and hydrazine replaced semicarbazide as the trapping agent. The standard curve for the assay was linear over blood alcohol concentrations of 0.05 to 0.50 g/dL. The major advantage of the ADH-glycine assay over the ADH-pyrophosphate assay is the shorter reaction time, ten minutes versus thirty minutes.

Whitehouse and Paul (1979) reported an enzymatic method that has been adapted to the Abbott Bichromatic Analyzer-l00. Fully automatic, the method can accommodate up to 192 assays per hour. It requires only 2.5 mL of plasma and therefore is applicable to analysis for ethyl alcohol in blood by finger stick.

Takel et al. (1985) described an enzymatic method for detecting ethyl alcohol in blood by use of membrane-bound microbial ADH (no EC number assigned). This enzyme catalyzes the reaction irreversibly and the rate of oxidation can be monitored by spectrophotometry of the reduction of the indicator dye. No pyridine nucleotides such as NA+ or NADP+ were used. The specific activity of membrane-bound ADH is 300-fold greater than cytosol NA-linked ADH (EC 1.1.1.1.) and its optimum pH is 4.0 as compared with pH 8.0 for cytosol ADH. Given these characteristics, the enzyme can be used to detect trace amounts of ethyl alcohol and the enzyme reaction can be performed in an acidic reaction mixture that includes the trichloroacetic acid used to deproteinize specimens of blood, plasma, or serum.

Drost and Maes (1983) evaluated a EMIT-st ethyl alcohol assay previously developed as a qualitative procedure. The day to day precision of the test with respect to the differences in absorbance (*delta A*) was evaluated, in order to establish its applicability for quantitative analyses. Mean values = ± SD (N = 10) for the *delta A* of the positive control and the cutoff calibrator were 146 ± 14 (CV = 9.6%) and 57 ± 5 (CV = 8.8%) respectively. The detection limit of the assay was 0.3 mg/mL ethanol. A series of spiked samples with ethanol concentrations in the range of 0.1 to 4.0 mg/mL were analyzed in triplicate by EMIT-st assay and by gas chromatography. For the EMIT-st assay, the response was only linear between 0.3 and 2.0 mg/mL ethanol. Concentrations higher than 2.0 mg/mL showed no pronounced difference in absorbance measurements. Serum samples (N = 54) of people involved in automobile driver alcohol blood checks were analyzed by EMIT-st and the results were compared to the corresponding gas chromatographic data. In the range of up to 2.0 mg/mL ethanol, a linear regression curve was calculated with a slope of 76.7, a *y*-intercept of 36.4, and a correlation coefficient of 0.79.

Degel and Paulus (1988) described a simple and rapid, but nevertheless precise and accurate method for measuring ethanol in serum, using the Roche Cobas Bio centrifugal analyzer and the EMIT-st serum ethanol assay reagent. Within-assay imprecision was 2.2% (CV), day-to-day imprecision was 2.5% (CV). The results correlated well with a commonly used gas chromatograph headspace method. Because of the rapidity and good practicability of this method, the authors concluded that the method is well suited for use in emergency care units of clinical chemistry laboratories.

Jortani and Poklis (1992) evaluated the enzymatic EMIT ETS PLUS ethyl alcohol assay which had been designed for use with the new Syva ETS PLUS analyzer and intended for the quantitative analysis of ethanol in human urine, serum, and plasma. The assay had a linear range up to 6.5 g/L and a low detection limit of 0.1 g/L. Results of the analysis of patient serum and urine specimens for ethanol by the EMIT assay correlated well with other methods. It was also found to be free of interference from small molecular weight alcohols, aldehydes, ketones, and glycols. The EMIT assay's linear range of up to 6.50 g/L ethanol was a major advantage over the ADx and aca assays; these assays were only linear to 3.00 g/L.

Sutheimer, Lavins, and King (1992) made a critical evaluation of the ETS-Plus Ethyl Alcohol Assay and concluded that it is simple to perform, sensitive enough to reliably detect ethanol above a concentration of 0.01 g/dL, and dynamic enough to reliably quantitate ethanol concentrations between 0.010 and 0.400 g/dL, correlating well with headspace gas chromatography. The technique is suitable for the analysis of relatively fresh (less than one month old) serum, plasma, urine, bile, vitreous humor, and gastric samples. With the aid of dilution, it is adaptable to the analysis of whole blood, relatively old specimens (more than three months old), viscous and highly pigmented plasma, bile, and the occasional extremely viscous vitreous humor specimens. In addition, samples can remain in the system's covered sample wheel compartment without significant (less than 10 percent) loss of ethanol concentration for up to two hours.

In addition, Jortani and Poklis (1993) evaluated the new upgraded ETS Plus urine and serum ethanol analyzer for analyzing ethanol in urine, serum, and plasma. The within-run precision of the ETS PLUS ethyl alcohol assay yielded a CV of 2.6% at a target value of 1.00 g/L (1.06 ± 0.03 g/L, N = 32) and a CV of 3.2% at a target value of 0.40 g/L (0.42 ± 0.01 g/L, N = 30). The linear regression analysis of thirty patient serum ethanol results by the ETS Plus and by gas chromatography yielded $y = 0.939 x + 0.03$ g/L. It was concluded that the software modifications in the new ETS Plus allowed the accurate quantitation of ethanol in serum.

Urry et al. (1993) evaluated the performance of the Techni-con Chem 1+ chemistry analyzer with the Syva EMIT ethyl alcohol assay in plasma and urine. The Chem 1+ was compared to a gas chromatograph method and it was determined that the Chem 1+ Analyzer demonstrated reliable performance of the EMIT ethyl alcohol assay of plasma and urine specimens.

In 1984, Abbott Laboratories introduced a radiative energy attenuation (REA) assay for the determination of ethyl alcohol on the TDx analyzer, a microprocessor-controlled automated fluorometer used for fluorescence polarization immunoassay for many therapeutically monitored drugs. In the REA method for ethyl alcohol, the enzyme-catalytic reactions of ADH and diaphorase result in the formation of reduced iodonitrotetrazolium (INT), a red color chromogen which has an absorbance peak of 492 nm. Because the chromogen's absorbance overlaps the excitation and emission spectrum of fluorescein (a fluorescent indicator added to the reaction) the fluorescence intensity decreases logarithmically with increasing concentration of reduced INT. The concentration of ethyl alcohol is therefore proportional to the degree of inner filter effect on the fluorophore. In addition, no cross-reaction toward methyl alcohol, isopropyl alcohol, or acetone at concentrations that might be expected in toxic situations occurred (Cary et al., 1984).

Recently, Abbott Laboratories reformulated the ethyl alcohol assay by replacing the iodonitrotetrazolium violet dye (INT) with a thiazolyl blue dye (MTT). The reason for this reformulation was to eliminate a probe wash step required after every run in the original method. In the reaction, the reduced MTT now yields a purple color with an absorbance at 565 nm. The new formulation significantly reduces the bias found by the analysis of postmortem blood with the original REA reagent system. Abbott Laboratories recommends a sensitivity limit for ethyl alcohol in postmortem blood by the REA method of 0.015 g/100 mL. Determination of ethyl alcohol in serum, fresh whole blood, fresh or postmortem urine, and vitreous humor by REA demonstrated no bias whatever (Cary, 1986).

Caplan and Levine (1986) performed a similar study to evaluate the two Abbott TDx REA ethyl alcohol assays, INT and MTT, and compared them to a reference method using headspace gas chromatography. Serum, plasma, urine, and whole blood were analyzed by the three methods. While statistical evaluation by least square regression analysis revealed good correlation, it was found that postmortem whole blood specimens, at high and low ethyl alcohol concentrations, showed a greater variability than did the other specimen types. For the other specimens, the discrepancies occurred only at the lower concentrations of ethyl alcohol. Of the two methods, the authors felt that although both TDx ethyl alcohol assays are acceptable methods, the MTT method performed somewhat better at lower ethyl alcohol concentrations for analyzing serum, urine, and fresh blood. It was recommended that a larger study is needed to determine a proper cutoff for reporting ethyl alcohol concentration in postmortem blood.

In a second study performed by Caplan and Levine (1987), 573 blood specimens from suspected driving while intoxicated individuals (DWI blood) and 532 postmortem blood specimens (PM blood) were analyzed by the REA method and a headspace gas chromatographic method (GC) currently used in their laboratory. Negative specimens (less than 10 mg/dL by GC) and positive specimens (greater than or equal to 10 mg/dL by GC) in each category were analyzed. Linear regression analysis comparing the REA values with the GC values was performed for each type of blood specimen. The equation obtained for DWI blood specimens was REA = 0.943 + 1.54; the equation for PM blood specimens was REA = 0.980 + 2.76. The correlation coefficient for each group was greater than 0.99. The data suggested that a limit of detection of 10 mg/dL could be applied for DWI blood specimens, while 20 mg/dL would be recommended as the limit of detection for PM blood specimens.

Prencipe and Iaccherii (1987) describe a new colorimetric method for measuring ethanol in plasma by use of a peroxidase-coupled assay system and alcohol oxidase (EC 1.1.3.13) from Pichia species. Absorptivity is low enough to give useful results within results without sample dilution. The absorbance of the blue dye that is formed is measured at 600 nm. The method is linear up to 4.0 g/L of ethanol. Within-run and between-run CVs were less than 2.45% and less than 1.92% respectively. Results correlate very well with those by gas chromatography (r = 0.9977). The procedure is also adaptable to automation.

Engelhart and Jenkins (2001) evaluated a disposable QED® saliva alcohol test to determine if the test would be useful for the determination of postmortem ethanol in cases where a rapid result was needed. QED tests were compared with ethanol levels determined by headspace GC analysis. Both salvia and vitreous humor specimens were used for the evaluation. QED tests were initially attempted using the oral fluids from fifty individuals. Of these cases, seventeen of the tests were valid with eight positive results. For twenty-three, the oral fluid was not attainable, and for ten cases, the sample was contaminated with blood making the tests invalid. The correlation between the oral fluid results and the blood headspace GC analysis was poor (r = 0.8345) over the range of 0.01–0.29 g/dL. Vitreous specimens were found to be the matrix of choice for analyzing postmortem cases using QED. Only six of 171 specimens were found to be unsuitable. The QED results correlated well with the headspace GC analysis (r = 0.9931, N = 165). When using ethanol levels > 0.02 g/dL (N = 126), an average vitreous GC/blood ratio of 1.16 correlated well with the average QED/blood ratio of 1.22. It was concluded that although the QED saliva test does not appear to be useful in determining postmortem saliva ethanol levels, it does provide accurate results when using postmortem vitreous humor as the testing matrix.

In the forensic laboratory, biochemical methods are not usually used for determining blood alcohol due to their lack of total specificity. Isopropyl alcohol and butyl alcohol interfere in the reaction. For forensic purposes, enzyme methods must be confirmed by an alternate technique (Garriott, 1983).

9.3 Gas-Chromatographic Methods

The most commonly used method for the forensic analysis of ethyl alcohol is gas chromatography. For the measurement of ethyl alcohol in biological fluids, several gas chromatographic methods, such as solvent extraction, protein precipitation, distillation, direct injection, or headspace techniques have been used (Jain and Cravey, 1972b; Gudzinowicz and Gudzinowicz, 1977; Wright, 1991; Tagliaro et al., 1992). Earlier methods involving the separation of ethyl alcohol from biological specimens usually utilized solvent extraction protein precipitation, and distillation. Recent methods involve direct injection and headspace techniques.

A Extraction techniques

One of the earliest methods was that of Cadman and Johns (1958) in which they reported a procedure using a Beckman GC-2 gas chromatograph equipped with a thermal conductivity detector (TCD) and a column containing 28 g of a mixture consisting of Flexol 8N8, diisodecyl phthalate, and polyethylene glycol 600 in a ratio of 15:10:3 by weight on 100 g of 42/60 mesh firebrick. The extraction technique consisted of pipetting 1 mL blood and 1 mL of n-propyl acetate into a 3-mL screwcapped vial containing 1 g of anhydrous potassium carbonate. The sample vial was mixed and shaken one minute on a mechanical mixer. The sample was centrifuged and a 35-mL aliquot of the n-propyl acetate was injected into the gas chromatograph. For purposes of quantitation, ethyl alcohol standards were prepared by adding measured amounts of ethyl alcohol to blood and the blood subsequently extracted and chromatographed under the same conditions as that of the unknown samples.

Lyon and Bard (1964) subsequently published a report using the same gas chromatograph as Cadman and Johns but utilized a column containing 15 g of the mixed liquid stationary phases (Flexol 8N8, diisodecyl phthalate, and polyethylene glycol in a ratio of 15:10:3) on 100 g of 30/60-mesh chromosorb. Extraction consisted of mixing the blood with calcium sulfate-sodium bisulfite mixture, then adding n-butanol. The tube was shaken and centrifuged. The n-butanol was removed and added to a tube containing anhydrous potassium carbonate, allowed to stand for five minutes, and an aliquot of the n-butanol injected into the gas chromatograph. Davis (1966) modified the method of Cadman and Johns using flame ionization detection and Steinberg et al. (1965) also modified the method using a column of 15-percent Hallcomid M-18 on 60/80 mesh, HMDS-treated Chromosorb W to effect separation of alcohols.

B. Distillation techniques

The method of Fox (1958) involved the separation of ethyl alcohol from biological specimens based on adding measured amounts of blood, urine, or tissue homogenate into a distilling flask containing 25 mL of water, 3 mL of 50-percent sodium tungstate solution, and 5 mL of 1.0 N sulfuric acid. The specimen was distilled and the distillate collected with a known amount of n-butanol added to the receiver flask. An aliquot of the distillate was then injected into a Perkin-Elmer Model 154B gas chromatograph equipped with a thermistor thermal conductivity detector. Two copper columns were employed: one, a 30/60 mesh C-22 firebrick, glycerol, and tricresyl phosphate (50:30:20) and the second firebrick, glycerol and tricresyl phosphate (60:18:11). Temperatures for column one and column two were 106°C and 84°C, respectively. The use of two columns allowed the separation of ethyl alcohol from methyl alcohol or formaldehyde when these mixtures were encountered. McCord and Gladsden (1964) used a similar method of distillation as that of Fox with protein precipitation, addition of a water-immiscible solvent, and subsequent distillation. It differs from the method of Fox in that the distillate was chromatographed without regard to its water content.

C. Direct-injection techniques

There are numerous direct injection techniques for the determination of ethyl alcohol in biological specimens by gas chromatography. These techniques may vary according to the preparation of the sample for testing and may consist of (1) direct injection of the sample, (2) protein precipitation and subsequent injection, or (3) dilution of the sample prior to injection. Probably the easiest and fastest is the injection of a diluted sample with an appropriate internal standard into a gas chromatograph equipped with a flame ionization detector. A number of suitable methods have been described (Maricq and Molle, 1959; Chundela and Janak, 1960; Wesselman, 1960; Machata, 1962; Parker et al., 1962; Bonnichsen and Linturi, 1962; Hessel and Modglin, 1964; Mather and Assimos, 1965; Curry et al., 1966; Finkle, 1971; Jain, 1971; Solon et al., 1972; Blume et al., 1973), all involving direct injection techniques.

Solon et al. (1972) and Baird (1973) described methods involving automated gas chromatographic analysis of ethyl alcohol in blood or urine. Solon used a Hewlett-Packard gas chromatograph, automatic liquid sampler, electronic integrator, and data processor with special software. Samples and calibrators are mixed in vials with n-propyl alcohol added as the internal standard. Vials are placed in position in the automatic liquid sampler, which is controlled by a subroutine in the data processor software which advances the samples to each of its thirty-six positions automatically. Vials in position one and two are filled with heparin, rinse solution. Position three is filled with a calibrator and the remaining positions are filled with unknown samples. The processor advances the sampler to position one and then to position three, where the standard is sampled and injected. The retention time and response factors relative to n-propyl alcohol are stored for later reference. The sampler then moves to position one to rinse the syringe and then to position four, unknown samples. The sample is injected and the data analyzed. The overall relative standard deviation was shown to be +1.00% and linearity was excellent in the range 0.015 to 0.26 g/dL. Baird described a modification of the method of Solon. Data reduction was ascertained by interfacing the Hewlett-Packard gas chromatograph and automatic liquid sampler with an Auto Lab System IV computing integrator. Other modifications included the use of a greater sample-internal standard dilution ratio

(1:8), computing results on a weight-to-volume basis, and different operating conditions.

Manno and Manno (1978) described an ultramicro method utilizing direct sample injection for the simultaneous identification and quantification of ethyl alcohol in blood and urine. Aliquots of whole blood or urine and an internal standard, 1-propyl alcohol, are mixed together in equal parts. One mL of the mixture is then injected into a gas chromatograph equipped with a flame ionization detector. The glass column, 3 mm i.d. by 2 m long, is packed with 0.2-percent Carbowax 1500 on 80/100 Carbopak C. The column is filled with a precolumn glass insert filled with a loosely packed silanized glass wool plug that acts as a trap for the nonvolatile protein material of the blood or urine samples. The optimal operating conditions for the gas chromatograph are: column temperature 120°C; injected temperature 100°C; carrier gas flow 20 mL/minute; hydrogen and air pressure set at optimal conditions for a hydrogen flame. When it is necessary to collect blood specimens in extremely small volumes, blood from a finger puncture can be collected in plain capillary tubes. One-half microliter of serum, plasma, or whole blood can be drawn into a 1.0-mL syringe from the capillary tube followed by 0.5 mL of internal standard. Contents of the syringe are then injected into the gas chromatograph. The peak area of the alcohol peak and the internal standard peak are measured and compared with known amounts of ethyl alcohol and internal standard and the concentration of ethyl alcohol present is calculated.

Livesey et al. (1995) developed a packed-column chromatographic procedure capable of simultaneous quantitation of methanol, ethanol, isopropanol, acetone and ethylene glycol. This method was subsequently updated to a rapid, sensitive, widebore capillary method. The packed-column system uses direct injection of 1 mL Na_2WO_4/H_2SO_4 deproteinized serum onto a 1.8 m × 2 mm (i.d) column packed with 80/100 HayeSep R. A linear temperature gradient from 90° to 205°C allows complete elution of all components within twenty minutes; minimum detection limits are 2 mmol/L. The widebore capillary method uses 0.1 mL of sample deproteinized by ultra filtration, injected onto a 30 m × 0.53 mm (id) 3-um Rtx-200 (Restek) column.

Baseline resolution to a minimum detection limit of 0.1 mmol/L of all compounds is achieved in five minutes with a linear temperature gradient from 40° to 250°C and dual internal standards of n-propanol and 1,2-butanediol. Traditionally most laboratories have used separate chromatographic conditions for analyzing alcohols and diols to avoid the system contamination seen with direct injection of whole blood (Jacobsen et al.,1992) or deproteinized serum (Cheung and Lin, 1987), researchers have used headspace for analysis of volatile alcohols (Brown and Long, 1988; Fraser, and MacNeil, 1989). Less volatile compounds such as ethylene glycol usually require derivatization before analysis. For laboratories receiving specimens that might contain alcohols and diols, a two system procedure is too time-consuming and labor-intensive; therefore a single packed-column chromatographic system capable of analyzing alcohols and diols without sample derivatization was initially developed. Subsequently, a more rapid and sensitive assay, utilizing a wide-bore capillary system was developed. Several problems were encountered in transferring the packed-column method to a wide-bore column. Column stationary-phase selections, sample preparation, choices of injection mode and technique, injection port septa, and type of syringe and needle style uses for injection are described.

O'Neal et al. (1996) described three gas chromatographic procedures for the determination of ethanol in postmortem blood using alternative internal standards to n-propanol. A direct injection procedure using t-butanol (IS) on 5-percent Carbowax 20M stationary phase in a Rtx (R)-BAC2 column, a headspace method using t-butanol (IS) and methyl ethyl ketone (IS) in a 1.2-percent Carbowax 1500 on 60/80 Carbopak C column. Tertiary butyl alcohol and methyl ethyl ketone were well resolved from ethanol, acetone, methanol and other commonly observed putrefactive volatiles using direct injection or headspace analysis. Coefficients of variation for the direct injection method were below 5 percent for ethanol and below 10 percent for the other volatiles. The LODs were 10 mg/L using either t-butanol or methyl ethyl ketone as internal standards. The use of t-butanol or methyl ethyl ketone as alternatives to n-propanol avoids the possibility of error in the quantitation of ethanol due to the presence of *n*-propanol as a putrefactive product in many postmortem specimens (Wigmore, 1993). Use of *t*-butanol or methyl ethyl ketone also allows for the identification of other volatiles that may aid in distinguishing antemortem ingestion from postmortem production of ethanol. Tertiary butyl alcohol (2-methyl-2-propanol), acetonitrile, and methyl ethyl ketone have been suggested as alternative internal standards to *n*-propanol since they have not been identified as putrefactive products in postmortem blood (O'Neal and Poklis, 1996).

D. Headspace techniques

Headspace techniques are based on Henry's law of physics, which states that the ratio of a dissolved substance in aqueous solution is dependent on temperature, pressure, and concentration in the aqueous medium. It follows, then, that volatile substances may be measured by analyzing the vapor, which is in equilibrium with a liquid specimen such as blood. Typically, the blood sample is placed into a vial with appropriate internal standard and sealed with a septum and allowed to stand, usually at 37°C, until equilibrium is reached. A sample of the headspace is removed from the vial by syringe and injected into a gas chromatograph.

Wallace and Dahl (1966) described a method in which sodium chloride was added to the samples in amounts greater than those required for saturation, to minimize the variations in the gas-liquid partition ratio of ethyl alcohol ordinarily caused by differences in dissolved solvents. According to the authors, the addition of the salt markedly increases the vapor pressure of ethyl alcohol in the biological samples and permits quantitative analysis of the vapor phase for ethyl alcohol without the preparation of complex standards. In the method, after addition of sodium chloride to a flask containing blood, the flask is capped with a rubber stopper and the contents equilibrated for five minutes. A 1-mL vapor sample is then injected into a column packed with 1.5 g Flexol 8N8, 1.5 g diisodecyl phthalate, and 1.5 g polyethylene glycol 600 per 100 g 100/120 mesh Chromosorb P. With the method described, 1 SD (N = 30) of a day-to-day quality control sample containing 0.098 g/dL ethyl alcohol concentration was 1.3.

Reed and Cravey (1971) in a search for a simple, rapid, specific, quantitative procedure for the analysis of ethyl alcohol from blood, investigated the advantages of headspace techniques that had been documented by Goldbaum et al. (1964); Duritz and Truitt (1964); Wallace and Dahl (1966); Bassette and Glendening (1968); and Glendening and Harvey (1969). The authors selected 1,4-dioxane as an internal standard (Biasotti and Bradford, 1969) and to reduce the variation in the vapor phase-liquid partition ratios of blood and other aqueous fluids, sodium chloride was used (Wallace and Dahl, 1966). Compared with a widely used distillation-oxidation method (Kozelka and Hine, 1941), this headspace technique provided comparable accuracy with the advantage of speed, simplicity, and specificity. The unknown blood sample is measured accurately by means of 1-mL tc pipette to a small beaker containing 1 mL of 1-percent aqueous 1,4-dioxane and the pipette is washed in and out several times while swirling the beaker. An aliquot of the mixture is added to a vial containing sodium chloride. The stopper bottle is equilibrated for eight minutes and 1.5 mL of vapor phase is injected in a 0.25-inch-by-8-feet stainless steel column packed with 40/60 firebrick impregnated with 28 percent by weight, the following mixtures: diisodecyl phthalate, Flexol 8N8, and Carbowax 600 in a ratio of 10:15:3 (Cadman and Johns, 1958).

Karnitis and Porter (1971) described a method which consists of equilibrating blood with *n*-propyl alcohol as the internal standard and then injecting the vapors into a 0.125-inch-by-6-feet stainless steel column packed with Porapak S. Concentrations were linear over the range 0.00 to 0.35 g/dL blood ethyl alcohol. Correlation of blood ethyl alcohol concentration results were excellent when compared with a distillation method (Shupe and Dubowski, 1952).

Dubowski (1976) described a new method for quantitating ethyl alcohol in equilibrated headspace gas of biological liquids by means of a solid-state metal-oxide semiconductor (MOS) detector. After equilibration of the sodium chloride-saturated specimen at 40°C in a closed vessel, a Taguchi MOS sensor is momentarily exposed to the headspace vapor. The resulting DC voltage change from baseline conditions accurately reflects the alcohol concentration of the liquid specimen, and can be read in direct alcohol-concentration units.

Jones (1977) described a method for the determination of blood alcohol concentration by headspace analysis using an electrochemical detector. A determination can be made within two minutes and only 0.1 mL of blood is required for analysis. The detector response was linearly related to ethyl alcohol concentration up to 0.30 g/dL. The accuracy of the method based on comparison with an enzymatic technique (Buijten, 1975) was high, the mean recovery being 102.2 percent of the attributed concentration. The Alcometer Evidential device used is based on an electrochemical ("fuel cell") principle for ethyl alcohol oxidation. The unit consists of a sampling head thermostated at 60°C between tests, containing the electrochemical detector and the aspirating sampling valve. A Set button serves to activate the sampling valve and discharge the fuel cell and a "Read" button releases the sampling valve (causing aspiration of a 0.6-mL test sample) and activates the fuel cell. The detector signal is displayed on a digital voltmeter in DC voltage, which may be calibrated to blood alcohol units. For the headspace analysis, the sampling head of the Alco-meter is fitted with a special nozzle connection to hold a Luer-fitting hypodermic needle in place of the mouthpiece normally used for breath alcohol. A blood sample of 0.1 mL is transferred into a 10-mL serum bottle and made airtight with a rubber septum. Samples are equilibrated in a water bath at 25°C for fifteen minutes. The vapor phase above each blood sample is adjusted to atmospheric pressure prior to headspace sampling. The sampling head with the hypodermic needle attached is allowed to pierce the rubber septum of the serum bottle containing the sample and the Set button is pressed to activate the sampling mechanism. Immediately afterward the Read button is pressed to aspirate the headspace vapor sample for analysis. The final reading on the digital voltmeter is recorded and is proportional to the alcohol concentration in the headspace vapor. The Set button is pressed to discharge the detector in preparation for a new test. The ease of the operation and rapid analysis time make the method ideal for mass screening for ethyl alcohol in forensic laboratories.

Today, the most widely accepted headspace sampling method is based on one that was developed by Machata (1972) using a Perkin-Elmer Multifract F-40 system. This system consisted essentially of a gas chromatograph equipped with a flame ionization detector and a special electro-pneumatic valve dosing system in addition to a conventional injection port for manual sampling; a precision thermostated turntable water bath; and control unit, recorder or printing integrator (or both). The principles of the system are three basic steps of headspace sampling: (1) equilibration, (2) pressurization, and (3) transfer of an aliquot of the headspace onto the column. After equilibrium is established in the vial, a needle connected to the carrier gas inlet is introduced through a rubber cap into the headspace of the vial. If the pressure in the vial is smaller than the carrier gas inlet pressure, part of the carrier gas flow will enter the vial and pressurize it until it reaches the inlet pressure. At this point the carrier gas supply is momentarily cut off for a specified time. This action causes the gas to flow from the vial into the column, barely injecting an aliquot of the headspace. Coefficients of variation below 3% have been reported. Detailed descriptions of the Multifract F-40, F-42, and F-45 are found in manuals published by the Perkin-Elmer Company, and more recently a detailed procedure was reported by Dubowski (1977).

In addition to the Multifract F-40, F-42, and F-45, the newest automatic headspace sampler is the Perkin-Elmer Model HS-100 mounted on a Sigma gas chromatograph. It combines the simplicity of CRT interaction with the versatility of the microprocessor-control, dual-channel gas chromatograph. The microprocessor control ensures precise thermostating and timing and also allows automatic unattended injection and analysis of up to 100 samples (Hurt and Welton, 1983).

Christmore et al. (1984) described solutions for two problems encountered in an automated headspace gas chromatograph method (Anthony et al., 1980). The first is the catalytic oxidation of ethyl alcohol by oxyhemoglobin, a process that is limited only by the amount of oxygen present in the sealed vial. This reaction was prevented by the addition of sodium dithionite. The second problem dealt with the lack of a suitable salting-out agent and led to the selection of ammonium sulfate which improved recovery of ethyl alcohol as well as enhanced the precision of the method.

Penton (1985) modified an autosampler technique previously used for liquid injection into a gas chromatograph to function as an automatic headspace sampler by replacing the syringe with a 100-mL gas-tight syringe and shortening the needle that normally enters the vial for sampling. In addition, instead of the 1.0 to 1.5 mL of liquid sample, the vials contained 200 mL of liquid. The vapor above the liquid was injected into the gas chromatograph. Since the autosampler was not thermostated, the effect of temperature change was examined by placing the gas chromatograph and autosampler in an environmental chamber and analyzing a sample at various temperatures. The author states that the results were in general agreement with those reported by others (Hauek and Terfloth, 1969; Machata, 1975) that in headspace determination of blood ethyl alcohol the internal standard corrects for temperature fluctuations.

A paper by Jones and Schubereth (1989) describes the analysis of ethanol in blood specimens from suspect drunk drivers and the associated quality assurance procedures currently used in Sweden for legal purposes. Aliquots of whole blood from two separate Vacutainer tubes were diluted with 1-propanol as the internal standard before analysis by headspace gas chromatography (HS-GC) with three different stationary phases: Carbopak B, Carbopak C, and 15 percent Carbo-wax 20 M. The actual HS-GC analysis, the integration of chromatographic peaks, the collection and processing of results, as well as the quality control tests involved the use of computer-aided techniques. The standard deviation of analysis (y) increased with concentration of ethanol in the blood specimen (x), and the above 0.50 mg/g the regression equation was $y = 0.0033 + 0.0153x$. A deduction is made from the mean analytical result to compensate for random and systematic errors inherent in the method. At BACs of 0.5 and 1.5 mg/g, the allowances made are 0.06 and 0.09 mg/g, respectively.

Macchia, et al. (1995) evaluated the suitability of headspace gas chromatography (GC) with a capillary column as a method for determining the ethanol content in different biological fluids. This procedure allows for the use of headspace GC not only as a reference method but also in routine diagnostics and monitoring work. The authors stated that recent literature reviewed reports, (prior to publication of this method), no standardized methodology that is at the same time suitable for ethanol determination in all routinely available biological fluids (blood, serum, plasma, urine, and saliva). Reproducibility studies for the biological fluids tested resulted in coefficients of variation that ranged from 0.8 to 2.9 percent and recoveries averaged 99 percent. Linearity was verified in the range of 0.01–20 g/L of ethanol in aqueous solutions using only a small sample volume (0.1 mL). Internal standard and sample manipulation was not necessary. A Dani 3800 GC (Carlo Erba, Milan, Italy) equipped with a flame-ionization detector (FID), an HS40 headspace analyzer (Perkin-Elmer, Norwalk, CT), an HP-FFAP (cross-linked FFAP) 50-m × 0.2-mm capillary column (0.33-mL film thickness), and an HP 3396 series-II integrator (Hewlett-Packard, Amsterdam, the Netherlands) was used. Headspace vials (20-mL) were subjected to the following parameters: The sample temperature was 75°C, and both the needle and transfer temperatures were 110°C. The GC cycle, thermostating, pressurization, injection, and withdrawal times were 9, 30, 3, 0.20, and 8.8 minutes, respectively. The samples were analyzed under the following conditions: The oven temperature was isothermal at 70°C, and the detector temperature was 150°C. The flow rate of the helium gas carrier was 200 kPa, and no auxiliary gas was used. Air and hydrogen were set for the best FID function. No internal standard was used.

9.4 Other Methods for Alcohol Analysis
A. High-performance liquid chromatography
An excellent review by Tagliaro et al. (1992) focused on the different chromatographic strategies for blood alcohol determination which can be adopted for clinical and forensic purposes. Particular attention was paid to gas chromatography and to high-performance liquid chromatography. These authors indicated that while the separation of aliphatic alcohols is easily accomplished by LC under reversed-phase conditions, the lack of an adequately sensitive detec-

tor has hindered the application of HPLC to blood alcohol determination. The first application of HPLC to blood analysis (Davis, Holland, and Kissinger, 1979) which used HPLC with electrochemical detection to determine precolumn-generated NADH from ADH-catalyzed EtOH oxidation. In this method, the use of HPLC improved the alcohol enzymic assay only indirectly, by improving the NADH measurement step, but leaving unchanged the inherent selectivity limits of the enzymic assays.

B. Gas chromatography—Mass spectrometry

Gas chromatography-mass spectrometry (GC-MS) has found little application for routine alcohol determinations in light of the fact that FID is not specific for ethyl alcohol. The specificity and accuracy of GC with FID for blood alcohol has never been seriously questioned. Mass fragmentography of ethanol in blood and urine, after GC on a porapak Q column, was carried out by Pereira et al. (1974) with a quadrupole mass spectrometer, using ions at m/z 31 and 45 for EtOH and 33 and 49 for [^{2}H$_5$]EtOH. As little as 5 ng of alcohol could be detected. Other methods (Bonnichsen et al., 1974; Liebich, 1982) provide for the determination of endogenous aliphatic alcohols as ethanol, *n*-propanol, *n*-butanol, isobutanol and isopentanol in serum and urine by gas chromatography-mass fragmentography and may be used to identify any spurious formation of these substances under certain conditions.

References

Anthony, R.M., Sutheimer, C.A. and Sunshine, I. Acetaldehyde, methanol, and ethanol by headspace gas chromatography. *J. Anal. Toxicol.* 4:43–45, 1980.

Baird, W.W. Paper presented to Pacific Coast Conference on Chemistry and Spectroscopy, San Diego, Nov. 1973.

Bassette, R. and Glendening, B.L. Analysis of blood alcohol by direct headspace sampling and gas chromatography. *Microchem. J.* 13:374, 1968.

Bechamp, M.A. Sur la fermentation de l'urine normale et sur les organismes divers qui sont capables de la provoquer. *C. R. Acad. Sci.* 61:374, 1865.

Biasotti, A.A. and Bradford, L.W. Quantitative determination of ethanol by gas liquid chromatography after collection from the vapor phase on anhydrous magnesium perchlorate. *J. Forensic Sci. Soc.* 9:65–74, 1969.

Blume, P., Berchild, K.M. and Cawley, L.P. A gas chromatographic analysis of ethanol with identifying confirmation. *Anal. Biochem.* 54:429–433, 1973.

Blystone, P.G. and Collins. H.L. Determination of blood alcohol levels using a direct readout spectrophotometer. Presented at the Semi–Annual meeting of the California Association of Criminalists. Monterey, Calif., May 1984.

Bonnichsen, R. and Linturi, M. Gas chromatography determination of some volatile compounds in urine. *Acta. Chem. Scand.* 16:1289, 1962.

Bonnichsen, R. and Theorell. H. An enzymatic method for the microdetermination of ethanol. *Scand. J. Clin. Lab. Invest.* 3:58, 1951.

Bonnichsen, R., Hedfjall, B. and Ryhage, R. Determination of ethyl alcohol by computerized mass chromatography. *Z. Rechtsmed.* 71:134–138, 1972.

Bradford, L.W. Concepts and standards of performance in the technique of alcohol analysis of physiological specimens. Reprinted from the *Proceedings of the Symposium on Alcohol and Road Traffic*, Indiana University, Indianapolis, 1958, pp. 61–79.

Brown, D.J. and Long, W.C., Quality control in blood alcohol analysis: Simultaneous quantitation and confirmation. *J. Anal Toxicol.* 12:279–83, 1988.

Buijten, J.C. An automatic ultramicro distillation technique for determination of ethanol in blood and urine. *Blutalkohol* 12:393–398, 1975.

Cadman, W.J. and Johns, T. Gas chromatographic determination of ethanol and other volatiles from blood. Read to Ninth Annual Pittsburgh Conference on Analytical Chemistry and Applied Spectroscopy, March 1958.

Caplan, Y.H. The determination of alcohol in blood and breath. In: Saferstein, R. (ed.), *Forensic Science Handbook*. Englewood Cliffs, NJ: Prentice-Hall, 1982, pp. 592–652.

Caplan, Y.H. and Levine, B. The analysis of ethanol in serum, blood, and urine: A comparison of the TDx REA ethanol assay with gas chromatography. *J. Anal. Toxicol.* 120:49–52, 1986.

Caplan, Y.H. and Levine, B. Evaluation of the Abbott TDx-radiative energy attenuation (REA) ethanol assay in a study of 1105 forensic whole blood specimens. *J. Forensic Sci.* 32:55–61, 1987.

Cary, P.L. Reformulated REA ethanol assay evaluated. *J. Anal. Toxicol.* 10:38–39, 1986.

Cary, P.L., Whitter, P.D. and Johnson, C.A. Abbott radioactive energy attenuation method for quantifying ethanol evaluated and compared with gas-liquid chromatography and the DuPont ACA. *Clin. Chem.* 30:1867–1870, 1984.

Cavett, J.W. The determination of alcohol in blood and other body fluids. *J. Lab. Clin. Med.* 23:543, 1938.

Cheng, F.S. and Christian, G.D. Enzymatic determination of blood ethanol, with amperometric measurement of rate of oxygen depletion. *Clin. Chem.* 24:621–626, 1978.

Christmore, D.S., Kelly, R.C. and Doshier, L.A. Improved headspace analysis. *J. Forensic Sci.* 29:1038–1044, 1984.

Chundela, B. and Janak, J. Quantitative determination of ethanol besides other volatile substances in blood and other body fluids by gas chromatography. *J. Forensic Med.* 7:153–161, 1960.

Committee on Medicolegal Problems American Medical Association. *Alcohol and the impaired Driver*. Chicago: American Medical Association, 1973.

Cravey, R.H. and Jain, N.C. Current status of blood alcohol methods. *J. Chromatogr. Sci.* 12:209–213, 1974.

Curry, A.S., Walker, G.W. and Simpson, G.S. Determination of ethanol in blood by gas chromatography. *Analyst* 91:742, 1966.

Davis, R.A. The determination of ethanol in blood or tissue by gas chromatography. *J. Forensic Sci.* 11:205–213, 1966.

Davis, G.C., Holland, K.L. and Kissinger, P.T. *J. Liq. Chromatogr.* 2:663, 1979.

Degel, F. and Paulus, N. A rapid and precise method for the quantitation of ethanol in serum using the EMIT-st serum ethanol assay reagent and a Cobas Bio centrifugal analyzer. *J. Clin. Chem. Biochem.* 26:351–353, 1988.

Drost, R.H. and Maes, R.A. Evaluation of the EMIT-st serum alcohol assay in toxicology. *Vet. Hum. Toxicol.* 25:412–414, 1983.

Dubowski, K.M. Method for alcohol determination in biological liquids by sensing with a solid-state detector. *Clin. Chem.* 22:863–867, 1976.

Dubowski, K.M. *Manual for Analysis of Ethanol in Biological Liquids*. U.S. Dept. of Transportation report No. DOT-TSC-NI ITSA-76-4, 1977.

Duritz, G. and Truitt. E.B. A rapid method for the simultaneous determination of acetaldehyde and ethanol in blood using gas chromatography. *Q. J. Stud. Alcohol* 25:498–510, 1964.

Engelhart, D.A. and Jenkins, A.J., Evaluation of an offsite alcohol testing device for use in postmortem forensic toxicology. *J. Anal. Toxicol.* 25:612–615, 2001.

Finkle, B.S. Ethanol-type C procedure. In: Sunshine, I. (ed.), *Manual of Analytical Toxicology*. Cleveland: CRC Press, 1971, pp. 147–149.

Fox. J.E. Fast chromatographic analysis of alcohols and certain other volatiles in biological material for forensic purposes. *Proc. Soc. Exp. Biol. Med.* 97:236, 1958.

Fraser, A.D. and MacNeil, W., Gas chromatographic analysis of methyl formate and application in methyl alcohol poisoning cases. *J. Anal Toxicol.* 13:73–6, 1889.

Garriott, J.C. Forensic aspects of ethyl alcohol. *Clin. Lab. Med.* 3:385–396. 1983.

Glendening, B.L. and Harvey. R.A. A simple method using headspace gas for determination of blood alcohol by gas chromatography. *J. Forensic Sci.* 14:136–145, 1969.

Goldbaum, L.R., Domanski, T.J. and Schloegel, E.L. Analysis of biological specimens for volatile compounds by gas chromatography. *J. Forensic Sci.* 9:63–71, 1964.

Gudzinowicz, B.J. and Gudzinowicz, M. *Analysis of Drugs and Metabolites by Gas Chromatography-Mass Spectrometry.* NY: Marcel Dekker, 1977, pp. 85–189.

Harger, R.N. A simple micromethod for the determination of alcohol in biological material. *J. Lab. Clin. Med.* 20:746, 1935.

Hauck, G. and Terfloth, H.P. Investigations on automatic blood alcohol determination according to the headspace method. *Chromatographia* 2:309–315, 1969.

Hessel, D.W. and Modglin, F.R. The quantitative determination of ethanol and other volatile substances in blood by gas-liquid partition chromatography. *J. Forensic Sci.* 9:255–264, 1964.

Hurt, S.G. and Welton, B. New microprocessor–controlled gas chromatographs. *Am. Lab.* 15:89–916, 1983.

Jacobsen, D. et al. Studies on methanol poisoning. *Acta Med Scand.* 212:5–10, 1992.

Jain, N.C. Direct blood injection method for gas chromatography determination of alcohols and other volatile compounds. *Clin. Chem.* 17:82–85, 1971.

Jain, N.C. and Cravey, R.H. Analysis of alcohol, part 1: A review of chemical and infrared methods. *J. Chromatogr.* Sci. 10:257–262, 1972a.

Jain, N.C. and Cravey, R.H. Analysis of alcohol, part 2: A review of gas chromatographic methods. *J. Chro-matogr. Sci.* 10:263–267, 1972b.

Jones, A.W. A rapid method for blood alcohol determination by headspace analysis using electrochemical detector. *J. Forensic Sci.* 22:283–291, 1977.

Jones, A.W. and Schuberth, J. Computer-aided headspace gas chromatography applied to blood alcohol analysis: Importance of online process control. *J. Forensic Sci.* 34:1116–1127, 1989.

Jortani, S.A. and Poklis, A. Emit ETS Plus ethyl alcohol assay for the determination of ethanol in human serum and urine. *J. Anal. Toxicol.* 16:368–371, 1992.

Jortani, S.A. and Poklis, A. Evaluation of the Syva ETS Plus urine drug and serum analyzer. *J. Anal. Toxicol.* 17:31–33, 1993.

Jung, G. and Ferard, G. Enzyme-coupled measurement of ethanol in whole blood and plasma with a centrifugal analyzer. *Clin. Chem.* 24:873–876, 1978.

Karnitis, L. and Porter, L.J. A gas chromatographic method for ethanol in vapors of biological fluids. *J. Forensic Sci.* 16:318–322, 1971.

Kirk, P.L., Garbor, A. and Parker. K.P. Determination of blood alcohol: Improvements in chemical and enzymatic procedures. *Anal. Chem.* 30:14–18, 1958.

Kozelka, F.L. and Hine, C.H. Method for the determination of ethyl alcohol for medicolegal purposes. *Ind. Engin. Chem. (Anal. Ed.)* 13:905, 1941.

Liebich, H.M., Buelow, H.J. and Kallmayer, R. Quantitation of endogenous aliphatic alcohols in serum and urine. *J. Chromatogr.* 239:343–349, 1982.

Livesey, J.F. et al. Simultaneous determination of alcohols and ethylene glycol in serum by packed or capillary column gas chromatography. *Clin Chem.* 41:300–305, 1995.

Lyons, H. and Bard, J. Gas chromatographic determination of lower alcohols in biological samples. *Clin. Chem.* 10:429–432, 1964.

Macchia, T. et al. Ethanol in biological fluids: Headspace GC measurement. *J. Anal. Toxicol.* 19:241–246, 1995.

Machata, G. Die Routineuntersuchung der Blutalkohol-konzentration mit der Gas-Chromatographie. *Mikrochim. Acta.* 4:691, 1962.

Machata, G. Determination of alcohol in blood by gas chromatography headspace analysis. *Perkin Elmer Clin. Chem. Newsl.* 4:29–32, 1972.

Machata, G. The advantages of automated blood alcohol determination by headspace analysis. *Z. Rechtstned.* 75:229–234, 1975.

McCord, W.M. and Gladsden, R.M. The identification and determination of alcohols in blood by gas chromatography. *J. Gas Chromatogr.* 2:38–39, 1964.

Manno, B.R. and Manno, J.E. A simple approach to gas chromatographic microanalysis of alcohol in blood and urine by a direct-injection technique. *J.Anal Toxicol.* 2:257–261, 1978.

Maricq, L. and Molle, L. Investigations on the determination of blood alcohol levels by gas chromatography. *Bull. Acad. Med. Belg.* (Ser. 6) 24:199–232, 1959.

Mather, A. and Assimos, A. Evaluation of gas-1iquid chromatography in assays for blood volatiles. *Clin. Chem.* 11:1023–1035, 1965.

O'Neal, C.L. and Poklis, A. Postmortem production of ethanol and factors which influence interpretation: a critical review, *Am. J. Forensic Med. Pathol.*, 17:8–20, 1996.

O'Neal, C.L. et al. Gas chromatographic procedures for determination of ethanol in postmortem blood using *t*-butanol and methyl ethyl ketone as internal standards. *Forensic Sci. Int.* 83:31–38, 1996.

Parker, K.D. et al. Gas chromatographic determination of ethyl alcohol in blood for medicolegal purposes. *Anal. Chem.* 34: 1234–1236, 1962.

Penton, Z. Headspace measurement of ethanol in blood by gas chromatography with a modified auto-sampler. *Clin. Chem.* 31:439–441, 1985.

Pereira, W.E. et al. The determination of ethanol in blood and urine by mass fragmentography. *Clin. Chim. Acta.* 51:109–112, 1974.

Poklis, A. and Mackell, M.A. Evaluation of a modified alcohol dehydrogenase assay for the determination of ethanol in blood. *Clin. Chem.* 28:2125–2127, 1982.

Prencipe, L., Iaccheri, E. and Manzati, C. Enzymatic ethanol assay: A new colorimetric method based on a measurement of hydrogen peroxide. *Clin. Chem.* 33:486–9, 1987.

Redetzki, H.M. and Dees, W.L. Comparison of four kits for enzymatic determination of ethanol in blood. *Clin. Chem.* 22:83–86, 1976.

Reed, D. and Cravey, R.H. A quantitative gas chromatographic method for alcohol determination. *J. Forensic Sci. Soc.* 11:263, 1971.

Shupe, L.M. and Dubowski, K.M. Ethyl alcohol in blood and urine. A simple photometric method for its forensic determination. *Am. J. Clin. Pathol.* 901, 1952.

Smith, H.W. The specificity of the desiccation method for determining alcohol in biological fluids. *J. Lab. Clin. Med.* 38:762–766, 1951.

Smith, H.W. Methods for determining alcohol. In: Curry, A.S. (ed.), *Methods for Forensic Science*, vol. 4. NY: Interscience, 1965, pp. 1–97.

Solon, J., Watkins, J. and Mikkelsen, L. Automated analysis of alcohols in blood. *J. Forensic Sci* 17:447–452, 1972.

Steinberg, M., Nash, J.B. and Walker, J.Q. Quantitation of alcohols using gas chromatography and a 15% Hallcomid column. *J. Forensic Sci.* 10:201, 1965.

Sunshine, I. and Nenad, R.A modification of Winnick's method for the rapid determination of ethyl alcohol in biological fluids. *Anal. Chem.* 25:653, 1953.

Sutheimer, C.A., Lavins, E. and King, T. Evaluation of the Syva ETS-PLUS ethyl alcohol assay with application to the analysis of antemortem whole blood, routine postmortem specimens, and synovial fluid. *J. Anal. Toxicol.* 16:119–124, 1992.

Tagliaro, F. et al. Chromatographic methods for blood alcohol determination. *J. Chromatogr.* 580:161–190, 1992.

Takel, H. et al. Enzymatic determination of serum ethanol with membrane–bound dehydrogenase. *Clin. Chem.* 31:1985–1987, 1985.

Urry, F.M. et al. Application of the Technicon Chem 1+ chemistry analyzer to the Syva EMIT ethyl alcohol assay in plasma and urine. *J. Anal. Toxicol.* 17:287–291, 1993.

Vasiliades, J., Pollock, J. and Robinson, C.A. Pitfalls of the alcohol dehydrogenase procedure for the emergency assay of alcohol: A case study of isopropanol overdosage. *Clin. Chem.* 24:383–385, 1978.

Wallace, J.E. and Dahl, E.V. Rapid vapor phase method for determining ethanol in blood and urine by gas chromatography. *Am. J. Clin. Pathol.* 46:152–154, 1966.

Wesselman, H.J. Quantitative determination of ethanol in pharmaceutical products by gas chromatography. *J. Am. Pharmacol. Assoc.* 49:320, 1960.

Whitehouse, L.W. and Paul, C.J. Micro-scale enzymic determination of ethanol in plasma with a discrete analyzer, the ABA–100. *Clin. Chem.* 25: 1399–1401, 1979.

Widmark, E.M.P. A micromethod for the estimation of alcohol in blood. *Biochem. Z.* 131:473, 1922.888.

Wigmore, J.G., The distribution of ethanol in postmortem blood samples. *J. Forensic Sci.*, 38:1019–1020, 1993.

Wright, J.W. Alcohol and the laboratory in the United Kingdom. *Ann. Clin. Biochem.* 28:212–217, 1991.

Chapter 10

Quality Assurance

Barbara J. Basteyns and Graham R. Jones, Ph.D.

The development and documentation of a comprehensive quality assurance plan is essential for all laboratories or agencies involved in forensic alcohol testing. Any plan will be unique to the individual organization and may be developed in response to state or federal regulations, state administrative codes, accreditation or certification requirements, guidelines from professional organizations or principles of good laboratory practice.

Any quality assurance protocol must monitor the total laboratory operation which may be divided into the following general areas: (1) pretesting criteria, (2) laboratory issues, (3) personnel requirements, (4) testing criteria, (5) external proficiency testing, (6) test reporting systems and (7) post-testing issues. The plan can be documented in a quality assurance protocol manual that lists the standards or guidelines and documents the laboratory compliance. The protocol should be reviewed at least annually. Adherence to a well established quality assurance protocol in the forensic laboratory will facilitate acceptance of analytical results for ethanol in biological specimens, as well as interpretation or opinions related to those findings when presented in court.

The majority of breath alcohol testing is performed in a non-laboratory environment by law enforcement personnel. As with blood or urine testing, rules for regulation of breath testing can usually be found in the individual state administrative codes. Although the conditions of testing and personnel requirements will be different, the same basic considerations of quality assurance should apply (Dubowski, 1994). Breath alcohol testing methods and quality control practices are discussed in Chapter 8.

Laboratory Information Systems (LIS) and personal computers allow the laboratory to store, process, update and retrieve information which can aid in establishing and maintaining the necessary documentation.

10.1 Pretesting Criteria

The laboratory has the responsibility for recommending or providing suitable specimen collection kits for the analysis of blood or urine ethanol in antemortem and postmortem samples. Collection kits should contain materials and instructions for use which provide adequate specimens collected with the proper anticoagulant and preservative in a manner designed to maintain their integrity and evidentiary value. If requests for reanalysis or testing for drugs other than ethanol are a common occurrence, it is advisable to collect multiple specimens so that a sealed, unopened specimen will be available for these purposes. All collection kits which will be transported by mail must include absorbent materials to contain the biological material should a spill occur during transit.

It is advisable to provide a test request form that documents subject, submitter and collection information. This same form can document receipt of the specimen in the laboratory, analytical results and review by the laboratory director.

Chain of custody, or the record of all persons having access to the specimen from collection to analysis, must be established in any subsequent court proceedings. If specimens are hand-delivered to the laboratory, a notation of the date and time of receipt should be made on the request form or in a separate custody log. Court rulings have established that the use of the U.S. Postal Service does not break the chain of custody. Specimens received by mail should only be opened by the analyst or person responsible for chain of custody specimens.

If specimen collection and analysis of the specimen are to be made in the same facility, it is advisable to secure the specimen in a locked box or secure refrigerator between collection and analysis. The lockbox should have restricted access to appropriate authorized personnel only.

The analyst must establish that the subject name on the request form and specimens agree, the specimen is sealed securely and the specimen was collected in a sample container of the kind recommended by the laboratory (or required by statute). If the above conditions are met, a notation on the number of specimens and their condition is recorded. Any deviations should be noted on the request form.

The seal on the specimen collection tube should not be broken until the specimen is assayed. All specimen vials should be secured in a limited access refrigerator when not being processed or sampled for analysis.

Criteria for rejection of specimens should be developed. Examples might include: insufficient specimen submitted to performing a reliable test; or a blood specimen that has coagulated due to exposure to heat. Criteria should also be established which may require special interpretation on laboratory reports such as possible contamination with embalming fluid or the presence of decomposition products.

10.2 Laboratory Issues

The laboratory space should provide an environment conducive to the production of high quality work.

Ideally, a forensic laboratory is located in a secure building with limited access. Adequate space for instrumentation, chemical hoods, biological safety cabinets, accessible safety showers and eyewashes, and controlled environmental parameters such as temperature and humidity should be provided. A secure, refrigerated specimen storage area with a temperature system that can be monitored and recorded is necessary to insure sample integrity. The laboratory should have appropriate solvent and acid storage cabinets as well as adequate storage for dry chemicals. All laboratories must develop a chemical safety plan as well as observe the provisions of the blood-borne pathogens guidelines (OSHA 1991).

10.3 Personnel Considerations

Personnel qualifications for alcohol analysts will vary dependent on laboratory, jurisdiction and job responsibilities. Typically, laboratory analysts will have a minimum of a B.S. in chemistry, medical technology or a related field of science. Analysts involved in impaired driving cases may require state certification. Interviews with potential employees should evaluate not only relevant laboratory experience but also assess whether the candidate possesses the communication skills necessary to provide expert testimony in court. It is also prudent to perform background checks for evidence of serious driving offenses or felony convictions which could compromise the person's credibility in subsequent court appearances.

Establishment of a training protocol (Figure 10.1) for those involved in forensic alcohol analysis should document the training schedule, criteria for evaluation, and continuing education parameters. The analyst should become familiar with the laws or administrative code regulating alcohol analysis as well as the licensure and certification requirements for personnel and laboratories.

The laboratory should maintain documentation of the successful completion of all training as well as records on continuing education and outside activities of personnel such as meetings, courses and presentations. Details should include a description of the course content, who gave the course, when, where, and the number of contact hours. These types of records can be easily kept in a form (e.g., com-

Method of Training

1. Analysts are trained in the use of a gas chromatograph with automatic injector and reporting integrator or data system. Analysts perform 100 ethanol assays (in duplicate) on specimens previously assayed by a certified analyst.

2. Analysts are given an in-house course on alcohol pharmacology and training in preparation for courtroom testimony. In addition, all new analysts make one or more trips to an actual trial with an experienced analyst.

3. As required, all analysts are certified through the appropriate local or state agency to perform analysis on forensic specimens collected from impaired drivers.

4. Where available, analysts participate in alcohol pharmacology and breath testing instrumentation and interpretation training courses provided by the local or state agency. In addition, they may participate in breath to blood correlation studies as part of training course for breath test operators.

5. Analysts should take advantage of additional training opportunities including workshops held by professional organizations or universities.

6. Where available, analysts should keep themselves apprized of changes to the local database of alcohol literature and indeed regularly review the relevant scientific literature.

7. All analysts should participate on a rotating basis in the analysis of specimens from local, state or commercial alcohol proficiency test providers.

Figure 10.1 Example toxicologist training summary for blood and urine ethanol/volatiles

puter database) that allows easy retrieval and editing by the analyst. These records can be used in court to demonstrate the qualifications of the analyst and strengthen their position as an expert witness.

Preparation for testimony in court should be an integral part of the analyst's training. This training will include familiarization with specific state statutes, certification procedures and regulations governing collection, analysis and reporting of forensic alcohol specimens. Courtroom procedures should be described in detail, and the analyst should be given the opportunity to participate in mock trials covering both direct testimony and cross examination procedures. It is critical that the analyst be capable of providing concise explanations of all quality assurance practices that are used to insure reliable laboratory results.

Training should also be provided in the area of alcohol pharmacology and interpretation of results if this type of testimony is routinely expected of alcohol analysts in a specific jurisdiction. It is helpful to accompany other analysts to court to observe testimony prior to his or her first appearance. The analyst should prepare a curriculum vitae which documents education, training, certification (if appropriate), professional experience, professional affiliations and relevant publications.

10.4 Testing Criteria
Any methods employed by the laboratory must be sensitive, specific, reliable and appropriate for use with the types of specimens to be assayed. Specific methods of analysis are discussed in Chapter 9.

A. Standard operating procedures manual
All methods used in the laboratory should be documented in a *standard operating procedures manual* (SOP). It is advisable to use a standard format for procedure manuals. For example, a guide for clinical procedures manuals that is also applicable to forensic procedures is published by the National Committee for Clinical Laboratory Standards (NCCLS GP2-A4).

Any procedure manual should contain the following sections: (1) a brief description of the principle of the method, (2) specimen requirements, (3) reagents used in the method, (4) equipment and supplies, (5) instrumentation, (6) standards and controls, (7) calibration procedures, (8) quality control procedures, (9) step-by-step directions, (10) required calculations, (11) result reporting procedures, (12) procedure notes or comments, (13) limitations of the method and (14) method references.

Specimen requirements address the preferred and acceptable specimens, required volume for analysis and recommended preservatives or anticoagulants. The reagents section should include source, method of preparation and stability. Any necessary equipment and laboratory supplies should be listed. The instrumentation and operating parameters should be detailed.

Sources and preparation of all standards and controls should be included. The step-wise documentation of the procedure should be written in a fashion that is clear to all potential users. Criteria for evaluation of control material should be included as well as action to be followed when conditions are not met. Procedure notes include any special precautions, or can address additional testing such as procedures to follow when volatiles other than ethanol are detected. The limitations sections should include the limit of detection, any known interferences and the lowest concentration reported as positive. The method should be reviewed on an annual basis by the laboratory director or designee. Any changes to the procedure made between review periods should be noted and initialed as they occur.

Any new method introduced into the laboratory must be evaluated for accuracy, precision and reliability preferably by comparison to an established reference method. Copies of all replaced methods should be retained for a period of time to correspond to any court testimony related to their use.

B. Standards and controls

Standards are preparations of known concentrations of the analyte to be measured which are prepared from material traceable to a certified source. They are used for instrument calibration and to verify linearity of the method. Controls are preparations which contain known amounts of the analyte in the same or similar matrix as the specimens. They are used to document accuracy, precision and lack of bias in the analytical procedure.

Ethanol standards can be prepared from 100-percent ethanol. This reagent is hygroscopic (i.e., it absorbs water rapidly) so only freshly opened bottles should be used for standard preparation. A high quality 95-percent ethanol, which is more stable, is equally suitable for standards. When calculating the volume of ethanol required for a standard, it is essential to correct for density of ethanol at the preparation temperature. Alternatively, the ethanol may be weighed directly into a vessel such as a volumetric flask. It is advisable to check all prepared standards versus a certified reference standard available from the National Institute of Standards and Technology (NIST SRM 1828) or Cerilliant (Certified Alcohol Standard Solutions). Standard concentrations are typically expressed in weight of ethanol per volume of specimen (g/100 mL or mg/100 mL). The concentrations of the standards should cover the range anticipated in the specimens, which typically is from zero to 0.60 g/100 mL. A minimum of three different standards and a blank containing no ethanol should be assayed with each set of specimens. It is also advisable to prepare a standard at the lowest reportable concentration.

Each new set of standards should be verified against the standards in current use as well as the certified reference material. Laboratories that use gas chromatographic techniques should also prepare a combination standard which contains other volatiles that may be detected in biological specimens such as acetone, methanol and isopropanol.

Although commercial ethanol controls are available, the use of in-house prepared controls allows more flexibility in matrix and range of concentrations than commercial preparations. Controls may be prepared by adding stock ethanol solutions to preserved whole blood, serum or urine, mixing thoroughly and freezing in small aliquots. In order to obtain reliable statistical data, a minimum of ten aliquots should be tested over a period of time to establish the mean, standard deviation and acceptable range for the controls. Frozen ethanol controls in biological materials are stable for at least eight months if the aliquots are tightly capped and the freezer maintains a constant temperature.

C. Evaluation of quality control criteria

Each laboratory should develop as part of their standard operating procedure manual a section on criteria for acceptance or rejection of laboratory results for ethanol analyses. For example, if samples are run in duplicate, it should be noted how closely the duplicate results must agree. Other criteria include the acceptable deviation of control results from the established target value, and the action to be taken in the event of a control failure. An aqueous blank specimen should always be assayed to document that nothing in the procedure will cause a false positive result. Standards are used to demonstrate linearity of the method. Controls prepared in the matrix to be assayed are typically used to document the within-run and between-run precision and accuracy of the method. The analysis of duplicate specimens can also demonstrate precision. All of this information can be used in court to support the validity of the laboratory result. Standard statistical methods and guidelines are available for evaluation and interpretation of laboratory results.

D. Instrument maintenance manuals

An instrument maintenance manual should be prepared for all laboratory instruments which documents routine preventive maintenance and repair. The document should include instrument name, model and serial number, date and initial of analyst, description of problem or routine maintenance and any corrective action or relevant comments.

E. Criteria for review and validation of results

Protocol should be established for review and validation of all ethanol results. Laboratory Information Systems (LIS) may provide instrument interface options for electronic transfer of results which can reduce possible transcription errors and may also have defined methods for result review and validation. Any system should provide comparison between results on instrument output, any worksheets and the final laboratory report. Quality control data should be reviewed for compliance with criteria indicated in the operating procedures manual and any necessary corrective action taken where minimum criteria have not been met. The laboratory worksheet should contain information on instrument conditions and all standards and control target concentrations for comparison to actual determined values.

10.5 External Proficiency Testing

Participation in external proficiency testing programs for ethanol is a critical part of any quality assurance program. Programs which evaluate blood and urine ethanol determinations are available from several sources (see References). It is desirable to participate in more than one program in order to receive frequent specimens to demonstrate current competence.

Participation in suitable proficiency programs should be documented in the quality assurance manual. A method for review and corrective action for any unsatisfactory performance should also be documented.

10.6 Test Reporting Systems

The accuracy and reliability of all test reporting systems is a necessary component of quality assurance. At a minimum, laboratory reports should be reviewed and signed by the analyst, although in many jurisdictions, review is undertaken by a second person, often the laboratory director or designee. The report should contain information about the period of time the specimen will be retained prior to disposal in case further analysis is required. The report should also include the laboratory name, address and telephone number. Electronic data transfer is becoming common in many forensic laboratories. Review methods and protocols should also be developed to monitor these systems.

10.7 Post-testing Issues

The laboratory policies on retention and storage of forensic alcohol specimens must preserve their integrity for retesting purposes. Some laboratories may be required to retain the specimen container in order to demonstrate the label and seal as part of the evidentiary proceedings. Any policy should address storage conditions, specimen identification and security issues.

Instrument output, laboratory worksheets and reports, internal and external proficiency testing results should be retained for as long as the results of the analysis may be required in court, which could be for many years. It may be desirable to reach an agreement with the state attorney or with the jurisdiction's district attorney's office as to the length of original record storage. Records may be electronically archived for long-term storage, although many jurisdictions still require the long-term archiving of the paper records. Any system should allow for ready access and retrieval of relevant information. Any laboratory or analyst's certification records must be maintained even if they are renewed on an annual basis in order to document past certification for any analysis in question.

A policy for amended or corrected reports should be established. All communications with clients should be documented in either a manual or computer log which will contain information on incoming or outgoing telephone calls and any communication by letter, fax or electronic means.

10.8 Computer Support

LIS and personal computers have become an integral part of laboratory operations. An LIS can provide documentation of many of the primary components of quality assurance such as requisition entry information, subject demographics, testing results, quality control information, result validation, report history and communication with clients. Some systems have the capability to provide audit information on all personnel who enter, validate or modify information. Systems can also provide instrument interface options which allow direct transfer of results from the laboratory instrument to the computer record. Quality control information can also be stored and statistical data retrieved to demonstrate analytical performance. LIS may also offer various management reports on workload statistics, origin of specimens and turnaround time which can be used to monitor aspects of the laboratory operation. They also offer opportunities to transmit results or reports electronically to clients by fax, modem or secure Internet link.

References

Dubowski, K.M. Quality assurance in breath-alcohol analysis. *J. Anal. Toxicol.* 18:306–311, 1994.

Forensic Toxicology Laboratory Guidelines, 2002. Joint publication of the Society of Forensic Toxicologists (SOFT; P.O. Box 5543, Mesa, AZ 85211-5543) and American Academy of Forensic Sciences (AAFS; Toxicology Section, P.O. Box 669, Colorado Springs, CO 80901-0669). Available for download from the SOFT web site (http://www.soft-tox.org).

Occupational Safety and Health Administration, 29 CFR Part 1910.1030: *Occupational Exposure to Bloodborne Pathogens*, December 6, 1991. (OSHA, 200 Constitution Avenue, NW, Washington, DC 20210; http://www.osha.gov).

Clinical Laboratory Technical Procedure Manuals; Approved Guideline, 4th ed. Lucia M. Berte, MA, MT(ASCP), (NCCLS, 940 West Valley Road, Suite 1400, Wayne, PA 19087-1898, e-mail: exoffice@nccls.org).

Reference Materials and Controls

National Institute of Standards and Technology (NIST, 100 Bureau Drive, Stop 3460, Gaithersburg, MD 20899; http://www.nist.gov). Standard Reference Material (SRM) 1828a (aqueous ethanol 95.6%, 2.003%, 0.0960%, 0.02309%).

Cerilliant (811 Paloma Drive, Suite A, Round Rock, TX 78664; http://www.cerilliant.com). NIST traceable aqueous ethanol solutions 0.010–0.40%.

Restek Corporation (110 Benner Circle, Bellefonte, PA 16823; http://www.restekcorp.com). NIST traceable aqueous ethanol solutions 0.015– 0.30%.

Bio-Rad Laboratories (Clinical Diagnostics Group, 4000 Alfred Nobel Drive, Hercules, CA 94547, e-mail: diagcs@bio-rad.com). Whole blood control (Tox 1, Tox 2) containing ethanol (bi-level), acetone, methanol and isopropanol.

Sigma-Aldrich (P.O. Box 14508, St. Louis, MO 63178-9916; http://www.sigmaaldrich.com). Human serum ethanol controls (E5258 0.20% and E5133 0.07%).

Proficiency Test Programs

College of American Pathologists (CAP; 325 Waukegan Road, Northfield, IL 60093; http://www.cap.org).

Whole Blood Alcohol Survey: Three sets of five whole blood specimens (AL1) or serum specimens (AL2) per year. Specimens may also contain acetone, methanol and isopropanol.

Toxicology Survey (T-series): Three sets of serum and urine specimens per year. Specimens contain drugs and some contain ethanol, drugs or both.

California Association of Toxicologists Toxicology Survey (address varies with member responsible for survey; http://www.cal-tox.org). Four urine or blood specimens per year with alcohol as a random constituent.

F.A.A. Aeromedical Institute Toxicology Survey (Proficiency Testing Program for Drug Analysis, CAMI, AAM-600, P.O. Box 25080, Oklahoma City, OK 73125; http://www.cami.jccbi.gov/AAM-600/Toxicology/600FOR.html). Four sets of blood or urine specimens per year; specimens contain may ethanol and other drugs.

National Highway Traffic Safety Administration Blood Alcohol Proficiency Testing Project (NHTSA, Safety and Environmental Technology Division (DTS-34), Volpe National Transportation Systems Center, Kendall Square (55 Broadway), Cambridge, MA 02142). Two sets of three whole blood specimens per year (primarily available to U.S. laboratories).

In addition to the above programs, many states operate their own regulatory blood alcohol proficiency test programs. Some of these may be available to out-of-state forensic laboratories.

Chapter 11

Collection and Storage of Specimens for Alcohol Analysis

William H. Anderson, Ph.D.

11.1 Introduction

The purpose of collecting a biological specimen and performing a forensic analytical assay for ethanol is to determine the significance, if any, of ethanol in a medicolegal investigation. The proper interpretation of the analytical result depends on several factors. In all cases the assay must be accurate, precise, and specific for ethanol; these concerns have been addressed in detail in other chapters of this book and will not be considered here. In addition, insight must be provided as to whether the measured concentration of alcohol is essentially the same as the concentration at the time of specimen collection. Questions concerning the potential loss or gain of ethanol from specimens analyzed at varying times after collection are an inevitable component of most cases involving alcohol. Postmortem specimens present an additional challenge: does the measured concentration of alcohol reflect the concentration at the time of death?

There are several complicating factors that must be considered in order to answer these seemingly simple questions. This chapter concerns itself with procedures and the rationale for their use that have been developed to properly collect and preserve biological specimens for ethanol analysis.

11.2 Loss of Ethanol

The loss of ethanol from biological specimens has been a concern and a matter of investigation for most of the history of modern forensic toxicology. To date, three major theories have been presented to explain ethanol losses from biological specimens (Brown et al., 1973). These include (1) evaporation, (2) enzyme mediated oxidation, and (3) action of microorganisms.

A. Evaporation

Ethanol is a volatile substance with a boiling point of 78.5°C. Its volatility and vapor pressure are the reasons for the successful measurement of ethanol in breath specimens. These same properties allow ethanol to be lost from biological specimens. Brown et al. (1973) demonstrated ethanol loss by evaporation when the specimen container closure was faulty. These results are consistent with the author's observation of ethanol loss from biological specimens and aqueous solutions when either no seal is present or the specimen container is not sealed adequately. Usually these problems arise from not completely closing screw-cap containers or not properly sealing a rubber stopper on a vacuum tube. Storage temperature has an obvious effect on potential losses by evaporation mechanism; the lower the temperature the less chance of loss. Prouty and Anderson (1987) reported an accelerated loss of ethanol in the special situation in which small specimens volumes (< 4 mL) were collected in containers designed to hold much larger specimen volumes (30 mL). The 30-mL tubes contained 250 mg of NaF. These authors attributed the loss to a salting-out effect. Experiments were designed in which blood bank blood was used to prepare a 0.200 g/dL ethanol standard. Aliquots of varying volumes (4, 8 and 28 mL) were pipetted into 30-mL vials containing 250 mg of NaF; in addition, the smallest volume (4 mL) was pipetted into vials without NaF. The ethanol concentrations were measured after twenty-four hours and after seventy-two hours of equilibration at 5°C. The results of this experiment are shown in Table 11.1. The small volume specimens placed into the vials containing 250 mg NaF exhibited a statistically significant loss of ethanol as compared to the 28-mL specimens containing NaF and the 4-mL specimens without the addition of NaF. Unfortunately, placing small volumes of blood, vitreous fluid, or urine in large specimen containers frequently occurs with postmortem specimens. It is a practice that should be avoided. The loss of ethanol by evaporation can be minimized by (1) using leak-resistant containers and tightly securing the closure, (2) storing the specimens in a refrigerator or freezer, and (3) placing specimens in a container that has a minimal air space above it. As described in the next sections, these recommendations are also sound advice for minimizing ethanol loss by other mechanisms.

B. Oxidation

Brown et al. (1973) first reported that ethanol could be oxidized to acetaldehyde in stored specimens. In a companion publication Smalldon and Brown (1973) described this process as an oxyhemoglobin-mediated oxidation that utilized the oxygen in the blood and in the air in contact with the blood. Initial losses by this mechanism were reported as 0.02 mg/dL/day at 4°C, 6 mg/dL/day at 37°C, and 43 mg/dL/day at 62°C. These losses appeared to be independent of the concentration of the ethanol in the specimens. In practice, specimens stored under normal laboratory conditions for eighteen months resulted in losses of 20–40 mg/dL of ethanol. This mechanism for ethanol loss was not inhibited by fluoride, but it was inhibited by sodium azide, dithionite, nitrite, and hydrogen sulphite. The loss was greatly dependent on temperature and could be eliminated by storing specimens at –20°C. These authors and Scaplehorn (1970) indicated that losses depended on the volume of air space in the container. Chang et al. (1984) reported similar losses in room temperature storage experiments of 3.0 and 6.75 years duration. The results of Brown and Smaldon (1973) would indicate that this mechanism of loss could be prevented or lessened by storing specimens at refrigerator or freezer temperatures, placing specimens in containers with minimal air space above them, and using azide as a preservative for long-term storage. The use of azide has not reached common practice in the United States. In a recent study, Dubowski et al. (1997) considered the stability of ethanol in human whole blood controls. These authors compared multilevel controls of ethanol that contained fluoride (1 percent) and anticoagulant, with and without sodium

Table 11.1
Results of Volume Experiments

Specimen	Volume	Flouride	Mean (mg/dL)[1]
Day 1	4 mL	Yes	190
Day 1	8 mL	Yes	200
Day 1	28 mL	Yes	206
Day 1	4 mL	No	198
Day 3	4 mL	Yes	165
Day 3	8 mL	Yes	185
Day 3	28 mL	Yes	198
Day 3	4 mL	No	201

[1]N = 6

Adapted from Prouty and Anderson, 1987.

azide. The azide-containing blood samples showed no alcohol losses. The azide free specimens had small losses over the one-year period of the study (< 5 percent). These authors concluded that for performance-test and control specimens the use of sodium azide is unnecessary and unwarranted. Winek and Paul (1983) reported no loss of ethanol when specimens were stored at room temperature for up to fourteen days.

C. Microbial action

It is generally recognized that many different microbes are capable of using ethanol as a substrate for metabolism (Harper and Corry, 1988; Dick and Stone, 1987; Brown et al., 1973; O'Neal and Poklis, 1996). Harper and Corry (1988) reported the rapid loss of ethanol from unpreserved samples containing high numbers of microbes. They also reported that these losses were much greater when there was a large air space present in the specimen container. This suggested to them that aerobic metabolism was more likely to cause a loss of ethanol than anaerobic metabolism. The loss of ethanol by this mechanism is generally not of major concern in specimens taken from living subjects by aseptic techniques. This is true because a high number of microbes are required to be present for significant ethanol losses to occur and because sodium fluoride is almost always used a preservative to prevent bacterial action. Sodium fluoride has been demonstrated to be effective in preventing ethanol loss from stored specimens (Brown et al., 1973; Winek and Paul, 1983; Dick and Stone, 1987; Amick and Habben, 1997). Dick and Stone (1987) reported the loss of ethanol from specimens from a living subject that had been preserved with 1 percent sodium fluoride and attributed the loss to microbial contamination. Strains of the bacteria *Serratia marcescens* and a *Pseudomonas sp.* were isolated from the specimens. These bacteria were capable of growing at ambient temperature in blood containing 1 percent sodium fluoride. The ability of these organisms to reduce the alcohol concentration of a specimen depended on the storage temperature and the sodium fluoride concentration. The recommendations from this study were that specimens be preserved with 2-percent sodium fluoride and that specimens be stored at refrigeration

temperatures. The loss of ethanol was inhibited by fluoride at 4°C. The authors attributed the presence of bacteria to contamination, which resulted from the use of an automatic pipetting device that contaminated the specimens from living patients with bacteria from postmortem specimens.

D. Recommendations to prevent ethanol loss

An examination of the described mechanism for ethanol loss from biological specimens leads to sound conclusions regarding methods to minimize losses. Blood specimens to be analyzed for ethanol should: (1) contain a chemical preservative, preferably 1-percent sodium fluoride in specimens from living subjects and 1-2 percent for postmortem specimens; (2) be placed in a container that minimizes the air space above the specimens; and (3) be refrigerated as soon as possible.

11.3 Ethanol Gain

An increase in concentration of ethanol in biological specimens is invariably associated with contamination of the specimen. This contamination may take the form of physical contamination or contamination with microorganisms that are capable of producing ethanol. The contamination may take place before, during, or after collection.

A. Physical contamination

Physical contamination is the simplest and most straightforward of the contamination mechanisms and will be discussed first. A recognized source of physical contamination is the use of alcohol containing swabs to disinfect the area of specimen collection in the living patient. This method of specimen contamination is well documented in the literature (Heise, 1959; Taberner, 1989; Goldfinger and Schaber, 1982) with appropriate admonitions against using alcohol swabs for this purpose. Aqueous povidone iodine solutions are often employed for this purpose and are as effective or more so than ethanol for the intended purpose (Ryder and Glick, 1986). The attention that this subject has received in recent years has greatly diminished this mode of contamination in specimens collected for alcohol-related traffic cases, but caution must still be employed when specimens are collected at a hospital for medical purposes and subsequently retrieved for a medical legal investigation. Much to the author's chagrin, he learned that ethanol-containing swabs were used in a local hospital to collect specimens for blood gas analysis. It is also possible to contaminate specimens with isopropanol in a similar fashion.

It is possible to contaminate postmortem specimens with embalming fluids. This type of contamination can occur when a body is embalmed prior to specimen collection or if contaminated syringes or other devices are used to collect the specimen. Although most embalming fluids do not contain ethanol, some do (see Chapter 6 for components of embalming fluids). In addition, all of these fluids contain volatile compounds that may interfere with the analytical process or the interpretive process of blood alcohol analyses. The practice of starting the flow of embalming fluid prior to specimen collection should be strictly avoided. This advice has been given but not always heeded for over forty years (Newbarr and Myers, 1954). Caution should be exercised even when specimens are collected in modern autopsy suites by competent forensic pathologists or pathology assistants. The syringes used for specimen collection should be clean and dry and not contaminated in any manner, including with water.

Another manner in which specimens become contaminated is collection via a transthoracic puncture or blind external chest stick. There is an acute danger of contamination by this technique in cases of trauma, but it can also occur in deaths with no trauma. This type of collection technique is prone to contamination via cardiac fluid or with stomach contents. Logan and Lindholm (1996) and Winek et al. (1995) have reported cases where contamination of this type has caused considerable difficulty. The author has observed purported blood samples collected in this manner that were orange in color, had a pH of 2.0, and smelled like orange juice. Collection of forensic blood specimens via an external chest stick is strongly discouraged.

B. Production of ethanol by microorganisms

Contamination of specimens with microorganisms that results in increases in ethanol concentrations in biological specimens is a more complex subject. It has been recognized for some time that ethanol can

be produced by many different microbes under favorable conditions (Corry, 1978). For significant alcohol to be produced, a microorganism capable of producing alcohol must be present in sufficient numbers, appropriate substrate must be available, and the temperature must be appropriate (Canfield et al., 1993; Corry, 1978).

Experiments with rodents have been performed which illustrate the potential for ethanol to be produced by microorganisms during the putrefaction process (Nicloux, 1935; Davis et al., 1972; Iribe et al., 1974). The data of Davis et al. (1972) is representative of the findings of these experiments. These authors studied the formation of ethanol in the bodies of intact conventional and germfree mice and in stored tissues which were removed immediately after sacrifice from conventional mice. "Conventional mice" refers to mice in which clean but not sterile conditions were used for collection and storage. All three groups were stored at 22°C in sterile, aerated, and humidified containers. Three mice were analyzed on subsequent days to determine the alcohol concentration of various organs. The data presented in Figure 11.1 illustrate the production of alcohol during the storage of conventional mice. Significant amounts of ethanol are detectable in as little as forty-eight hours. While following a general trend to increase with time, there are periods when the alcohol concentration would fall from day to day. There was also a wide range of concentrations among the three individual mice on any given day. The data for ethanol formation in stored organs is also presented in Figure 11.1. The pattern of alcohol formations is quite different from that of the intact mice. Maximal concentrations were achieved much quicker and then rapidly declined in this group as compared to the stored intact mice. There was no alcohol formation in the germ free mice. These data are in general agreement with those of Iribe et al. (1974), who also studied the neoformation of alcohol in decomposing mice. These authors studied the formation of ethanol in mice that had been drowned and stored in water and a second group that had been strangled and allowed to decompose in air. Significant ethanol was detected in both groups with maximal concentrations of approximately 160 mg/dL reached in 8–10 days when the temperature was 25°C. When the tem-

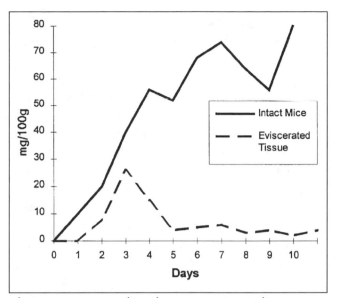

Figure 11.1 *Mean ethanol concentration in liver specimens of decomposing intact mice and decomposing eviscerated liver specimens as a function of time*

perature was 17°C, maximal concentrations were reached 2–5 days later and were somewhat less. After the maximum concentration was reached, the concentrations gradually declined to insignificant concentrations. The data of Davis et al. (1972) and Iribe et al. (1974) are in agreement and illustrate that ethanol can be produced during the putrefaction process, and that the amount of ethanol produced depends on the incubation period, the storage conditions, and the temperature.

The formation of ethanol in human cadavers has been suspected and documented for some time. One of the earliest reports was from Nicloux (1936) who examined several bodies at various postmortem intervals, 17 days–3.5 months, and detected alcohol in concentrations of 40–132 g/100 g in all tissues that were examined. It appeared that certainly three of the five had not consumed alcohol prior to death. Bonnichsen et al. (1953) presented several cases in which it seemed likely that ethanol was a postmortem artifact. These data are presented in Table 11.2. This is one of the earliest reports in which microorganisms capable of producing ethanol were isolated, identified, and thought to be the cause of the observed alcohol concentration. Isolated organisms included *Streptococcus faecalis*, *Candida albicans*, *Saccharomyces sp.*, *Escherichia coli*, *Klebsiella sp.* and *Clostridium perfringens*. The distribution of alcohol in these cases is inconsistent with the known distribution of ethanol after consumption. These authors suggested that multiple specimens might be necessary to properly interpret alcohol concentrations in postmortem specimens. They especially recommended urine as a complementary specimen, for ethanol production in glucose-free urine was deemed unlikely. Plueckhahn (1967) presented evidence from detailed experiments that illustrated the production of ethanol by microorganisms. This author also looked at decomposing specimens and the

Table 11.2
Ethanol Concentration in Various Tissues and Fluids

Tissue	(mg/100g)			
	Case 1	Case 2	Case 3	Case 4
Stomach contents	310	23	***	17
Blood	19	164	0	235
Liver	26	***	***	112
Brain	21	24	31	38
Urine	0	6	***	***
Kidney	***	39	79	107
Muscle	***	***	***	0
Heart	***	***	***	0
Spleen	***	***	***	111
Pleural fluid	230	***	***	***

*** = not performed
Data from Bonnichsen, 1953.

production of ethanol in stored specimens. Several organisms were identified in postmortem specimens and proven to be capable of generating alcohol when inoculated into postmortem specimens. A synopsis of his conclusions from this work as related to the effect of microorganisms is as follows: blood alcohol levels at autopsy are valid up to forty-eight hours after death if simple principles are observed in collection and storage of samples; false blood alcohol levels greater than 200 mg/dL can be generated in autopsy blood samples which are not correctly stored; high blood alcohol levels may develop during putrefaction; alcohols other than ethanol may occur in significant quantities in putrefying bodies; specimens should be stored below 6°C. Plueckhahn and Ballard (1968) and Blackmore (1968) presented additional data identifying additional microorganisms capable of producing alcohol in postmortem specimens. Blackmore (1968) agreed with Bonnichsen et al. (1953) as to the significance of urine as a specimen of choice to evaluate the potential of postmortem generation of alcohol. The subject of ethanol production by microorganisms has been thoroughly reviewed by Corry (1978) and is essential reading for anyone interested in this topic. Currently, it is universally recognized by all toxicologists that ethanol can be produced in decomposing specimens. An overview of the topic has been more recently presented by Mayes (1987), Gilliland and Bost (1993) and O'Neal and Poklis (1996). The latter review thoroughly covers most topics concerning postmortem generation of ethanol.

C. Recognition of postmortem generation of alcohol

The detection of postmortem generation of alcohol has relied on several basic concepts: (1) review of the case history; (2) the concentration of the ethanol; (3) the condition of the specimen; (4) determining that the distribution of ethanol in various tissues and fluids is inconsistent with that in the living subject; (5) detecting the presence of other aliphatic alcohol, acetaldehyde or other volatiles; and (6) culturing postmortem specimens and determining the identity and ethanol-producing capability of any microorganisms that are detected.

A review of the case history is an essential step in the assessment of an alcohol result. For example, significant alcohol in a child or infant, or in any case in which history does not indicate the probability of alcohol consumption should be viewed with caution. Trauma victims may also be prime candidates for postmortem generation of alcohol (Moriya and Hashimoto, 1996 and Moriya and Ishizu, 1994).

There have been attempts to define the maximum amount of alcohol that can be produced by microorganisms with the ultimate goal of determining an alcohol concentration at which one can state without equivocation that alcohol was consumed. Alcohol concentrations of 0.15-0.20 g/dL have been proposed as cutoff concentrations for determining that alcohol was consumed (Bogusz el al., 1970, Spitz and Fisher, 1980). However, Canfield et al. (1993) reported two examples in which these concentrations were exceeded. It should be noted that all of the cases reported on by Canfield et al. were from fatal air crashes. This increases the likelihood of contamination of the specimens. Levine et al. (1993) provided information that at 0.04 g/dL and above, the probability that alcohol was consumed is very high.

The condition of the specimen is an obvious criterion for possible contamination. If the specimen has a bad odor and is discolored, postmortem generation of alcohol is a distinct possibility but not a certainty (Canfield et al., 1993). As previously mentioned, Bonnichsen et al. (1953) and Blackmore (1968) have recommended that urine be used as a complementary specimen to blood in putrefied bodies. The concentration of ethanol in the urine is often negative or much less than that of the concentration in blood or tissue specimens. Zumwalt et al. (1982) analyzed blood and other specimens from 130 decomposing bodies and developed an objective scale for assessing the degree of decomposition, using the acronym "SMELLBAD". They corroborated the utility of urine as an alternate specimen, but pointed out that urine is often not available for postmortem investigation. They presented data to indicate that vitreous fluid is much less contaminated with microorganisms than blood or tissue. The data presented in Table 11.3 support their conclusions that vitreous fluid and urine are very useful to assess the potential

Table 11.3
Cases with Presumed Endogenous Ethanol

	EtOH (mg/dL)		
Case#	Blood	Vitreous	Urine
1	10	neg	***
2	10	neg	***
3	10	neg	***
4	10	neg	***
5	20	***	neg
6	20	***	neg
7	20	neg	***
8	20	neg	neg
9	30	neg	***
10	30	neg	***
11	40	neg	***
12	40	neg	***
13	40	neg	***
14	50	neg	***
15	50	neg	***
16	50	neg	***
17	50	neg	***
18	60	neg	neg
19	70	neg	***
20	110	neg	neg
21	120	***	neg
22	130	neg	***
23	220	***	neg

*** = not performed

for postmortem generation of ethanol. More recent reports have reinforced the utility of vitreous humor and urine as specimens of choice in evaluating postmortem ethanol concentrations (Caplan and Levine, 1990; Levine et al., 1993). Although urine is a very useful specimen, it must be recognized that significant amounts of ethanol can be produced in urine specimens that are contaminated with yeast and also have a high glucose content (Saady et al., 1993).

Decomposition of tissue can produce aliphatic alcohols other than ethanol, acetaldehyde, acetone, and other volatile compounds (Bonnichsen, 1953; Mayes, 1987). The identification of these products has been recommended as a method of determining whether postmortem generation of ethanol has occurred (Kuhlman et al., 1991; Gilliland and Bost, 1993; Mayes et al., 1992). Canfield et al. (1993) have pointed out that the issue may not be as straightforward as it seems. These authors cite cases of postmortem generation of ethanol without the production of other volatiles and cases in which other volatiles were detected without any apparent production of ethanol. In this author's opinion, the presence of other aliphatic alcohols or acetaldehyde in decomposing tissues indicates that some microbiological action has likely taken place and that alcohol results from a single postmortem specimen should viewed with caution. The distribution of ethanol in various fluids and tissues has been studied. Backer (1980) has presented often cited ranges of blood:fluid and blood:tissue ratios. Concentration ratios in decomposing bodies often are very different than the expected ranges. These ratios are often used to assess the likelihood of postmortem production of ethanol (Kuhlman et al., 1991; Gilliland and Bost, 1993; Mayes et al., 1992; Zumwalt et al., 1982).

The detection and identification by microbiological techniques of microorganisms that are capable of producing ethanol in postmortem specimens has been suggested and recommended by Harper and Corry (1988) as a way to determine if postmortem generation of alcohol has occurred. These authors presented elegant experimental details to accomplish this task. Recently, Kupfer et al. (1999) have presented a PCR-based identification of postmortem microbial contamination. Difficulties with this approach are: (1) microorganisms multiply and then decline throughout the storage interval for a specimen and a culture at any one time does not represent the history of the specimen; (2) laboratory conditions do not exactly mimic the conditions to which the body has been subjected; and (3) the expertise to routinely perform this type of procedure does not exist in routine postmortem toxicology laboratories. This approach is seldom used in laboratories in the United States while all the other techniques are routinely utilized.

11.4 Preservation of Biological Specimens

Sodium fluoride has historically been used to prevent microorganisms from causing the loss or gain of ethanol in biological specimens (Newbarr and Myers, 1954). The stability of ethanol concentrations in specimens collected via sterile techniques in living subjects is well documented (Glendening et al., 1965; Brown et al., 1973; Corry, 1978; Dick and Stone, 1987; Winek and Paul, 1983). The concentration of fluoride has varied over time between 0.25–1 percent. The author recommends that 1-percent sodium fluoride be used for preservation of all specimens. The concentration of fluoride used in specimens from living subjects may not be adequate for postmortem specimens, as a result, higher concentrations have been recommended (i.e. 2 percent) (Dick and Stone, 1987). Sodium fluoride has been shown to inhibit most microorganisms except *Candida albicans* (Chang and Kollman, 1989 and Blume and Lakatua, 1973). This reports indicated that at room temperature sodium fluoride did not prevent the production of some ethanol. If the specimens were kept at refrigeration temperature, no ethanol was produced. On the other hand several recent reports indicate that 1-percent sodium fluoride is effi-

cacious in inhibiting *C. albicans* in urine specimens (Jones et al., 1999; Sulkowski et al., 1995; Lough and Fehn, 1993). Other chemical preservatives have been recommended (Bradford, 1966; Smalldon and Brown, 1973; Harper and Corry, 1988), but sodium fluoride is used almost exclusively in the United States. Regardless of the chemical preservative, maintaining the specimens in a refrigerator or freezer will prevent significant post-collection generation of ethanol.

A. Collection of specimens from living subjects

The collection of specimens from living subjects requires attention to detail but is straightforward and relatively simple. Each legal jurisdiction may have specific requirements concerning the collection of specimens from living subjects; obviously, these requirements should be followed exactly as specified. The procedural details listed below are general in nature and are based on the scientific concerns addressed in this chapter.

1. Blood is collected from one of the cubital veins of the forearm.
2. The disinfectant used to clean the arm should not contain ethanol, isopropanol, or other volatile compounds. Povidone iodine solutions have proven effective for this purpose.
3. Sodium fluoride (1 percent) is effective as a preservative.
4. Most driving legislation that concerns ethanol requires the analysis of whole blood. Potassium oxalate or EDTA will suffice as an anticoagulant. Vacuum collection tubes with preservative and anticoagulant that have met the tests of legal challenges are commercially available.
5. After properly labeling the tube with all legally required information, the specimen, a laboratory request form, and a chain of custody form should be sealed in an appropriate container.
6. The specimens and accompanying documents should be sent to the laboratory as soon as possible.
7. On receipt by the laboratory, specimens should be refrigerated by the laboratory and after analysis kept in a frozen or refrigerated state.

B. Collection of postmortem specimens

A blood specimen is always desirable as a postmortem specimen. The collection site of the blood specimen has been a topic of much debate. Early concerns about diffusion of ethanol from the stomach into heart blood (Turkel and Gifford, 1957) prompted concerns about heart blood as a reliable specimen for alcohol analysis, although Plueckhahn and Ballard (1967) dispute the likelihood of this occurring. Harper and Corry (1988) expressed similar reservations about heart blood because it is more likely to be affected by microbiological contamination. On the other hand, Plueckhahn (1967) found no statistical difference between heart blood and femoral blood as related to alcohol content. Similar conclusions were reached by Prouty and Anderson (1987). Briglia et al. (1992) found no statistical difference in heart and femoral blood, but found large differences between heart and femoral blood in individual cases. All of the authors did report considerable differences in concentration of various blood sites in certain conditions (i.e., putrefaction, incomplete absorption of alcohol at the time of death, small specimens in tubes designed for larger specimens, trauma and so on) and in some cases no satisfactory explanation could be offered. These reports all emphasize the need to precisely state the origin of a postmortem blood specimen. Blood from the central cavity (heart, aorta, vena cava and so forth) is routinely collected for drug and alcohol screening in most forensic centers. In cases of suspected contamination or putrefaction, blood from a peripheral site (preferably a femoral vessel), vitreous fluid, and urine are useful, and often necessary complements to central cavity blood specimen. In light of current knowledge, it is recommended that fluid specimens be preserved with 1.5-2 percent sodium fluoride. Specimen collection by thoracic puncture often leads to controversy about potential contamination. It is preferable to take specimens from peripheral sites if no autopsy is performed. Tissue specimens may provide insight into the distribution of alcohol at the time of death as well as insight into the potential for postmortem generation of alcohol. We recommend freezing tissues on receipt. It should be recognized that a positive result from a single isolated tissue specimen from putrefied bodies offers little value in assessing the role of ethanol in an investigation. All specimens should be refrigerated if stored for a period of time before sending to the laboratory. In order to maintain the specimens in the same condition as when received, laboratories should refrigerate specimens on receipt and store them in a frozen state.

11.5 Conclusions

The task of collecting proper specimens in medical legal investigations requires an understanding of the chemical and microbiological process that may affect an analytical result. However, observing a few simple criteria will provide sufficient safeguards to preserve most specimens for a valid alcohol determination. Simply stated, avoid contamination, use proper sized containers, use proper preservatives, and store specimens at appropriate temperatures. In specimens properly collected and preserved from living subjects, the interpretation of results is relatively straightforward. Many additional factors must be considered when interpreting ethanol concentrations in postmortem specimens. Forewarned is forearmed!

References

Amick, G.D. and Habben, K.H. Inhibition of ethanol production by Saccharomyces cerevisiae in human blood by sodium fluoride. *J. Forensic Sci.* 42:690–692, 1997.

Backer, R.C., Pisano, R.V. and Sopher, I.M. The comparison of alcohol concentrations in postmortem fluids and tissues. *J. Forensic Sci.* 25:327–331, 1980.

Blackmore, D.J. The bacterial production of ethyl alcohol. *J. Forensic Sci. Society* 8:73–78, 1968.

Blume, P. and Lakatua, D.J. The effect of microbial contamination of the blood sample on the determination of ethanol levels in serum. *Am. J. Clin. Path.* 60:700–702, 1973.

Bogusz, M., Guminska, M. and Markiewicz, J. Studies of the formation of endogenous ethanol in blood putrefying invitro. *J. Forensic Med.* 17:156–168, 1970.

Bonnichsen, R. et al. Development of ethanol in blood samples and human organs during forensic chemical practice. *Acta Pharmacol. et Toxicol.* 9:352–361, 1953.

Bradford, L.W. Preservation of blood samples containing alcohol. *J. Forensic Sci.* 11:214–216, 1966.

Briglia, E.J., Bidanset, J.H. and Dal Cortivo, L.A. The distribution of ethanol in post–mortem blood specimens. *J. Forensic Sci.* 37:991–998, 1992.

Brown, G.A. et al. The blood, part 1: Important variables and interpretation of results. *Analyt. Chim. Acta* 66:271–283, 1973.

Canfield, D.V., Kupiec, T. and Huffine, E. Postmortem alcohol production in fatal aircraft accidents. *J. Forensic Sci.* 38:914–917, 1993.

Caplan, Y.H. and Levine, B. Vitreous humor in the evaluation of postmortem blood ethanol concentrations. *J. Anal. Toxicol.* 14:305–307, 1990.

Chang, J. and Kollman, S.E. The effect of temperature on the formation of ethanol by Candida albicans in blood. *J. Forensic. Sci.* 34:105–109, 1989.

Chang, R.B. et al. The stability of ethyl alcohol in forensic blood specimens. *J. Anal. Toxicol.* 8:66–67, 1984.

Corry, J.E.L. Possible sources of ethanol ante- and post-mortem: Its relationship to the biochemistry and microbiology of decomposition. *J. Appl. Bacteriology* 44:1–56, 1978.

Davis, G.L., Leffert, R.L. and Rantanen, N.W. Putrefactive ethanol sources in post-mortem tissues of conventional and germ free mice. *Arch. of Path.* 94:71–74, 1972.

Dick, G.L. and Stone, H.M. Alcohol loss arising from microbial contamination of drivers' blood specimens. *Forensic Sci. Int.* 34:17–27, 1987.

Dubowski, K.M., Gadsden, R.H. Sr. and Poklis, A. The stability of ethanol in human whole blood controls: An interlaboratory evaluation. *J. Anal. Toxicol.* 21:486–491, 1997.

Gilliland, M.G.F. and Bost, R.O. Alcohol in decomposed bodies: Postmortem synthesis and distribution. *J. Forensic Sci.* 38:1266–1272,4, 1993.

Glendening, B.L. and Waugh, T.C. The stability of ordinary blood alcohol samples held various periods of time under different conditions. *J. Forensic Sci.* 10:192–200, 1965.

Goldfinger, T.M. and Schaber, D. A comparison of blood alcohol concentration using non-alcohol and alcohol-containing skin antiseptics. *Ann. Emerg. Med.* 11:665–667, 1982.

Harper, D.R. and Corry, J.E.L. Collection and storage of specimens for alcohol analysis. In: Garriott, J.C. (ed.), *Medicolegal Aspects of Alcohol Determination in Biological Specimens.* Littleton, MA: PSG Publishing, 1988, pp. 145–169.

Heise, H.A. How extraneous alcohol affects the blood test for alcohol. Pitfalls to be avoided when withdrawing blood for medicolegal purposes. *Am. J. Clin. Path.* 32:169–170, 1959.

Iribe, K. et al. Relations between production of alcohol from body fluid and LDH activity in decomposition of corpses. *Reports National Research Institute of Police Science*, Tokyo 27:8–11, 1974 (in Japanese, English summary).

Jones, A.W. et al. Storage at 4 degrees C or addition of sodium fluoride (1%) prevents formation of ethanol in urine inoculated with Candida albicans. *J. Anal. Toxicol.* 23:333–336, 1999.

Kuhlman, J.J. et al. Toxicological findings in federal aviation administration general aviation accidents. *J. Forensic Sci.* 36:1121–1128, 1991.

Levine, B. et al. Interpretation of low postmortem concentrations of ethanol. *J. Forensic Sci.* 38:663–667, 1993.

Kupfer, D.M. et al. PCR-based identification of postmortem microbial contaminant: A preliminary study. *J. Forensic. Sci.* 44:592–596, 1999.

Logan, B.K. and Lindholm, G. Gastric contamination of postmortem blood samples during blind–stick sample collection. *Am. J. Forensic Med. Pathol.* 17:109–111, 1996.

Lough, P.S. and Fehn, R. Efficacy of 1% sodium fluoride as a preservative in urine samples containing glucose and Candida albicans. *J. Forensic Sci.* 38:266–271, 1993.

Mayes, R.W. The postmortem production of ethanol and other volatiles. In: *Proceedings of the 24th International Meeting of the International Association of Forensic Toxicologists*, G.R. Jones and P.P. Singer, Banff, Canada, 1987.

Mayes, R.W. et al. Toxilogic findings in the USS Iowa disaster. *J. Forensic Sci.* 37:1352–1357, 1992.

Moriya, F. and Hashimoto, Y. Endogenous ethanol production in trauma victims associated with medical treatment. *Nippon Hoigaku Zasshi.* 50:263–267, 1996.

Moriya, F. and Ishizu, H. Can microorganisms produce alcohol in body cavities of a living person? A case report. *J. Forensic Sci.* 39:883–888, 1994.

Newbarr, F.D. and Myers, R.O. Special aspects and practical considerations of the medicolegal autopsy. In: Gradwohl, R.B.H. (ed.), *Legal Medicine.* St. Louis: C.V. Mosby, 1954, pp. 20–67.

Nicloux, M. Neoformation d'alcool ethylique dans le cadavre humain en voie de putrefaction. *Compte Rendu des Seances de la Societe de Biologie*, Paris 121:975–978, 1936.

Nicloux, M. Sort de l'alcool dans le cadavre d'un mammifere alcoolise. Neoformation d'alcool chez les animaux temoins. *Comptes Rendus des Seances de la Societe de Biologie*, Paris 120:1306–1309, 1935.

O'Neal, C.L. and Poklis, A. Postmortem production of ethanol and factors that influence interpretation. *Am. J. Forensic Med. Pathol.*, 17:8–20, 1996.

Plueckhahn, V.D. The significance of blood alcohol levels at autopsy. *Med. J. of Aust.* 2:118–124, 1967.

Plueckhahn, V.D. and Ballard, B. Factors influencing the significance of blood alcohol levels at autopsy. *Med. J. of Aust.* 1:939–943, 1968.

Prouty, R.W. and Anderson, W.H. A comparison of postmortem heart blood and femoral blood ethyl alcohol concentrations. *J. Anal. Toxicol.* 11:191–197, 1987.

Ryder, K.W. and Glick, M.R. The effect of skin cleansing agents on ethanol results measured with the DuPont automatic clinical analyzer. *J. Forensic Sci.* 31:574–579, 1986.

Saady, J.J., Poklis, A. and Dalton, H.P. Production of urinary ethanol after sample collection. *J. Forensic Sci.* 38:1467–1471, 1993.

Scaplehorn, A.W. Home Office Centr. Res. Establ. Rep. No. 35, 1970.

Smalldon, K.W. and Brown, G.A. The stability of ethanol in stored blood, part 2: The mechanism of ethanol oxidation. *Analyt. Chim. Acta* 66:285–290, 1973.

Spitz, W.U. and Fisher, R.S. *Medicolegal Investigation of Death.* Springfield IL: Charles C. Thomas, 1980, 567–568.

Sulkowski, H.A., Wu, A.H. and McCarter, Y.S. In-vitro production of ethanol in urine by fermentation. *J. Forensic Sci.* 40:990–993, 1995.

Taberner, P.V. A source of error in blood alcohol analysis (Letter). *Alcohol and Alcoholism* 24:489–490, 1989.

Turkel, H.W. and Gifford, H. Erroneous blood alcohol findings at autopsy. *JAMA* 64:1077–1079, 1957.

Winek, C.L. and Paul, L.J. Effect of short-term storage conditions on alcohol concentrations in blood from living human subjects. *Clin. Chem.* 29:1959–1960, 1983.

Winek, C.L. Jr., Winek, C.L. and Wahba, W.W. The role of trauma in postmortem blood alcohol determination. *Forensic Sci. Int.* 74:213–214, 1995.

Zumwalt, R.E., Bost, R.O. and Sunshine, I. Evaluation
    of ethanol concentrations in decomposed bodies. *J.
    Forensic Sci.* 27:549–554, 1982.

Chapter 12

Reporting of Laboratory Results

James C. Garriott, Ph.D.

Results of analyses for ethyl alcohol are used regularly in the courts for various types of litigation (as in prosecution of the drinking driver), in medicine, for evaluation and treatment of the patient, and in other forensic settings, such as evaluation of cause of death in autopsy cases.

Since legal limits for driving under the influence are defined by the concentration of alcohol in the blood or breath, it is essential to report findings uniformly and accurately, as well as to include adequate documentation of chain of custody for acceptability in courts of law.

12.1 Analysis Specificity

Any forensic analysis for ethyl alcohol must be performed by a procedure that is specific for ethyl alcohol, to the exclusion of any other interfering substances. Methods and methodologic considerations have been discussed in Chapters 8 and 9. Although oxidation and enzyme procedures have long been used for ethyl alcohol determinations, and are currently used in many clinical laboratories, these methods do not involve separation of the analyte prior to measurement, and are not totally exclusive.

The methods now uniformly accepted for forensic alcohol analysis utilize gas liquid chromatography. It is generally accepted that the only other volatile substances present in the blood of human sub-jects at concentrations similar to those encountered for ethyl alcohol, and with the potential for eluting from the column in the same retention time range as ethyl alcohol or with sufficient volatility to potentially interfere with breath analysis are: acetone, acetaldehyde, methanol, isopropanol, and paraldehyde (Mason and Dubowski, 1974). Although a few others have been reported (e.g., acetonitrile, ethyl chloride), these are highly toxic, and would be encountered rarely under special circumstances only. Thus any forensic method for ethyl alcohol must properly separate these potentially interfering agents, to rule out any possible coelution in gas chromatography or interference by cross-reactivity when using enzyme or oxidation techniques.

12.2 Uniformity of Reporting Blood
A. Blood

In the United States, designation of ethyl alcohol concentrations in blood is usually in conformance with state laws. Since most statutes express alcohol concentration in "percent weight/volume" concentration units, the blood concentration is expressed as grams (of ethyl alcohol) per 100 milliliters of blood, and often, "wt/vol" is written after this result. Another commonly used concentration unit is milligrams per deciliter, or mg/dL, mostly used by clinical laboratories. This unit of concentration is easily converted to grams per 100 mL by dividing by 1,000.

If the units are to be expressed as weight/weight (wt/wt), a slight correction must be made to convert the volume in milliliters to weight in grams. Thus one divides the figure in wt/vol by 1.055, the average specific gravity of blood (American Medical Association, 1968; Jones, 1992).

In Scandinavia and Germany, the concentration unit "per mille" is often used. This designation is by weight, and refers to milligrams of alcohol per gram of blood, or grams of alcohol per 1,000 grams (kilogram) of blood. This unit is approximately equivalent to the percent wt/vol when the former is divided by ten. However, a slight correction factor is necessary, because one milliliter of blood weighs on average 1.055 grams (e.g., 0.10% wt/vol = 0.948%. [per mille]) (Widmark, 1981; Jones, 1992). Examples of reporting unit variations used are given in Table 12.1.

The units discussed above use conventional metric units. Beginning in July, 1986, the *Journal of the American Medical Association* (*JAMA*), following recommendations of the American National Metric Council, began reporting all drug concentrations in conformance with the *Système International d'Unitès* (SI) (International System of Units), adding conventional units in parentheses to aid in the transition. Beginning July 1, 1988, SI units were used exclusively in *JAMA*, and its nine AMA specialty journals (Lundberg, 1986; Lundberg, 1988). However, in both the United States and in Western Europe, forensic scientists and journals have not followed the lead of the medical journals, and metric units continue to be used universally for forensic alcohol reporting. The *JAMA* as well as the *New England Journal of Medicine* (*NEJM*) have now reverted to the use of conventional metric units with SI units expressed secondarily (in parentheses) (*JAMA*, Instructions for Authors, Jan, 2003; *NEJM*, Instructions for Submission). Nevertheless, forensic scientists, as well as physicians, should be prepared to use and interpret the international (SI) units for alcohol concentrations.

The SI unit for alcohol (as with other drugs) bears no resemblance to the conventional metric units now used. The SI unit for alcohol is expressed as millimoles per liter (mmol/L) and signifies the number of molecular weight units of alcohol (1 mole) per liter of volume. The molecular weight of alcohol is 46.07. The conversion factor becomes 217.1, for converting the customary legal alcohol concentration unit of grams percent (or gm/dL), and 0.2171 to convert mg/dL. Thus, 0.10 percent (wt/vol) of ethyl alcohol in blood is equivalent to 21.71 mmol/L (See Table 12.2) (Lundberg, 1986).

Caution must be used when converting clinical alcohol values for forensic purposes, since hospitals and clinical laboratories almost always use plasma or serum for alcohol analysis. These fractions of blood contain more water than blood proportionally, and therefore have higher concentrations of alcohol than whole blood (see Chapter 5).

B. Breath

Formerly, measured breath alcohol concentrations were reported as blood concentrations by use of a conversion factor of 2,100:1, presuming that 2,100 mL of alveolar breath contained the same quantity of alcohol as 1.0 mL of blood. Variabilities in this ratio can exist, however, and it is now considered more accurate to report breath alcohol as an actual mass to volume unit in breath. In the U.S., alcohol concentrations as determined by breath testing are reported

Table 12.1
Concentrations of Alcohol (Ethanol) in Whole Blood for Legal Purposes

Concentration Unit	Country	Legal Limit
Percent weight/volume (% w/v)	United States[*]	0.08–0.10 g/100 mL
Milligrams per 100 milliliter (mg/dL)	Great Britain	80 mg/100 mL
Milligrams per milliliter (mg/mL)	Netherlands	0.50 mg/mL
Milligrams per gram (mg/g)	Sweden	0.20 mg/g
Milligrams per gram (mg/g)	Norway	0.20 mg/g

[*] 33 states including the District of Columbia have lowered the legal limit for driving to 0.08 g/100 mL (0.08 g/dL)

Source: Insurance Institute for Highway Safety, 2003; A.W. Jones, 2003.

Table 12.2
Units for Expressing Ethyl Alcohol Concentrations

Conventional metric units

0.10% (wt/vol) = 0.10 g/100 mL of blood =
100 mg% = 100 mg/dL = 1,000 ppm =
0.0948% (wt/wt) = 0.948 %. (per mille, mg/g,
g/kg, wt/wt) = 1.00 g/L

SI units

0.10% (wt/vol) = 21.71 mmol/L (46.07 = mol wt
of ethyl alcohol)

---

as grams per 210 liters of breath. For most purposes, this quantity is equivalent to a blood concentration in g/100 mL. Thus, 0.15 g/210 L as a breath concentration would be the same as 0.15 g/dL or g/100 mL of blood, assuming a blood/breath ratio of 2,100:1. More recent research indicates that a ratio 2,300:1 provides a more accurate correlation of breath with blood alcohol concentrations, although even higher ratios may apply, generally giving the advantage to the subject when interpreting a breath alcohol as a blood value (See Jones, Chapter 3). In Britain, use of this factor results in a legal standard of 35 μg/100 mL of breath, equivalent to the legal limit for blood concentration of 80 mg/100 mL of blood (Jones, 1995).

12.3 Chain of Custody

Principles of chain of custody of evidence are discussed in Chapter 10. The chain of custody must be clearly documented when reporting results of forensic alcohol examinations. Generally, the laboratory's official chain of custody begins with the arrival of the sample in the laboratory. The report of the analysis should include the date and time of arrival of the sample (most conveniently by a date stamp on the report form); the deliverer's signature or initials, the receiving person's signature, a brief description of the evidence, date of completion, and results. Of course, the units of measurement should be clearly indicated (e.g., "the blood contained 0.15 % wt/vol ethyl alcohol").

12.4 Other Considerations for Reporting Results

It is often desirable to further elucidate the criteria used for alcohol analysis. The method used for the analysis can be referred to simply as "gas chromatography" or "headspace gas chromatography." Since many laboratories use their own procedures or their own modifications of published procedures, it is not practical to refer to a specific procedure in reporting results. However, the laboratory should always be prepared and willing to provide a copy of the actual procedure used, if the laboratory analysis is to be used in litigation. The accuracy and confidence limits of the procedure used should also be known. For example, if a laboratory reports a blood alcohol of 0.11 g/dL and the method shows large variability or has poor accuracy or precision, this single blood alcohol analysis may not be sufficient prima facie evidence for conviction of driving while intoxicated in a state whose limit for intoxication is 0.10 g/dL.

It also may be desirable to define the limits of detectability for the analyte, alcohol. A negative result may be reported if the amount found was less than 0.01 g/dL or in some cases 0.02 g/dL. If such limits are used as laboratory policy, this should also be stated.

References

American Medical Association Committee on Medicolegal Problems. *Alcohol and the Impaired Driver. A Manual on the Medicolegal Aspects of Chemical Tests for Intoxication*. Chicago: American Medical Association, 1968.

Insurance Institute for Highway Safety. *DUI/DWI Laws as of July 2002, State Law Facts, 2002*. Arlington, VA: Insurance Institute for Highway Safety, November, 2002.

Jones, A.W. Blood and breath alcohol concentrations. *Brit. Med. J.* 305:955, 1992.

Jones, A.W. Blood alcohol concentration, measures of. In: Jaffe, J. (ed.), *Encyclopedia of Drugs and Alcohol*. NY: MacMillan, 1995, pp 164–167.

Lundberg, G.D., Iverson, C. and Radulescu, G. Now read this: The SI Units are here. *JAMA* 255:2329–2338, 1986.

Lundberg, G.D. SI unit implementation: The next step. *JAMA* 260:73–76, 1988.

Mason, M.F. and Dubowski, K.M. Alcohol, traffic, and chemical testing in the United States: A resume and some remaining problems. *Clin. Chem.* 20: 126–140, 1974.

Widmark, E.M.P. *Theoretical Foundations and the Practical Application of Forensic-Medical Alcohol Determination*. Berlin: Wein, Urban and Schwartzenberg, 1932. (English translation published as *Principles and Applications of Medicolegal Alcohol Determination*. Davis, CA: Biomedical Publications, 1981.)

Chapter 13

Alcohol Effects and Driver Impairment

Herbert Moskowitz, Ph.D.

13.1 Introduction

Forensic professionals are most frequently called on to discuss the effects of alcohol in court cases involving motor vehicle driving. This chapter will summarize the literature on the epidemiological and behavioral experimental studies dealing with driving related behavior. It should be noted, however, that alcohol plays a major influence in mortality and morbidity in other areas of activity. For example, in the *Sixth Special Report to the U.S. Congress on Alcohol and Health* (1987), it was noted that in 1980 there were more than 25,000 motor vehicle deaths attributable to alcohol, more than 21,000 to violence, more than 3,000 attributable to falls and 1,500 roughly in fires. In a 1993 paper Ralph Hingson and Jonathan Howland performed an extensive review of the literature and found that studies on alcohol involvement in falls, drowning and burns indicated that between 21 to 77 percent of the fatals had been drinking and between 18 and 53 percent of the injured had been drinking. Thus, there is evidence for massive overrepresentation of alcohol in many areas of non-intended injury. Unfortunately, the mechanism by which alcohol produces these increased injuries and fatalities in these situations has not been as thoroughly investigated as has the effects of alcohol in motor vehicle collisions. The forensic professional called to comment on the role of alcohol in non-motor vehicle accidents has to examine a much broader range of material than will be covered in this chapter. For example, memory is affected by alcohol and is an important component of aircraft control, but this chapter, which is devoted to motor vehicle related impairments, will have no discussion of that.

It was 1904 when a journal first reported an association between alcohol use and automobile collisions. More than six decades later, the U.S. Department of Transportation (1968) presented a report to Congress on alcohol and highway safety that stimulated a national program to reduce drinking and driving. The 1968 report estimated 25,000 alcohol-related driving deaths and 800,000 alcohol related collisions in the U.S. annually. Although the ensuing thirty-plus years of countermeasures have shown a significant drop in alcohol-related driving, collisions, and fatalities, alcohol still remains the single leading factor in serious injuries and fatalities on the road. Our most reliable source of information on alcohol-related crashes comes from the Fatality Analysis Reporting System (FARS, 1997) of the National Highway Traffic Safety Administration (NHTSA). In 1982, 56.7 percent of fatal collisions had alcohol involvement, a figure that dropped to 39.9 percent by 1996 (Burgess and Lindsey, 1998). These figures are conservative since they do not take into account hit-and-run collisions, which studies indicate have a preponderance of intoxicated drivers.

13.2 Alcohol Use while Driving

The decrease in the alcohol-related fatality rate is paralleled by a corresponding decrease in the number of drivers on the roads with alcohol present. The latter is determined by roadside surveys and studies where drivers are randomly stopped and requested to submit a breath sample under promises of confidentiality. Lund and Wolfe (1991) compared nationwide roadside surveys performed in 1973 and 1986 and reported that drivers on the road with a positive blood alcohol concentration (BAC) declined by more than 25 percent. Voas et al. (1998) reported on a 1996 National Roadside Survey showing continued decline with positive BACs on the road decreasing 53 percent from 1973. These figures refer to weekend, nighttime drivers between the hours of 10:00 P.M. and 3:00 A.M., which is when the greatest frequency of drinking-driving occurs. In the period from 1973 to 1986, the decline in drivers on the road was roughly equivalent for all blood alcohol levels. However, in 1996 the decline from 1986 was almost wholly in drivers below BACs of 0.05 grams per deciliter (g/dL). The decline for drivers above 0.05 g/dL was statistically insignificant, suggesting a problem in convincing the remaining heavy drinkers not to drive. The decline in drinking-driving was greatest among under-twenty-one-year-olds, perhaps because many countermeasure programs had been aimed at this age group. The most resistant group to changing drinking-driving behavior has been the 21–34 age group. The large decrease in alcohol-related driving occurred during a twenty-three-year period (1973–1996) in which average per capita alcohol consumption in the United States decreased by only 15 percent. Additional evidence that drinking and driving has declined in the United States is shown by the decrease in the number of arrests for driving under the influence of alcohol (DUI) from 1,921,100 in 1983 to 1,467,300 in 1996, despite increased law enforcement activities (Greenfield, 1998). Clearly, both attitudes and behavior regarding drinking and driving have been changed. A major influence on the attitudes of the public and legislators regarding drinking and driving has been studies which have established the probability of collisions at different BAC levels. The dominant belief of the public and public officials from the turn of the century to the 1940s was that alcohol-related traffic collisions were the consequence of gross intoxication and massive excessive drinking.

13.3 Alcohol and Accidents

The development of portable breath testing devices in the 1950s permitted a quantitative approach to examining the relationship between BAC levels and crash probabilities. Utilizing the then new technology, several case control epidemiological studies were performed worldwide. The largest such study occurred in Grand Rapids, Michigan, and compared breath alcohol levels in roughly 6,000 crash-involved drivers with roughly 7,600 non-accident-involved control drivers (Borkenstein et al., 1964). For a year, with police cooperation, research personnel raced to the sites of most traffic collisions in Grand Rapids. Assisted by agreement from the State Attorney General on the confidentiality of information and testing results, the researchers were able to persuade most drivers to provide both a breath sample and a completed questionnaire. At similar sites non-accident-involved control drivers were stopped by police officers. They were asked to provide breath samples and fill out a questionnaire, again with agreements for confidentiality. The probability of involvement in a collision was then determined for each BAC level by comparing the relative number of collision-involved drivers at that BAC level in the crash group with the relative number of non-collision-involved drivers at that BAC level in the control group.

The Grand Rapids study indicated that the relationship between the probability of causing an accident and the BAC level was a sharply rising exponential function. At 0.10 g/dL BAC there was a roughly 600 percent increase in crash causality compared with the crash rate for drivers with 0 g/dL BAC. At 0.15 g/dL BAC the increased crash causality was 2,500 percent. It was discovered that the effects of alcohol in increasing crash causality was not uniform for all individuals. Young drivers, age sixteen and seventeen, increased crash causality almost 500 percent with BAC levels below 0.04 g/dL. At every BAC level, both drivers under twenty-one and over seventy years of age had greater crash causality than drivers age 25–45. There was also a variation in collision causality with alcohol level as a function of the frequency with which drivers consumed alcohol. Drivers drinking daily had a lower crash frequency at every BAC level compared to drivers drinking once a week or less frequently. It should be noted that we are discussing the probability rate of causing an accident at a given BAC level among different drinking classifications. While the probability of causing a collision is greater at any given BAC level for infrequent drinkers, these drinkers drink less frequently and therefore are less likely to be involved in collisions. Heavy drinkers drink more frequently and thus are more likely to be involved in collisions, and have a greater crash rate, even though at any given BAC level at each drinking episode, they are less likely to be involved in an accident than infrequent drinkers.

One aspect of the Grand Rapids report, which created some confusion, was the statement that it found no increase in crash causality for alcohol levels below 0.04 g/dL compared to zero BAC. In fact, the report suggested that drivers might even do better at those lower levels. However, this aspect of the statistical analysis of the Grand Rapids data was rebutted by many researchers including Allsop (1966) Hurst (1973) and others. Their criticism of the Grand Rapids study was based on the failure of the study to compensate for factors other than alcohol which determine crash rates between the zero BAC group and the positive BAC groups. Collision probabilities at each BAC level are calculated by comparing the rate of crashes among drivers with no alcohol (i.e., zero BAC) with the rate of crashes among drivers at various BAC levels. For a valid comparison, it is required that the zero BAC alcohol group share similar characteristics, at least, in all characteristics which influence the rate of collisions, to the positive BAC group other than the level of alcohol. For example, in the Grand Rapids study, the zero BAC group had a greater proportion of both young and older drivers compared to the proportion of the young and older drivers in the positive alcohol groups. Both young and older drivers have much higher crash rates per mile even without alcohol present than do drivers age 25–55. There was a larger proportion of 25–55-year-olds in the positive BAC level groups than there was in the zero BAC group. Other group differences that are important in affecting crash rates include educational level, number of miles driven, occupational level, and frequency of drinking, which were all unequally distributed among BAC groups. Deter-

mining the relationship between BAC level and crash probability in complex epidemiological studies requires controlling for the relative presence of all the group differences which affect crash rates. This in turn requires more sophisticated statistical techniques than were used by the Grand Rapids study.

What is required in order to have a meaningful comparison is to have common characteristics in the drivers in the zero BAC group as in the higher BAC level group. The Grand Rapids data report was reanalyzed by Allsop (1966), Hurst (1973) and Zylman (1973). An example of such reanalysis is shown in Figure 13. 1 (Hurst, 1973) indicating the relative probability of crash involvement as a function of BAC level, but separately for five classifications of drinking frequency. Relative probability refers to the probability of crash involvement for each subgroup (e.g., daily drinkers) in comparison to the overall crash probability of all drivers at zero BAC being defined as a probability of one. Several interesting findings can be noted in the figure. For drivers at the zero BAC level there is a wide discrepancy in accident rates, by a ratio of more than 3:1. At zero BAC level daily drinkers had the lowest accident rate compared to weekly, monthly, or yearly drinkers. This paradoxical finding is easily explained. There is

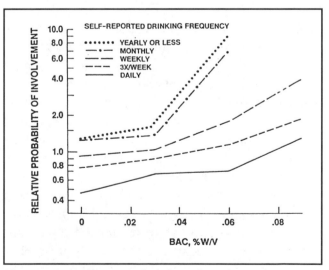

Figure 13.1 *Relative probability of crash involvement by self-reported drinking frequency. Reprinted from* Journal of Safety Research, *Vol. 5, No. 3, Hurst,* Epidemiological aspects of alcohol in driver crashes and citations, ©1973, with permission from Elsevier Science.

a large correlation between age and drinking frequency. Young or old drivers tend not to drink daily,
and yet these drivers have a higher accident rate than
25–55-year-olds who might be drinking daily.

It should also be noted that once we have separated the drinking frequency groups, for each category of drinking frequency the probability of involvement in collision increases with any departure
from zero BAC. In addition, the rate of increase of
collision probability with increasing BAC is greatest
for the least frequent drinkers and slower for the
most frequent drinkers. Properly analyzing epidemiological data in a situation where the dependent
variable (collision rate or collision probability) is
determined not only by varying levels of alcohol, but
by age, sex, drinking frequency, drinking history,
education, annual driving mileage and so on requires
complex analytical techniques. Techniques such as
logistic regression and so on were less available in
1964.

After an interlude of almost forty years, the U.S.
Department of Transportation sponsored another
major epidemiological study of alcohol influence on
crash probability, collecting data from two cities,
Long Beach, California and Fort Lauderdale,
Florida, each for more than a twelve-month period.
A preliminary report of the study by Moskowitz,
Blomberg, Burns, Fiorentino and Peck (2002) was
presented at the 16th International Conference on
Alcohol, Drugs and Traffic Safety. In both cities,
teams of officers and researchers went to the scene
of traffic collisions to obtain breath alcohol samples
and to complete questionnaires for the involved drivers. This occurred for eight hours, from late afternoon to early morning, seven days a week. The study
sample included more than 4,900 crash drivers and
over 10,000 control drivers.

The study design represented an improvement
over prior studies, such as the Grand Rapids Study,
in that the control drivers were sampled at the same
site and time and in the same direction of travel as
the original crash drivers. Two control drivers were
obtained for each crash driver one week later. A notable improvement in the study's design was that,
unlike any other prior epidemiological study, extensive efforts were made to capture as many hit-run
drivers as police exertions could obtain. Moreover,

through the use of passive alcohol sensors, BAC estimates were obtained even for drivers who refused to
participate. These factors proved important since
more than 69 percent of the apprehended hit-run
drivers had positive BACs, typically in the higher
ranges.

Moreover, almost 50 percent of the crash drivers
who refused to participate had positive BACs in contrast to fewer than 16 percent of the control drivers
who refused to participate. This study revealed a
major methodological problem in all the preceding
epidemiological studies of alcohol involvement in
crashes. If it had not been for the apprehension of
some 20 percent of the hit-runs, enabling estimates
of alcohol presence among the hit-run drivers, and
the use of the passive alcohol detectors to determine
alcohol presence in drivers who refused to participate, it was estimated that more than 46 percent of
all drivers involved in crashes who had positive
blood alcohol would not have been detected.

In addition to these improved sampling procedures obtaining information on the presence of alcohol in crash and control drivers, the new study applied logistic regression analysis to adjust the control and crash samples for variation in age, sex,
drinking practice history and so on. Thus, an improved analysis was obtained of the probability of
crash involvement as a function of BAC. The results
indicated that crash probability increased for alcohol
involved drivers at all BAC levels including .01 g/dL
onward. Further, the crash probabilities by BAC
were considerably greater for accident involvement
than in any other prior study. The final complete report is expected to be published in 2003 by the U.S.
Department of Transportation.

13.4 Single-Vehicle Collisions

The Grand Rapids study reported that the probability
of a single vehicle collision at various BAC levels
was greater than that of a multiple-vehicle collision.
That finding was supported by reports in the 1950s
and 1960s that roughly 70 percent of fatally injured
drivers in single-vehicle collisions had alcohol
present (NHTSA, 1997). In 1996, 53.7 percent of fatally injured single vehicle collision drivers had alcohol present. This contrasts sharply with the 1996
figure for fatally injured drivers in multiple-vehicle

crashes, where only 21.9 percent had alcohol present. Since the probability of involvement in a multiple car collision is determined by the behavior of two or more drivers, the lower alcohol multiple-vehicle collision rate is likely a result of the avoidance ability of the non-alcohol impaired driver. Zador (1991) argues that only single-vehicle crashes provide a true measure of the contribution of alcohol to increasing the rate of crash involvement, due to the avoidance component of the nonimpaired driver in multiple vehicle collisions. Zador examined the probability of fatal alcohol-related single vehicle crashes as a function of driver age and sex using data from the FARS files of the National Highway Traffic Safety Administration. Both age and sex were important components of alcohol-related fatal collision rates. For the fatal alcohol collision rate, ignoring the age and sex factors, Zador determined that 0.02–0.04 g/dL BAC increased fatal crash involvement by 40 percent. BACs between 0.05 and 0.09 g/dL increased fatal crash involvement by 1,100 percent. BACs between 0.10 and 0.14 g/dL increased fatal collision probability by 4,800 percent, and at or above 0.15 g/dL, fatal collision rates increased by 38,000 percent. Thus, the role of alcohol in fatal crash causation is even greater than the Grand Rapids report suggested for all collisions.

13.5 Subjective Measures of Impairment

Impairment is defined here as any change in performance level from that exhibited at zero BAC. Impairment is not the same as intoxication. Dictionaries note two or more definitions of intoxication (*Webster's*, 1976). One definition is poisoning or any abnormal state produced by a chemical agent. Other definitions use terms such as "drunk," "inebriation," "strong excitement of mind or feelings," and "enthusiasm, frenzy or madness." These latter definitions of intoxication are consistent with the use of the term by the lay public. If the lay public's definition of intoxication is used, which implies obvious signs of lack of judgment, self-control and motor skills, there is less correlation to either collision rate or impaired driving than is found with BAC level. Widmark, 1981, reported on the experience in Sweden of testing drivers arrested for behaviors suggesting being under the influence of alcohol. Swedish law required

these drivers to be tested at the police station by physicians on a seven-item behavioral test battery. Even at 0.15 BAC physicians assessed only 50 percent of the arrested drivers as being under the influence. In fact, the physicians considered all drivers as under the influence only when arrested drivers were above 0.26 g/dL. There were many cases in Widmark's monograph of individuals arrested for aberrant driving who were at a BAC level above 0.20 g/dL, yet were declared by physicians as not under the influence. Similar results were reported by Perper et al. (1986). Eighty-seven patients entering an alcohol treatment program with positive blood alcohol concentrations were administered a behavioral test battery. Twenty-four percent of the subjects at a 0.20 g/dL or higher showed no evidence of intoxication. Twenty-six percent of the patients with BACs of 0.30 g/dL or higher passed many behavioral tests, although not all. Urso (1981) had physicians grade patients in a Pittsburgh hospital emergency room on several simple behavioral tests and judge them as either intoxicated or nonintoxicated. Patients considered nonintoxicated had blood samples obtained on discharge from the emergency room. Those patients who were evaluated as being sober, but who nevertheless had alcohol present, were found to have a mean BAC level of 0.272 g/dL. One patient declared nonintoxicated had achieved a 0.54 g/dL BAC level. It is not only physicians who have difficulty assessing intoxication. Police officers have a similar problem. The probability of a police officer (Borkenstein, Trubitt and Lease, 1963) detecting drivers on the road whose BACs are above the legal limit is estimated to be far below 1 percent. Moreover, even in situations in which the officer has a direct personal interaction, behavioral intoxication may not be apparent. Wells et al. (1997) examined police ability to detect impairment at a series of sobriety checkpoints in North Carolina. When drivers were cleared by the police as presumably not under the influence, researchers requested breath samples for BAC analysis under a pledge of confidentiality. The findings for the released drivers were compared with the arrested drivers. Eighty-seven percent of drivers between 0.05–0.079 g/dL were not arrested; 62 percent of those between 0.08–0.99 g/dL were not arrested; 64 percent of those between 0.10–0.119 g/dL were not arrested, as were 62 percent of those at or above 0.12 g/dL. Clearly it is difficult for trained observers, police or physicians, to determine whether alcohol impairment is present in a driver relying only on simple observations or verbal interrogations.

13.6 Driving Abilities Impaired by Alcohol

As noted above, many drivers do not exhibit obvious intoxication even at high BACs, which contrasts with their impairment under alcohol when tested on objectively measured driving-related performance tasks. Examples of such tasks are driving simulators, instrumented vehicles on closed courses or laboratory tasks. Eighty-five to 90 percent of drivers in the region of 0.08–0.10 g/dL are successfully identified when using the U.S. Department of Transportation recognized sobriety tests, developed by Burns and Moskowitz (1977). Individuals tested under the influence of alcohol in hospitals, police stations, or roadside situations are not subjected to the demand for skills performance that driving requires. Moreover, some individuals appear to compensate for a short time for some alcohol-produced deficits.

It is perhaps the motion picture industry that has created the impression that alcohol impaired driving is associated with intoxication, such as gross motor impairment. Human factors failure, defined as the skills required in a man-machine interaction situation, is the dominant or major cause of 90 percent of auto collisions. In an Indiana University study of accident causation factors, Treat (1980) found decision and recognition errors (improper lookout, distraction, improper evasive action, inattention and excessive speed) as the causal factor in the majority of the accidents. Performance errors were a factor in roughly 10 percent of the collisions. Only looking at motor impairment in drivers under the influence of alcohol to determine if they are impaired drivers misses the effects of alcohol on cognitive factors such as attention, recognition, and decisions, the major collision factors. Thus, a study in Birmingham, England of accident causation factors (Clayton, 1972) reported that 90 percent of the alcohol-related cases fell into the categories of either perceptual error, decision error, or excessive speed. Excessive speed could perhaps be best described as a judgment error.

Epidemiological studies such as the Grand Rapids study, which used case control methods where crash participants are compared with noncrash control drivers, are extraordinarily expensive to perform. They require police and research teams to rush to the scenes of collisions and gather data. Thus, the last half-century has seen only a dozen case control studies of alcohol factors in traffic crashes throughout the world. Other epidemiological studies are those that rely on secondary sources of data such as police reports or coroners' reports. However, the epidemiological studies are complemented by the thousands of experimental studies examining the effects of alcohol at various BAC levels on driving-related skills performance in laboratories, driving simulators, closed courses, and even occasionally in instrumented cars on the public highway. An extensive review (Moskowitz and Robinson, 1988) of the experimental scientific literature on driving-related skills under alcohol levels of 0.10 g/dL or lower concluded that there is near universal impairment of most skills required for driving, even at low BACs. In contrast to the variability of subjective assessment of intoxication or impairment of individuals under the influence of alcohol, the experimental literature reveals impairment of nearly all significant man-machine interaction skills, differing only in the magnitude of the impairment as a function of BAC level, and the BAC level at which impairment first became significant. Of the behavioral variables examined in the Moskowitz and Robinson (1988) review, the ability to divide attention was the behavioral function most frequently impaired at the lowest BAC levels.

Division of attention is a description of the brain's ability to monitor and respond to more than one source of information or task at the same apparent time. Most skills performance tasks in modern society, such as driving, flying, or performing industrial work, typically require this ability. As Stephens and Michaels (1963) have noted, driving is primarily a timed-shared activity between a compensatory tracking task (i.e,. car control) and a visual search and recognition task for potential dangers. This chapter will not discuss the debate on whether this ability represents a simultaneous monitoring of two tasks or a rapid shifting between the time-shared activities. But it has been increasingly clear that one of the major requirements for a safe traffic system is keeping the mental workload required for driving within the limits of human capacity. Any stressor such as alcohol, drugs, or fatigue, which limits the capacity of the human brain to rapidly monitor the various aspects of the driving task, will serve to decrease the safety margin. A study by Moskowitz, Burns and Williams (1985) demonstrated that divided attention performance was impaired for all subjects in the study at a 0.015 g/dL BAC level, roughly the equivalent of consuming between one-half and three-fourths of a can of beer. Since mental workload and its distribution, which is involved in the ability to divide attention, is a component of nearly all studies, it is important to isolate the effects of alcohol on divided attention from the effects on the components of the task which are the constituent members of the divided attention task. For example, Chiles and Jennings (1969), in a series of studies performed for the Federal Aviation Administration, examined the effects of alcohol on performance in a compensatory tracking task while the subjects were simultaneously but intermittently, required to perform a series of subsidiary tasks. The study was performed at BACs near 0.10 g/dL. Because the subsidiary tasks were intermittent the authors were able to analyze tracking performance with and without the presence of the subsidiary task. They noted that "the results of these tests showed that for no measure of the several measures of tracking was tracking significantly affected by alcohol when tracking was performed by itself" (Chiles and Jennings, 1969, p. 8). On the other hand, tracking was impaired by alcohol when the subject was concurrently performing the subsidiary task. The authors concluded that "a decrease in the ability of the subjects to timeshare the performance of tasks, requiring the exercise of different psychological functions may be the most detrimental effect of alcohol on trained subjects. Motor effects may be somewhat less important" (p. 9). A study by Moskowitz and Sharma (1974) examined the issue further. This study examined the effect of three levels of alcohol, including placebo, on the ability to detect lights in peripheral vision under three conditions of mental workload of central vision. The subjects sat facing a 204-degree visual arc

with a central fixation light surrounded by thirty-two peripheral lights at six-degree intervals.

There were three central visual conditions with the fixation light being either unblinking, blinking at a low rate or blinking at a fast rate. The subjects were required to fixate their central vision on this light and, at a tone signal presented every twenty seconds, report the number of light blinks during that period. At the same time, they were required to report whenever a peripheral light signal appeared at any of the thirty-two peripheral points. The alcohol dosages used produced mean BAC levels of 0.0 g/dL for placebo, 0.06 g/dL for the lower dose, and 0.09 g/dL for the higher alcohol dose. Figure 13.2 presents the percent of failures in detecting peripheral lights as a function of the angle at which the peripheral light was present. The angles are counted inward from a pretest measurement of each subject's static peripheral limit. As the top graph suggests, when the central fixation light was not blinking, there was no effect of the two active alcohol doses on the ability of subjects to detect the light presentations in peripheral vision. However, the second and third graphs demonstrate that when the central fixation light required a mental load (i.e., the subjects were required to count the blinking fixation light and simultaneously detect peripheral lights) alcohol produced a large and significant impairment of the ability to detect the peripheral light. Note that increasing the alcohol dose produced a greater degree of impairment and that increasing the mental workload also produced a greater increase in the impairment produced by alcohol. The two factors interacted. Thus, the number of errors in counting the fixation blinks increased with alcohol dosage and with greater mental workload.

The Moskowitz and Sharma (1974) study failed to demonstrate impairment of peripheral vision at roughly 0.10 g/dL BAC unless a subsidiary test was present. The result agrees with the Chiles and Jennings (1969) study, which similarly failed to find impairment of a tracking task at 0.10 g/dL without a subsidiary task. Both studies illustrate why there is frequent lack of agreement between studies on behavioral functions under alcohol in the older literature, where investigators were unaware of the potential effects of alcohol on cognitive function. Experi-

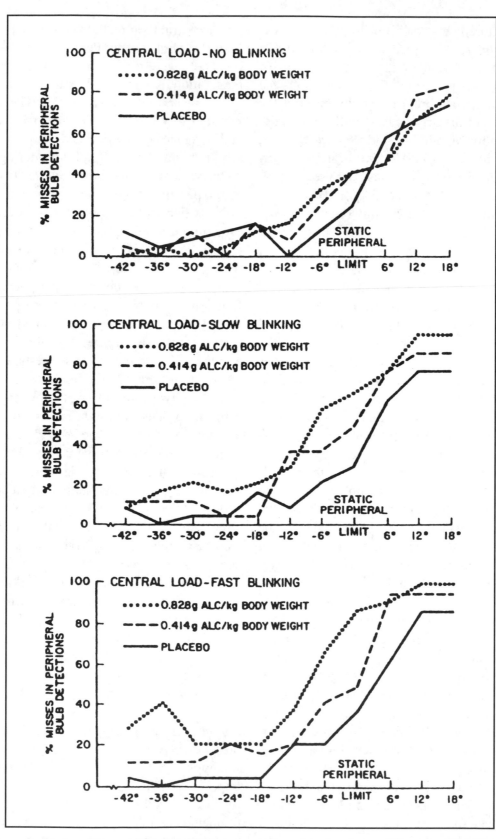

Figure 13.2 *Percentage of undetected peripheral light presentations (Moskowitz and Sharma, 1974.) Reprinted with permission from* Human Factors, *Vol. 16, No. 2, p. 177. ©1974 by the Human Factors and Ergonomics Society. All rights reserved.*

mental studies of behavioral function under the influence of alcohol have to be designed so that the behavioral functions being examined are isolated from other behavioral functions that are also affected by alcohol.

An example of the problems that can occur with the failure to carefully control variables in a behavioral study on alcohol can be seen in a study by Adams and Brown (1975), who reported that they found impairment of glare recovery at a BAC level of 0.01 g/dL, a level of alcohol which would result from consuming no more than a half can of American beer. Subsequently, a study by Sekuler and MacArthur (1977) found no impairment of glare recovery at a 0.09 g/dL BAC. Sekuler and MacArthur demonstrated that the Adams and Brown report of impairment was due to the effect of alcohol on the subjects' difficulty in acquiring the brightness comparison target used as a measure of glare recovery, rather than the direct effect of alcohol on glare recovery. Thus, what was purported to be a study of glare recovery turned out to be a study of visual search, a more complex behavior involving attention and perception, rather than the biological change in sensory receptor function involved in glare recovery. Sekuler and MacArthur were not disputing that Adams and Brown had demonstrated visual performance impairment at 0.01 g/dL BAC. Their point was that Adams and Brown had mistaken the behavioral function which produced the impairment under alcohol.

These studies illuminate why much of the earlier literature examining impairments produced by alcohol on behavior resulted in contradictory findings. The extent of literature now available in human factors is primarily a product of research during and since World War II. Even more recent is an understanding of the breadth of cognitive factors in skill performance. This contrasts with earlier emphasis on simple sensory processes and motor skills. As noted above, it is precisely the cognitive deficits under the influence of alcohol that appear to be paramount in the majority of alcohol-related accidents. Not coincidentally, it is these cognitive factors that are the most sensitive to the impairments of alcohol.

The review by Moskowitz and Robinson (1988) on the effects of low levels of alcohol on driving-re-

lated behavior summarized studies on reaction time, tracking, concentrated attention, divided attention, information processing, visual functions, perception, psychomotor skills, and performance in simulators and on the road. The report obtained more than 500 studies from a random sampling of computer literature databases. From these 500 studies, 177 were selected for incorporation in the report because they met such scientific criteria as performing statistical analysis, having sufficient information that the BAC at the time of behavioral testing could be determined, and the presence of placebo treatment. Of the 177 studies, 158 reported impairment of one or more behavioral skills at one or more BAC levels.

Only nineteen studies failed to report impairments at the levels examined, which ranged from 0.01 g/dL BAC to 0.10 g/dL and above. Of the nineteen negative studies of alcohol effects, sixteen were studies of reaction time. A total of thirty-seven studies examined reaction time, twenty-one of which found evidence of impairment by alcohol and sixteen did not. Reaction time studies were the only studies that failed to consistently and overwhelmingly—almost unanimously—demonstrate impairment by alcohol. No systematic study of the variation in results from reaction time experiments has been undertaken to explain the variability. However, it was noted that the reaction time experiments involving complex situations tended to show more impairment, whereas the simpler experiments with fewer demands for cognitive functioning tended to be more resistant to impairment by alcohol. Since the driving task is intrinsically a complex task, as we have noted earlier, studies on simple reaction time under the influence of alcohol appear irrelevant. More to the point, many of the complex reaction time studies, which are more analogous to driving situations, are relevant. It is noteworthy that it is these studies that are most likely to show evidence of impairment under the influence of alcohol.

Since there is frequent reference to simple and complex reaction times in legal context, it is important to note that what researchers have in mind when they refer to simple or complex reaction time is not what lay public or attorneys or even traffic engineers conceive as simple. For psychologists studying reaction time, a simple situation is one where the subject is told in advance what the signal is that he or she should respond to, when it will occur, and what the response should be. Thus, a typical simple reaction time experiment would involve a subject sitting at a table, resting her or his hand on a button, and concentrating on a light bulb that is lit at specified times, often preceded by a warning sound. The button is pressed when the light appears. The necessity of controlling the vehicle in its lane and heading, precludes total devotion of the driver's mental capacity to attend to an object such as a traffic signal in front of him. Moreover, neither traffic signals nor other vehicles have the degree of certainty as to time of appearance and state of condition that the light bulb signal has in a simple reaction time experiment. There is nothing in driving that is comparable to what a psychologist would consider a simple reaction time experiment. There is obviously considerable variability in the mental workload demand of the complex reaction time situations that arise in driving. It is precisely the mental workload demand of driving that is most susceptible to the effects of alcohol. Tracking studies under the influence of alcohol were one of the earliest areas studied. Tracking is analogous to car control in driving. A subject uses a controlling device such as a steering wheel to follow a target that moves on a TV monitor or in actual driving follows the contours of the road. Tracking is the essence of what most people have in mind when they conceive of car control. Moskowitz (1973) reviewed the literature of tracking under the influence of alcohol and concluded that there was variability in alcohol effects depending on whether the tracking task was compensatory or pursuit. A compensatory tracking task has the operator observing only a single input, the error or the difference between the desired position and the actual position of a controlled element. The controlled element is moved to reduce this error. A pursuit tracking task has the observer viewing both the desired target and the position of the controlled element and the latter is moved to follow the moving target. Compensatory tracking tasks performed alone have generally failed to find alcohol impairment, except at very high BACs. Most studies examining pursuit tracking, or those that have combined either pursuit or compensatory tracking with some concurrent or subsidiary

tasks, have found impairments at BAC levels of 0.05 g/dL or higher.

As early as 1959, Drew, et al. (1959) demonstrated impairment of tracking at 0.02 g/dL and higher alcohol levels in a fairly complex driving simulator. The Moskowitz and Robinson report examined twenty-eight more recent tracking studies, where the tracking task was accompanied by some additional task, and found that the BAC level at which impairment occurred was as low as 0.02 g/dL. Higher alcohol levels were required to produce tracking impairment when the tracking task was presumably by itself. In the Moskowitz and Robinson review, there were an additional twenty-eight studies of psychomotor performance, and again, the BAC level at which impairment was found varied primarily depending on the skill levels required for the motor performance. Standing steadiness, a test frequently used in police sobriety tests, albeit with eyes closed, exhibited impairment at BACs below 0.05 g/dL. If an instrument was available to measure the body sway, it picked up changes in skill levels which simple visual observation failed to uncover.

Twenty-eight visual function studies were reviewed, all of which found impairment. At the lowest BAC levels impairment was found in studies of ocular motor control and eye movement. However, the magnitude of impairment was frequently small and unlikely to produce significant impairment of driving functions. The same comment can be made of visual functions such as acuity, convergence, blink rate and so on which only demonstrate impairment at relatively high BAC levels. Visual functions with greater cognitive content exhibited impairments at lower levels. Belt (1969) used eye movement recordings in drivers on the road and demonstrated that BACs as low as 0.04 g/dL produced changes in the distribution of eye fixation. Increasingly, drivers concentrated their fixation within a smaller central visual field and more rarely had wider angle fixation. Similar results have been found by other investigators, including Buikhuisen and Jongman (1972), who reported that drivers in a driving simulator exhibited a form of tunnel vision with fewer visual excursions to the periphery. Moskowitz, Zeidman and Sharma (1976) found a similar shift in distribution in eye fixation, but also an increase in fixation duration.

Thus, not only did alcohol change the manner in which the driver used his or her eyes, as for example in visual search of the environment, but alcohol slowed the ability to process information, requiring longer fixation on an object in order to perceive its nature. A consequence of the longer duration was that fewer fixations were possible in driving a given distance at a given speed and, as a result, less could be seen. Drivers are literally looking less, because each look under the influence of alcohol takes longer, and therefore they can make fewer looks in any given time or passing a given distance on the road. Further demonstration of the impairments produced by alcohol on visual perception is found in Hicks (1976) where drivers under the influence of alcohol were unable to discern the meaning of road signs until they were at closer distances as compared to driving unimpaired. Most visual measures are impaired by 0.10 g/dL BAC or higher. However, many visual functions are impaired at any measurable level of alcohol, and these tend to be those more related to cognitive functions. In the behaviors examined above, there has been no discussion of a behavior frequently reported in police reports, namely judgment. Police frequently report signs of impaired judgment under alcohol, such as aggressive behavior, irrational behavior and speeding.

Unfortunately, in the confines of a laboratory, it has usually been difficult to produce an objective measure of judgment. However, in a study by Cohen et al. (1958) the issue was examined using English bus drivers. The drivers, who were experienced in traveling through narrow streets, were required to maneuver a bus through a narrow gap between two upright posts. The two posts were placed at varying spacing and the drivers were initially asked to judge from some distance whether they could drive through the space, and then asked to proceed to do so. After drinking six ounces of whiskey, there was a small change—six-tenths of an inch—in the separation required for a driver to successfully drive the bus through the posts' gap. However, there was a large and significant change in the number of times drivers attempted to drive their bus between the two posts when the posts were closer together than the

width of the bus. Cohen suggested that alcohol did little to impair the drivers' ability to see the distance between the posts or the motor ability to drive; rather, the effect was on the judgment of drivers as to their ability to perform the task. In the Moskowitz and Robinson (1988) survey, thirty-five studies examined the effects of alcohol on various behaviors at 0.04 g/dL and lower. All thirty-five demonstrated impairment, suggesting that there is no threshold below which the presence of alcohol does not produce impairment in some behavioral area.

A literature review on the effects of low doses of alcohol on driving related skills was published by Moskowitz and Fiorentino (2000) to serve as a follow-up on the previously discussed Moskowitz and Robinson report. This more recent review of the literature summarized 112 studies published from 1981 to 1997, which had been screened for scientific acceptability, including the inclusion of placebo treatments, the ability to determine BAC at the time of behavioral testing, and adequate statistical significance. In this more recent review 27 percent of the studies report finding impairment by .039 g/dL BAC, 47 percent by .049 g/dL and 92 percent by .079 g/dL. Thus, far more studies reported impairment at lower levels than the 1988 review by Moskowitz and Robinson. The difference may be accounted for by improvements in the methods and instruments used by researchers in the past decade and a half and by the more frequent examination of multiple BAC levels within a single study, rather than as in earlier studies where only one BAC level was examined. Some studies reported impairment at BACs as low as less than .01 g/dL BAC. The areas showing greatest sensitivity to alcohol impairment were on-the-road and simulator studies of driving, divided attention tasks and measures of drowsiness. The least sensitive behavioral areas were simple reaction time and studies of critical flicker fusion. In between were tasks such as vigilance, tracking, perception, visual functions and cognitive tasks.

The conclusion of the 2000 study was that the review of the literature provided strong evidence that some driving related skills were impaired with any departure from zero BAC. By .05 g/dL the majority of studies reported impairment of some skill by alcohol. As noted earlier in the Moskowitz and Robinson review, it is clear that alcohol effects differ by behavioral area, which explains why some drivers involved in serious accidents due to cognitive defects can appear unintoxicated to casual observers.

An additional study published in 2000 by Moskowitz, Burns, Fiorentino, Smiley and Zador (2000) examined the performance of 168 subjects in a driving simulator and a divided attention task. The subjects were placed into four age groupings from 19–70 years, three drinking practices categories of very light, moderate and very heavy, and two sex categories of male and female. The moderate and heavy drinkers were tested on the behavioral test battery at BACs of 0.0, .02, .04, .06, .08 and .10 percent. The light drinkers were tested at the same BACs, except for the highest level, .10 percent, as preliminary testing indicated that many light drinkers became ill at that level.

Across all categories of subjects, performance became significantly impaired on the test battery at the lowest BAC level, .02 percent. Both the magnitude of impairment and the number of behavioral areas impaired increased as the BAC level examined was increased.

Interestingly, differences in the magnitude of impairment by alcohol between categories of age, sex and drinking practice were small, inconsistent in direction and did not reach statistical significance. The subjects were representative of perhaps more than 90 percent of the drinking population. However, due to requirements for subject protection, no subjects were tested under the age of nineteen nor were any alcoholics included as subjects. With these constraints in mind, at any given BAC it was impossible to distinguish, age, sex or drinking practice differences. And all categories showed significant impairment beginning at the lowest level tested, .02 percent.

13.7 Rate of Alcohol Consumption

A factor that influences the degree of impairment produced by alcohol is the rate at which consumption has been undertaken by the driver. In a study by Moskowitz and Burns (1976) four groups of subjects drank alcohol at different rates to achieve a 0.10 g/dL peak BAC level. The duration over which they drank ranged from fifteen minutes to four hours. The

group that consumed the greatest amount of alcohol was the group that took the longest period of time to achieve 0.10 g/dL, since as they were consuming the alcohol, they had to compensate for the metabolism that was proceeding in their body. Thus the amount of alcohol consumed was correlated directly with the duration of time to reach the desired 0.10 g/dL BAC level. Nevertheless, the most impaired individuals were in the group that drank the fastest, even though they drank the least. The least impaired was the group that drank the most, because they drank it at a slower rate.

13.8 Alcohol and Fatigue

A new area of research in the last decade has been the effect of alcohol on sleepiness in drivers. Particular attention has been paid to studying the alcohol effects on sleep, even after the BAC level has dropped to zero. For example, in Roehrs et al. (1994), subjects were given two alcohol treatments and one placebo treatment on separate days. An alcohol treatment designed to peak at 0.06 g/dL was given at 7:30 A.M., an alcohol treatment designed to peak at 0.04 g/dL was given at 10:30 A.M. Thus, by 3:30 P.M., all subjects were at zero BAC. Subjects were examined on a sleep latency test, which measured sleepiness by determining the time it takes to fall asleep. Subjects were tested at two hour intervals beginning at 9:30 A.M. until 9:30 P.M. Subjects exhibited a decreased sleep latency (i.e., a shortened time to fall asleep) throughout the entire period when alcohol was present, as well as in the 3:30 P.M. period when the BAC had dropped to zero, in comparison with the placebo treatment day.

A comparable study by Walsh et al. (1991) examined the sedating effect of an alcohol treatment ingested at 9:30 P.M., which produced a mean BAC of 0.069 g/dL at 11:20 P.M. and which dropped to 0.019 g/dL at 3:20 A.M. Sleep tendencies under alcohol were compared with sleep tendencies under placebo. Sleep latency was tested at two-hour intervals from 11:00 P.M. to 5:30 A.M. The subjects were divided into two subcategories, alert individuals and sleepy individuals, based on their mean latency to fall asleep on the placebo treatment day. Subjects who were designated sleepy exhibited extremely short latency to falling asleep even on the placebo trial. No effect could be discerned for alcohol on the alcohol trial session of the "sleepy" subjects. However, subjects who normally took longer to fall asleep, who were termed alert on placebo treatment days, demonstrated increased sleep tendencies for the entire testing period under alcohol. The experiment suggests that the sedating effect of alcohol interacts with other characteristics of the subject.

In a study by Roehrs, et al. (1989), subjects were examined on sleep latency after consuming either alcohol or placebo and either having a one-hour nap or no nap. There were four conditions: alcohol plus no nap, alcohol plus a nap, placebo plus no nap and placebo plus a nap. The alcohol was consumed at 9:00 A.M. and the one-hour nap began at 10:00 A.M. For all four experimental conditions, the latency to sleep onset was examined every two hours from 12:00 to 6:00 P.M. The alcohol dose, which produced a peak BAC of 0.04 g/dL, significantly reduced the time to fall asleep. On the other hand, the one hour nap increased the time to fall asleep. The effect of the alcohol was to counteract the effects of the nap, so that subjects who had both alcohol and a nap were similar in the sleep tendencies of the no nap subjects under placebo.

Evidence that these laboratory studies are relevant to real life driving situations can be found in a study by Hicks et al. (1998). The authors examined accident rates for the years 1989 to 1992 for the state of New Mexico for the week before the changes to and from daylight savings time and the two weeks after the changes in daylight savings time. There was an increase in the number of alcohol-related traffic crashes during the seven days following daylight savings changes. It was found that the proportion of crashes, which were alcohol related, rose sharply in the first week after daylight savings time changes, whereas the proportion of alcohol-related accidents in the week before and the second week after daylight savings time changes were the same.

13.9 Alcohol and Aggression

The last decade has seen a sharp increase in reports of aggressive driving on the road. The increase in the phenomenon of road rage appears to be following the increased congestion on our highways. While no hard epidemiological evidence exists to specify the correlation between aggressive driving and the presence of alcohol, there is an extensive and impressive literature from the laboratory demonstrating increased aggressive behavior under alcohol. Numerous epidemiological studies specify a role for alcohol in violent crimes of assault, rape and murder. Bushman and Cooper (1990) performed a meta-analysis of thirty experimental studies and concluded that the evidence supported the conclusion that alcohol did in fact cause aggression. These studies used male subjects described as social drinkers. The review noted that the likelihood that any given experiment demonstrates aggressiveness under alcohol was modulated by other conditions. There have been volumes written on the relationship between alcohol and aggression. For example, Brain (1986) presented evidence from both human and animal experimental studies and human clinical and epidemiological studies of a causal relationship between alcohol and aggressive and violent behaviors. The authors, nevertheless, insisted that these are modulated, both by the individual characteristics of the subjects, which are predispositional factors and the situational factors, such as, increased traffic density on the road. There are various theories as to why there is a pharmacological effect of alcohol on aggression. Studies such as Mulvihill et al. (1997) support the notion that one contributing factor is that alcohol reduces the ability to inhibit behavior in humans. At this point in history (2003), our understanding of the factors leading to aggressive behavior in individuals under alcohol is limited. While there is an overwhelming preponderance of evidence demonstrating that alcohol causes increased aggression, as a function of predisposing and situational variables, the mechanism for this relationship is unknown and fairly strongly debated. Unfortunately, little is known of the role of alcohol in inducing aggression in driving except for single reports of specific episodes. I could find no literature for motor vehicle accidents, which analyze the crash data with respect to aggressive behavior under alcohol.

13.10 Alcohol and Degree of Injury

The discussion above has concerned the behaviors that underlie greatly increased probability of crashes, injuries, and deaths when drivers use alcohol on the road. However, there is another aspect of alcohol that accounts for the large toll of injuries and fatalities—the role of alcohol in determining the severity of the injury received in a collision. This is distinguished from the role of alcohol in the causation of the injury, which is what we have been discussing above. In 1985 the Committee on Trauma Research of the National Research Council on the Institute of Medicine noted that "use of alcoholic beverages predisposes to more severe and extensive injury than would be experienced by nondrinkers, given impact of the same severity." "Alcohol beverage use that produces even moderate or low blood alcohol concentration can significantly increase the fatality rate associated with cardiac injury and the debilitating effects associated with CNS damage" (Committee on Trauma Research, 1985, p. 57). There is an extensive literature supporting the National Research Council's report, including both epidemiological and experimental studies with animals. Examples of epidemiological studies include Waller et al. (1986) examining over a million traffic crash reports in North Carolina from 1979 to 1983 and controlling for a wide variety of factors such as crash severity, type of vehicle, speed, car weight, driver age and sex, seatbelt use and so forth. They estimated that overall the presence of alcohol increased the probability of being killed in an accident 225 percent over that of a similar non-alcohol-involved driver. Evans and Frick (1993) used data furnished by FARS regarding two-car crashes where at least one driver was killed. Again, a variety of control factors such as relative weight and impact areas were covariates in the analysis. It was determined that the presence of a BAC of 0.10 g/dL roughly doubled the risk of death from a given impact and a BAC of 0.25 g/dL tripled the probability of death. These epidemiological studies were supported by animal experiments where animals underwent a standardized force with and without alcohol and demonstrate increased trauma with alcohol (e.g., Brodner et al., 1981), as well as studies in patients experiencing trauma who exhibited altered biochemical processes when alcohol was present (cf. Woolf et al., 1990).

References

Adams, A.J. and Brown, B. Alcohol prolongs time course of glare recovery. *Nature* 257:481–483, 1975.

Allsop, R.E. *Alcohol and Road Accidents*. (Road Research Laboratory Report No. 6) 1966, Harmondsworth, England: Road Research Laboratory.

Belt, B.L. *Driver Eye Movement as a Function of Low Alcohol Concentrations*. Columbus, OH: Driving Research Laboratory, Ohio State University, 1969.

Borkenstein, R.F. et al. *The Role of the Drinking Driver in Traffic Accidents*. Bloomington, IN: Department of Police Administration, Indiana University, 1964.

Borkenstein, R.F., Trubitt, H.J. and Lease, R.J. Problems of enforcement and prosecution. In Fox, B.H. and Fox, J.H. (eds.), *Alcohol and Traffic Safety,* Public Health Service Publication No. 1043. Washington, DC: United States Government Printing Office, 1963, pp. 137–188,

Brain, P.F. (ed.). *Alcohol and Aggression*. Beckenham, Kent: Croom Helm Ltd., 1986.

Brodner, R.A., Van Gilder, J. C. and Collins, Jr., J.F. Experimental spinal cord trauma: Potentiation by alcohol. *J. Trauma* 21:124–129, 1981.

Buikhuisen, W. and Jongman, R.W. Traffic perception under the influence of alcohol. *Quarterly J. Studies on Alcohol* 33:800–806, 1972.

Burgess, M. and Lindsey, T. *Alcohol Involvement in Fatal Crashes—1996*, Technical Report DOT HS 808-686. Springfield, VA: National Highway Traffic Safety Administration, 1998.

Burns, M. and Moskowitz, H. *Psychophysical Tests for DWI Arrest*, Report No. DOT HS-802-424. Washington, DC: National Highway Traffic Safety Administration, U.S. Department of Transportation, 1977.

Bushman, B.J. and Cooper, H.M. Effects of alcohol on human aggression: An integrative research review. *Psychological Bulletin* 107:341–354, 1990.

Chiles, W.D. and Jennings, A.E. *Effects of Alcohol on Complex Performance*, Report No. AM 69-14. Oklahoma City: Federal Aviation Medicine, Civil Aeromedical Institute, 1969.

Clayton, A.B. An accident-based analysis of road-user errors. *J. Safety Research* 4:69–72, 1972.

Cohen, J., Dearnaley, E.J. and Hansel, C.E.M. The risk taken in driving under the influence of alcohol. *British Medical J.* 6/21:1438–1442, 1958.

Committee on Trauma Research, Commission on Life Sciences, National Research Council, and the Institute of Medicine. *Injury in America: A Continuing Public Health Problem*. Washington, DC: National Academy Press, 1985.

Drew, G.C., Colquhoun, W.P. and Long, H.A. *Effect of Small Doses of Alcohol on a Skill Resembling Driving*. Medical Research Council Memorandum, No. 38, London, Her Majesty's Stationary Office 1959.

Evans, L. and Frick, M.C. Alcohol's effect on fatality risk from a physical insult. *J. Stud. Alc.* 54:441–449,1993.

Greenfeld, L.A. *Alcohol and Crime: An Analysis of National Data on the Prevalence of Alcohol Involvement in Crime,* NCJ 168632. Washington, DC: U.S. Department of Justice 1998.

Hicks, G.J., Davis, J.W. and Hicks, R.A. Fatal alcohol-related traffic crashes increase subsequent to changes to and from daylight savings time. *Perceptual and Motor Skills* 86:879–882, 1998.

Hicks, J.A. An evaluation of the effect of sign brightness on the sign reading behavior of alcohol impaired drivers. *Human Factors* 18:45–52, 1976.

Hingson, R. and Howland, J. Alcohol and non-traffic unintended injuries. *Addiction* 88:877–883, 1993.

Hurst, P.M. Epidemiological aspects of alcohol in driver crashes and citations. *J. Safety Research* 5:130–148, 1973.

Lund, A.K. and Wolfe, A.C. Changes in the incidence of alcohol-impaired driving in the United States, 1973–1986. *J. Stud. Alc.* 52: 293–301, 1991.

Moskowitz, H. Laboratory studies of the effects of alcohol on some variables related to driving. *J. Safety Research* 5:185–199, 1973.

Moskowitz, H. and Burns, M.M. Effects of rate of drinking on human performance. *J. Stud. Alc.* 46: 482–485, 1976.

Moskowitz, H., Burns, M.M. and Williams, A.F. Skills performance at low blood alcohol levels. *J. Stud. Alc.* 46:482–485, 1985.

Moskowitz, H. and Robinson, C.D. *Effects of Low Doses of Alcohol on Driving-Related Skills: A Review of the Evidence*, Technical Report DOT HS 807-280. Springfield, VA: National Highway Traffic Safety Administration, 1988.

Moskowitz, H. and Sharma, S. Effects of alcohol on peripheral vision as a function of attention. *Human Factors* 16:174–180, 1974.

Moskowitz, H., Ziedman, K. and Sharma, S. Visual search behavior while viewing driving scenes under the influence of alcohol and marijuana. *Human Factors* 8:417–432, 1976.

Moskowitz, H. and Fiorentino, D. *A Review of the Literature on the Effects of Low Doses of Alcohol on Driving-Related Skills*, DOT HS 809-028. National Highway Traffic Safety Administration, 2000.

Moskowitz, H. et al. *Driver Characterisitics and Impairment at Various BACs*, Technical Report DOT HS 809-075. Springfield, VA: National Highway Traffic Safety Administration, 2000.

Moskowitz, H. et al. Methodological issues in epidemiological studies of alcohol crash risk. In: *Proceedings of the 2002 Montreal, Canada, International Conference on Alcohol, Drugs and Traffic Safety*, 2002.

Mulvihill, L.E., Skilling, T.A. and Vogel-Sprott, M. Alcohol and the ability to inhibit behavior in men and women. *J. Stud. Alc.* 58: 600–605, 1997.

National Highway Traffic Safety Administration. *Traffic Safety Facts 1996: A Compilation of Motor Vehicle Crash Data from the Fatality Analysis Reporting System and the General Estimates System*, DOT HS 808-649. Washington, DC: Author, 1997.

Perper, J.A., Twerski, A. and Wienand, J.W. Tolerance at high blood alcohol concentrations: A study of 110 cases and review of the literature. *J. Forensic Sciences* 31:212–221, 1986.

Roehrs, T. et al. Residual sedating effects of ethanol. *Alcsm Clin. Exp. Res.* 18:831–834, 1994.

Roehrs, T. et al. Sedating effects of ethanol after a nap. *Alc. Drugs & Driv.* 5/6:351–356, 1989.

Sekular, R. and MacArthur, R.D. Alcohol retards visual recovery from glare by hampering target acquisition. *Nature* 270:428–429, 1977.

Shinar, D., Treat, J.R. and McDonald, S.T. *Accident Analysis and Prevention* 15:175–191, 1983.

Stephens, B.W. and Michaels, R.M. Time sharing between compensatory tracking and search-and-recognition tasks. *Highway Research Record* 55:1–16, 1963.

Treat, J.R. A study of precrash factors involved in traffic accidents. *The HSRI Research Review*, Volume 10, No. 4/Volume 11, No. 1. Ann Arbor, MI: University of Michigan Highway Safety Research Institute, 1980.

U.S. Department of Human Services; Sixth Special Report to the U.S. Congress, *Alcohol and Health*, 1987.

U.S. Department of Transportation. *Alcohol and Highway Safety: A Report to the Congress from the Secretary of Transportation*. Washington, DC: Author, 1968.

Urso, T., Gavaler, J.S. and Van Thiel, D.H. Blood ethanol levels in sober alcohol users seen in an emergency room. *Life Sciences* 28:1053–1056, 1981.

Vaos, R. et al. Drinking and driving in the United States: The 1996 National Roadside Survey. *Accident Analysis and Prevention* 30:267–275, 1998.

Waller, P.F. et al. The potentiating effects of alcohol on driver injury. *JAMA* 256:1461–1466, 1986.

Walsh, J.K. et al. Sedative effects of ethanol at night. *J. Stud. Alc.* 52:597–600, 1991.

Wells, J.K. et al. Drinking drivers missed at sobriety checkpoints. *J. Stud. Alc.* 58: 513–517, 1997.

Widmark, E.M.P. *Theoretical Foundations and the Practical Application of Forensic-Medical Alcohol Determination*. Berlin: Wein, Urban and Schwartzenberg, 1932. (English translation published as *Principles and Applications of Medicolegal Alcohol Determination*. Davis, CA: Biomedical Publications, 1981.)

Woolf, P.D. et al. Alcohol intoxication blunts sympatho-adrenal activation following brain injury. *Alcsm Clin. Exp. Res.* 14:205–209, 1990.

Zador, P.L. Alcohol-related relative risk of fatal driver injuries in relation to driver age and sex. *J. Stud. Alc.* 52:302–310, 1991.

Zylman, R. Youth, alcohol, and collision involvement. *J. Safety Research* 5:58–72, 1973.

Chapter 14

Epidemiological Basis of Alcohol-Induced Psychomotor Performance Impairment (PMPI)

Barbara R. Manno, Ph.D. and Joseph E. Manno, Ph.D.

14.1 Introduction

Psychomotor performance impairment (PMPI) occurring after consumption of alcoholic beverages is widely recognized and accepted by many among the lay public, medical, and forensic communities. It is also accepted that PMPI occurs in a dose-related manner. Although subjective observations may be made concerning PMPI, it is necessary that strong, objective, scientifically-based PMPI findings are available to support civil and criminal litigation in alcohol-related cases, legislative action, as well as public education programs.

There are newsworthy instances of alcohol-related incidents in private and commercial transportation which illustrate the need for such knowledge. One of the most notable occurred in 1989, when the crude oil tanker *Exxon Valdez* crashed on Bligh Reef in Prince William Sound, off the shore of Alaska. The ship carried 1.2 million of gallons of crude oil—a fifth of which spilled into the water. Over 37,000 birds and animals were killed and the local fishing industry was severely affected (Hunt and Witt, 1994; O'Harra, 1989). To these losses was added the cost of immediate operations for cleanup of the crude oil and losses to the future environment and commerce of the area for years to come. This does not include loss to the shipping line, the work force of the refinery that was to receive the oil, or the consumer who would have used the processed oil products or the fish sold by the fisherman. This is but one case of many which could have been cited. It can easily be seen that a domino effect occurs when an otherwise potentially responsible individual drinks alcoholic beverages before, during or while operating a motorized conveyance or machinery.

In the 1970s the National Transportation Safety Board (NTSB) began documenting alcohol and drug abuse in transportation accidents. It became clear by the 1980s that problems existed in all forms of transportation with little corrective action being undertaken. The NTSB, in 1983, recommended to the Department of Transportation (DOT) that it issue rules to prohibit the use of alcohol and other drugs for a specified period before duty, while on duty and to require toxicological testing on all employees responsible for train operation. The final rule, "Control of Alcohol and Drug Use in Railroad Operations," was issued in 1985 by the Federal Railroad Administration (FRA) of the DOT. The rule required alcohol and drug testing in three instances: after accidents, for reasonable cause and for pre-employment evaluation. Subsequently in 1988, the DOT issued drug testing rules for persons working in safety sensitive occupations in all areas of commercial transportation (Hall, 1995; Sweedler, 1992). Before these actions by the DOT, the legal definition of driving impairment from alcohol prevailed at ≥ 0.10 g/dL and information gathering and accident investigation rested primarily with local and state law enforcement agencies. Additionally, the vast majority of the alcohol-driving epidemiological data was gleaned from noncommercial vehicular and pedestrian accidents. Recognition of the myriad of problems associated with alcohol's role in accidents has resulted in the lowering of the legal limits of intoxication to 0.08 g/dL in most states. Further lowering of the legal definition of intoxication or impairment at a BAC of 0.04 g/dL is defined for commercial vehicle operators and persons in safety-sensitive positions as indicated above. See Chapter 20 (Alcohol Testing in the Workplace) for more detailed discussion of the development of workplace testing laws and program. Hunt and Witt (1994) have succinctly summarized the status of alcohol-related accidents and fatalities, making the following points: the leading cause of death in the United States in 1989 for 5–34-year-olds in traffic crashes; alcohol contributed to approximately one-half of the 44,000 driver fatalities and, of these, more than 50 percent were impaired drivers; accident risk is estimated to be eight times higher for a drunk driver with the risk rising precipitously when the blood alcohol concentration (BAC) reaches or exceeds 0.08 g/dL. Alcohol involvement in other vehicular accidents ranges from 10 percent in general aviation accidents to 69 percent in recreational boating accidents.

Greater emphasis on the economic, environmental and human consequences of motor vehicle accidents and the role played by alcohol has dictated that PMPI must be well-researched and carefully documented. Therefore, it is incumbent upon us to understand how the multitude of individual studies can be related to one another to support the concept of alcohol-induced PMPI. This should provide assistance in case development and is the foundation for design of new studies to prove or disprove PMPI with alcohol and other drugs, either alone or in combination. It also offers a base on which to develop educational programs and other measures to reduce alcohol involvement in accidents.

14.2 Establishing the Relationship

The general format for seeking the relationship of alcohol-PMPI is outlined in Figure 14.1. The initiation of such documentation (Step 1) usually begins with the casual observation that alcohol appears to be a common factor associated with changes in an individual's ability to perform psychomotor tasks

(e.g., driving an automobile). Figure 14.1 defines the process as a seven-step procedure.

Step 2 (Figure 14.1), of necessity, asks the question "How many events (crashes, mishaps, accidents and so on) in the target population involve drinking drivers?" If the answer is "few" then there obviously need be no further expenditure of effort on the problem. Ideally, on the other hand if many events involve drinking drivers then the population and events involving drinking drivers should be reevaluated and compared with a similarly matched population of non-drinking drivers or other indicators. If no difference in the two groups is shown then no problem may exist. If a positive response is attained, further investigation is required. This step may also proceed based only on the degree of alcohol involvement documented in the accidents studied. Fortunately, initial investigators (Holcomb, 1938) chose automobile (personal injury) accident cases to investigate and found that 25 percent of the drivers had blood alcohol concentrations greater than or equal to 0.10 g/dL. It was also shown that sample populations of non-crash drivers were positive for alcohol in only 2 percent of the cases. More recent studies (Pendleton, 1986) explored the circumstances of 1,260 driver fatalities and found that 51 percent of the drivers were legally intoxicated (BAC > 0.10 g/dL). The role of alcohol compared with the total number of traffic fatality rates per 100 million vehicle miles traveled in the United States, 1977–98 is represented in Figure 14.2 (Yi, 2000). Figure 14.3 shows alcohol-related fatality rates per 100,000 population, registered vehicles, and licensed drivers in the United States, 1977–98 for the same period (Yi, 2000).

While the end result may be the same (i.e., a vehicular-personal injury, fatality or property damage), distinction between the nuances defining the alcohol-impaired driver may be necessary. This is required in order to describe cause and effect relationships surrounding the accident and for assignment of responsibility in a legal environment.

We are concerned in Step 4 (Table 14.1) with the question, "Is the accident of the drunk driver related to PMPI or can it be that other factors such as vehicular, environmental, or human are involved?" Other factors or variables are defined in Table 14.1

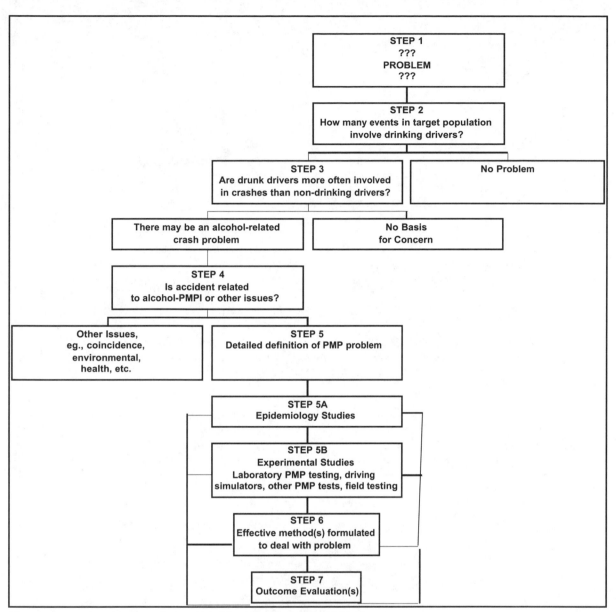

Figure 14.1 *Decision tree for establishing alcohol-related PMPI*

Table 14.1
Variables in Accident Reseach

Categories	Definition
Vehicular	Relationship to design, construction and operating characteristics of vehicle.
Environmental	Operating conditions, traffic conditions, time of day, weather, road surface conditions and so forth
Human	Characteristics of driver—physical, social, psychological, length of time driving, driving experiences, age or other related descriptors which measures which may affect driver's ability to perform driving or other tasks.

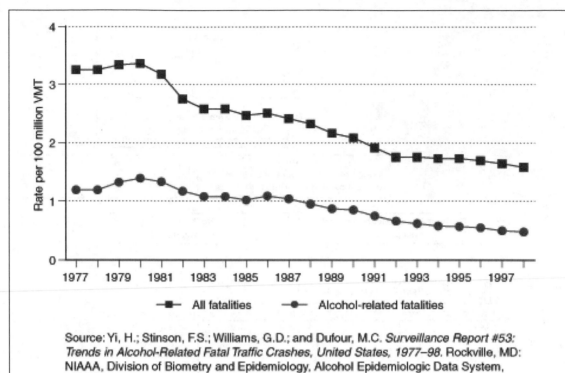

Source: Yi, H.; Stinson, F.S.; Williams, G.D.; and Dufour, M.C. *Surveillance Report #53: Trends in Alcohol-Related Fatal Traffic Crashes, United States, 1977–98.* Rockville, MD: NIAAA, Division of Biometry and Epidemiology, Alcohol Epidemiologic Data System, December, 2000.

Figure 14.2 Total and alcohol-related traffic fatality rates per 100 million vehicle miles traveled (VMT), United States, 1977–78 (Yi, 2000)

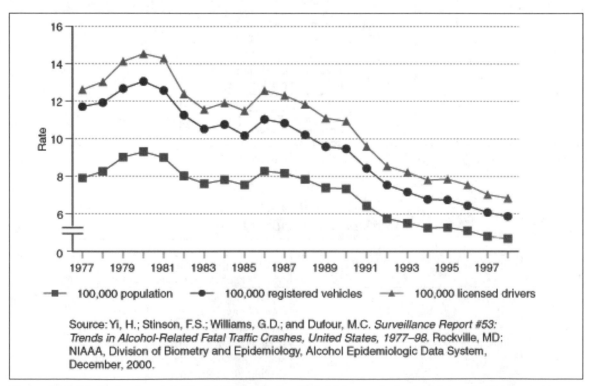

Source: Yi, H.; Stinson, F.S.; Williams, G.D.; and Dufour, M.C. *Surveillance Report #53: Trends in Alcohol-Related Fatal Traffic Crashes, United States, 1977–98.* Rockville, MD: NIAAA, Division of Biometry and Epidemiology, Alcohol Epidemiologic Data System, December, 2000.

Figure 14.3 Alcohol-related traffic fatality rates per 100,000 population, registered vehicles and licensed drivers, United States, 1977–78 (Yi, 2000)

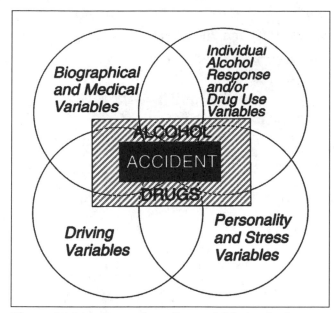

Figure 14.4 *Major confounding variable impinging on interpretation of drunk driving assessment*

and Figure 14.4. If other factors are contributory to accident causation, it may serve the purpose of the accident researcher to pursue these at a later time. In our case we are limited to discussion of alcohol-induced PMPI and shall proceed to Step 5 of Figure 14.1. This general approach could serve to direct many avenues of study.

Once the relationship has been superficially established that alcohol may be involved as a causative factor in vehicular accidents, the problem must be defined with as much detail as is feasible. This may be approached as shown in Figure 14.1, Steps 5A and 5B. Step 5A consists of epidemiological studies of accidents, where attempts are made to draw a correlation between the presence or absence of alcohol in accident cases. This should also involve subcategorization of the data based on the BAC of the driver or other involved persons. Step 5B, Experimental Testing, is represented by data from laboratory studies of animals and humans using various scientifically sound and validated testing devices and designs. The purpose of this step is to provide an

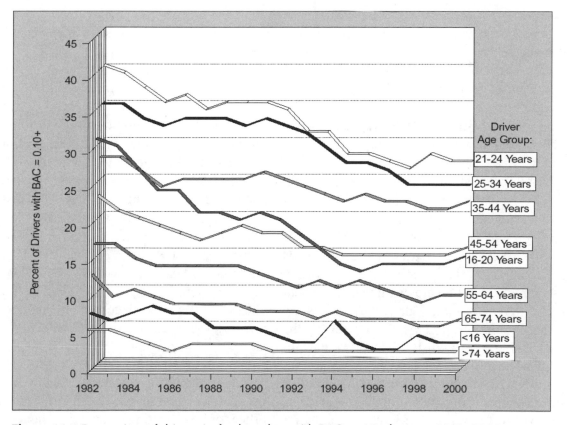

Figure 14.5 *Proportion of drivers in fatal crashes with BAC = .10+ by age, 1982–2000 (NHTSA, 2001)*

Table 14.2
Alcohol Involvement for drivers in fatal crashes, 1991 and 2001 (NHTSA, 2001)

Drivers Involved in Fatal Crashes	1991		2001		Change in Percentage, 1991-2001
	Number of Drivers	Percentage with BAC 0.08 g/dl or Greater	Number of Drivers	Percentage with BAC 0.08 g/dl or Greater	
Total Drivers					
Total*	54,391	27	57,480	21	-22%
Drivers by Age Group (Years)					
16–20	8,002	23	7,963	18	-22%
21–24	6,748	38	6,016	33	-13%
25–34	14,151	36	11,534	28	-22%
35–44	9,482	28	11,201	25	-11%
45–64	9,153	17	13,005	17	0%
Over 64	5,471	7	6,421	6	-14%
Drivers by Sex					
Male	40,731	30	41,711	24	-20%
Female	12,825	16	14,867	13	-19%
Drivers by Vehicle Type					
Passenger Cars	31,102	27	27,287	23	-15%
Light Trucks	14,702	30	20,595	23	-23%
Large Trucks	4,291	3	4,749	1	-67%
Motorcycles	2,816	44	3,245	29	-34%

*Numbers shown for groups of drivers do not add to the total number of drivers due to unknown or other data not included.

environment where controlled studies may be performed using selected variables which may be included or excluded during testing. The experimental studies include alcohol consumption coupled with individual response, behavior-testing devices or both. The studies also include testing under controlled conditions using actual driving experiments or field tests (See Chapter 13). Step 6 (Figure 14.1) addresses the formulation of methods to deal with the problem and will not be discussed here since it is beyond the scope of the present work.

Step 7 (Figure 14.1) is directed toward evaluation of effectiveness of educational instruments implemented to alter the outcome of the problem. Table 14.2 and Figure 14.5 are examples of accident statistics on alcohol-related driving fatalities by BAC. Other important variables when assessing the drivers in fatal crashes with BAC = 0.10+ g/dL include total number of drivers, driver age, sex and vehicle type (NHTSA, 2001). Figure 14.5 shows this data for the years from 1982 to 2000 (NHTSA, 2000). Steps 5A, 5B, 6 and 7 of Figure 14.1 are dynamic in nature and affect each other once started.

Constant and continuing evaluation is a feature of these steps.

It may be generalized that the incidence of alcohol-related accidents is under-reported. Previously, in the United States and, to a lesser extent in other countries, there was no uniform reporting responsibility either by official agency or reporting format. This began to change with the initiation of the Fatal Accident Reporting System (FARS) in 1975 by the National Highway Traffic Safety Administration of the Department of Transportation (NHTSA, 1991). The distinctions between FARS and its newer National Accident Sampling System (NASS), Crashworthiness Data System (CDS) and General Estimates System (GES) are detailed in Table 14.3. Table 14.4 compares alcohol involvement among drivers by their survival status. Table 14.5 compares alcohol involvement among pedestrians and pedicyclists (NHTSA, 2002a).

Under-reporting of alcohol-involved accidents occurs for several reasons. Many times the arresting officer or investigating official does not question the presence of alcohol in either the accident victim or

Table 14.3
NHTSA Databases Established to Address Accident Statistics

Database	Date Established	Data Sources
Fatal Accident Reporting System (FARS)	1975	Only most severe accidents reported. Based upon census of fatal traffic crashes with fifty states, Puerto Rico, District of Columbia. Crash must involve motor vehicle traveling on a traffic way customarily open to the public and must result in the death of a person (vehicle occupant or a nonmotorist) within thirty days of crash. Standard reporting format includes ninety different coded data measures reported on three forms (accident, vehicle-driver ,and person).
National Accident Sampling System (NASS)	1979	Complementary to FARS. Based on all police reported crashes including nonfatal and property damage.
Crashworthiness Data System (CDS)	1988	Collects detailed data on approximately 7,000 crashes involving light passenger vehicles each year. Supports research crash safety; biomechanics of trauma; development of test equipment, procedures and criteria; supports motor vehicle and passenger safety standards; and consensus information programs.
General Estimates System (GES)	1988	Less detailed data collection than CDS. Samples approximately 45,000 police reported traffic crashes (all types). Does not investigate crashes. Provides data to assess state of and trends in traffic safety.

vehicle-operator until hours after the incident. By the time the question arises, the BAC is greatly reduced or the alcohol may have disappeared from the blood of the subject. In many instances, the presence of alcohol is never questioned (Jones and Joscelyn, 1978; Pendleton, 1986). The police officer may choose not to report a suspicion of increased driver BAC because of increased documentation requirements, amount of time required for subsequent court appearances or fear of personal lawsuits growing out of the report. With the addition of commercial and safety sensitive testing coupled with society's increased lack of tolerance for drinking and driving, we are beginning to see more reports of instances of testing for reasonable cause. For example, in 2001 security personnel at the Miami, Florida airport reported the odor of alcohol emanating from two pilots reporting for their flights. Upon the immediate return of the flight to the gate before takeoff, it was found that both pilots exceeded the 0.04 g/dL limit established by the DOT and America West company policies. It was reported that in fact the breath tests indicated one pilot had a BAC of 0.091 g/dL and the other had a BAC of 0.084 g/dL which also exceed Florida's legal limit for operation of machinery (U.S.A. Today, 2002; cnn.com, 2003).

In spite of these apparent omissions, the BAC reporting rate has become more consistent in the recent past and indicates a change in accident statistics for fatally injured drivers (up from 54 percent to 73 percent) and for surviving drivers (from 16 percent up to 25 percent [NHTSA, 1991; Perrine et al., 1989]). The problems in reporting would suggest that due to the nonhomogeneous nature of data collection, a distinct under estimation of the magnitude of the alcohol-treated mishaps has existed. This is not a new suggestion but tends to be lost when reading epidemiological studies of hundreds or even thousands of accidents.

In an effort to provide more extensive data collection and statistical reports, NHSTA has revised their method of estimating missing information about blood alcohol concentration for persons involved in fatal crashes (NHTSA, 1998). Accordingly more detailed information on the new multiple imputation method including detailed tabulations of alcohol in various demographic categories (age, sex, time of day and so forth) is now available (NHTSA, 2002b,c). This is discussed in more detail later in this chapter.

Table 14.4
Alcohol Involvement among Drivers in Fatal Crashes by Their Survival Status: A Comparison of Estimates Using the New and Old Methods, 1982–2000* (NHTSA, 2000a)

Year	Killed		Survived		Total	
	New	Old	New	Old	New	Old
1982	55	53	29	28	41	39
1983	54	51	28	27	39	38
1984	51	49	27	25	38	36
1985	49	48	23	23	35	34
1986	50	48	25	23	36	34
1987	48	47	23	23	34	33
1988	47	47	22	22	33	33
1989	46	46	20	21	31	32
1990	46	46	23	21	33	32
1991	45	44	21	21	31	31
1992	43	42	19	19	30	29
1993	41	40	18	18	28	27
1994	38	37	18	16	27	25
1995	39	38	16	16	26	25
1996	38	37	16	16	26	25
1997	36	35	15	15	24	24
1998	36	35	15	15	24	23
1999	36	35	14	14	24	23
2000	37	36	16	15	26	24

*Based on 1982-1999 Final FARS Files and 2000 Annual Report File

Table 14.5
Alcohol Involvement among Fatally Injured Pedestrians and Pedacyclists: A Comparison of Estimates Using the New and Old Methods, 1982–2000* (NHTSA, 2000a)

Year	Pedestrians		Pedalcyclists	
	New	Old	New	Old
1982	42	41	22	20
1983	42	40	18	20
1984	40	39	18	18
1985	40	39	15	18
1986	39	39	17	18
1987	38	38	19	21
1988	37	37	18	19
1989	39	39	18	19
1990	38	38	20	21
1991	38	38	24	24
1992	39	38	20	22
1993	38	37	22	23
1994	36	36	20	21
1995	37	37	23	24
1996	38	38	22	23
1997	35	34	22	23
1998	38	37	24	24
1999	38	37	26	26
2000	38	37	25	26

*Based on 1982-1999 Final FARS Files and 2000 Annual Report File

14.3 Working through the Ambiguities

A number of terms have been used to label the study of drinking and operation of motorized vehicles (e.g., automobiles, trucks, boats, motorcycles, bicycles and airplanes) and other mechanized equipment (Laurence, Snortum and Zimring, 1988). Included in the list of descriptors are drunken driving, drunk driving, drinking driving behavior, DUI, DWI and alcohol-impaired driving. No single term is completely accurate in defining the act of vehicular (or other equipment) operation after consumption of alcohol and one's ability to perform the associated tasks without ensuing problems. While "drinking driver" and "drunk driver" quite often can be described based on such things as BAC, behavior, drinking pattern, and other issues, the terms are often used synonymously. For simplicity, the term,

drunk driver, is used to identify this class of drivers and the related issues in this work because it is universally understood. It is noted that NHTSA now defines "alcohol involvement" in their data collection and analysis. NHTSA designates a fatal crash as alcohol-related or alcohol-involved if either a driver or non-motorist (usually a pedestrian) had a measurable or estimated blood alcohol concentration (BAC) of 0.01 g/dL or above. It further defines a nonfatal crash as alcohol-related or alcohol-involved if police indicate on the police accident report that there is evidence of alcohol present. The code does not necessarily mean that a driver or non-occupant was tested for alcohol (NHTSA, 2002b).

Table 14.6.
Alcohol Involvement (Percentage) in Fatal Crashes and Fatalities by Crash BAC and Imputation Method, FARS 1982–2000* (NHTSA, 2002)

Year	Fatal Crashes		Fatalities	
	BAC=.01+	BAC=.10+	BAC=.01+	BAC=.10+
1982	59 (57)	49 (46)	60 (57)	49 (46)
1983	57 (55)	48 (45)	58 (56)	48 (45)
1984	56 (53)	45 (43)	56 (54)	46 (43)
1985	53 (52)	42 (41)	53 (52)	43 (41)
1986	54 (52)	43 (41)	54 (52)	43 (41)
1987	52 (51)	41 (40)	52 (51)	41 (40)
1988	50 (50)	41 (40)	51 (50)	41 (40)
1989	49 (49)	40 (39)	49 (49)	40 (39)
1990	50 (49)	41 (40)	51 (50)	41 (40)
1991	48 (48)	40 (38)	49 (48)	40 (38)
1992	47 (46)	38 (36)	47 (45)	38 (36)
1993	45 (43)	36 (35)	45 (44)	36 (35)
1994	43 (41)	35 (32)	43 (41)	34 (32)
1995	42 (41)	34 (33)	42 (41)	34 (32)
1996	42 (41)	34 (32)	42 (41)	34 (32)
1997	40 (38)	32 (30)	40 (39)	32 (30)
1998	40 (39)	32 (30)	40 (39)	32 (30)
1999	40 (38)	32 (30)	40 (38)	32 (30)
2000	41 (40)	33 (31)	41 (40)	33 (31)

(*Based on 1982-1999 Final and 2000 Annual Report (AR) Files)
(Values in parentheses represent estimates from the **old** imputation methodology)

Before proceeding, it is necessary that certain other key terms used throughout epidemiology literature be defined. The word, epidemiology, refers to the science that deals with the incidence, distribution and control of disease in a population, or the sum of the factors controlling the presence or absence of a disease or pathogen. Epidemic refers to affecting or tending to affect many persons within a community, area or region at one time. In the strict sense, epidemiology would not readily apply to the study of the alcohol PMPI. However, the principles established by investigators in epidemic research may be applied to the problems associated with our topic. Retrospectively, demography may better define the type of study reported concerning the alcohol-PMPI work. Predominantly, the reports are statistical studies of the characteristics of human populations, especially with reference to size and density, growth, distribution, migration and vital statistics and the effect of all of these on social and economic conditions, which is demographic data.

Accident for a long period of time referred only to automobile accidents. Interestingly enough, with technological developments in the more recent past, additional data are becoming available on both operators and passengers of motor vehicles, aircraft, motorcycles, bicycles, as well as industrial and pedestrian accidents and alcohol. Operation of mechanical devices, however simple, requires psychomotor control as well as maintenance of behavioral control. All reports center about a common point—the occurrence of an accident. Authors vary with their definition of accident. Here it is interpreted as a sudden event or change occurring without intent or

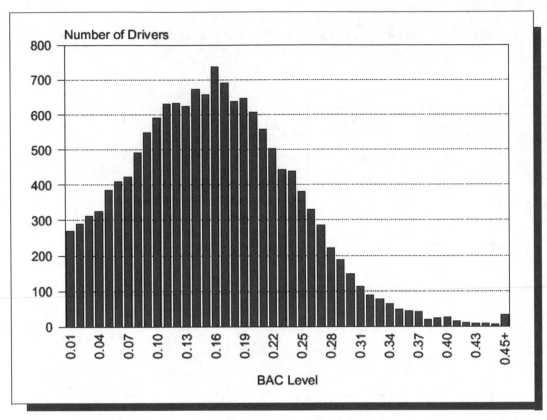

Figure 14.6 *Distribution of BAC levels for drivers involved in fatal crashes with BAC 0.01 or higher (NHTSA, 2001)*

volition through carelessness, unawareness, ignorance or a combination of causes and producing a negative or detrimental event. The keys to this definition are sudden event or change without intent and producing a negative or detrimental result.

The new reporting formats and broader definitions permit inclusion of data other than automobile accidents since alcohol-accident research is now including operation of other vehicles or devices (e.g., commercial and private trucks, airplanes, motorcycles, pedestrians, snowmobiles, bicycles and industrial accidents) (Baker and Fisher, 1977; Birrell, 1971; Davis and Smith, 1982; Dietz, 1974; Erikkson and Bjornstig, 1982; Haddon et al., 1961; McCarroll et al., 1962; Plueckhahn, 1978; Irwin, 1983; Klein et al., 1994; Billings et al., 1973; Ryan, 1974; NHTSA, 1993 a,b). These new inclusions in alcohol-PMP reports are applicable to understanding alcohol-PMP because they involve cases other than the historical forensic criminal application to automobile drunk driving (i.e., civil litigation). With the addition of

these new case types, the reporting affects a larger population of accident perpetrators and victims.

It soon becomes apparent to the reader that even the word impairment as used in alcohol-PMPI reports can be ambiguous. **Impairment** in common and scientific usage refers to something being made or becoming worse or being diminished in value, excellence and so forth. Alcohol-accident epidemiology uniformly applies a legal definition of impairment or one defined by law. **Legal impairment** means that at a given blood concentration of alcohol the individual is considered to be "impaired." Impaired is further described by descriptive terms such as "drunk," "driving while intoxicated (DWI)" or "driving under the influence (DUI)." In the United States, federal and many state BAC limits for driving have been set at ≥ 0.08 g/dL; however, it is set at ≥ 0.04 g/dL for underage drivers and workplace testing. The blood alcohol value will vary with the state or country in which the law is applicable. On the other hand, **pharmacologic impairment** refers to the blood concentration of alcohol whereby certain body functions, behavioral patterns, or as in our work here, PMP is altered. The blood concentrations at which alcohol produces legal and pharmacologic impairment may differ significantly. For example, in 1994, eleven states in the United States established a BAC of ≥ 0.08 g/dL to define legal impairment from alcohol (Johnson and Walz, 1994). By the end of the year 2000, state laws in thirty states made it a criminal offense to operate a motor vehicle with a BAC of 0.10 g/dL. One state and Puerto Rico did not have illegal per-se BAC levels (NHTSA, 2001). By 2001, all states and the District of Columbia had twenty-one-year-old minimum drinking age laws (NHTSA, 2001). Currently (2003) thirty-two states and the District of Columbia have adopted 0.08 g/dL. Other countries, such as Great Britain and Sweden, define legal impairment at a BAC of 0.08 g/dL. The threshold BAC for pharmacologic impairment may be as low as 0.02 g/dL. According to some researchers neuromuscular responses are impaired at 0.04 to 0.05 g/dL; vision at levels below 0.10 g/dL; simple and complex tracking at levels between 0.05 to 0.10

g/dL; and attention, at levels as low as 0.03 g/dL (Jones and Joscelyn, 1978; see Chapter 15). The basis for impairment in epidemiological literature pivots around the various state and federal legal definitions of BAC. This remains the case today.

NHTSA (1998; 2002a,b) introduced the new multiple-imputation procedure for estimating missing blood alcohol concentration for the FARS report now that the threshold for legal impairment in the United States is established at ≥ 0.08 g/dL. Before 2001, estimation of alcohol involvement was made in the three categories: 0.00, 0.01–0.09, and ≥ 0.10 g/dL. The new method estimates alcohol involvement in the new categories: 0.00 g/dL (no alcohol), 0.01 g/dL (impaired) and 0.08+ g/dL (intoxicated). It also stated that the new method has the ability to report alcohol involvement at any BAC concentration. Table 14.6 demonstrates the rates of alcohol involvement and intoxication in fatal crashes as estimated by the two procedures. The standard error of the estimated alcohol involvement (percentage) in fatal crashes by BAC ranged from 0.2692 to 0.4155

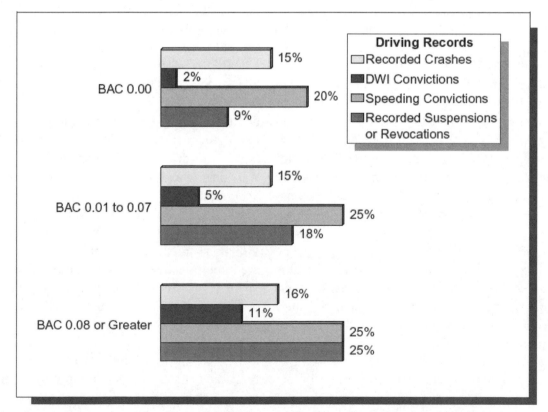

Figure 14.7 *Previous driving records of drivers killed in traffic crashes, by blood alcohol concentration, 2001 (NHTSA, 2001).*

(NHTSA, 2001). Although useful and meeting a legal definition, impairment remains implied rather than explicit because data collection has been subjective rather than objective in nature or has been statistically manipulated to provide estimated missing BAC. No apparent consideration has been established to marry the limits of detection and quantitation for the variety of chemical alcohol methods used by laboratories to the NHTSA categories for data grouping. From a practical medicolegal standpoint, it remains a difficult and costly task for the participants in a trial wherein an individual has a BAC at concentrations reported below 0.04 g/dL.

Figure 14.6 shows the distribution of BAC of drivers involved in fatal crashes in 2001 (NHTSA, 2002c). It indicates that 80 percent of the drivers who had been drinking (BAC ≥ 0.01 g/dL) and were involved in fatal crashes had a BAC above the legal definition of intoxication of 0.08 g/dL. This leaves 20 percent of the drivers with BAC between 0 and 0.079 g/dL open to interpretation by "experts" based on alcohol pharmacology research literature with little data at lower BACs on the actual role of bad driving and other factors.

PMP can be influenced by a number of variables. A term commonly confused and even interchanged with PMP is behavior. PMP refers to performance of tasks involving muscular action believed to ensue from prior conscious mental activity. Behavior is a less-tangible variable which is more encompassing and which has several definitions depending on its direct application. A general meaning of behavior is the manner in which a person responds in reaction to social stimuli, or to inner need, or to a combination thereof. An operant psychologist may define behavior as an activity of a defined organism (humans, in this case), especially observable activity when measurable in terms of quantifiable effects on the environment whether arising from internal or external stimuli. A more general meaning which applies is anything which an organism does that involves action and response to stimulation. A grossly general definition states that behavior is the response of an individual, group, or species to a broad range of factors constituting its environment. An officer of the law or court may choose to depend on the meaning of behavior which states that it is the treatment

shown by a person toward another or others, especially in his conformity with or divergence from the norms of good manners or social decorum.

In the final analysis it is very difficult in alcohol-PMPI epidemiological research to completely isolate any given variable discussed above. The interplay of major variables on the drunk driver is illustrated in Figure 14.4. In carefully reviewing existing epidemiologic reports, it becomes readily evident that all variables shown in Figure 14.4 impinge on each other to produce their respective and collective alterations in the response of the drunk driver, as alcohol does. In addition, the impact of sociological and demographic variables such as alcohol consumption patterns, recidivism, repeated DWI offenses, driving records, age and sex of drivers and effects of DWI treatment programs must be given consideration (Baker and Spitz, 1970; Bako et al., 1977; Brown, 1978; Filkins et al., 1970; Hagger and Dax, 1977; McGuire, 1978; Maisto et al., 1979; Maki and Linnoila, 1976; Rosenberg et al., 1974; Shaffer et al., 1977; Shultz and Layne, 1979; Whitlock et al., 1971; Davis, 1974; Pelz, 1975; Perrine, 1975, 1976; Waller, 1972, 1973).

Recidivism and repeated DWI offenses are referred to separately. Recidivism is a tendency to return to bad habits after some intervening attempt to alter one's habits through alcohol treatment or learning programs. It is therefore critical that laboratory and field testing be performed in addition to epidemiologic research in studying alcohol-PMPI of humans who drive or ride in motor vehicles or who walk near where motor vehicles are operated. Figure 14.7 represents data from drivers killed in traffic crashes based on their previous driving records. It is readily apparent that DWI convictions, speeding violations and previous suspensions and revocations are important variable in crashes (NHTSA, 2002c).

After discussing the variables which may influence the drunk driver and the multiple, sometimes confusing definitions of parameters to be studied, a commonality can be found which strongly indicts alcohol as an offending variable in PMPI. The fact remains that after investigation of thousands of motor vehicle accidents, alcohol has been present in the blood of many drivers in amounts greater than described as the minimum concentration for legal

PMPI. Since legal impairment is easily demonstrated at blood alcohol concentrations higher than those described for pharmacologic impairment, it follows that a societal problem exists involving the drunk driver. For example, Figure 14.7 shows the number of drivers killed in traffic crashes by BAC in 2001. At BAC at 0.00 g/dL only 2 percent of drivers' records are associated with DWI. This increases to 5 percent in the category of 0.01 to 0.07 g/dL BAC and 11 percent at BAC ≥ 0.08 g/dL. There remains a disparity between the legal and pharmacologic definitions of impairment based on the BAC of the drivers. This is especially true since younger driver in some states are required to be judged at lower BAC (as low as 0.04 g/dL) than adults (0.08 g/dL) except where the workplace standards apply to adults (BAC ≥ 0.04 g/dL) (NHTSA, 2002d).

14.4 Chronological Development of Epidemiology Database

A strong case is made for the need to understand how the epidemiological studies are germane to PMPI. This is implied when reference to these same epidemiological studies is made with increased emphasis on alcohol's impact on the human and financial aspects of accidents and health care delivery, the general economy as well as its ramifications in the law enforcement and judicial systems. Close examination of epidemiological studies leaves one with the impression that the customary cohesiveness of the scientific method is lacking when assessing the contribution of alcohol to PMPI. This literature is represented with few exceptions by a series of mostly isolated noncontrolled collections of demographic information concerning accidents and alcohol. The notable exceptions are summarized below. This presentation format was selected because there were no sufficient commonalities between the studies to use a more traditional tabular comparison. Additionally, it provides the reader with a brief overview of the material contained within a given reference which in some instances may be difficult to obtain otherwise.

A. North American studies

Heise (1934) [Pennsylvania, U.S.A.]. Analysis of BAC of drivers, passengers, pedestrians including hit-and-run drivers from 199 consecutive automobile accidents where victims required hospitalization. Alcohol accidents were more numerous than those that were not alcohol related. Alcohol was present more often in accidents involving injury or death of two people per accident versus one person per accident in non-alcohol crashes. Average BAC = 0.21 g/dL; pedestrian accidents, driver BAC = 0.14 g/dL; drinking pedestrian accidents, BAC = 0.20 g/dL; majority of accidents involving young and old people were alcohol related. If driver was sober then passenger was usually sober; those with high BAC also had passenger with equally elevated BAC. Weekends showed peak in alcohol related accidents (Sunday showed 3:1 increase in accidents with alcohol, with number of injuries or death increasing to 8:1). This disproportion was not observed on weekdays. Overall higher accident rate occurred during early evening (dark) hours. Alcohol-user related cases peaked higher at 6:00–7:00 P.M. Correlation was between alcohol-accident not darkness-accidents. Early morning accidents were non-alcohol related. Conclusions: (1) considering a person sober if he can walk and talk is of little value in assessing alcohol related statistics, (2) high incidence of weekend and night, male alcohol-related accidents, (3) drinking pedestrian often involved while children-old people struck often by sober drivers.

Holcomb (1938)[1] [Evanston, Illinois, U.S.A.]. BAC tests were performed at crash scene. Compared BAC of drivers involved in personal injury crashes versus drivers (control) regularly using same roadways. Twenty-five percent of crash drivers compared to 2 percent of noncrash drivers were legally drunk.

Lucas et al. (1955) [Toronto, Canada]. Study conducted from approximately 6:30–10:30 P.M. daily except Sundays (December 1951 through November 1952) involving 433 drivers of nonfatal, personal injury or property damage crashes. Fifteen percent of drivers were legally intoxicated by United States standards (i.e., BAC of > 0.10 g/dL).

Haddon and Braddess (1959) [Westchester County, New York, U.S.A.]. Studied driving fatalities between 1950–1953. Found that about 70 percent of driver fatalities in single vehicle crash had BAC > 0.10 g/dL. Fifty-five to 65 percent of subjects were too intoxicated to drive; 35–54 percent had BAC > 0.15 g/dL.

Hadden et al. (1961) [New York City (Manhattan), U.S.A.]. Studied fifty cases of fatally injured pedestrians, eighteen years and older, compared to similarly exposed persons not involved. Controls were obtained at accident site, same day of week and time of day, same age and sex as accident cases (200 subjects). Descriptive results: Accidents tended to occur in major shopping and business districts. Time of accidents: 6:00–12:00 P.M. (51 percent); 3:00 P.M.–3:00 A.M. (73 percent); 6:00–9:00 A.M., smallest percentage involved in accidents; and 41 percent died within six hours of accidents. Weather (rain) was not a significant factor. Mean age of fatality = 58.8 years, nonfatal injury age = 48.4 years, control = 41.6 years. There is an age-associated risk of involvement as well as age-related risk of fatal outcome involved. Data also suggest correlation of increased risk to the elderly with little or no BAC and middle-aged high BAC. Those involved were more often foreign born, not married, lower socioeconomic level as compared with matched control. Involved persons were within short distance of their homes.

Alcohol first becomes evident in the 0.01–0.04 g/dL BAC range. Percentage of people surviving less than six hours by BAC: 0.00 g/dL = 26 percent; 0.05 g/dL = 47 percent; 0.10 g/dL = 42 percent; 0.15 g/dL = 32 percent. Control BAC: 0.00 g/dL = 67 percent; 0.05 g/dL = 16 percent; 0.10 g/dL = 8 percent; 0.15 g/dL = 6 percent. Alcohol (BAC)-related fatalities were significantly different whether compared to site matches or age-sex matched controls.

McCarroll and Haddon (1962)[1] [New York City (Manhattan), U.S.A.]. Matched control taken at times and places of fatal crashes. Seventy-three percent of accident-responsible drivers had been drinking to some degree compared with 26 percent similarly exposed but noninvolved drivers. Forty-six percent of accident responsible group (eighty-six) had BAC >0.025 g/dL contrasted to negative BAC of

larger control groups (N = 516). Alcohol fatalities occurred closer to home than non-alcohol-involved drivers. No fatally injured subject lived outside city. Males were overrepresented in case group; non-married cases had higher BAC than married cases. Fatally injured cases and controls were matched by age and socioeconomic status. No association between accident involvement and vehicle age was evident. Suggest relationship of alcoholism may be a factor in alcohol-involved cases with very high BAC.

Borkenstein et al. (1964)[1] [Grand Rapids, Michigan, U.S.A.]. Nonfatal crashes studied. BAC tested on-scene; daily all hours. Data collected at scene for period July 1962–June 1963. Data collected seven days per week, twenty-four hours a day on 5,985 drivers. Randomly selected control groups (N = 7,590 drivers) from drivers using roadway at times and places of all types of crashes. Approximately 6 percent of drivers had BAC > 0.10 g/dL. Note that the value was lower than Lucas et al. (1955) report probably because Lucas study was done during evening hours. Data on 300 crashes classified as "fatals and driver injured" and 404 crashes labeled "other visible injury" show that approximately 9 percent of drivers had BAC > 0.10 g/dL. Results from this controlled study show that higher BACs were much less prevalent among non-crash drivers than crash-involved drivers.

Neilson (1969)[1] [California, U.S.A.]. Single and multivehicle crash study done between 1962–1968; BAC on motor vehicle fatalities. Forty-five percent of all fatally injured drivers in crashes had BAC > 0.10 g/dL. About 60 percent of fatalities had BAC of 0.10 g/dL when involved in single vehicle crashes. Thirty to 35 percent of multivehicle crash drivers had BAC > 0.10 g/dL. Pedestrian data shows 40 percent of fatalities had BAC > 0.10 g/dL. Data of Waller et al. (1970) and Neilson (1969) are consistent with each other.

Waller et al. (1970)[1] [California; U.S.A.]. BAC on motor vehicle fatalities studied from 1950–1967; single vehicle and multivehicle crashes. Approximately 50 percent of all fatally injured drivers involved in crashes had BAC > 0.10 g/dL. Sixty percent of single vehicle fatalities had BAC >0.10 g/dL; 30–35 percent multivehicle fatalities had BAC > 0.10 g/dL. Data summary excludes deaths occurring more than six hours after accident. Pedestrian data = 35 percent fatalities had BAC > 0.10 g/dL. The data is consistent with findings of Neilson (1969).

Baker and Spitz (1970)[1] [U.S.A.]. Study based on autopsy and police reports. Control or cause of bias of BAC in drinking driving considered in this crash study. Period studied was January 1, 1964 through December 31, 1968 (N = 328 subjects; 305 auto drivers, twenty-two truck drivers, one taxi driver). No limit placed on length of time between crash and death. Crash site information included a variety of road conditions (urban, rural roads and highways). BAC performed on all drivers who died less than six hours of crash. Results have been analyzed according driver responsibility, age of driver killed versus those surviving multivehicle collisions, length of survival, microscopic liver findings by age and BAC, presence of arteriosclerotic heart disease. No correlation found between driver responsibility and disease or physical disability. Decreased ability of older drivers to survive crashes caused them to be over represented in fatality-crash statistics. Delayed death resulting from crashes occurred more often among older drivers (sixty-plus years) than younger drivers.

Filkins et al. (1970)[1]; **Zylman et al.** (1975)[1] [Detroit, Wayne Co., Michigan, U.S.A.]. Single and multivehicle crashes studied in years 1967–1969; BAC influence on motor vehicle fatalities. BAC performed on 309 subjects; 96 percent of subjects survived less than six hours. Forty to 50 percent of drivers tested had BAC > 0.10 g/dL; 29–43 percent of drivers had BAC > 0.15 g/dL; 16–28 percent had BAC of > 0.20 g/dL.

Perrine et al. (1971)[1]; **Haddon et al.** (1961)[1]; **Jones and Joscelyn** (1976)[1] [U.S.A.]. Pedestrian fatalities. Thirty-one to 43 percent of subjects tested had BAC in excess of 0.10 g/dL. Twenty-five to 37 percent had BAC in excess of 0.15 g/dL.

Perrine et al. (1971)[1] [Vermont, U.S.A.]. Single and multivehicle crash studies in years 1967–1969; BAC data on motor vehicle fatalities. Bias of study given consideration. Controls were drivers using roads at same times and places as fatal crashes. About 65–70 percent of drivers fatally injured in single vehicle accidents had BAC > 0.10 g/dL. About 40 percent of fatalities in multivehicle acci-

dents had BAC > 0.10 g/dL. Less than 4 percent of control of noncrash drivers had BAC > 0.10 g/dL. High BAC was rarely observed in noncrash drivers compared with crash-involved drivers.

Waller (1972)[1]; **Zylman** (1974)[1] [U.S.A.]. Retrospective data analyzed from police reports. Forty percent of "responsible" drivers in multi vehicle crash had BAC > 0.10 g/dL; only 10 percent of "non-responsible" drivers > 0.10 g/dL; 64 percent of drivers with 0.00 g/dL BAC found responsible for crash.

Joscelyn and Treat (1973)[1] [U.S.A.]. Multidiscipline team approach to study of accident causes. Lists alcohol impairment as the prime cause of 7 percent of all types of accidents investigated and a prime or contributing cause of 16 percent of crashes studied by them. Impairment considered to be at BAC > 0.08 g/dL.

Clark and Clark (1973)[1] [Washtenan, Michigan, U.S.A.]. Fatal crashes studied in years 1968–1973. Statistics on crashes involving drivers and adult pedestrian. Fifty to 60 percent of fatally injured adult drivers had BAC > 0.10 g/dL; 40 percent of fatally injured adult pedestrians had BAC > 0.10 g/dL.

Billings, Wick et al. (1973) [U.S.A.]. Postmortem studies showed that 10–35 percent of pilots killed in U.S. aircraft accidents had measurable BAC at time of death.

Ellingstad and Westra (1974) [South Dakota, U.S.A.]. Fatal crashes studied (1972–1973). Forty to 50 percent of driver fatalities had BAC > 0.10 g/dL.

Zeller (1975) [U.S.A.]. U.S. Air Force had 4,200 accidents as well as low-magnitude occurrences defined as "incidents" between 1962–1973. These included eighty-nine instances wherein alcohol, drugs or both were associated in some degree. Association was defined as "presence of empty bottles in clothing to known ingestion of alcohol or drugs." The eighty-nine cases involved ninety-one aircraft and 269 people. Of these, sixty-six aircraft were destroyed; 128 people known to have been killed, missing or presumed dead. Forty of the eighty-nine occurrences were in 1962–1967, forty-nine occurred in 1968–1973. Alcohol was reported to have been the most frequently used drug (25/89). Not all accidents reported involved aircraft damage or members of the primary flight crews but rather crew members. These individuals were injured or killed while performing their duties or involved in other air or ground (flightline) mishaps.

Florendo (1975)[1] [Los Angeles, U.S.A.]. Fatal crashes studied in 1972–1974. About 50 percent of driver fatalities had BAC > 0.10 g/dL.

Spencer and Ferguson (1975)[1] [Fairfax, Virginia, U.S.A.]. Fatal crashes studied. 60 percent of driver fatalities had BAC > 0.10 g/dL.

Jones and Joscelyn (1976) [New Orleans, U.S.A.]. Fatal crashes studied (1972–1973). Fifty to 55 percent of driver fatalities had BAC > 0.10 g/dL. Twenty-five to 30 percent of pedestrian fatalities had BAC > 0.10 g/dL.

Jones and Joscelyn (1976); **Hurst** (1970; 1974)[1]; **Lucas et al.** (1955) [U.S.A.]. Review of crash predictability based on presence of alcohol. Lucas (1955) introduced a risk term called hazard; defined as the involvement of drivers in any BAC interval relative to the drivers in the lowest BAC interval measured. Hurst (1970, 1974) applied this term to controlled studies in conjunction with probability theory (i.e., Bayes' law) to calculation of probability of drivers being involved in a crash if a given BAC is reached relative to probability of crash involvement at zero (or lowest measured) BAC. Risk begins to increase very rapidly at BAC near 0.08 g/dL and increases rapidly at high BAC (i.e., BAC > 0.15 g/dL).

Farris et al. (1976)[1] [Huntsville, Alabama, U.S.A.]. Nonfatal, personal injury crashes, daily all hours; BAC on drivers at scene (2/3) or at hospital (1/3). Controls used road at same time and place as crashes. Thirteen percent of 596 drivers in nonfatal, personal injury crashes had BAC > 0.10 g/dL. Control group consisted of 804 noncrash drivers using roadway at times and places of 314 personal injury crashes.

Baker and Fisher (1977) [U.S.A.]. Retrospective study of ninety-nine fatal motorcycle crashes from police and medical examiner records. BAC determined in sixty-two motorcycle drivers; two-thirds had measurable amount of alcohol, one-half had ≥ 0.10 g/dL BAC; high concentrations most commonly found in 20–34 years of age group. Police mentioned alcohol in only nine cases. BAC distribution of motorcycle drivers was similar to those in fatally injured drivers of cars and trucks in state of Maryland.

Jones and Joscelyn (1978); **Traffic Injury Research Institute** (1975)[1] [Canadian National Survey (1973)]. BAC on motor-vehicle fatalities. BAC on 1,111 subjects; 1,006 died within six hours of crash; 44 percent had BAC > 0.11 g/dL. Forty-nine percent had BAC equal to Canadian legal limit for impairment (0.08 g/dL).

Riddick and Luke (1978) [District of Columbia, U.S.A.]. Noncontrolled postmortem study of 604 cases examined from Medical Examiner's Office, District of Columbia. Study had a population bias because cases included death by natural causes, homicide, suicide, traffic accidents, nontraffic accidents, and cause-of-death-unknown. In the forty-four traffic accidents, twenty-two deaths—of which twelve (50 percent)—were alcohol-associated. Cases were biased because death due to trauma and younger age groups were included.

McGuire (1978) [U.S.A.]. Controlled behavioral study. Classroom and behind-the-wheel with alcohol. One year record of 876 court-referred, first-offender, drinking drivers who graduated from a "Don't Drink and Drive" program compared with 802 drivers exposed to usual court procedures of probation and fine (control group). Found that the control group had 78 percent more alcohol-related violations, 23 percent more moving violations, 40 percent more license suspensions, and 34 percent more accidents. Discusses importance of study design in accident research.

Jalazo et al. (1978) [Pennsylvania, U.S.A.]. A noncontrolled study of arrested drivers which explored the relationship between BAC at time of screening with self-reported alcohol use and clinical judgement of recent drinking. Moderate correlation with Breathalyzer measurements of BAC was shown. Conclusion: self-reports and clinical judgement of alcohol consumption are unreliable.

Ryan and Mohler (1979) [U.S.A.]. Data from 1963 showed that in 43 percent of fatal civil aviation accidents that the pilots had BAC ≥ 0.15 g/dL. This value slowly declined each year until 1976 when it was 13 percent. Studies of fatalities (N = 1,345) occurring between 1969 and 1974 showed 26.7 percent had alcohol present with 19.5 percent represented by pilots. The authors point out that the "eight-hour abstinence" rule went into effect on December 5, 1970.

The data from the early cases reported since December, 1970 indicated that the eight-hour rule impacted on social drinkers but appeared to be less effective on "hardcore" heavy drinkers. Information on the human factors profile of civil aviation fatalities is included.

Shultz and Jayne (1979) [Arkansas, U.S.A.]. Study of DWI and public drunkenness offenses in "dry" rural setting; noncontrolled. BAC tended to be higher in young persons arrested for DWI and public drunkenness than in older people.

Maisto et al. (1979) [Tennessee, U.S.A.]. Retrospective, controlled evaluation; single and multiple offenders. Control group: random sampling of all drivers in state; test group: random sampling of single and multiple DWI offenders. Some demographic data (e.g., race, sex, type of offense). Conclusion: average interval decreases between convictions for DWI offenses (first and second, two years; second and third, seventeen months; third and fourth, eleven months; fourth and fifth, eight months).

Sonderstrom et al. (1979) [Maryland, U.S.A.]. Difficulties in diagnosis and management of roadway trauma involving presence of alcohol; noncontrolled study. Forty-eight percent of roadway trauma patients had positive BAC; 78 percent of positive BAC were > 0.10 g/dL (i.e., prima facie or presumptive evidence of DWI in most states at time of study).

Lundberg et al. (1979) [California, U.S.A.]. Prospective and retrospective components to study. Includes drug and alcohol data; controlled study. Behavior of driver observed and recorded. Compared observed alcohol odor on subject against analysis of BAC, only 56 percent of odor-detected cases were positive on analysis. Pooled data from thirteen laboratories used. Conclusions: data include observations on persons with psychoactive drugs, alcohol or both present in blood. Data not well separated in order to draw conclusions on alcohol alone; otherwise, study well presented. Observation notes rarely included in literature reports to substantiate "impaired function" change.

Weston (1980) [New Mexico, U.S.A.]. Psychological autopsy. Noncontrolled work. Thirty-nine percent of automobile driver fatalities and 40 percent of pedestrian fatalities had some blood alcohol present. Alcohol was involved in 39–74 percent of several types of violent crime. Psychological autopsy was used to prepare profiles of drivers in vehicular accidents. Drivers were grouped by behavioral characteristics likely to contribute to accident. Behavioral disorders where alcohol played a role were judged to be present in 28 percent of serious and fatal accidents studied.

MMWR (December 10, 1982) [U.S.A.]. Data analysis from Fatal Accident Reporting System (FARS). Based on crude death rate. In 1981, FARS shows alcohol played important role in highway fatalities in young drivers. Young driver fatalities (DWI) involved 4,738 persons. Accidents involving young drivers totaled 9,310. Forty-nine percent of young drivers with known alcohol involvement were more likely to be killed than those with zero or unknown alcohol involvement. Also shows data on distribution of crashes by BAC age.

Lloyd and Venus (1983) [Texas, U.S.A.]. Noncontrolled study. Speeding accounted for 24 percent of fatalities. Forty percent of fatally injured people were nondrivers. Decrease in fatalities occurred with enactment of 55-mph speed limit. DWI was a contributing factor in 24 percent of all fatal accidents and 28 percent of all rural fatalities. An increase of young fatalities and DWI was observed in the ten-year period 1970–1980.

Mason and McBay (1984) [North Carolina, U.S.A.]. This is an extensive report on alcohol, marijuana and other drug use in 600 fatally injured drivers in North Carolina, 1978–1981. Alcohol detection (79.3 percent) occurred more often than was any other drug for which testing was done. BAC testing of 85.5 percent of all drivers was positive for alcohol and 67.8 percent of drivers of all drivers had BAC ≥ 0.10 g/dL. Data included on other drugs.

Pendleton et al. (1986) [Texas, U.S.A.]. Results of study comparing medical examiners findings with investigating officer's conclusion concerning alcohol as a contributing factor to accidents involving 1,260 fatally injured drivers. Fifty-one percent of DWIs had BAC > 0.10. Data collection covered fifteen Texas counties for the period January 1, 1983–December 31, 1984. Legal limit for intoxication in Texas is > 0.10 g/dL BAC. Average BAC = 0.114 g/

dL in 1,260 driver fatalities studied, 80 percent of accident reports did not cite alcohol as contributing factor to accident; however, average BAC of these was 0.096 g/dL. Statistics cited: Driver age: 26-to-30-years age group most involved. Males more involved than females; most accidents occurred between 11:00 P.M.–3:00 A.M. on Sunday, Saturday, and Thursday. State police reported alcohol involvement in fatal accidents more often than local authorities. Data are consistent with national statistics.

Compton (1988) [U.S.A.]. Reports that drugs have been detected in 10–22 percent of crash-involved drivers. Drugs alone (no alcohol) were found in only 2–15 percent of these drivers. High levels of alcohol were found in combination in drug using drivers (53–77 percent). While drug presence in drug-alcohol using does not always imply driver impairment, alcohol when present with drugs may have been responsible for the crash. The authors noted the primary problem when interpreting data involving alcohol and drug combinations is the difficulty of separation of drug or alcohol effects or their combined effects.

Johnson and White (1989) [U.S.A.]. Self-reported data were collected for 18–21-year-olds (N = 556 men and women) at two points in time to assess the prevalence of DUI from alcohol and marijuana. Factors evaluated were driving after drinking and amount of alcohol consumed, risk-taking or impulsive orientation, negative intrapersonal state, stress and use of alcohol and other drugs as coping mechanisms. Determined that a minimum level of drinking and driving occurs at least once for most young people; frequency of substance abuse correlated with frequency of driving while intoxicated. Among other issues their findings suggest that impaired driving is associated with risk-taking behavior and is most often engaged in by persons who frequently use alcohol and drugs to cope with their problems. They point out that their data may be somewhat biased due to data gathering based on self-reporting of alcohol and drug use; however the trends are probably valid.

NHTSA (1993b) [U.S.A.]. Nine percent of motorcycle operators involved in fatal crashes in 1992 had at least one prior conviction for DUI compared with only 4 percent of passenger vehicle operators.

Comparison of statistics from 1992 showed that 35.5 percent of fatally injured motorcycle operators had BAC ≥ 0.10 g/dL while light truck, passenger car and large trucks were represented at 25.5, 21.7 and 1.4 percent, respectively. Of the fatally injured motorcycle operators, 35.6 percent had a BAC ≥ 0.10 g/dL. Additionally, 12 percent had BAC between 0.01–0.09 g/dL. Fatalities in 30–34-year-olds > 35–39-year-olds > 25–29-year-olds (52.9, 46.6 and 44.1 percent, respectively). More than one-half or 52.4 percent of 1,016 motorcyclists died in single vehicle crashes were intoxicated and more than two-thirds (67.7 percent) of those killed on weekend nights were intoxicated. Statistics revealed that motorcycle operators killed at night were approximately three and one-half times more likely to be intoxicated than those killed during the daytime (51.4 percent compared to 15.4 percent). Helmet use was lower in intoxicated motorcycle operators compared with sober operators.

Johnson and Walz (1994) [U.S.A.]. Beginning in 1983, the states of Oregon and Utah passed laws making it illegal per-se to drive with a BAC of ≥ 0.08 g/dL. Maine joined the list in 1988 followed by California (1990), Vermont (1991), Kansas and North Carolina (1993) and New Mexico, New Hampshire and Florida in 1994. All other states retain the BAC ≥ 0.10 g/dL. Data comparisons made between measures of alcohol-related fatal crashes over a two-year period before and after legislation suggests that decreases occurred following implementation of the legislation. While states did not show statistically significant declines in all thirty measures, they did show declines in several measures in each instance. Four states demonstrated decreases as follows. Alcohol > 0.10 g/dL: California (–4 percent), Oregon (–11 percent), Vermont (–31 percent). Any alcohol: Oregon (–9 percent), Vermont (–36 percent). Police-reported driver alcohol involvement: Oregon (–13 percent), Utah (–30 percent). Estimated alcohol involvement: Oregon (–11 percent), Vermont (–40 percent).

Klein, Morgan and Weiner (1994) [U.S.A.]. The report develops a significant number of geodemographic descriptors concerning rail-highway accidents which were collected using Claritas, a commercially available market research tool. Data indicates that rail-crossing driver fatalities exhibited rates of alcohol involvement about two times (24.4 percent) that of drivers in other intersection crashes (12.8 percent) however they were about the same as for drivers in all fatal crashes (26.1 percent). The statistics mentioned for all fatal crashes includes data from a combination of single vehicle and multiple vehicle crashes. Young drivers (21–24 years) had the highest rates of alcohol involvement, followed by 25–34-year-old drivers when looking at all three fatal crash categories (rail-crossing, intersection and all crashes).

Cerrelli (1995) [U.S.A.]. Occurrences of fatal crashes are more likely to occur with a high correlation (0.942) by time and day of week. A similar variation occurred as the proportion of intoxicated drivers were involved in fatal crashes. Injury crashes occurred independent of time and day of the week.

B. International citations

Underwood Ground (1975) [Great Britain]. Case report of forced landing of small aircraft with three people aboard after engine stall at low altitude. Pilot was an experienced commercial airline pilot. Two deaths and one injury occurred. BAC of pilot of 0.149 g/dL and urine-alcohol content of 0.139 g/dL.

Plueckhahn (1978) [Australia]. Noncontrolled, retrospective study. For period January 1967–June 1978, studied 344 vehicular fatalities. Victims, seventeen-plus years of age, died within four hours of accident. Victim drivers, 17–50 years old, totaled 147. Fifty-four percent of 147 victims had BAC > 0.10 g/dL at autopsy, thirty-five male pedestrians (60 percent) had BAC > 0.15 g/dL and 80 percent of pedestrian accidents occurred between 6:00–10:00 P.M. Fewer women road traffic victims observed.

Brown (1978) [New Zealand]. Comparison of alcohol-crash statistics with availability of alcohol. Noncontrolled study of the effects of a beer distribution strike on occurrence of alcohol-related incidents. Reduction in number of incidents on weekends and on total number; however, no long-term effects observed.

McDermott and Strang (1978) [New Zealand]. Historical review. Experience over three years post-legislation on compulsory blood alcohol tests. Of 21,863 male driver casualties, 27.1 percent had BAC legal limit (0.05 g/dL) and 13.7 percent had BAC > 0.15 g/dL. BAC of 9,187 female driver casualties was > 0.05 g/dL with 3.7 percent > 0.15 g/dL. Nondrivers had a slightly lower incidence of elevated BAC. Again, confirmed greater drinking involvement of males and city versus country driving data.

McDermott (1978) [Australia]. Discusses alcohol-driving legislation; BAC-driving incidence; relates BAC incidents to variables of sex, geography, religion, ethnicity and recidivism; role of medical community in prevention program.

Robinson (1979) [Ireland]. Deals with presence of drugs in specimens from impaired-driver cases. Impaired driver defined in law. Includes primarily drugs of abuse, alone or in combination with alcohol. Diazepam was most common of all drugs detected.

Honkanen et al. (1980) [Finland]. Controlled, prospective study. Blood serum drug screen and BAC on 201 drivers performed within six hours of road accident. Control drivers randomly selected at service stations totaled 325. Questionnaire on subject's health and use of drugs completed. Fifteen percent of drivers and 13 percent of controls admitted taking drugs during previous twenty-four hours. Two percent of both drivers and controls had taken psychotropic drugs, however, analysis revealed 5 percent of patients and 2.5 percent of controls were positive for this type of drug. Diazepam was found in sixteen of eighteen subjects positive for psychotropic drugs. Fifteen percent of drivers and 1 percent of controls were positive for alcohol. Conclusion: Drug use in Finland is lower than other Western countries; illness appears to be a greater risk hazard. Interview (i.e., self-reporting) not a reliable method to determine psychotropic drug use. Diazepam may increase accident risk but alcohol still most important risk factor.

Landauer (1981) [Australia]. Literature review. Study involves diazepam literature, however, some alcohol information surfaced.

Galloway and Patel (1981) [Scotland]. Prospective study. Of 1,566 road traffic victims studied, 41 percent were drivers, 36 percent passengers and 23 percent were pedestrians. Seventy-six percent were discharged after treatment and 24 percent required additional in-patient care. Forty-six percent of accidents occurred between midnight and 8 A.M. One-third occurred on Saturdays and Sundays. Men under thirty-five years old were over-represented as drivers and passengers. Three-fourths of male drivers were between 17–35 years old. Age of pedestrians and women passengers were similar. One-half of pedestrian total were over thirty-five years old. Automobile crashes were more frequent than motorcycle than bus crashes, in that order. Nineteen percent of road accident victims and 19 percent of other accident victims had detectable levels of ethanol. Data shows male pedestrians were often highly intoxicated; also large number of road accident cases in general showed presence of intoxicating levels of alcohol.

Simpson et al. (1982) [Ontario, Canada]. Review with emphasis on young people and alcohol-crashes. Good presentation of variables in epidemiological studies and the state of existing alcohol data.

Crompton (1982) [England]. Autopsy study of 208 cases with data on type vehicle, age, sex and alcohol involvement. Data suggest that majority of fatal accidents occur before the alcohol levels in the urine and blood have reached equilibrium (i.e., during the phase of rising blood alcohol). Evidence also shows that young chronic alcoholics rather than occasional drinker are at cause in road accidents. Passenger with BAC approximately 0.100 g/dL is at great risk especially if driver is also drinking. Accidents appear to occur within half-hour of drinking. Suggest an hour "sobering period "thereby bypassing rising BAC phase and the overconfident and impulsive phase because drinker would be on falling side of BAC curve.

Cimbura et al. (1982) [Canada (Ontario)]. Fatally injured drivers and pedestrians (N = 484) studied for presence of drugs and alcohol in blood and urine, occasionally on vitreous humor, stomach contents and liver. Alcohol was found in 57 percent of drivers and other drugs in 26 percent of the drivers. Psychoactive drugs were present in blood of 9.5 percent of drivers in concentrations that could adversely affect driving ability. Marijuana and diazepam accounted for the majority of psychoactive drugs present.

McDermott and Hughes (1982) [Australia]. Noncontrolled study of driver and nondriver accident casualties. County had compulsory alcohol testing for all road crashes. Twenty and one-half percent of both driver and nondriver fatalities had alcohol levels in excess of legal driver limit (0.05 g/dL). Driver (9.8 percent) and nondriver (6.4 percent) samples had BAC > 0.15 g/dL; 27.4 percent male and 9.2 percent female drivers exceeded the BAC limit; 18.7 percent city and 25 percent of country drivers exceeded BAC limit. Greatest decrease in DWI immediately following implementation of increased penalties for DWI.

Reports based on both retrospective and prospective epidemiological data collection indicate that a strong relationship exists between alcohol consumption, BAC and the occurrence of automobile and other accidents. The legal threshold for PMPI is reported to be approximately 0.08 g/dL alcohol in blood with other pharmacologic and functional thresholds showing impairment at BACs < 0.08 g/dL (See Chapter 15). These observations have been reported with the advent of both breath analysis devices and automobiles (Heise, 1934; Jones and Joscelyn, 1978). More recent studies have shown a reduction in some measures of alcohol involvement in driver fatalities between 1990–1992 (Johnson, 1994; NHTSA, 2001).

Careful examination of epidemiological reports indicates that prospective studies would most likely yield more useful information because uniform questions concerning the accident circumstances would be asked at the time of the accident investigation. Retrospective studies on the other hand require addressing a battery of standard questions from multiple non-homogeneous sources at a future point in time often far removed from the accident event. This obviously leaves interpretation of data open to question in many instances if it may be used at all.

One can no longer isolate the drunk driver in analyzing crash data but must include data not only on motor craft other than automobiles but also pedestrian and passenger data. We also need to assemble data on workplace accidents as well. In doing so, one discovers that the numbers swell and the implication of alcohol's involvement in accidents is strengthened. Hard and fast evidence linking alcohol and PMPI that would apply uniformly to every driver with PMPI is lacking for a single conclusion to be made in every conceivable situation. Therefore, each case must be investigated and carried to its final resolution based on a large number of descriptive variables.

Unfortunately as the use of mind altering drugs of all pharmacologic classes becomes more prevalent, the issues of application and interpretation of the alcohol data is further clouded. A relatively few reports appear in the epidemiological literature at present on drug-related as compared with alcohol-related motor vehicle accidents (Finkle et al., 1968; Zeller, 1975; Mason and McBay, 1984; Garriott et al., 1977; Honkanen et al., 1980, 1976; Jick et al., 1981; Job, 1982; Landeau, 1981; Lundberg et al., 1979; Marks, 1982; Robinson, 1979; Turk et al., 1974; Cimbura et al., 1982; Simpson et al., 1982; Bastos and Galante, 1976; Davis, 1974; Compton, 1988). Not only is the lack of information on drug-induced PMPI a confounding variable in accident research and case interpretation, the lack of a data base concerning the combined effects of alcohol and drugs is adding more confusion (Figure 14.2). However, a trend toward drug-PMPI and drug-alcohol interaction leading to increased PMPI is emerging. As Compton (1988) has noted, the primary interpretative problem when drugs and alcohol are both present is whether to attribute functional effects in the subject to either drug or alcohol or their combination. This remains a problem today.

14.5 The Twenty-First Century: What Has Been Learned from Epidemiological Research?

Traffic fatalities in alcohol-related crashes rose by 0.4 percent from 17,380 in 2000 to 17,448 in 2001. However, this represents a 13-percent reduction in 2001 from the 20,159 alcohol-related fatalities reported in 1991. It has been estimated that alcohol was involved in 41 percent of fatal crashes and in 7 percent of all crashes reported in 2001. That translates to an average of one alcohol-related fatality every thirty minutes. Injuries in crashes where police reported alcohol present involved 275,000 people. This represents an average of one person injured ap-

proximately every two minutes. In 2000, approximately 1.5 million drivers were arrested for driving under the influence of alcohol or narcotics. The arrest rate for this group of drivers is one arrest for every 130 licensed drivers in the United States. Thirty-five percent of all traffic fatalities in 2001 occurred in crashes in which at one driver or nonoccupant had a BAC of ≥ 0.08 g/dL (NHTSA, 2001).

Results of other demographic indicators have also be reported by NTHSA (2001) coupled with the above information gives us descriptors with which to identify those most likely to be in alcohol-involved crashes. These are summarized below (NHTSA, 2002c).

Highest intoxication rates for drivers by age
- 21–24 years (33 percent)
- 25–34 years (28 percent)
- 35–44 years (25 percent)

Intoxication rate for drivers by vehicle type
- Highest: Motorcycle operators (29 percent)
- Lowest: Large truck operators (1 percent)
- Same: Light trucks and passenger car drivers (23 percent)

Safety belt use by drivers
- 23 percent of fatally injured drivers (BAC = ≥ 0.08 g/dL)
- 33 percent of fatally injured impaired drivers (BAC = between 0.01 and 0.07 g.dL)
- 53 percent of fatally injured sober drivers

Prior conviction for driving while intoxicated
- Drivers with a prior conviction are ten times more likely to be fatally injured than sober drivers.

Intoxicated pedestrians killed in crashes by age
- 36 percent of all pedestrians ≥ 16 years killed in traffic crashes were intoxicated.
- 7 percent of pedestrians ≥ 65 years were intoxicated.
- 52 percent of pedestrians 35–44 years were intoxicated.

Pedestrian fatalities
- 41 percent drivers, pedestrians or both were intoxicated.
- 33 percent of pedestrians were intoxicated compared to 15 percent of drivers.

- 6 percent of instances both driver and pedestrian were intoxicated.

BAC ≥ 0.08 g/dL

- 80 percent (11,802/14,706) drivers who had been drinking had BAC ≥ 0.01 g/dL.
- All involved in fatal crashes had BAC ≥ 0.08 g/dL.

Impact of minimum drinking age laws

- Number of lives saved rose from 14,816 in 1994 to 20,970 in 2001. See Figure 14.8.

14.6 Summary

The simple correlation of the high incidence of BAC above the legal limit in drivers having accidents indicates that a significant problem exists. We can only conclude that alcohol is present in a large number of drivers in amounts greater than legally permissible based on the epidemiology literature, especially in driver populations involved in accidents. In the majority of these persons, alcohol has been present in amounts exceeding the currently accepted legal and pharmacologic thresholds for PMPI. However, the epidemiology data alone cannot solely identify alcohol as the causative or contributive factor in any single accident scenario. The scientific support of the BAC threshold for pharmacological and legal designation of alcohol (or drug or both) PMPI remains with the experimental studies where other variables such as environment, amount of alcohol consumed, or temporal relationship between alcohol use and accidents or crash conditions, and BAC and PMPI can be ascertained under controlled conditions (see Chapter 15). These laboratory and field investigations, discussed in the next chapter, in concert with the epidemiology studies also permit improved prospective design and standardization of testing procedures. The data may be used to correlate blood alcohol concentration with general and functional impairment which may occur. As these collective efforts become more sophisticated they will permit development of educational programs directed toward drivers who drink and drive. They will also aid the forensic community in adjusting the definitions of legal impairment and subsequent law

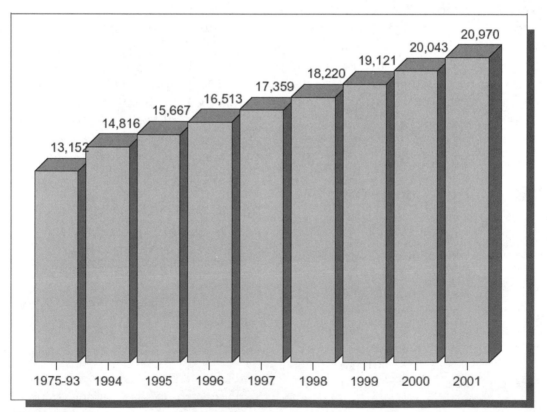

Figure 14.8 Cumulative estimated number of lives saved by minimum drinking age laws, 1975–2001 (NHTSA, 2001)

changes as necessary and knowledgeable interpretations of PMPI in individual alcohol associated cases. We have witnessed this process beginning with Heise's work in the 1930s, progressing to the establishment of the federal legal definition of impairment established as ≥ 0.08 g/dL as we have moved into the twenty-first century, as well as the DOT workplace guidelines set at ≥ 0.04 g/dL. At the same time, we have observed a significant downward trend in the number of fatalities in alcohol-involvement in fatal crashes. The knowledge gained since the 1930s with alcohol-related driving accidents serves as an excellent prototype for future studies which are necessary to define other drug and alcohol PMPI issues.

References

American Medical Association Committee on Medicolegal Problems. *Alcohol and the Impaired Driver. A Manual on the Medicolegal Aspects of Chemical Tests for Intoxication.* Chicago: American Medical Association, 1970.

Baker, S.P. and Fisher, R.S. Alcohol and motorcycle fatalities. *Am. J. Public Health* 67:246–249, 1977.

Baker, S.P. and Spitz, W.M. Age effects and autopsy evidence of disease in fatally injured drivers. *JAMA* 214:1,079–1,088, 1970.

Bako, G., MacKenzie, W.C. and Smith, E.S.O. Case–control study of recidivist drivers involved in fatal highway accidents in Alberta in 1970–72. *Can. Med. Assoc. J.* 116:149–151, 1977.

Bastos, M.L. and Galante, L. Toxicological findings in victims of traumatic deaths. *J. Forensic Sci.* 21:176–186, 1976.

Billings, C.E. et al. Effects of Ethyl Alcohol on Pilot Performance. *Aerospace Med.* 44:379–382, 1973.

Birrell, J.H.W. A comparison of the postmortem blood–alcohol levels of drivers and passengers compared with those of drinking drivers who killed pedestrians. *Med. J. Aust.* 2:945–948, 1971.

Borkenstein, R.F. et al. *The Role of Drinking Driver in Traffic Accidents.* Bloomington: Indiana University, Dept. of Police Administration, 1964.

Brown, R.A. Some social consequences of partial prohibition in Auckland, New Zealand. *Drug Alcohol Depend.* 3:377–382, 1978.

Cerrelli, E.C. *Crash, Injury and Fatality Rates By Time of Day and Day of Week.* NHTSA Technical Report DOT–HS–808194, January 1995.

Cimbura, G. et al. Incidence and toxicological aspects of drugs detected in 484 fatally injured drivers and pedestrians in Ontario. *J. Forensic Sci.* 27:855–867, 1982.

Clark, D.C. and Clark, F.A. *Analyses of Washtenaw County Alcohol Safety Action Program Crash Criteria Measures.* Ann Arbor: University of Michigan, Highway Safety Research Institute, 1973.

CNN. October trial for ex-pilots accused of drinking before flight, August 6, 2002 (http://cnn. law. printhi...?cpt?&expire=–1&url=3711580&fb= Y&partnerID–201; printed 2/11/03).

cnn.com. Judge bars viewing of tape in case of pilots accused of being drunk. http://www.cnn.com/2002/LAW/10/24/pilot.hearingtapes. Printed 2/11/2003.

Compton, R.P. *Use of Controlled Substances and Highway Safety: A Report to Congress.* NHTSA Technical Report DOT–HS–807261, March 1988.

Crompton, M.R. Alcohol and fatal road traffic accidents. *Med. Sci. Law* 22: 189–194, 1982.

Davis, J.H. Carbon monoxide, alcohol and drugs in fatal accidents in Dade County, Florida, 1956–1968. *Clin. Toxicol.* 7:597–613, 1974.

Davis, S.. and Smith, L.S. Alcohol and drowning in Cape Town. A preliminary report. *S. Afr. Med. Tydskr.* 62:931–933, 1982.

Dietz, P.E. and Baker, S.P. Drowning: Epidemiology and prevention. *Am. J. Public Health* 64:303–312, 1974.

Ellingstad, V.S. and Westra, D.P. *Analytic Study, part 1: An Analysis of Total Project Impact*. Vermillion, SD: University of South Dakota, Department of Psychology, 1974.

Eriksson, A. and Bjornstig, U. Fatal snow mobile accidents in Northern Sweden. *J. Trauma* 22:977–982, 1982.

Farris. R., Malone. T.B. and Lilliefors, H. *A Comparison of Alcohol Involvement in Exposed and Injured Drivers*. Phases I and II. National Highway Traffic Safety Administration Technical Report DOT-HS-801–826, 1976.

Filkins, L.D. et al. *Alcohol Abuse and Traffic Study: A Study of Fatalities, DWI Offender. Alcoholics and Court-Related Treatment Approaches*. Final Report U.S. Dept. of Transport, National High way Safety Bureau Contract No. FH-11-6555 and FH-11-7129, 1970.

Finkle, B.S., Biasotti, A.A. and Bradford, L.W. The occurrence of some drugs and toxic agents encountered in drinking driver investigation. *J. Forensic Sci.* 13–236–245, 1968.

Florendo, R.M. *An Analysis of Ultimate Performance Measures, 1974*. LA: County of Los Angeles, Alcohol Safety Action Project, 1975.

Galloway, D.J. and Patel, A.R. Road traffic accident–related morbidity as seen in an accident and emergency department. *Scot. Med. J.* 26:121–124, 1981.

Garriott, J.C. et al. Incidence of drugs and alcohol in fatally injured motor vehicle drivers. *J. Forensic Sci.* 22:383–389, 1977.

Haddon, W., Jr. and Bradess, V.A. Alcohol in the single vehicle fatal accident. *JAMA* 169:1587–1593, 1959.

Haddon, W. et al. A controlled investigation of the characteristics of adult pedestrians fatally injured by motor vehicles in Manhattan. *J. Chron. Dis.* 14:655–678, 1961.

Hagger, R. and Dax, F.C. The driving records of mutli–problem families. *Soc. Sci. Med.* (A) 11:121–127, 1977.

Hall, J.E. Alcohol and other drug use in commercial transportation. In: *Schaffer Library of Drug Policy* [Internet]. [cited 2003 February 11]. [about 7p.] Available from: http://www.druglibrary.org./schaffer/MISC.driving/s1p1.htm, printed 2/11/2003.

Harger R.N., Lamb, E.B. and Hulpieu, H.R. Rapid chemical test for intoxication employing breath; new reagent for alcohol and procedure for estimating concentration of alcohol in body from ratio of alcohol to carbon dioxide in breath. *JAMA* 110: 779–785, 1938.

Heise, H. Alcohol and automobile accidents. *JAMA* 103:739–741, 1934.

Holcomb, R.L. Alcohol in relation to traffic accidents. *JAMA* 3:1076–1085.

Honkanen, R.L., Ertama, L., Linnoila, M. et al. Role of drugs in traffic accidents. *Br. Med. J.* 281:1,309–1,312, 1980.

Honkanen. R. and Visuri, T. Blood alcohol levels in a series of injured patients with special references to accident and type of injury. *Ann. Chir. Gynecol.* 65:287–294, 1976.

Hunt, W.A. and Witt, E.D. Behavorial Effects of Alcohol Ingestion: Implications for Drug Testing. *Toxic Substances J.* 13:41–49, 1994.

Hurst, P.M. Epidemiology aspects of alcohol and driver crashes and citations. In: Perrine, M.W. (ed.), *Alcohol, Drugs and Driving*, NHTSA Technical Report DOT–HS–801–096, 1974.

Hurst, P.M. Estimating the effectiveness of blood alcohol limits. *Behav. Res. Hwy. Safe.* 1:87–99, 1970.

Irwin, S.T., Patterson, C.C. and Rutherford, W.H. Association between alcohol consumption and adult pedestrians who sustain injuries in road traffic accidents. *Br. Med. J.* 286:522, 1993.

Jalazo, J., Steer. R.A. and Fine, E.W. Use of breathalyzer scores in the evaluation of persons arrested for driving while intoxicated. *J. Stud. Alcohol* 39:1304–1307, 1978.

Jick, H. et al. Sedating drugs and automobile accidents leading to hospitalization. *Am. J. Public Health* 71:1,399–1,400, 1981.

Job, R.F.S. Does diazepam affect driving ability? *Med. J. Aust.* 1:89–91, 1982.

Johnson, M.D. and Walz, M.C. *A Preliminary Assessment of the Impact of Lowering the Illegal Per Se Limit to 0.08 in Five States.* NHTSA Technical Report DOT–HS–808–207, December, 1994.

Johnson, V. and White, H.R. An investigation of factors related to intoxicated driving behaviors among youth. *J. Stud. Alcohol* 50:320–330, 1989.

Jones, R.K. and Joscelyn, K.B. A systems approach to the analysis of transportation law. *Transp. Law J.* 8:71–89, 1976.

Jones, R.K. and Joscelyn, K.B. *Alcohol and Highway Safety: A Review of the State of Knowledge.* NHTSA Final Report DOT-HS-5–01217, 1978.

Joscelyn, K.B. and Treat, J.R. *A Study to Determine the Relationship between Vehicle Defects and Crashes.* Bloomington: Indiana University, Institute for Research in Public Safety, 1973.

Klein, T., Morgan, T. and Weiner, A. *Rail-Highway Crossing Safety: Fatal Crashes and Demographic Descriptors* NHTSA Technical Report DOT-HS-808196, November 1994.

Landauer, A.A. Diazepam and driving ability. *Med. J. Aust. L.* 624–626,1981.

Laurence, M.D., Snortum, J.R. and Zimring, F.E. A note on terminology. In: Laurence, M.D., Snortum, J.R. and Zimring, F.E. (eds.), *Social Control of the Drinking Driver.* Chicago: The University of Chicago Press, pp xvii–xviii, 1988.

Lloyd, L.E. and Venus, P. Death and Texas roads: The picture worsens for young adults. *Tex. Med.* 79:53–56, 1983.

Lucas, G.W.H. et al. Quantitative studies of the relationship between alcohol levels and motor vehicle accidents. In *Proceedings of the Second International Conference an Alcohol and Road Traffic.* Toronto: Garden City Press Cooperative, 1955.

Lundberg, G.D., White, J.M. and Hoffman, K.I. Drugs (other than or in addition to ethyl alcohol) and driving behavior: A collaborative study of the California Association of Toxicologists. *J. Forensic Sci.* 24:207–215, 1979.

Maisito, S.A. et al. Driving records of persons convicted of driving under the influence of alcohol. *J. Stud. Alcohol* 40:70–77. 1979.

Maki, M. and Linnoila, M., Characteristics of driving in relation to the drug and alcohol use of Finnish outpatients. *Mod. Probl. Pharmacopsychiatry* 2: 11–21, 1976.

Marks, V. Drugs and driving. *R. Soc. Health J.* 102: 205–210. 1982.

Mason, A.P. and McBay, A.J. Ethanol, marijuana and other drug use in 600 drivers killed in single-vehicle crashes in North Carolina, 1978–1981. *J. Forensic Sci.* 29:987–1026, 1984.

McCarroll, J. et al. Fatal pedestrian automotive accidents. *JAMA* 180:127–133, 1962.

McCarroll, J.R. and Haddon, W., Jr. A controlled study of fatal automobile accidents in New York City. *J. Chron. Dis.* 15:811–826. 1962.

McDermott, F. Control of road trauma epidemic in Australia. *Ann. R. Coll. Eng.* 60:437–450, 1978.

McDermott, F. and Strang, P. Compulsory blood alcohol testing of road crash casualties in Victoria: The first three years. *Med. J. Aust.* 2:612–615. 1978.

McDermott, F.T. and Hughes, E.S.R. Compulsory blood alcohol testing of road crash casualties in Victoria: The second three years (1978–1980). *Med. J. Aust.* 1:294–296, 1982.

McGuire, F.L. The effectiveness of a treatment program for the alcohol-involved driver. *Am. J. Alcohol Abuse* 5:517–525, 1978.

MMWR. Reduction in Alcohol-Related Traffic Fatalities: United States, 1990–1992. *MMWR* 42(47): 905–909,1993.

MMWR. Patterns of alcohol use among teenage drivers in fatal motor vehicle accidents United States 1977–1981. *MMWR* 32:344–347, 1982.

Neilson, R.A. *Alcohol Involvement in Fatal Motor Vehicle Accidents. California 1962–1968.* San Francisco: California Traffic Safety Foundation, 1969.

NHTSA. *Traffic Safety Facts 1992. A Compilation of Motor Vehicle Crashes Data from the Fatal Accident Reporting System and the General Estimates System.* NHTSA Technical Report DOT-HS-808-022, September 1993a.

NHTSA. *Traffic Safety Facts 1992. Motorcycles* (U.S. G.P.O.: 1993-343-273:80140). Washington, DC: National Center for Statistics and Analysis, Research and Development, 1993b.

NHSTA. *Multiple Imputation of Missing Blood Alcohol Concentration (BAC) values in FARS.* Technical Report DOT-HS-808-816, October 1998.

NHTSA. *Traffic Safety Facts 2000: A Compilation of Motor Vehicle Crash Data from the Fatality Analysis Reporting System and the General Estimates System.* NHTSA Technical Report DOT-HS-809-337, 2001.

NHTSA. *Estimates of Alcohol Involvement in Fatal Crashes. New Alcohol Methodology.* NCSA document number DOT-HS-809-450, 2002a.

NHTSA. *Transitioning to Multiple Imputation: A New Method to Impute Missing Blood Alcohol Concentration (BAC) values in FARS,* NHTSA Technical Report DOT-HS-809-403, January 2002, Revised June, 2002, Revised October, 2002b.

NHTSA. *Traffic Safety Facts 2001: Alcohol.* NHTSA Technical Report DOT–HS–809–470 (2002c).

NHTSA. *State Alcohol Related Fatality Rates,* NHTSA Technical Document DOT–HS– 809–528, December 2002d.

O'Harra, D. Pilots in treacherous waters. *Anchorage Daily News*, April 02, 1989. http://www.adn.com/ evos/stories/EV395.html; printed 2/11/03.

Pelz, D.C., McDole, T.L. and Schuman, S.H. Drinking–driving behavior of young men in relation to accidents. *J. Stud. Alcohol* 36:956–972. 1975.

Pendleton, O.J., Hatfield, N.J. and Bremer, R. *Alcohol Involvement in Texas Driver Fatalities: Accident Reports versus Blood Alcohol Concentration.* College Station, TX: Texas Transportation Institute, Texas A&M University System, 1986.

Perrine, M.W. Alcohol and highway crashes. *Mod. Probl. Pharmacopsychiatry* 11:22–41, 1976.

Perrine, M.W. Alcohol involvement in highway crashes: A review of the epidermiologic evidence. *Clin. Plast. Surg.* 2.11–34, 1975.

Perrine, M.W. and Huntley, M.S., Jr. *Influences of Alcohol Upon Driving Behavior in an Instrumental Car.* NHTSA DOT-HS-800-625. 1971.

Perrine, M.W., Waller, J.A. and Harris, L.S. *Alcohol and Highway Safety: Behavioral and Medical Aspects.* NHTSA Technical Report DOT–HS–800–599, 1971.

Plueckhahn, V.D. Alcohol and road safety: Geelong experience 1967 to 1978. *Med. J. Aust.* 2:615–625, 1978.

Plueckhahn, V.D. Alcohol consumption and death by drowning in adults: A 24 year epidemiological analysis. *J. Stud. Alcohol* 43:445–452. 1982.

Riddick, L.R. and Luke, J.C. Alcohol-associated deaths in the District of Columbia—A Postmortem study. *J. Forensic Sci.* 23:493–501, 1978.

Robinson, T.A. The incidence of drugs in impaired driving specimens in Northern Ireland. *J. Forensic Sci. Soc.* 19:237–244, 1979.

Rosenberg, N., Laessig. R.H. and Rawlings. R.R. Alcohol. age and fatal traffic accidents. *Q. J. Stud. Alcohol* 35:473–489, 1974.

Ryan, L.C. and Mohler, S.R. Current Role of Alcohol as a Factor in Civil Aircraft Accidents. *Aviation Space Environ. Med.* 50:275–279, 1979.

Shaffer. J.W. et al. Social adjustment profiles of female drivers involved in fatal and nonfatal accidents. *Am. J. Psychiatr.* 134:801–804, 1977.

Shultz, S.D. and Jayne, N.R., Jr. Age and BAC when arrested for drunken driving and public drunkenness. *J. Stud. Alcohol* 40:492–495, 1979.

Simpson, H. M., Mayhew, D.R. and Warren, R.A. Epidemiology of road accidents involving young adults: Alcohol. drugs and other factors. *Drug Alcohol Depend.* 10:35–63, 1982.

Soderstrom, C.A. et al. Alcohol and roadway trauma: Problems of diagnosis and management. *Am. Surg.* 45:129–137, 1979.

Spencer, J.A. and Ferguson, W.S. *An Analysis of Ultimate Performance Measures to Determine Total Project Impact of the Fairfax County Alcohol Safety Action Project.* Richmond, VA: Highway Safety Division of Virginia, Virginia Highway Traffic Research Council, 76-R29. 1975.

Sweedler, B.M. Alcohol and other drug use in the railroad, aviation, marine and trucking industries–progress has been made. In: *Proceedings of Alcohol, Drugs and Safety, T-92,* Cologne, Germany, 1992.

Traffic Injury Research Foundation of Canada. *Analysis of Fatal Traffic Crashes in Canada, 1973. Focus: The Impaired Driver.* Ottawa: Traffic Injury Research Foundation of Canada, 1975.

Turk, R.F., McBay, A.J. and Hudson, P. Drug involvement in automobile driver and pedestrian fatalities. *J. Forensic Sci.* 19:90–97, 1974.

Underwood Ground, K.E. Impaired pilot performance: Drugs or alcohol. *Aviation Space Environ. Med.* 50:1284–1288, 1975.

U.S.A. Today. Alcohol, drug violations rare among airline employees, FAA says. *U.S.A. Today,* July 3, 2002 http://www.U.S.A.today.com/travel/news/2002/2002–07–03–faa–reax.htm, printed 2/11/03)

Waller, J.A. Current issues in the epidemiology of injury. *Am. J. Epidemiol.* 98:72–76. 1973.

Waller, J.A. Factors associated with alcohol and responsibility for fatal highway crashes. *Q. J. Stud. Alcohol* 33:160–170. 1972.

Waller, J.A. et al. Alcohol and other factors in California highway fatalities. In *Proceedings of the 11th Annual Meeting of the American Association for Automotive Medicine.* Charles C. Thomas, Springfield, Ill. 1970.

Weston, J.T. Alcohol's impact on man's activity: Its role in unnatural death. *Am. J. Clin. Pathol.* 74: 755–758, 1980.

Whitlock, F.A. et al. The drinking driver or the driving drinker? Alcohol, alcoholism and other factors in road accidents. *Med. J. Aust.* 2:5–16, 1971.

Widmark, E.M.P. Alcoholic excretion in urine and a simple clinically applicable method for diagnosing alcoholic intoxication in drivers. *Ups. Lakaref. Forh.* 19:241–273, 1914.

Widmark, E.M.P. *Die theoretischen Grundlagen und die praktische Verwendbarkeit der gerichtlich–meizinischen Alkoholbestimmung.* Berlin: Urban and Schwarzenberg, 1932.

Yi, H. et al. *Surveillance Report #53: Trends in Alcohol–Related Fatal Traffic Crashes, United States, 1977–98.* Rockville, MD: NIAAA, Division of Biometry and Epidemiology Alcohol Epidemiogic Data System, December, 2000. (http://www.niaaa.nih.gov/gallery/epidemiology/farfig2c.htm; printed 2/14/2003)

Zeller, A.F. Alcohol and other drugs in aircraft accidents. *Aviation, Space Environ. Med.* 46: 1271–1274, 1975.

Zylman, R., Blomberg, R.D. and Preusser, D.F. *A Review of the Literature on the Involvement of Alcohol in Pedestrian Collision Resulting in Death and Injury.* NHTSA Technical Report DOT-HS-801-413, 1975.

Zylman, R. A critical evaluation of the literature on "alcohol involvement" in highway deaths. *Accid. Anal. Prevent.* 6:163–204, 1974.

Endnote

1. Abstracted from Jones and Joscelyn, 1978.

Chapter 15

Experimental Basis of Psychomotor Performance Impairment

Joseph E. Manno, Ph.D. and Barbara R. Manno, Ph.D.

Whose heart is filled with anguish and sorrow? Who is always fighting and quarreling? Who is the man with bloodshot eyes and many wounds?

It is the one who spends long hours in the taverns, trying out new mixtures.

Don't let the sparkle and the smooth taste of strong wine deceive you. For in the end it bites like a poisonous serpent; it stings like an adder. You will see hallucinations and have delirium tremens, and you say foolish, silly things that would embarrass you no end when sober. You will stagger like a sailor tossed at sea, clinging to a swaying mast.

And afterwards you will say, "I didn't even know it when they beat me up . . . Let's go and have another drink."

Proverbs 23:29–35 (*The Living Bible*, 1971)

15.1 Introduction

The effects of alcohol (ethanol) on human performance were probably first observed when it was discovered that fruits left for a period of time developed an unusual odor and flavor and their consumption led to sensorium and behavioral changes. The paraphrased quotation above from earlier bible translations reaffirms the early recognition of man's problems associated with consumption of alcohol. Schmiedeberg (1902), using more detailed scientific terminology, described these changes in sensorium, behavior and appearance. He described the alterations as loud and profuse speech and vivacious acts, increased pulse rate, engorgement and flushing of the skin over the whole body, and a sensation of warmth. Schmiedeberg further dispelled the accepted concept that alcohol acts as a stimulant and introduced the concept which is now widely accepted that alcohol acts as a depressant. The loss of inhibitions at low blood alcohol concentration (BAC) is a result of removal of inhibitions due to depression of the central nervous system (CNS). Subsequent deepening of the depressant effects attributed to alcohol is more outwardly recognizable as the BAC increases (Forney and Harger, 1965).

A translation of Schmiedeberg's description (1908) of the behavioral and physiologic effects of alcohol on an individual is still an appropriate depiction of alcohol's effects. Schmiedeberg explained that the typical person first loses the finer grades of attention, judgment, reflection, and the ability to comprehend. Applied to a soldier, he explains that the soldier becomes more courageous because he observes danger less and thinks or reflects on it less. The public speaker is not tormented and influenced by the closeness of his audience and is further deluded into speaking more freely, is more animated, has a higher opinion of his thoughts and judgment beyond that which he would exhibit in a sober state.

On attaining the state of sobriety, the individual most often regrets his performance in the delusional state. Schmiedeberg further compares the drunken person with the sober one in describing the drunken individual's self-attributes of increased physical strength. The person will attempt to demonstrate this great strength, thus wasting his energies without consideration of the potential for the harmful consequences of his actions. In contrast, the actions of the sober person are represented by a more thoughtful, cautious demeanor (Forney and Harger, 1958).

The effects of alcohol ingestion continue to be described with a variety of ambiguous terms such as "drunk," "intoxicated," "under the influence," "inebriated," "tipsy," "wacked," "shot" and other equally colorful terms that are easily understood in a social setting. It is generally accepted that the ingestion of alcohol produces decrements in human performance above a certain BAC and the number varies between individuals. Describing the effects of alcohol in terms of psychomotor performance impairment for medical legal purposes becomes more complex because it is necessary to relate these effects to a specific adverse event that could also readily occur without the presence of alcohol. Because it would not only be difficult, but costly to determine if a specific individual had significant psychomotor performance impairment based on observations and limited testing by the arresting police officer, most states and countries have defined a BAC which can be used as prima facie evidence that the individual in question is or was under the influence of alcohol (Pilchen, 1988; Garriott, 1996; Chapter 12). These blood and breath alcohol concentrations range between 0.05 g/dL and 0.1 g/dL. Congress passed a Federal incentive grant in 1998 as part of the Transportation Equity Act for the 21st Century (TEA-21) to encourage states to adopt a 0.08 g/dL BAC per se concentration as illegal (23 U.S.C., Section 163). In 2000, they further passed (0.08 g/dL BAC for all drivers twenty-one years of age and older as the national standard for impaired driving as part of the Department of Transportation's appropriations for fiscal 2001. In order to provide incentive for state legislatures to adopt the lower BAC level, part of the plan that provided for a graded loss of federal highway construction funds if the new lower BAC was

not adopted by the dates specified (NHTSA, January, 2003). It is lower still (0.04 g/dL) as a result of the US Department of Transportation regulations for commercial vehicle operators and related persons in safety sensitive positions (14CFR 61; 49CFR 382; 49CFR655; Dubowski and Caplan, 2003). These numbers provide a basis for establishing general BAC ranges wherein a specific individual should not operate a motor vehicle or perform hazardous duties. It is imperative that it is understood that it is not possible or acceptable practice to conclude human impairment based on random urine alcohol concentration values. Therefore, no interpretative urine alcohol limits have been set.

Prior to the advent of the industrial revolution and the introduction of mechanized manufacturing and vehicular travel there was little concern about alcohol-induced psychomotor performance impairment. Mechanization brought with it the development of high-speed transportation as well as the introduction of faster, more intricate, and complicated manufacturing equipment and processes. Mechanization continues to require performance with more care on the part of operators and workers in order for completion of simple and complex tasks, without harm to either themselves or others.

Science, technology, and economic and public policy coexist in a dynamic milieu and often do not keep pace with one another. The psychomotor performance impairment associated actions of an individual after consumption of alcohol have been known for centuries; however, the chemical tests for alcohol were not available until the mid- to late 1800s (Bouchardt and Sandras, 1847; Subbotin, 1891). On the other hand, the ability to reliably detect and quantitate alcohol in body fluids, tissue and breath were not described until over a half century later (Widmark, 1914, 1922). Consequently, the need to scientifically establish cause and effect relationships of alcohol-induced psychomotor performance impairment and the BAC was not recognized until the early twentieth century and is discussed elsewhere (see Chapter 14). While not all facets of the alcohol-induced psychomotor performance impairment problem have been completely explored, there is sufficient research with alcohol that the testing paradigms used for alcohol provides an excellent model for research associated with other mood altering or CNS acting drugs or chemicals.

Before focusing the discussion on the alcohol-human factors related to psychomotor performance impairment, the reader is reminded of the less rigid or definable variables impacting event or study interpretation. There are four major event categories that are confounding to both accident or workplace scene investigations and interpretation of laboratory, simulator, on-the-road-testing or workplace incident studies. These are vehicular, environmental, crash, and human factors (Figures 15.1 to 15.4). No single category is exclusive unto itself with regard to other causative factors. There are several sub-factors within a major factor category and these can also interact in more than one major category (e.g., environmental conditions and human factors that may be common to both). Epidemiology studies (Chapter 14) may easily implicate any or all of these variables as investigation of their role in causation of accidents and crashes proceeds. The primary problem with these noncontrolled variables that occur in the laboratory simulator, during on-the-road-testing or in environmental studies is that they cannot be designed to mimic the actual accident setting. Therefore, they complicate interpretation of the data due to their absence. For example, the subject in any type of prospective driving performance research study may feel more secure because they are aware that their safety has been considered. Consequently, the true impact of a specific outcome may be lessened (Compton, 1988). Manno and Manno (1988; Chapter 14) have previously discussed how these major factors can interact to further complicate accident investigation, interpretation of events, and relationship of research data to an alcohol impaired person. Therefore, it is difficult for the scientist to offer simple explanations relating psychomotor performance changes induced by alcohol or drugs. Many of the alcohol-psychomotor performance relationships are established by public policy and statute. Although these are based on scientific research and epidemiological research, they are not always adequate to establish a scientific basis for the causation

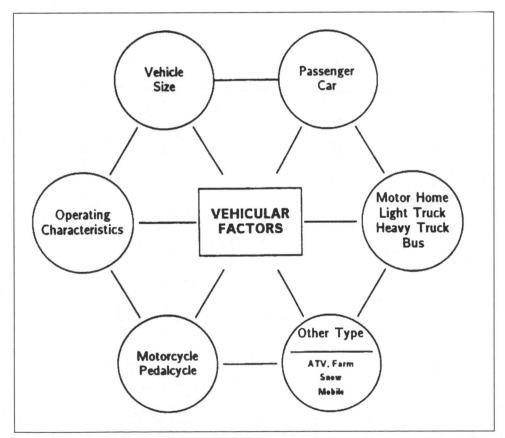

Figure 15.1 *Confounding variables: Vehicular factors influencing accidents*

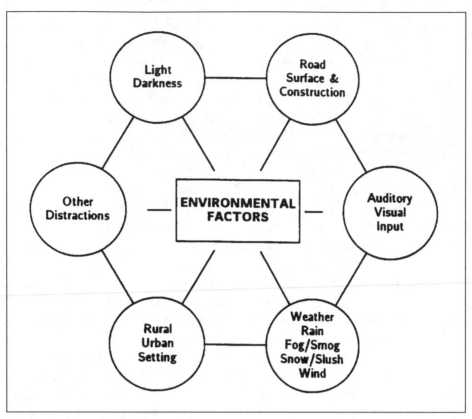

Figure 15.2 *Confounding variables: Environmental factors influencing accidents*

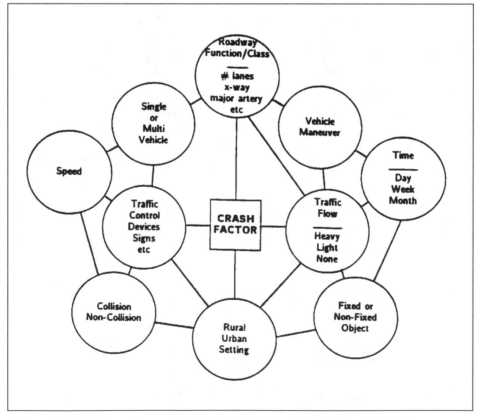

Figure 15.3 *Confounding variables: Crash factors influencing accidents*

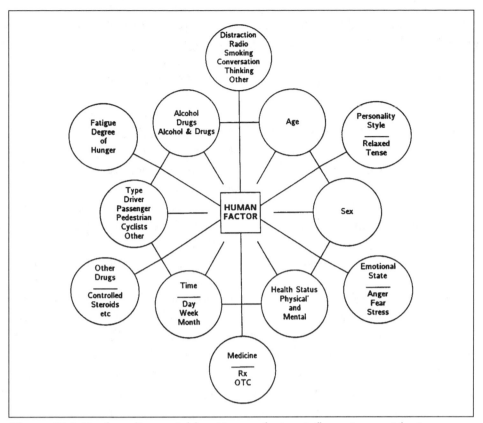

Figure 15.4 *Confounding variables: Human factors influencing accidents*

of a specific accident. The need for more rigid guidelines has grown more rapidly than the ability of science to provide an algorithm that can include all the factors.

15.2 Observation and Measurement of Alcohol Performance Impairment

The establishment of legal alcohol intoxication (i.e., DWI or alcohol-associated accident causation) is determined by a series of events. It begins with the stopping of a driver by a law enforcement officer because of the driver's unusual or illegal driving behavior or as part of a postaccident investigation. Those items that are relevant to this chapter deal with eyewitness or law enforcement descriptions of the behavior of the implicated person before, during and after the incident, as well as other scene details.

The behavioral changes accompanying alcohol intoxication are similar to those previously described. Observed behavioral and performance signs include: alcohol odor on the breath, flushed appearance, muscular incoordination, speech difficulties (slurred or mispronunciation of words), disorderly

or out-of-the-ordinary conduct, unusual mental changes, dizziness, tremors, sleepiness, nausea and vomiting (AMA, 1970).

Law enforcement officers are given the charge to be able to recognize and detect an intoxicated individual. A number of deviations from normal driving have been described to assist in this identification and are listed below (AMA, 1970).

1. Unreasonable speed (high).
2. Driving in spurts (slow, then fast, then slow).
3. Frequent lane changing with excessive speed.
4. Improper passing with insufficient clearance, also taking too long or swerving too much in overtaking and passing (i.e., overcontrol).
5. Overshooting or disregarding traffic control signals.
6. Approaching signals unreasonably fast or slow, and stopping or attempting to stop with uneven motion.

7. Driving at night without lights. Delay in turning lights on when starting from a parked position.
8. Failure to dim lights to oncoming traffic.
9. Driving in lower gears without apparent reason, or repeatedly clashing gears.
10. Jerky starting or stopping.
11. Driving unreasonably slow.
12. Driving too close to road shoulders or curbs; or appearing to hug the edge of the road or continually straddling the centerline.
13. Driving with windows down in cold weather.
14. Driving or riding with head partly or completely out of the window.

These behavioral descriptors are commonly used and understood by the general population as being associated with alcohol and intoxication. When observed by a law enforcement officer, they can be used to provide probable cause to stop an individual driving a motor vehicle for further investigation. After further interaction between the law enforcement officer and driver, the suspected individual may be subjected to additional behavioral testing to evaluate possible psychomotor performance impairment. Based on the outcome of the behavioral testing, the officer may request that a breath or blood alcohol test (or both) be performed to determine if the individual is legally intoxicated. The behavioral test battery normally includes the Standardized Field Sobriety Test (SFST) which is discussed later in this chapter. NHTSA has sponsored research to develop a DWI detection guide for law enforcement officers that listed twenty cues and the probabilities of a driver demonstrating one of these cues would have a BAC ≥ 0.10 g/dL (Harris, 1980a,b). Similarly, Stuster (1997) identified twenty-four driving cues predictive of DWI at ≥ 0.08 g/dL.

In order to scientifically document the effects of alcohol on behavior and performance, it has been necessary to utilize the tools provided by psychology psychometrics, medicine and toxicology. A goal of the forensic scientist is to assemble an organized body of knowledge concerning alcohol related psy-

chomotor performance impairment and be knowledgeable in its application. This allows the forensic scientist to establish a scientific basis for any conclusions or opinions that relate to determining accident causation or establishing DWI in a driver. In pursuing this goal we must be able to distinguish scientific from nonscientific explanations (i.e., an *a priori* belief, faith or common sense). In making these distinctions it is necessary to use scientifically acceptable research paradigms and technology when designing and conducting research, and to interpret the results of the study based on acceptable statistical methodology.

The effects of alcohol on performance have been examined in the laboratory, in closed course field investigations and with on-the-road testing using a variety of testing methods. The experimental design varies among the individual studies. Their primary and common goal has been the attempt to address human factors associated with where alcohol is exerting its effects; how alcohol may be producing its effects; when the effects may come into play; what, if any, relationship exists between body fluid and tissue alcohol concentrations; what environmental, psychological, medical, physiological and pharmacological (drugs or other chemical) factors coexist; and which may interact to induce more profound psychomotor performance alterations resulting from drug or chemical interactions; and to provide reliable interpretation of test results.

Observed behavior of the subject in the laboratory and on-the-road-testing studies can provide additional information that permits corroboration, refinement, or rejection of psychomotor performance changes. These recorded observations also help demonstrate the broad scope of individual variation in performance (no-response; response; varying degrees of response) in alcohol-related incidents. Ideally, these studies should be performed in a controlled environment in order to control for variables and thereby permit use of the findings in a statistically valid predicative manner. This would allow the data to be more relevant to individual situations and assist in assignment of responsibility or proportional causation in alcohol-related accidents that result in property damage accidents, injuries or fatalities. These investigations use a wide range of testing protocols including simple tasks, complex tasks and multi-tasking paradigms. The variety of approaches permit extrapolation of data relating to psychomotor performance to the varying degrees of complexity of operator tasks in general or everyday living and working environments.

Another aspect of understanding and interpreting psychomotor performance studies is the observation of an individual's behavior at different doses of alcohol or at different BACs. Testing at different doses of alcohol or at different BACs may appear to be a redundancy, however, it should be remembered that the rates of alcohol absorption and distribution varies considerably among people. The studies discussed have assisted in establishing the blood alcohol concentrations (BAC) at which significant readily observable alterations in psychomotor performance have occurred.

Alcohol also affects the functions of various organ systems of the body (e.g., cardiovascular, renal, and hepatic and so on). However, our discussion shall focus only on the neuropsychological, neurobehavioral, neuropharmacological and neurotoxicological aspects of the central nervous system (CNS) which have an impact on task performance and work that are significantly affected by alterations in psychomotor performance components. Accordingly, the discussion is designed to provide the reader with an overview of reports that demonstrate alcohol-induced psychomotor performance impairment based on observed behavior, laboratory studies, field tests and on-the-road testing. Ultimately, the objective is the application of the research data to determine if alcohol is involved in producing psychomotor performance impairment encountered in daily life or the workplace. The literature cited in this chapter is not inclusive but rather is representative of available reports and provides an overview of the primary considerations as applied to the alcohol-psychomotor performance impairment problem. The supporting epidemiological work is discussed in Chapter 14.

15.3 Psychomotor Performance Testing

The laboratory component of alcohol related psychomotor performance testing is directed towards either a description of the mechanism by which alcohol exerts its effect or the site of action (system, tissue, cellular or subcellar location) where the effects of alcohol occur. After determining the task to be studied (e.g., driving a car), the task is dissected into its components to determine which body systems contribute to its completion. For example, operation of a motor vehicle (automobile, train, plane, cycle and so forth) requires information concerning the operator's reaction time, eye-hand-foot coordination, response to visual and auditory stimuli, attendance to completion of simple and complex tasks, learning, and ability to follow directions, to mention a few. To measure alcohol induced changes in an individual's response for any of these systems, we must first establish which body systems or functions are affected by the alcohol and what other factors may temporally interact to alter these responses. Alcohol effects on these functions of psychomotor performance are listed in Tables 15.1 and 15.2. Other information that is necessary to establish accurate and meaningful BAC-psychomotor performance impairment cause and effect relationships are:

- the dose of alcohol administered calculated from the volume of the beverage consumed and the alcohol concentration of the beverages;
- an estimation of the volume of distribution (Vd) of alcohol in that individual based on an estimation of their lean body mass. Events that can alter the Vd should also be considered (i.e., blood loss, fluid administration and so on);
- the time period during which the beverage was consumed and its temporal relation to the accident (of particular importance is the determination of the time from ingestion of the last drink to the time of the adverse event and an estimation of the amount and type of food present in the stomach at that time);
- the time at which the blood and breath specimens were collected for testing and the temporal relationship to the time of the accident;
- the analytical method used to test the specimen and its established precision and accuracy. (i.e., gas chromatography versus an enzymatic test; infrared (IR) based breath testing versus oxidation breath testing);

Table 15.1
Skills: Reaction Time and Coordination, Reflexes and Cerebration

These body functions are necessary for performing tasks such as driving or flying. The blood alcohol (g/dL) at which observations were made and a brief description of the alteration are also shown.

BAC	Response	Effect
	Reaction Time and Coordination	
0.02	Impairment threshold	
0.05	Handwriting legibility, time required for writing, fine motor coordination, accuracy	Impaired
	Complex motor tasks requiring coordination	Impaired
0.08	Reaction to optical and acoustical stimuli	Impaired
0.10	Simple visual reaction time	Slowed
	Reflexes	
0.05	Simple or well-practiced skills	Unimpaired
	Sensory threshold	Increased
	Pain threshold	Increased
	Motor reactivity of conditioned reflexes	Increased
	Respiratory conditioned reflex	Slowed
	Excitatory reactions (remove inhibitions)	Favored
0.05–0.10	Body sway	Increased
	Emotional responsiveness and alteration of emotional level	Reduced
	Cerebration	
0.03–0.06	Motor function (function dependent)	Impaired
0.10	Fluency of work, production and conformity to standards of performance	Reduced
BAC is subject variable	Creative ability	No inspiration
	Intellectual function and dexterity	Impairment disappears as alcohol disappears from blood
Occurs in alcoholism	Wechsler IQ test	Deteriorates for various higher mental activities over ten-year period of alcoholism; **not observed with acute alcoholism**

- the type of specimen collected (i.e., serum, whole blood, plasma, urine; mixed expiratory air, alveolar air and so forth);
- social drinking history of the individual (i.e., daily, weekly, rarely);
- knowledge of alcohol pharmacokinetics that apply at the particular BAC;
- the presence of other drugs or chemicals; and
- the individual's general health condition at time of any incident.

Investigators can be more accurate and precise in correlating the temporal and quantitative relationship of alcohol to psychomotor performance impairment as a causative factor in any given accident if they have access to as many of the details discussed above as possible. In the absence of an accurately

Table 15.2
Skills: Work Performance and Special Senses (Vision, Smell, Taste and Hearing)

BAC	Response	Effect
	Work Performance	
	High skill/attentiveness	More impaired by alcohol than low skill/heavy physical work
0.02	Telegraphers threshold	Deterioration
0.06	Simulated work of immediate demand or prolonged nature	Not changed
0.075	Telegraphy	56–72 percent impaired
0.10	Long work requirements	Deterioration
	Special Senses **Vision**	
0.03	Voluntary convergence	Impaired
As concentration increases	Binocular vision at 0.5 meters, gives rise to diplopia	Lost
0.04 (Phase I) Severe Intoxication (Phase II)	Positional nystagmus (biphasic)	2 phases separated by 1–2 hrs; stage I (immediate) lasts 3–4 hrs during alcohol intake; stage II lasts 5–15 hrs and sometimes present after alcohol gone from blood
0.05–0.15	Fusion and convergency	Markedly impaired
0.06	Far to near vision accommodation	Reduced by 0.10–0.20 sec
0.08	Visual acuity	Lost
0.10	Euphoria	
0.10	Stereoscopic vision	Decreased
	Dark adaptation	Transitory
Low levels	Fusion frequency	Decreased
Low levels	Color distinctio n	Fails
	Olfactory and Taste	
	Olfactory threshold	
	Appetite/satiety	Increase parallels rise and fall of olfactory threshold
	Auditory	
	Distraction	Greater
0.15	Perception	No change

measured alcohol concentration in breath or blood, it is extremely difficult if at all possible, to accurately (within 95% confidence limits or beyond a reasonable doubt) estimate the BAC from observed or measured psychomotor performance impairment. This situation can occur when an individual fails the SFST and refuses a chemical test for intoxication. In these situations, despite the high degree of correla-tion of the signs measured by SFST to BACs of 0.08 and 0.10 percent, the SFST should not be used to es-tablish a BAC.

The various experimental tests used for measur-ing psychomotor performance have been scientifi-cally designed to evaluate the functional responses while attempting to maintain a high degree of con-trol over as many variables (independent and dependent) as possible. This may only be accomplished in a controlled laboratory setting where reproducible dosing schedules, testing sessions, and an optimal environment for testing without external factors such as weather, mechanical, noise and so on can be maintained. An independent variable in such studies is one that is selected and whose value has been assigned by the investigators (e.g., doses of alcohol to be administered). In order to test the independent variable, the behavior (response) or dependent variable is measured. Manipulation of the independent variable (alcohol) dictates that at least two levels of active drug and one of inactive drug (placebo) should be used as the independent variables. Typical dependent measures that are applied in performance testing are behavioral, physiological and self-reported measures. Behavior measures are indicated by measurement of actual subject behavior. The response may be described by measures such as frequency of responding, latency of response, and number of errors. Physiological measures monitor the subject's bodily functions (for example, heart rate, blood pressure, and electrical activity of the brain or respiratory rate). These measures provide information concerning the subject's state of arousal (physical and mental activity). The drawback to using physiological measures is the risk of making incorrect conclusions because one must often infer psychological states from physiological measures or observations. An example in forensic work would be the use of a lie detector test to determine if an individual is telling the truth or not. The test is conducted by monitoring changes in respiratory rate, skin conductivity and heart rate and correlating changes in these to the subject's response to questions. These physiological measures are used to assist in determining if a subject is stating true answers to questions. There are a number of subjective tests available which can be used for subjects to self-evaluate their responses to a given drug or situation. These are usually graded on a numerical score (0 = no dizziness to 5 = the dizziest that I have ever been in my life). The score may be quantified by marking along a line between two mood extremes. Some of the tests are the Hopkins symptom checklist, Cornell Medical Index, Side Effects Questionnaire, Stanford Sleepiness Scale, Self-rated Performance evaluation

to name a few. Several caveats are necessary when using this type of measure. If a retrospective response has been required, the subject may or may not have been accurately responding. He or she may be under- or over-grading the response or giving the investigator what they think the investigator may want to hear or the subject's memory may have been clouded by time and intervening events. In a prospective response, the subject's answer is based on speculation on future performance which may or may not ever occur. The same caveat should be observed in both types of reports.

Test subject safety can be more optimally addressed in descending order of laboratory over field testing over on-the-road testing studies as a causal relationship is developed between the variables because the investigator is in control of the research environment. Closed course investigations are performed in a semi-protected testing environment offering advantages over using real equipment (e.g., automobiles, airplanes and so on) in a realistic course but without such interferences as vehicular or pedestrian traffic. Closed course studies overlap both simulation and on-the-road-testing to some degree.

Simulation (re-creation of the real-world situations) in the laboratory setting affords yet another degree of control over extraneous variables present in on-the-road-testing or real-life scenarios. Simulation studies permit the investigator to easily alter some testing parameters to re-create what would be too hazardous to interject into on-the-road-testing paradigms. There is overlap between simulation in laboratory testing, closed course and on-the-road-testing settings.

There remains a question concerning the direct applicability of simulator, field and on-the-road-testing study data to actual vehicular operation in the presence of alcohol or other drugs (Holloway, 1995). It may never be possible to resolve the issues surrounding direct application of the data to a real-life event. In the meantime, protocols for psychomotor performance investigations must be continuously refined and pursued. Simply put, if we want to determine if alcohol alters reaction time, it would be necessary to use a timed test with a visual or auditory stimulus and a mechanism to quantitatively measure the subject's response. The test would be done both in the presence and absence of alcohol using a sufficient number of subjects to provide statistically valid results. The alcohol, including the placebo, would be administered in the same manner to all subjects in the study with all subjects hopefully having followed pre-test instructions with regard to such issues as food intake and drug or alcohol use. The experimental design (testing protocol) should be controlled for the homogeneity of subject population (e.g., sex, age, weight, health), dosing amount, dosing schedule, specimen collection and handling, testing intervals and recording of data. The resulting data would then be subjected to powerful statistical analysis to establish the mathematical probability that the hypothesis advanced at the initiation of the study has been proved at a significant level (i.e. that it is not a random observation or a predictable occurrence).

Objective behavioral and performance effects of alcohol or any drug are best studied as prospective experiments. They should incorporate a control group as well as an experimental group. More specifically, these investigations should be composed of a control or placebo (alcohol-free) dose and at least two alcohol doses to provide minimal experimental conditions. Control groups are of two types. One type occurs when each subject serves as his or her own control (testing before and after alcohol). The other occurs when a placebo dose is administered. These two types of control groups may be used in combination in the same study.

Experimental dosing design should provide a mechanism to stabilize subject response due to prior knowledge of the dose of drug or placebo that they received in order to obviate placebo-responders. Design stabilization is accomplished by studies identified as randomized single or double blind studies. In the randomized single blind format, the subject knows if he or she is to receive placebo or alcohol but not dosing order. A randomized double blind study is one where both investigator and subject are blind to dosing order of placebo and alcohol. Some investigators have also kept the subject blind to dosing design by not indicating to the subject he or she would receive placebo as well as alcohol in the study. Today with the oversight role of the Institutional Review Boards for Human Experimentation

(IRB) in human research studies, the total blind approach must be justified before the IRBs will approve the study protocols. The same is true of behavioral studies incorporating a type of deception or certain types of reward system. The term crossover study is also applied. Crossover refers to dosing using more than one dose of alcohol plus placebo given in a mixed order. Bordens and Abbott (1991) have provided a more detailed discussion of behavioral research. This permits statistical evaluation of the data to determine dose or dosing order effects of the testing agent exists. In reviewing the alcohol laboratory testing literature, one will encounter two types of testing, psychometrics and psychomotor. Psychometric testing refers to the development and administration of psychological and intelligence testing instruments. The tasks evaluate motor function only, cognitive function only or the interaction of both functions. Psychomotor testing refers to performance of tests requiring both motor and cognitive function and is applied to tasks determining motor only, cognitive only or cognitive-motor function. Despite some researchers criticism of this type of experimental design, it does offer the opportunity, if used properly, to assess the individual subject as his own control (based on before alcohol dosing BAC-test response), and the individual subject response over time (based on placebo versus active doses). The rationale for this dosing paradigm is to control for dosing order effects and group response. This permits the investigator to control the design to eliminate or assess the effect of fatigue over the testing period. This is a standard pharmacological research design for drug dosing when determining the relationship of drug coupled with the pharmacokinetics of the drug under examination.

The scientific literature is replete with individual studies and reviews reporting the outcome of a variety of designs, both simple and complex in nature, which are supportive of the negative cause and effect relationship of alcohol and performance. The dose of both as a function of the quantity of alcohol administered and the number of doses investigated varied widely among studies.

Alcohol impairment research has taken new direction since the mid-1980s. One important new direction is toward investigations of psychomotor performance at BAC ≤ 0.05 g/dL. Emphasis has been directed at alcohol-induced impairment involving those skills necessary for maintenance of safe and productive travel, recreation, work and interpersonal relationships. These types of studies have shown psychomotor performance impairment as low as 0.015 g/dL and increasing as BAC increases (Moskowitz et al., 1985; NHTSA, 2000). This, however, is not a new idea since Goldberg reported as early as 1948 that experienced drivers in graded road tests were impaired by as much as 25–30 percent at BAC of 0.04–0.06 g/dL. These BACs were lower than were previously thought necessary to produce driving impairment.

A second direction more recently found in the area of alcohol psychomotor performance research is the attempt to develop a mechanism by which the many and varied alcohol performance studies can be analyzed for their common features. This research is providing a mechanism whereby the strength and credibility of larger study groups may be utilized in the place of many studies with smaller populations thereby offering more reliable data interpretation and application tools for actual events wherein alcohol-induced psychomotor performance impairment may have been a major or complicating factor. Representative of these types of studies are those of Levine et al. (1975); Moskowitz and Robinson (1988); Linnoila et al. (1986); Mitchell (1985); Kruger (1990, 1993); Vogel-Sprott (1993); Kruger et al. (1990); Holloway (1994, 1995); Stuster and Burns (1999); and Moskowitz and Fiorentino (2000).

The third direction that investigators have begun to evaluate is the reliability of the assessment measures used in alcohol, drug and other situational, behavioral and subjective research. Representative work in this third important area of alcohol impairment research has been published by Baker et al. (1985); Martin et al. (1993); Nagoshi and Wilson (1988, 1989); Nagoshi et al. (1991); Vogel-Sprott et al. (1985, 1987); Wilson and Nagoshi (1987); Parrott (1991a,b,c); Finnigan and Hammmersley (1992); Kaplan et al. (1985); Holloway (1994, 1995); Stuster and Burns (1999); and Moskowitz and Fiorentino (2000).

A. National Advanced Driving Simulator (NADS)

The National Advanced Driving Simulator (NADS), developed by NHTSA and located at the University of Iowa's Oakdale Research Park in Iowa City, Iowa, offers high-fidelity, real-time driving simulation. This sophisticated, state of the art driving simulator consists of a large dome in which entire cars and the cabs of trucks and buses can be mounted. Along with other electronic and mechanical features that produce effects permitting the driver to feel acceleration, braking and steering cues as if he were actually driving a real car, truck or bus. The NADS contains several subsystems that work in real time to provide a repeatable, natural and undistorted representation of the visual, motion, auditory and control feel sensory cues associated with the driving environments. Using this simulator, crash scenarios can be presented to the driver in an entirely safe and acceptable manner while permitting electronic gathering and storing of driver response data (NHTSA, 2003).

B. Roadside testing or field sobriety testing (FST)

A variety of field sobriety tests (FST) were used by law enforcement officers in the United States before the work of Tharp, Burns and Moskowitz (1981) to detect impairment and to develop probable cause to arrest individuals. The FSTs, are used to assess coordination, balance and dexterity. These functions have been found to decrease as BAC increases. Some versions of FSTs include a test of a person's ability to perform simultaneous, simple tasks. One's ability to perform simple task also has been found to decrease as the BAC increases (Wilkinson, Kime and Purnell, 1974).

Before discussing the scientific literature on field sobriety testing, it is necessary to describe three of the components of standardized field sobriety test battery (SFST): horizontal gaze nystagmus (HGN), walk-and-turn (WAT) and one-leg stand (OLS). The discussion is limited to test performance and how the test is affected by alcohol.

Nystagmus is described as a "bouncing" eye motion that is displayed in two ways: (1) pendular nystagmus, where the eye oscillates equally in two directions, and (2) jerk nystagmus, where the eye moves slowly from a fixation point and then is rapidly corrected through "saccadic" or fast motions. Normally when the eyes follow an object moving left and right, the lateral rectus muscle (contraction pulls the eye away from the nose) and the medial rectus muscle (contraction pulls the eye toward the nose) contract and relax appropriately so the movement is smooth. (Spence and Mason, 1987). If the contraction and relaxation of these two muscles is not coordinated, then the eye movement is jerky and results in nystagmus.

Several types of nystagmus have been described, however, we are interested in alcohol gaze nystagmus (AGN) and more specifically horizontal gaze nystagmus (HGN). HGN refers to jerky eye movement from left to right or right to left, hence horizontal gaze nystagmus. Vertical gaze nystagmus (VGN) also can occur but it is not measured as part of the SFST. Alcohol, a central nervous system depressant, affects motor control systems for the eye and produces the uncoordinated contraction and relaxation of the two muscles. HGN represents involuntary movement therefore the individual exhibiting HGN cannot control eye movement, is unaware of its occurrence and has no vision loss (Dietrich, 2003). It has been concluded that HGN is the most powerful of the three tests comprising the SFST. HGN can also occur from ingestion of other drugs that produce CNS depression and from disease states that affect nerves and muscles.

The walk-and-turn (WAT) test is an easy to administer, divided-attention test. The subject is given oral instructions to take nine-steps, heel-to-toe, along a straight line. After taking the nine steps the subject must execute a one-foot turn and return in the same manner in the opposite direction. The examiner looks for seven indicators of impairment while the subject performs the test. The indicators are: (1) subject cannot maintain balance while listening to instructions; (2) begins test before the instructions have been completed; (3) stops to regain balance while walking; (4) does not touch heel-to-toe; (5) uses arms to maintain balance; (6) loses balance during turn; and (7) takes incorrect number of steps. Sixty-eight percent of persons who fail two or more of these indicators will have a BAC of ≥ 0.10 g/dL (NTL, 2003). Impairment from alcohol ingestion

will occur in the WAT. Other drugs and certain disease states can also produce impairment in the WAT.

One-leg stand (OLS) is another relatively easy to administer test of divided attention performance. The subject is directed to stand with one foot held approximately six inches off the ground and to count aloud by thousands (one thousand-one, one thousand-two . . .) until told to put the foot down. The subject is timed for thirty seconds. There are four indicators of impairment for the OLS that include (1) swaying while balancing; (2) using arms to balance; (3) hopping to maintain balance; and (4) putting foot down. Sixty-five percent of persons failing two or more indicators on the OLS will have a BAC ≥ 0.10 g/dL (NHTSA, 1983). Impairment from alcohol ingestion will occur in the OLS. Other drugs and certain disease states can also produce impairment in the OLS.

The NHTSA (1977) in 1977 commissioned a research investigation to determine the best methods of detecting impaired drivers using FSTs. This work validated earlier observations regarding the relationship between alcohol consumption and HGN, WAT and OLS tests and the ease with which the tests could be administered at the roadside. In 1981, the HGN, WAT and OLS were standardized thereby ensuring that law enforcement officers could expedite administration of the tests in an easy, effective and uniform manner. The research showed that when the SFST was administered by a trained and experienced law enforcement officer, it was accurate 83 percent of the time as an indicator when an individual's BAC ≥ 0.10 g/dL. It was this work that established that the WAT, HGN and OLS tests when used together, as the SFST, as a roadside screening test, was a useful aid for law enforcement officers in their decision making process in suspected DWI. The SFST is considered to be a battery of tests that include the walk-and-turn, (WAT), horizontal gaze nystagmus (HGN), and one-leg stand (OLS). The test battery should be administered in a standardized manner by a trained law enforcement officer. The tests comprising the SFST are individually well documented in the medical (neurology) and driving performance literature (Burns and Moskowitz, 1977). The WAT, HGN and OLS have a combined predictability of 83.3 percent at 0.08 g/dL BAC. Individually, the WAT, HGN and OLS have a predictability factors of 68, 77 and 65 percent, respectively. Table 15.3 summarizes the major work validating the SFST. Although initial work (Stuster and Burns, 1998) indicates that the SFST using two indicator scores for HGN may be useful to indicate impairment at 0.04 g/dL, it is imperative that the FST be more fully evaluated at that level as well as re-evaluated with carefully designed laboratory and roadside studies at incremental BACs between 0.00–0.07 g/dL.

The three tests are strongest when they are used together to produce a cumulative score. The sum of the failed indicators along with other evidence associated with the case in question is used to determine if the individual is impaired. The greater the sum of the indicators failed, the stronger is the indication of impairment (NTL, 2003).

The three components of the SFST evaluate CNS integrity of brain regions that are associated with maintaining balance and motor function. These tests are considered to be sensitive indicators of the types of behaviors that they evaluate. The tests may be representative of alterations in CNS function due to the presence of CNS drugs or neuropathologic conditions. They are easily administered and require limited training of personnel administering the test battery.

As indicated in Table 15.3 the NHTSA (1983) study again showed that the HGN was the most predictive component of the SFST, however, a higher predictability was attained when all three component scores were combined (Stuster and Burns, 1998). It was stated that law enforcement officers administering the SFST were given three choices to describe motorist's BAC the 1998 study. The categories were: (1) BAC above or below 0.08 g/dL; (2) BAC above or below 0.04 g/dL; and (3) BAC above 0.04 g/dL but below 0.08 g/dL. Law enforcement officer estimates of BAC $\geq$ 0.08 g/dL were accurate 91–94 percent of the time, depending on rejection or acceptance of some of the false positives. Law enforcement officer estimates of BAC < 0.08 g/dL but > 0.04 g/dL were accurate 94 percent of the time when deciding to arrest and 80 percent of the time in relevant cases overall. Based on this work it was implied that the SFST could be used with slight modifi-

cation to adequately discriminate above or below BACs of 0.08 g/dL but that further work is necessary to fully validate the SFST at BACs of 0.04 g/dL. We agree that additional validation studies are required at BAC of 0.04 g/dL. We strongly recommend that validation studies are also needed to strengthen the roadside SFST as a significant evidence-gathering tool for use by law enforcement officers to support their actions when stopping a motorist suspected of DWI. However, some caveats are important in applying the SFST. For example, the HGN should not be tested in the direct, bright glare of headlights of a car in order to obtain a consistent and more nearly accurate result. Since the reliability of the HGN depends on a cumulative score, its reliability would be diminished if it were used on an individual who was blind in one eye or the OLS on people with a leg injury or a missing leg. Testing with these two instruments to evaluate visual response and balance as performance indicators will lead to erroneous decisions (Stuster and Burns, 1999).

The SFST is used by law enforcement officers in all states but not in all jurisdictions. Two potential issues with the SFST battery are brought to the reader's attention. The first issue is related to adjudication of a DWI when failure of a SFST battery is the only evidence for legal action to be brought against the suspected driver. The second issue is related to whether the data on which testimony is given has been peer reviewed and is accepted by the appropriate scientific community.

On the question of adjudication of a DWI based solely on a failed SFST. It should be remembered that the intended purpose of the SFST battery is to establish a probable cause for measuring the actual breath or blood alcohol concentration. If an individual refuses the administration of a chemical test, the SFST or a FST cannot be used to establish beyond a reasonable doubt that the actual BAC was in fact equal to or above the legal designation for DWI.

The SFST has been shown to have high degree of reliability when paired with measured BACs of 0.04 g/dL, 0.08 g/dL, and 0.10 g/dL. Although the tests are sensitive, there are many confounding variables such as the presence of other drugs, physical and medical illnesses, including neurological and mental diseases states, experience of the law en-

Table 15.3
The Historical Development and Validation of Standardized Field Sobriety Test (SFST)

BAC in the referenced studies was expressed as breath or blood alcohol concentrations based upon chemical tests used.

Year	tests	BAC (g/dL)	Percent Accuracy[1]	Comments	References
1977	HGN[2] WAT[3] OLS[4]	≥ 0.10	76	Variety of FST used. Established that HGN, WAT, and OLS identified to be most sensitive test. No validation of tests or consistency of administration but easy to use at roadside.	Burns and Moskowitz, 1977
	others (e.g., finger-to-nose, maze-tracing, backward-counting)	≥ 0.10			
1981	HGN	≥ 0.10	83	Validated SFST[5]; standardized test administration for easy, quick, efficacy and uniformity at roadside.	Tharp, Burns and Moskowitz, 1981
	WAT	≥ 0.10			
	OLS	≥ 0.10			
1983	HGN	≥ 0.10	77	Concluded HGN most powerful tool of group.	NHTSA, 1983
	WAT	≥ 0.10	68		
	HGN + WAT	≥ 0.10	80		
	OLS	≥ 0.10	65		
1986	HGN	≥ 0.10	92	Administered by trained and experienced LEO.[6]	Dietrich, 2003
1987	SFST	≥ 0.10	96	Administered by trained and experienced LEO.	Dietrich, 2003
1998	SFST	≥ 0.08	91–94	Need *four* positive HGN clues.	Stuster and Burns, 1998
	SFST	≥ 0.04	94	Need *two* positive HGN clues.	Stuster and Burns, 1998

[1] Percentage of time LEO correctly predicted BAC from SFST performance
[2] Horizontal gaze nystagmus
[3] Walk-and-turn
[4] One-leg stand
[5] Standardized field sobriety test (HGN, WAT and OLS)
[6] Law enforcement officer

forcement officers and the testing environment that can lead to false prosecution for DWI when the only evidence is the SFST results. These variables preclude the use of the SFST in lieu of a chemical test for alcohol to establish per se evidence that the alleged drinking driver had a BAC ≥ 0.08 g/dL at the time of the incident. The development of reliable and easy to administer chemical tests that can measure alcohol concentration in breath and saliva should eventually replace the SFST for establishing probable cause for evidentiary breath testing. Such procedures are already in use by the Department of Transportation (Dubowski and Caplan, 2003). An excellent review of the SFST for the forensic scientist can be found in the prosecutor's manual (Dietrich, 2003). The SFST has met the challenge under both *Frye* and *Daubert* rulings. Dietrich (2003) presents an excellent discussion with case law citations on the topic.

Regarding the second issue, when giving testimony scientific experts are asked if the data has been peer reviewed and accepted by the appropriate scientific community. When an expert reviews the literature reporting the DWI epidemiologic data and the progressive reports of the validation literature for the SFST it is rarely found in the peer reviewed scientific literature. It rather is available as final reports from government sponsored grants and contract final reports, usually the U.S. Department of Transportation, National Highway Traffic Safety Administration and published as government documents. It is pointed out that peer reviewed, as it is used for scientific studies, refers to articles submitted to scientific journals which are anonymously reviewed or judged by one or more scientists who are knowledgeable in the area of the topic. The critique with recommendations for acceptance, acceptance with suggested modifications or nonacceptance for publication is made back to the journal editor for action. These reviewers judge not only the writing skills of the authors but all aspects of scientific design, data analysis and conclusions of the work based on the actual work performed. The reviewers are asked by the journal to declare if a conflict of interest exists between reviewer and authors before acting in the referee capacity. The studies that are required to document the need and validity of a test like the SFST are costly and time-intensive; therefore, it falls to government agencies to sponsor this type of research. It is not clear whether the sponsoring agency subjects the experimental design to true peer review before or after the work is done. Submission of the final report to a peer-reviewed scientific journal would meet this need and would be available to others in the worldwide literature. The government reports are not included in currently available databases or easily obtained through specialty libraries. In many instances because these reports are not in the databases, scientists are often not aware of their existence and value.

C. Impairment when BACs are between 0.00 and 0.079 g/dL

Moskowitz and Robinson (1988) reviewed 177 alcohol-psychomotor performance impairment studies, 89 percent reported psychomotor performance impairment of one or more skills. Impairment was found in thirty-five studies at ≤ 0.04 g/dL BAC. However, the majority of investigations reported psychomotor performance impairment at less than 0.07 g/dL BAC (Figure 15.5). Since the majority of BAC studied only one level performance of BAC, it was suggested that the numbers most likely reflected

an underestimation of the level for beginning psychomotor performance impairment. See Chapter 13 for further discussion.

Reaction time, coordination and reflexes are terms that describe tasks requiring dexterity and a timed response to a stimulus. Bjerver and Goldberg (1950) used a driving task involving parallel parking of an automobile, driving out of a garage and turning the auto around on a narrow road to determine alcohol performance effects. The test is considered to be a complex task and showed that performance time for these functions were lengthened at a 0.04 g/dL BAC. Bschor (1953) reported that the threshold for impaired coordination occurs at BAC as low as 0.02 g/dL. Using the tests such as the Romberg test and mechanical devices it has been shown that individuals demonstrate impaired body stance evidenced by significantly increased body sway (ataxia) at 0.10 g/L BAC while others have reported impairment at BAC of approximately 0.04–0.05 g/dL (Franks et al., 1976; Fregley, Bergstedt and Graybiel, 1967; Goldberg, 1943; Idestrom and Cadenius, 1968; Kiplinger et al., 1974; Manno et al., 1991; McWilliams, 1993). Body sway increases as the BAC increases until it develops into a stagger and stops at the higher levels where the individual is significantly impaired to preclude standing and moving. In spite of the predominance of reports supporting the development of ataxia as a function of BAC, some investigators have reported that if experienced drinkers are motivated it is possible to overcome this effect. Psychomotor performance impairment has been overcome by this type of drinker at BACs as high as 0.20 g/dL (Laves, 1955; Prag, 1953).

Moskowitz and Robinson (1988) concluded that simple reaction time is not a sensitive measure of impairment. It was further suggested that most experiments using simple reaction time did not demonstrate any alcohol effects. Because of the simple reaction time tasks use repetitive testing of a single known stimulus and single known response, it is stated that these tasks (simple reaction time) are unrelated to reaction time demands of actual driving (Moskowitz and Fiorentino, 2000).

Components of graphologic testing such as handwriting legibility, time required for writing, fine motor coordination and accuracy are impaired at

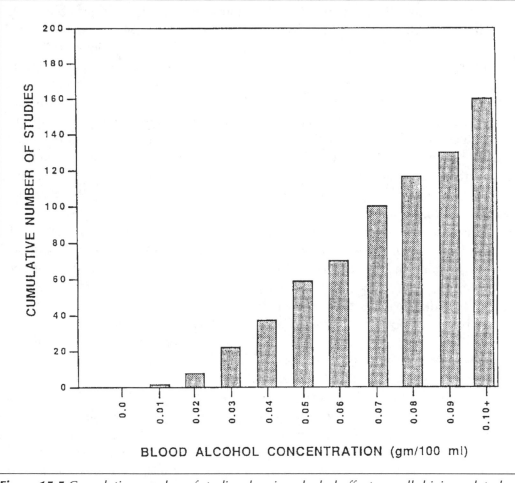

Figure 15.5 *Cumulative number of studies showing alcohol effects on all driving-related skills (Moskowitz and Robinson, 1988)*

BAC of 0.05 g/dL. The threshold of impairment for telegraphers was 0.02 g/dL BAC with 56–72 percent showing impairment at 0.075 g/dL BAC (AMA, 1970).

Integrated skilled behavior of the drinker becomes more impaired as the BAC increases with the individual demonstrating hasty, careless and disorganized performance (Wallgren and Barry, 1970). Several studies have shown that drinkers show decreased ability to perceive rapidly changing events (Wallgren and Barry, 1970; Buikhuisen and Jongman, 1972; Ehrensing et al., 1970; Cappell et al., 1972). The perception of the passage of time has been reported to be increased and slowed in the presence of low amounts of alcohol (Wallgren and Barry, 1970; Goldberg, 1943). The ability of the alcohol drinker to estimate the degree of his own psychomotor performance impairment is underestimated (Wallgren and Barry, 1970; Goldberg, 1943).

One study of alcohol effects on time-shared tasks such as flying is reported to have demonstrated impairment at a BAC of 0.04 g/dL. Loss of overall flying proficiency as described by complex tasks such as flying a Link trainer over a U-shaped course with the trainer programmed to present the operator with changes in heading (direction), altitude and air speed have been reported. This early work showed that the loss in overall flying proficiency occurred at BAC of 0.05 g/dL (Aksnes, 1954). Billings (1972) reported similar results (0.05 g/dL BAC) using flying as the time-shared or complex task as the evaluation tool. Modell and Mountz (1990) demonstrated the effects of alcohol on specific piloting skill at low BAC. Ability to perform complex psychomotor tasks during the absorptive phase after alcohol ingestion is reduced at BAC as low as 0.015 g/dL. Impairment in tracking of radiofrequency signals, airport-traffic-control vectoring, traffic observation and avoidance, and aircraft descent has been associated with BAC in the range of 0.03 to 0.05 g/dL (Ross and Mundt, 1988; Billings et al., 1973). Additionally, impairment of short-term memory, decreases in tracking performance during whole-body motion, target tracking, and complex tracking has been reported (Tang and Rosenstein, 1967; Ryback, 1970). Modell and Mountz (1990) discuss current Federal Aviation Administration regulations that prohibit any crewmember of a civil aircraft from flying within eight hours after consumption of any alcoholic beverage, while under the influence of alcohol, or while they have 0.04 percent by weight or more alcohol in the blood (Modell and Mountz, 1990; Dubowski and Caplan, 2003). The results of performance studies clearly demonstrate piloting skills impairment at and below the permissible limit (Garriott, 1993).

Drivers have been tested using other modes of vehicular transportation (e.g., Huber, 1955). Huber's studies (1955) were designed to evaluate the accuracy of driving attention, memory, reaction time and ability to handle a vehicle. He found that the motorcycle riders were impaired in their ability to judge speed and that their reaction time was impaired at BAC of 0.05 g/dL. More recently Stuster (1993) developed a motorcycle DWI detection guide for NHTSA. Later studies indicate that alcohol has a greater impact on motorcycle operation than on other modes of transportation. Garriott (1993) indicates that studies by Robinson using a motorcycle simulator reported increased psychomotor performance impairment decrement as BAC increased from 0.038–0.059 g/dL. Watson et al. (1992) has found that motorcycle drivers arrested for DWI had significantly lower BAC than a comparable group of car/truck drivers.

Forney et al. (1961) used a testing format resembling a Gymkhana sports car event in a closed course study. At 0.04 g/dL BAC, they were able to demonstrate intra-subject variability yielding results ranging from impairment to no impairment.

At BAC less than 0.05 g/dL the drinker is generally stimulated due to alcohol's ability to lift inhibitions thereby making risk-taking behavior more likely. On the other hand alcohol begins to produce a depression at concentrations above 0.05 g/dL BAC. At the same time an individual's moods and emotions are biphasic at the lower BAC and show interpersonal variation (Barry, 1974). The expression of aggressive tendencies generally increases at 0.10 g/dL BAC (McLelland et al., 1968; Cherek et al., 1985).

Skilled drivers driving on a special track have been tested for their driving skills including braking, starting, stopping and starting and backing. Their driving skill was decreased 25–30 percent with no improvement resulting with subsequent testing at BAC between 0.03–0.045 g/dL (Bjerver and Goldberg, 1950). Cohen, Dearnley et al. (1958) demonstrated that at BAC between 0.04–0.06 g/dL highly skilled bus drivers did not show an increased willingness toward risk taking as the BAC increased. However, there was more confidence shown by the drivers about performance at more difficult tasks. This has been interpreted as an indication of impaired self-judgment of driving skill with increasing BAC.

In evaluating subjects with light to heavy alcohol consumption habits the decrement in driving skills was present at BAC as low as 0.03 g/dL. The off-road testing which consisted of a theoretical garage area, parking test, alley and road tests demonstrated that one-half of the drivers had significant impairment at BAC = 0.08 g/dL. Seventy percent of the drivers at 0.05 g/dL, and 80 percent of heavy drinkers had diminished skill at BAC between 0.05 g/dL with 100-percent impairment at 0.15 g/dL (Coldwell, Penner et al., 1958). Excellent correlation between clinical and statistical psychomotor performance impairment is shown in this work.

Levine et al. (1975) analyzed forty-one of 179 English literature studies that met a number of criteria of which the primary factor was their ability to calculate dose of alcohol (mg/kg). All performance task data were grouped by their requirement for performance. These included in the cognitive domain, selective attention, in the perceptual-sensory domain, perceptual speed and in the psychomotor domain, control precision. The importance of this work in ascending order of effect when examining performance in this more global way is that at BAC of 0.4–0.5 g/kg, psychomotor tasks were impaired 8–10 percent; cognitive tasks were impaired 10–15 percent; and perceptual-sensory tasks were impaired 15–20 percent. On the other hand, when specific abilities were assessed, perceptual speed and control precision tasks were impaired 8–10 percent and selective attention tasks were impaired by as much as 35–40 percent. The greatest impairment was in evidence at one hour after alcohol administration. Moskowitz and Robinson (1988) reviewed the U.S. literature for the years of 1940–1985 in a similar manner. Their work categorized impairment (parameter most affected, lowest g/dL BAC for impairment) by reaction time (complex reaction time, 0.03 g/dL), tracking (compensatory, 0.02 g/dL), vigilance (delayed feedback, 0.06 g/dL), divided attention (primary task, 0.02 g/dL), information processing (decision time, 0.02 g/dL), visual function (oculomotor, 0.01 g/dL), perception (decision time, 0.01 g/dL), psychomotor (steadiness, 0.02 g/dL) and driving (emergency, 0.03 g/dL). Holloway (1995) pointed out that the review by Levine (1975) was based on a small study sample number and variance at each dose level causes the authors' performance-dose curve fitting technique to be questioned. Moskowitz and Robinson (1988) further recognize that a major limiting factor in data interpretation was the lack of details concerning actual doses of alcohol tested (i.e., limited dose ranges used and incidences where only one dose was studied contrary to the accepted minimal recommendations of two doses plus a control for a dose-response study). We concur with Moskowitz and Robinson (1988) concerning the limitations placed on data interpretation, especially the early alcohol and driving reports. There are four principle explanations for these limitations in experimental design. The first is the lack of sufficiently sensitive, reproducible alcohol analytical methods to quantify BAC, therefore, it was easier to report the data based on the dose of alcohol administered. The second explanation is that once a legal definition was set then the work clustered around the established or defined BAC to provide sufficient descriptive information to explain why crashes were occurring at that particular blood/breath alcohol concentration. Thirdly, the more recent advances in statistical tools coupled with improved computer hardware capability permits the researchers to evaluate a number of variables, such as multiple doses, inter- and intra-subject variability, pharmacokinetics and pharmacodynamics as a function of time after dosing. It should be re-emphasized here that the fourth factor is the significant variation in BAC existing among individuals at a given time when one examines the calculated dose of alcohol administered versus actual BAC attained in the subjects. This is despite the researcher and the subjects carefully adhering to all instructions dictated by the research protocols. It is difficult to impossible to control for some of these variations, therefore, the subject sample size for a given study is difficult to predict and significance is lost when evaluation is on BAC. These studies are people and time intensive and expensive to complete. Therefore, researchers may tend to report their data based on dose of alcohol administered rather than BAC attained.

Linnoila et al. (1986) based their work on the relationship between alcohol-induced psychomotor performance impairment on specific functions and driving related skills. They found that at moderate BAC, several perceptual-motor functions that are components of driving skill may be altered. These specific driving skill parameters were: attention to activities in the driver's peripheral visual field; range of scanning of the visual field; estimation of vehicular speed; and driver's ability to focus on a target. Based on simulated driving tasks, impairment of tracking was affected at BAC as low as 0.03 g/dL and driving-simulator performance was impairment at BAC as low as 0.05 g/dL. Their findings further suggested that at BAC < 0.05 g/dL that impairment of tasks requiring divided attention, a high information load, and/or high stimulus-response complexity were the most likely affected tasks. The importance of Linnoila et al's (1986) work is that laboratory studies of alcohol-induced impairment begin at BAC of 0.025–0.03 g/dL. This is well below the range of BAC 0.05–0.08 g/dL that has been reported based on the epidemiological literature. Linnoila's group points out that the difference between the ranges may be attributed to such factors as practice, familiarity with task, and context-specific tolerance, time of day tested, age or sex. These are also some of the terms that can be grouped together to explain inter-subject variation to alcohol's effects on not only performance but also in the pharmacological response of humans in general.

In spite of Mitchell's (1985) contention that the data does not support the findings of alcohol-induced impairment at BAC < 0.05 g/dL, the research published by Linnoila (1986), Kruger (1993), Holloway (1995); Honneger et al. (1970); Perrine et al. (1974); Billings and Wick (1972); Gruner et al. (1964); and Stuster and Burns (1998) supports the hypothesis that impairment begins at levels below BAC 0.05 g/dL. However, the risk factor for involvement in a nonfatal and fatal accident is not elevated below BAC 0.05 g/dL (Figures 15.6 and 15.7; Garriott, 1993). This data also supports the hypothesis that impairment below BAC 0.05 g/dL may be task or test specific or obscured in actual accidents by inter-subject and environmental variables. At BACs ≤ 0.05g/dL establishing alcohol's role in accident causation requires more careful review of environmental, vehicle and driver variables specific to the accident (AMA, 1970). It must be cautioned that at BACs below 0.030 g/dL additional attention must be given to the precision and accuracy of the analytical technique used to quantify the BAC. At BACs ≤ 0.01 g/dL the possibility of endogenous alcohol production must be considered (Jones, 1996).

Behavior at lower BAC (< 0.05 g/dL), as discussed above, appears to be stimulatory but is the result of the depressant effects of alcohol on an individual's inhibitions (Perrine et al., 1974). Above 0.05 g/dL, the depressant affects begin to become progressively more prominent as evidenced by the outward clinical signs of behavioral changes. Some individuals become more aggressive while others become more docile and friendly (Forney and Harger, 1965; Perrine et al., 1974; McLelland, 1972; Cherek, et al., 1985). Emotional responsiveness and alteration of emotional level is reduced in the BAC range of 0.05–0.10 g/dL (Barry, 1974; AMA, 1970). The direction (positive or negative attributes) and intensity of emotional and behavioral changes vary by subject and are dictated by behavioral norms of the individual in the absence of alcohol (AMA, 1970). That is, the proportion of negative behavior indicating aggression, antagonism, disagreement and so on tends to increase in the presence of alcohol. Visualize a group of people with their position in the group represented by the rings in a target. The central position in the group is the bull's eye. Each ring describes the relationship of each individual relative to the central position or bull's eye. Group position of the individual bears on the number of the subject's negative reactions (i.e., central group position increases the negative reaction but isolated positions are not increased in the presence of alcohol) (AMA, 1970). In other words, if a drunken individual is in a central position where he senses that his comfort zone is in peril he will display negative behavioral traits. If the drunken person is not in the central position and is distant to the central position in a group he will be less likely to display negative behavioral traits. His comfort zone has not been significantly invaded.

Increased risk taking behavior has been demonstrated in laboratory studies with alcohol using card games and monetary wagers (Wallgren and Barry, 1970). Subjects described as having introverted and extroverted personalities and groups whose drinking habits could be categorized as light or heavy also demonstrated increased risk taking characteristics when drinking (Newman and Fletcher, 1940; Drew et al., 1958; Cutter et al., 1973; Goodwin et al., 1973). Three studies either did not present the BAC attained by their subjects although Cutter et al. (1973) did classify his subjects as having a moderate consumption of alcohol. Drew et al. (1958) and Newman and Fletcher (1940) reported BAC ranges of 0.02–0.08 g/dL and 0.05–0.15 g/dL, respectively.

It is interesting that between 0.05–0.10 g/dL BAC subjects in driving simulator studies showed no appreciable change in the number of slow or indecisive response to traffic lights. Rather the number of completely erroneous decisions was significantly increased (Lewis and Sarlanis, 1969). This study is particularly interesting because the subjects report that their performance in this investigation improved while they were under the influence of the alcohol. In discussing this response and the significant increase in the "GO" response in the presence of alcohol, Lewis and Sarlanis (1969) state that the subjects showed a greater breakdown of self-control and clearness of thinking than they displayed in the absence of alcohol.

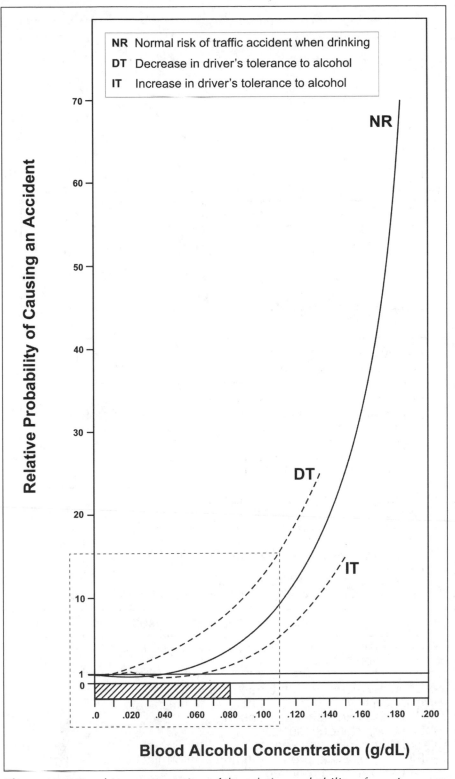

Figure 15.6 *Graphic representation of the relative probability of causing an accident as a function of breath alcohol concentration. Data redrawn from the Grand Rapids study (Borkinstein, 1974) and Jones (1988) which used breath alcohol quantitation. The solid line (NR) represents the Grand Rapids study data and the broken lines DT (decreased tolerance to alcohol) and IT (increased tolerance to alcohol).*

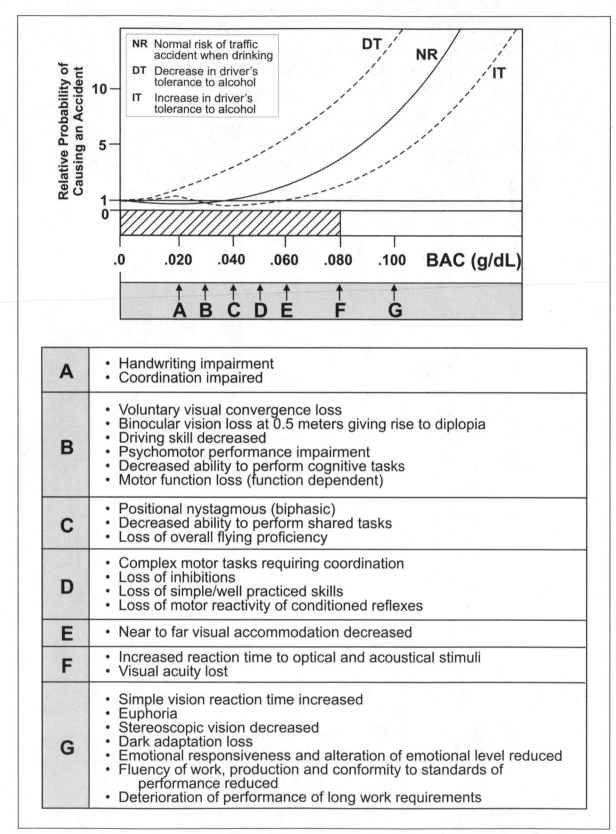

Figure 15.7 *Graphic enlargement of the boxed area of Figure 15.6. The letters with arrows (A–G) under BAC correspond to the letters in the table below the graph and shows where performance impairment onset has been reported with reference to BAC.*

D. Impairment at BAC ≥ 0.10 g/dL

Reflexes, such as those necessary to maintain one's balance, become more profoundly affected with increasing ataxia evident between 0.05–0.10 g/dL. The body sway at 0.10 g/dL is significantly increased (Franks et al., 1976; Fregly et al., 1967; Goldberg, 1943; Idestrom and Cadenius, 1968; Kiplinger et al., 1974; McWilliams et al., 1993; Manno et al., 1992). Although it has also been reported that below a BAC of 0.10 g/dL, body sway is not significantly altered, our studies have shown that ataxia is quantitatively increased in persons who have 0.07 g/dL BAC (Manno, et al., 1992; McWilliams et al., 1993). Persons consuming alcohol have been described as more tired and less vigorous at a BAC of 0.10 g/dL than at 0.05 g/dL (Warren and Raynes, 1972).

Forney and Harger (1965; 1971) in summarizing alcohol influence on reaction time indicate that the average normal reaction to light stimuli in the absence of alcohol is approximately 0.29 second and to sound stimuli, approximately 0.19 second. BACs of 0.10–0.20 g/dL have been found to prolong reaction time by 10–50 percent. However, reaction to optical and acoustical stimuli is reported to be impaired at BAC = 0.08 g/dL with simple visual reaction time slowed at 0.10 g/dL BAC (AMA, 1970). Simulated driving investigations at BAC 0.03–0.10 g/dL have also shown that errors in reaction time and response to turn signals are increased (AMA, 1970). Muellar's work (1954) demonstrated that at 0.10 g/dL BAC reaction time was lengthened by 80 percent and an individual displayed easily recognizable appearance of intoxication at 0.15 g/dL. He also showed that 20 percent of his subjects had impaired reaction times only at BAC 0.15–0.20 g/dL. It should be pointed out that Mueller used a small subject population (N = 10) with little details of the drinking patterns or habits of his subjects. His findings, however, support the concept that reaction time is slowed in the presence of alcohol and simply indicates that inter-subject variation relative to BAC should be only one of the considerations when applying reaction time to performance interpretation.

Elements of work and intellectual input to performance can be described by motor function, work flow and productivity, and the ability to follow direc-tions. Psychomotor function which is function dependent is impaired in the range of BAC of 0.03–0.10 g/dL. Complex motor tasks requiring coordination become impaired at a BAC of 0.05 g/dL (AMA, 1970). Work fluency, production and conformity to standards of performance have been observed to be decreased at a BAC of 0.10 g/dL (Wechsler, 1941). Tasks or work performance requiring a high degree of skill and attentiveness are more impaired by alcohol than tasks requiring a low level of skill and those associated with heavy physical work (Lundgren, 1947). Testing alcohol effects on attention and concentration ability using driving simulators to produce correct response to turning (accuracy test) indicated that the faculties of drivers needed for driving are impaired at BAC > 0.10 g/dL (Elbel, 1951a,b; Gruner, 1955; AMA, 1970; Wallgren and Barry, 1970). Additionally, test subjects displayed impaired self-criticism and judgment. This is supported by data that shows that work requiring long periods of performance deteriorates at 0.10 g/dL BAC. The lack of inspiration that varies by subject has been used to describe alcohol's affect on creative ability (Froster, 1949). Intellectual function and dexterity which is impaired in the presence of alcohol is restored as alcohol disappears from blood while chronic alcoholics studied over a ten-year period demonstrated significant deterioration of intellectual ability for various higher mental activities as tested on the Wechsler IQ test. The intellectual deterioration was not observed with acute alcoholism (Wechsler, 1941).

Perception of auditory stimuli shows no change, but distraction is greater in subjects at 0.15 g/dL BAC (AMA, 1970). Others have shown that auditory acuity is not usually effected at < 0.10 g/dL BAC (Pihkanen and Kauko, 1962) and discrimination of sound volume and intensity is decreased (Jellinek and McFarland, 1940).

Alcohol-induced changes also occur in the special senses of vision, hearing, smell and taste. Of these senses vision and hearing are more intimately associated with performance tasks than are taste and smell. The olfactory threshold for odors and appetite and satiety could be important in recognition of environmental influences surrounding completion of various performance tasks (e.g., driving, flying and various performance tasks (e.g., driving, flying and work). The ability to detect odor such as smoke or chemicals if affected by alcohol could prevent an individual from recognizing developing dangers. Appetite and satiety could affect work progress and performance especially in the alcoholic individual. The olfactory threshold and appetite and satiety of a subject support this scenario since it has been shown that these responses parallel the rise and fall of the olfactory threshold (Wallgren and Barry, 1970).

Vision is one of the most important senses necessary for safe and reliable execution of the majority of vehicular and work related performance tasks. Changes in the physiological components of vision are important indicators to explain performance changes related to BAC (Tables 15.1 and 15.2). While voluntary convergence begins to become impaired as low as 0.03 g/dL BAC most of the other reported significant changes occur at BAC (0.05 g/dL. The loss of binocular vision at 0.5 meter gives rise to development of diplopia as the BAC increases (Brecher, 1955; Forney and Harger, 1965; AMA, 1970).

Visual fusion and convergency is markedly impaired between 0.05–0.15 g/dL BAC. Decreased fusion frequency has been reported to occur at low BAC (AMA, 1970). Far to near vision accommodation is reduced by 0.10–0.20 sec at 0.06 g/dL BAC (Forney and Harger, 1965; AMA, 1970).

Static visual acuity (stationary objects) is lost at ≤ 0.08 g/dL with dynamic visual acuity impaired at > 0.10 g/dL BAC (Newman and Fletcher, 1941). Stereoscopic vision is affected at 0.10 g/dL BAC. Goldberg (1943) using flicker-fusion studies has reported that in the presence of alcohol a greater light intensity is required to initiate the response in the test than when tested in the absence of alcohol. Also, detectable visual impairment response occurred between 0.015 g/dL BAC for alcohol abstainers to 0.055 g/dL for heavy drinkers. This has been estimated to be about 0.5 to 2 ounces of whiskey for a 150-pound person or 2–3 cocktails may reduce visual acuity at BAC > 0.05 g/dL (Forney and Harger, 1965). Others have shown decreased visual acuity occurring at low BAC (Marquis et al., 1957; Miles, 1924; Bloomberg and Wassen, 1959).

Positional nystagmus in the presence of alcohol is biphasic with stage I beginning at 0.04 g/dL BAC. Stage I occurs immediately and lasts 3–4 hours during alcohol intake and is separated from stage II by 1–2 hours. Stage II, seen in severe intoxication, lasts 5–15 hours and is sometimes present after alcohol has dissipated from the blood (Barry, 1974).

Mortimer (1963), in simulator investigations under normal day and night driving conditions as well as glare conditions, has reported that low BAC produced significant changes in glare conditions and that the higher BAC significantly influenced day, night and glare condition performance. The range of BAC in this work was 0.01–0.07 g/dL.

A person's ability to detect a low contrast target under mesopic levels of illumination was studied in young adults (21–30 years old) and upper middle-aged individuals (50–60 years old). Significant and comparable impairment at 0.08 g/dL BAC was found in both groups of test subjects (Lewis and Sarlanis, 1969; Lewis, 1972). Little or no impairment was observed in these subjects at 0.06 or 0.04 g/dL BAC.

Other visual functions are impaired at BAC > 0.08 g/dL (Lewis et al., 1969; Lewis, 1972; Mortimer, 1963; Moskowitz, 1974; Newman and Fletcher, 1941) including impairment of light-dark adaptation at BAC of 0.15 g/dL (Forster and Starck, 1959). Glare resistance is impaired at 0.15 g/dL BAC, however, there appeared to be intersubject variation (Newman and Fletcher, 1940). Alcohol impairs color discrimination also (Schmidt and Bingel, 1953; Wallgren and Barry, 1970).

Studies of simple tracking ability, concentration and attention have been reported as producing no effect on tracking at BAC ≤ 0.10 g/dL and at > 0.10 g/dL (Chiles and Jennings, 1969; Colquhoun, 1962; Talland et al., 1964). In contrast, complex pursuit tracking indexed on a moving target produces impairment at BAC between 0.05–0.10 g/dL (Binder, 1971; Levine et al., 1973; Mortimer, 1963; Richter and Hobi, 1975; Kiplinger et al., 1974; Manno et, 1992). Simple simulator steering tests have shown a correlation between BAC and loss of vigilant steering capability at BAC between 0.05–0.15 g/dL. Later studies substantiated these findings by showing decreased accuracy in steering between 0.02–

0.08 g/dL BAC. Steering accuracy is described as a linear decrease as the BAC increased (Drew et al., 1959).

Mellanby (1919, 1920) described work wherein it was found that discrepant results were observed when BAC was measured as a function of the ascending or descending BAC. From this finding it has been postulated that psychomotor performance impairment is more impaired on the ascending rather than descending limb of the BAC curve. This has been referred to as the "Mellanby effect" (See Garriott, Chapter 2). Lewis and Sarlanis (1969) also studied the psychomotor performance on the ascending and descending limbs of the BAC and showed similar psychomotor performance impairment based on measures of breath alcohol. Others have not been able to replicate the Mellanby effect correlating it with performance changes. Forney and Harger (1965; 1971) addressed some of the issues explaining that when applying the Mellanby effect to interpretation of alcohol values and accidents in relation to psychomotor performance impairment that several important facts must be considered. Venous blood and breath are the preferred specimens for determining the concentration that reflects the concentration at the target site (i.e., the brain). It has been established that alcohol concentration in alveolar air is more closely correlated to arterial BAC than to the venous blood BAC. They further advise that the majority of the reports that have not substantiated the Mellanby effect collected venous blood from antecubital sites for alcohol testing. They postulate that the Mellanby effect is due to discrepancies between venous and arterial blood during the alcohol absorptive and post absorptive periods rather than a true psychomotor performance impairment effect.

Tolerance to some of the psychomotor performance impairment effects of alcohol can occur as discussed by Garriott (1993). Figure 15.6 is a modification of the Grand Rapids study (Borkenstein, 1974) and the work of Jones (1988). Jones illustrated the shift in the relative probability of nontolerant and tolerant drinkers becoming involved in crashes as compared to the subjects from the Grand Rapids study. It can be seen that at the same BAC, nontolerant drinkers (DT) are more likely to be involved in crashes (Figures 15.6 and 15.7) than toler-

ant drinkers (IT) (Figures 15.6 and 15.7) or average drivers (NR) (Figures 15.6 and 15.7). Chesher and Greely (1992) compared impairment in experienced and light drinkers. The result varies with the type of test parameters and with different studies. Laurell et al. (1990) in an on-the-road-testing investigation of alcohol effects in light and heavy drinkers showed higher psychomotor performance impairment in all subjects at ≤ 0.10 g/dL BAC and that no difference between the light- and heavy-drinking groups occurred. Rosen and Lee (1976) compared psychomotor performance impairment in alcoholics, heavy drinkers and social drinkers. Social drinkers demonstrated gross signs of intoxication at ≤ 0.10 g/dL BAC while heavy drinkers and alcoholics showed almost none of the same symptoms. It was concluded that all groups were equally impaired on cognitive performance measures and had equivalent performance levels while sober thereby negating any chronic deficits in the alcoholic subjects.

Coldwell et al. (1958) testing subjects with light to heavy drinking habits observed that driving skills began to be impaired as low as 0.03 g/dL with 70 percent of the subjects impaired at 0.05 g/dL; one-half of the drivers were significantly impaired at 0.08 g/dL; and 80 percent of the heavy drinkers were impaired at 0.05–0.12 g/dL BAC. Non-drinking skills were lost to all subjects as the BAC neared 0.15 g/dL indicating that regardless of drinking history all drivers showed psychomotor performance impairment as their BAC increased.

Naville et al. (1950) using drivers with varying skill levels could only perform purely automatic operations at 0.15–0.20 g/dL BAC. He showed that all drivers in his studies demonstrated psychomotor performance impairment at BAC > 0.10 g/dL. Newman et al. (1941a,b) had reported earlier that drivers with BAC of 0.15–0.20 g/dL were impaired in their ability to drive.

15.4 Application of Performance Information to DWI

In the determination of alcohol associated accident causation, it is clear from the above discussion that psychomotor performance impairment occurs at varying blood levels of alcohol even as low as 0.015 g/dL BAC depending on the function tested. It is also present at the time of an accident. This dichotomy can either be explained or resolved by recognizing that the probability of an accident happening likely will increase because of the increased psychomotor performance impairment that occurs at increasing BACs. There are a number of points that could be used as a basis for implicating psychomotor performance impairment as a function of BAC.

What is the relative probability that an individual who drinks and drives will be involved in an accident? Stated another way, what is an individual's risk factor for involvement in an accident after drinking alcohol? This can be approached from the epidemiology studies as discussed earlier (Manno and Manno, 1996, Chapter 14). Jones (1988) has summarized data from the well-known Grand Rapids survey of over 13,000 drivers and supplemented by other studies, such as the Vermont study of 1,184 drivers, show clearly that higher BACs are well correlated with a higher risk of being involved in a crash (Figures 15.6 and 15.7). The risk begins to increase very rapidly around 0.08 g/dL and becomes extremely high as the BAC reaches very high levels. The risk of involvement in a fatal crash for those with a BAC of 0.10 g/dL was twelve times as high as for those who had not been drinking at all, and there was more than a twenty-fold greater probability of involvement in any crash at BACs over 0.15 g/dL (Hurst, 1974; Borkenstein et al., 1974; Jones and Joscelyn, 1978).

Figures 15.6 and 15.7 also demonstrates the risk factor for becoming involved in an auto crash of drivers with various BACs. Curves DT and IT are designed to illustrate differences in alcohol tolerance levels, DT shows the effect of reduced tolerance such as seen in inexperienced drinkers and IT the effect of increased tolerance, with somewhat reduced risk (Jones, 1988; Garriott, 1993).

Figure 15.6 also shows that the relative probability of being involved in an accident is between five- and ten-fold greater when a person has a BAC of approximately 0.10–0.12 g/dL. At a BAC of 0.14 g/dL the risk is increased to about twenty-fold greater. A BAC of approximately 0.180 g/dL BAC increases the probability of involvement to greater than fifty-fold than with no alcohol (Perrine et al., 1988).

Tables 15.1 and 15.2 summarize the psychomotor performance laboratory, simulator and on-the-road-testing studies by reaction time and coordination reflexes, cerebration, work performance and special senses (i.e., vision, hearing, olfactory and taste). The data is arranged by category as a function of BAC within the category, giving the skill or performance indicator measured and the resultant effect.

Table 15.4 illustrates the ethanol equivalents needed to produce a given BAC, what behavior would likely to be displayed by the drinker, and the corresponding relative accident risk. Others have critically evaluated variables such as driver population, age, and other factors in a similar manner to assess their contribution to alcohol psychomotor performance impairment (Perrine et al., 1988). Table 15.4 also provides laboratory performance effects, intoxication indicators, observable performance effects and risk factor for accident involvement as functions of ethanol equivalents and BAC. The three alcohol effect measures do not change after one to two ethanol equivalent (0.015 g/dL BAC) and there is no greater accident risk than if alcohol was not present. At two to three ethanol equivalents (0.03 g/dL BAC) minimal effects are detectable in the three types of measures. At four to six ethanol equivalents (0.09 g/dL BAC) laboratory performance decrements are statistically significant and indicate impairment in most tests studied; observable performance decrements are evident which makes the individual appear to be drunk and 7–8 times more at risk of being involved in an accident. At 0.18 g/dL BAC (9–12 ethanol equivalents) laboratory tests consistently demonstrate psychomotor performance impairment, the individual consistently appears drunk, and the accident risk factor is more than fifty times greater (NHTSA, 1978).

When estimating the number of alcohol equivalents consumed for forensic purposes, exact pharmacokinetic formulas (Dubowski, 1976) should be used and should take into consideration the number equivalents consumed, the period of time during which the alcohol was consumed, and the lean body weight of the individual. Average values should be avoided and calculations should reflect the 95% confidence limits for metabolism. Rough estimates of the ethanol equivalents necessary to produce the BAC can be estimated using the "rule of fifteen." In our own experience, for example, this simple algorithm has been useful in discussing cases and retrospectively or prospectively screening cases prior to deciding for lengthy litigation by estimating BAC at the time of an accident. It is based on a hypothetical 150-pound (70-kilogram) man, approximate time of blood collection (if known), and approximate time of the accident. It should be recognized from Dubowski's work (1976) that the approach offers a very general assessment tool and that the drop of BAC by 0.015 g/dL per hour is an average rate of BAC decline. The range for twenty-five males was 0.011–0.022 g/dL BAC. Dubowski also showed the same range (0.011-0.022) of decline for fifteen females with an average of 0.018 g/dL BAC decline per hour. The "rule of fifteen" should always be accompanied with the estimated BAC range that shows individual variation.

Holloway (1995) has reviewed a number of studies in order to compare across a number of alcohol psychomotor performance functions and reanalyzed the data using linear regression procedures. The graphic representation of his findings plotted the percent of persons responding as effect versus the BAC in mg percent (mg/dL). Data subjected to analysis were intoxication level, psychosocial functions, automatic behaviors and performance, controlled behaviors and performance and simulator performance. He concluded that the psychosocial functions and automatic performance effects were almost identical in incidence of significant reports. Comparison of controlled performance shifts does not indicate greater alcohol sensitivity but it does suggest that alcohol is uniformly more efficient at altering the number of effected responses across doses. In comparing performance using driving and flight simulators he found a pattern of response similar to the other alcohol-related effects categories. Al-

Table 15.4
General Assessment Guide for Rating an Individual's Impairment Level and Risk Factor for Accident Involvement Based on Blood Alcohol Concentration (g/dL), Ethanol Equivalents or Both

Ethanol Equivalents	Blood Alcohol Concentration (g/dL)	Usual Intoxication Indicator	Laboratory Performance Effects	Observable Performance Effects	Relative Probability of Accident[1]
1	0.015	subclinical	none	none	1:1
2	0.030	subclinical	minimal	minimal	1:1
3	0.045	subclinical	detectable	observable in inexperienced drinkers	1.5:1
4	0.060	euphoria	consistent in certain tests	observable with careful observation	2.0–2.5:1
5	0.075	euphoria	consistent in most tests	observable in most nonchronic drinkers	4.5:1
6	0.09	euphoria excitement	consistent in most tests	individual appears "drunk"	7:1
7	0.120	euphoria excitement	consistent in all tests	individual appears "drunk"	12:1
8	0.150	excitement	consistent in all tests	individual appears "drunk"	25:1
9	0.180	confusion[2]	consistent in all tests	individual appears "drunk"	>50:1

[1] Ratio expressed as presence of positive BAC : absence of BAC
[2] At BAC 0.18–0.30 g/dL intoxication indicator is confusion.
At BAC 0.25–0.40 g/dL intoxication indicator is stupor.
At BAC 0.35–0.50 g/dL intoxication indicator is coma.
At BAC > 0.45 g/dL intoxication indicator is death.

though his work compares the number of reports of effects and not the magnitude of the effect, it is worth noting that the direction of response effect increases as the BAC increases regardless of the category of behavioral response studies.

Often it is difficult to reconcile differences between the scientific and the legal definitions of the BAC necessary for DWI/DUI to have occurred and to explain how an accident may have occurred, especially at the low BAC. Klitzner (1994) applying a systems approach to DWI and fatal crashes utilized the human factors approach to understanding traffic accidents. This approach indicates that there is a varying level of driver competence over time and a varying level of environmental demand over time. When the driver competence falls below environmental demand, the DUI or DWI arrest or alcohol-related crash occurs.

Table 15.5 summarizes the information available demonstrating the BAC at which a variety of performance measures have caused performance impairment. No reports of performance measures were found below lowest BAC represented by the blackened area for the respective measure. Like many of the studies discussed in this chapter, one should not assume that those BACs below the highest indicated in the table have actually been tested.

The effectiveness of this directed alcohol and driving research is shown in Figure 15.8. The line represents the yearly fatality rate per million vehicle miles (MVM) traveled between 1966 and 1995 (Stuster and Burns, 1998). Fatalities declined from approximately 5.5 per MVM in 1966 to 3.0+ per MVM in 1976 where it stabilized until the introduction of the SFST and DWI detection training in 1980. Since that time the fatality rate continued to

Table 15.5

The junction of the black and white areas shows the lowest BAC concentration where onset of impairment has been reported. The white area represents the BACs associated with onset of impairment.

Performance Measure	Blood Alcohol Concentration (g/dL)									
	.01	.02	.03	.04	.05	.06	.07	.08	.09	.10 +
PMP tasks				■	■	■	■	■	■	■
Cognitive tasks				■	■	■	■	■	■	■
Perceptual-sensory Tasks				■	■	■	■	■	■	■
Complex reaction time			■	■	■	■	■	■	■	■
Tracking (compensatory)		■	■	■	■	■	■	■	■	■
Vigilance (delayed Feedback)							■	■	■	■
Divided attention (primary task)		■	■	■	■	■	■	■	■	■
Information processing (decision time)		■	■	■	■	■	■	■	■	■
Visual function (oculomotor)	■	■	■	■	■	■	■	■	■	■
Perception (decision time)	■	■	■	■	■	■	■	■	■	■
Psychomotor (steadiness)		■	■	■	■	■	■	■	■	■
Impaired Tracking			■	■	■	■	■	■	■	■
Divided attention + high information load and/or High stimulus-response complexity				■	■	■	■	■	■	■
Ataxia body sway				■	■	■	■	■	■	■
Risk taking changes (light drinker)		■	■	■	■	■	■	■	■	■
Risk taking changes (heavy drinker)				■	■	■	■	■	■	■

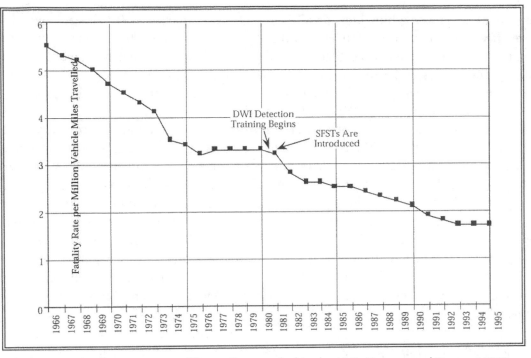

Figure 15.8 Fatality rates per million miles traveled in the U.S. (Stuster and Burns, 1998)

decline to just below 2.0 per MVM. According to Stuster and Burns (1998), an average of more than 155 people die each day from motor vehicle crashes in the U.S. It is estimated that 41 percent or sixty-four of the people dying daily in these crashes have been drinking alcohol.

Since the first edition of this book, significant information relating to the involvement of alcohol in traffic accidents has been gained. The most significant findings relate to driving with blood alcohol concentrations at levels below 0.10 g/dL. Some of this information is from reanalysis of existing FARS data, but new research has also been conducted using breath alcohol testing technology that has been developed in recent years. Most of this research indicates that impairment can occur at lower BACs and suggests that statutes regulating drinking and driving should be changed to reflect lower standards. Because of this new information and because of fund restriction for non-implementation, many states have reduced their standard for driving under the influence of alcohol from 0.10 g/dL to 0.08 g/dL. It would not be surprising if the "legal standard" was lowered further in the coming years to reflect a standard for all drivers of 0.04 g/dL BAC as is currently dictated for commercial drivers, pilots and persons in safety sensitive positions. Since driving is a privilege that requires a license, it is not unreasonable to set limits on a permissible BAC based on epidemiological data relating BAC to accident causation.

New technology has also been developed and implemented that allows for the easy and accurate measurement of alcohol in breath and oral fluids. These point-of-care testing (POCT) devices provide new tools for not only conducting on the road research associated with alcohol involvement, but can also be used to make an assessment of impairment by a police officer or an evaluation of alcohol toxicity by a paramedic or physician. These devices can also assist the driver in determining if his or her BAC is "legal," but should not be used in an effort to drink to a "safe level." Any POCT device used must be approved by the Food and Drug Administration and the users must comply rigidly with use and care instructions for the devices to be used at stated precision and accuracy levels. The program developed by the U.S. Department of Transportation that uses a two-step chemical test can serve as a model for the use of these devices. The U.S. Department of Transportation program prescribes a POCT device to be used initially. If the POCT result is 0.04 percent or greater, then the individual is tested further using evidentiary breath testing or a blood test. POCT devices can readily be used by police officers or other personnel and effectively replace the Standardized Field Sobriety Test that is currently used for establishing probable cause for evidentiary breath testing.

The use of lower standards for DWI also has far reaching implications in civil litigation associated with motor vehicle accidents involving driver alcohol consumption. At BACs greater than 0.10 g/dL, the probability of accident association with a BAC increases in a logarithmic manner with probabilities increasing rapidly as the BAC increases. At lower BACs, between 0.005 g/dL and 0.05 g/dL (0.005 g/dL selected as a potential endogenous level), many other factors must be considered in order to determine the effect of alcohol on accident causation. Some of these factors include:

- **Accuracy and precision of the method**. BACs can be measured by a variety of techniques. If the results are to be applied to a specific individual in a specific accident, the limits of the test must be taken into consideration.
- **Chain of custody**. BACs conducted in a medical facility for diagnostic and medical treatment purposes may not have the traditional chain of custody documentation. A review of the medical record and laboratory data should be conducted if there is any concern that the test result matches to a specific individual.
- **Tolerance**. At lower BACs an individual who regularly consumes alcohol may have developed some degree of tolerance to psychomotor impairment at lower BACs.
- **Accident reconstruction**. At lower BACs it becomes critical to determine what happened to cause the accident. It is important to determine the amount of contribution from the drivers with positive BACs in order to make a conclusion regarding alcohol involvement.

15.5 Conclusions

In summarizing this chapter we feel that several conclusions and recommendations can be made.

- Both controlled research and epidemiological studies relating the effects of alcohol and driving support the 0.1 percent and 0.08 percent legal set-points for having alcohol impairment.
- Initial research using lower BAC levels have indicated trends associated with some degree of impairment below 0.08 percent. These data support programs such as the DOT 0.04 percent BAC restriction for commercial transportation workers. A similar program could be implemented for the general public with penalties similar to speeding (i.e., graded fines based on the BAC) to reinforce public awareness of potential negative outcomes of drinking and driving. Such a program could identify drivers before they developed tolerance to the point of having a BAC above the legal limit.
- More research at lower BAC with statistically valid conclusions must be conducted to determine the effects of lower BACs as a component of accident causation as it applies to a single event.
- With the development of easy-to-administer, accurate and precise POCT for alcohol, consideration should be given to the use of these tests in lieu of the SFST for the establishment of probable cause for evidentiary breath or blood testing for alcohol.
- Increased public education should be conducted regarding the inability of the average person to visually recognize signs of impairment at BACs around and below 0.1 percent, particularly in experienced drinkers. This program should include education regarding the self use of POCT devices for measuring BAC and the importance of the BAC as the only valid measure to assess impairment.
- Additional responsibility should be placed on establishments that serve alcoholic beverages to insure that patrons do not drive if they have achieved a BAC in the impairing range. This could be partially accomplished by providing POCT devices, paid for by a cover charge, for measurement of the BAC. Physicians and pharmacists already have this responsibility as it applies to prescription medication that may produce negative psychomotor effects. Alcohol is a drug that produces psychomotor impairment. It is delivered to patrons in known doses and pur-

veyors should have some responsibility for public protection since the customers, by the definition of alcohol impairment and the development of tolerance to alcohol, cannot accurately make the judgment as to when they are impaired.

References

Aksenes, E.G. Effect of small doses of alcohol upon performance in a link trainer. *J. Aviat. Med.* 25: 680–688, 1954.

American Medical Association, Committee on Medicolegal Problems. *Alcohol and the Impaired Driver. A Manual on the Medicolegal Aspects of Chemical Tests for Intoxication.* Chicago, IL: American Medical Association, 1970.

Barry, H. III. Motivational and cognitive effects of alcohol. In: Perrine, M.W. (ed.), *Alcohol, Drugs and Driving*, technical report DOT–HS–801–096. National Highway Traffic Safety Administration, 1974, pp. 71–96.

Billings, C.E. and Wick, R.L. *Effects of Alcohol on Pilot Performance During Instrument Flight,* technical report FAA–AM–72–4. Federal Aviation Administration, 1972.

Billings, C.E. et al. Effects of ethyl alcohol on pilot performance. *Aerosp. Med.* 44:379–382, 1973.

Binder, A. An experimental approach to driver evaluation using alcohol drinkers and marihuana smokers. *Accident Analysis and Prevention* 3:237–256, 1971.

Bjerver, K. and Goldberg, L. Results of practical road tests and laboratory experiments. *Quart. J. Stud. Alc.* 11:1–30, 1950.

Blomberg, L.H. and Wassen, A. Preliminary report on the effect of alcohol on dark adaptation determined by an objective method. *Acta Ophthalmol.* 37:2, 1959.

Bordens, K.S. and Abbott, B.B. *Research Design and Methods: A Process Approach.* Mayfield Publishing Co., Mountain View, CA., 1991.

Borkenstein, R.F. et al. The role of the drinking driver in traffic accidents: The Grand Rapids Study, 2nd Edition, *Blutalkohol* 11, Suppl. 1:1–132, 1974.

Bouchardt, M.M. and Sandras, Dela digestion des boissons alcooliques et de leur role dans la nutrition physique. *Ann. Chem. Physique.* Ser. 21:448–457, 1847.

Brecher, G.A., Hartman, A.P. and Leonard, D.D. Effect of alcohol on binocular vision. *Am. J. Ophthalmol.* 39:44–52, 1955.

Bschor, F. Beobachtungen uber ein Funktionales prinzip bei der psychomotrischen leistungsminderung in den verschiedenen phasen der akuten alkoholintoxikation (Observations concerning a functional principle in the decrease of psychomotor performance during various phases of acute alcohol intoxication). *Deutsch. Z. ges gerichtl. Med* 41:273, 1953.

Buikhuisen, W. and Jongman, R.W. Traffic perception under the influence of alcohol. *Quart. J. Stud. Alc.* 33(3):800–6, 1972.

Burns, M. and Moskowitz, H. *Psychophysical Test for DWI Arrest*, DOT–HS–802–424. National Highway Traffic Safety Administration, Department of Transportation, 1977.

Cappell, H. et al. Alcohol and marihuana: a comparison of effects on a temporally controlled operant in humans. *J. Pharmacol. Exp. Ther.* 182(2):195–203, 1972.

Cherek, D.R., Steinberg, J.L. and Manno, B.R. Effects of alcohol on human aggressive behavior. *J. Stud. Alc.* 46(4):321–8, 1985.

Chesher, G. and Greely, J. Tolerance to the effects of alcohol. *Alcohol, Drugs and Driving,* 8:93–106, 1992.

Chiles, W.D. and Jennings, A.E. *Effects of Alcohol on Complex Performance.* Report No. AM 69-14. Oklahoma City: Federal Aviation Administration, Office of Aviation Medicine, Aeromedical Institute, 1969.

Cohen, J., Dearnaley, E.J. and Hansel, C.E.M. The risk taken in driving under the influence of alcohol. *Brit. Med. J.* 1:1438, 1958.

Coldwell, B.B. et al. Effect of ingestion of distilled spirits on automobile driving skill. *Quart. J. Stud. Alc.* 19:590–616, 1958.

Colquhoun, W.P. Effects d'une faible dose d'alcohol et certains autres facteurs sur la performance dans une tache de vigilance. *Bulletin du Centre d'Etudes et Recherches Psychotechniques* 11:27–44, 1962.

Compton, R.P. *Use of Controlled Substances and Highway Safety: A Report to Congress*, DOT-HS-807-261. National Highway Transportation Administration, Department of Transportation, 1988.

Cutter, S.G., Green, L.R. and Harford, T.C. Levels of risk taken by extraverted and introverted alcoholics as a function of drinking whiskey. *British Journal of Social and Clinical Psychology* 12:83–89, 1973.

Dietrich, J.J. *Horizontal Gaze Nystagmus: The Science and the Law: A Resource Guide for Judges, Prosecutors and Law Enforcement.* Alexandria, VA: American Prosecutors Research Institute, National Traffic Law Center. http://www.nhtsa.dot.gov/people/injury/enforce/nystagmus/ntlc.html. Printed 3/7/2003.

Drew, G.C., Colquhoun, W.P. and Long, H.A. *Effect of Small Doses of Alcohol on a Skill Resembling Driving*, Med. Res. Council Memorandum 38. London: H.M. Stationery Office, 1959.

Dubowski, K.M. Human pharmacokinetics of alcohol. *Alcohol Tech. Rep.* 5:5–7, 1976.

Dubowski, K.M. and Caplan, Y.A. Alcohol testing in the workplace. In: Garriot, J.C. (ed.), *Medicolegal Aspects of Alcohol*, 4th ed. Tucson, AZ: Lawyers & Judges Publishing Company, 2003.

Ehrensing, R.H. et al. Effect of alcohol on auditory and visual time perception. *Quart. J. Stud. Alc.* 31(4): 851–60, 1970.

Elbel, H. Bedeutung, Nachweis und Beurteilung der Alkoholwirkungen im Verkehr (Significance, proof and evaluation of the effects of alcohol in traffic). *Med. Welt* (Stuttgart) 20:1151–1154, 1951b.

Elbel, H. Bedeutung, Nachweis und Beurteilung der Alkoholwirkungen im Verkehr (Significance, proof and evaluation of the effects of alcohol in traffic). *Med. Welt* (Stuttgart) 20:1106–1108, 1951a.

Forney, R.B. et al. Performance in Gymkhana sports car event with low levels of blood alcohol. *Traffic Safety-Research Review.* 5:8–12, 1961.

Forney, R.B. and Harger, R.N. The alcohols. In: DiPalma, J.R. (ed.), *Drill's Pharmacology in Medicine,* 3rd ed. NY: McGraw-Hill, 1965, pp. 210–231.

Forney, R.B. and Harger, R.N. The alcohols. In: DiPalma, J.R. (ed.), *Drill's Pharmacology in Medicine*, 4th ed. NY: McGraw-Hill, 1971, pp. 275–302.

Franks, H.M. et al. The relationship between alcohol dosage and performance decrement in humans. *J. Stud. Alc.* 37(3): 284–97, 1976.

Fregly, A.R., Bergstedt, M. and Graybiel, A. Relationships between blood alcohol, positional alcohol nystagmus and postural equilibrium. *Quart. J. Stud. Alc.* 28:11–21, 1967.

Froster, G. Alkohol Och Diktning (Alcohol and creative writing). *Tirfing* 43:33, 1949.

Garriott, J.C. Pharmacology and toxicology of ethyl alcohol. In: Garriott, J.C (ed.), *Medicolegal Aspects of Alcohol*, 3rd ed. Tucson, AZ: Lawyers & Judges Publishing Company, Inc., 1996a.

Garriott, J.C.. Reporting of laboratory results. In: Garriott, J.C (ed.), *Medicolegal Aspects of Alcohol*, 3rd ed. Tucson, AZ: Lawyers & Judges Publishing Company, Inc., 1996b.

Garriott, J.C. Current science and issues in forensic aspects of alcohol. In: Garriott, J.C (ed.), *Medicolegal Aspects of Alcohol Determination in Biological Specimens.* Tucson, AZ: Lawyers & Judges Publishing Company, Inc., 1993, pp 293–307.

Goldberg, L. Quantitative studies on alcohol tolerance in man. The influence of ethyl alcohol on sensory, motor and psychological functions referred to blood alcohol in normal and habituated individuals. *Acta Physiol. Scand.* 16:5:1–128, 1943.

Goodwin, D.W., Powell, B. and Stein, J. Behavioral tolerance to alcohol in moderate drinkers. *Amer. J. Psychia.* 122:93–94, 1973.

Gruner, O. Alkohol und Aufmerksamkeit. Ihre Bedeutung im Motorisierten Verkehr (Alcohol and attention: its significance in motorized traffic). *Deutsch. Z. ges gerichtl. Med* 44:187, 1955.

Harris, D.H. Visual detection of driving while intoxicated. *Human Factors* 22:725–732, 1980a.

Harris, D.H. et al. *The Visual Detection of Driving while Intoxicated.* Washington, DC: Department of Transportation, National Highway Traffic Safety Administration, publication No. Report DOT-HS-7-1538, 1980b.

Holloway, F.A. *Low Dose Alcohol Effects on Human Behavior and Performance: A Review of Post–1984 Research.* Washington, DC: Department of Transportation, Federal Aviation Administration, Office of Aviation Medicine Technical Report DOT/FAA/AM-94/24, 1994.

Holloway, F.A. Low-Dose alcohol effects on human behavior and performance. *Alcohol, Drugs and Driving* 11:39–56, 1995.

Honneger, H., Kampschulte, R. and Klein, H. Storung der Sehscharfe fur bewegte Objekte durch (Alcohol disturbance of visual acuity for moving objects.) *Alkohol. Blutalkohol* 7:31–44, 1970.

Huber, O. Studies on alteration of driving ability of motorcyclists after moderate intake of alcohol. *Deutsch. Z. ges. gerichtl. Med.* 44:559, 1955.

Hurst, P.M. Epidemiological aspects of alcohol and driver crashes and citations. In: Perrine, M.W. (ed.), *Alcohol, Drugs and Driving,* technical report DOT HS 801-096. National Highway Traffic Safety Administration, 1974.

Idestrom, C.M. and Cadenius, B. Time relations of the effects of alcohol compared to placebo. Dose-response curves for psychomotor and perceptual test performances and blood and urine levels of alcohol. *Psychopharmacologia* 13:189–200, 1968.

Jellinek, E.M. and McFarland, R.A. Analysis of psychological experiments on the effects of alcohol. *Quart .J. Stud. Alc.* 1:272–371, 1940.

Jones, R.K. and Joscelyn, K.B. *Alcohol and Highway Safety 1978: A Review of the State of Knowledge,* DOT–HS–803–714. Washington, DC: National Highway Traffic Safety Administration, Department of Transportation, p.207, 1978.

Jones, A.W. Enforcement of drink-driving laws by use of "per se" legal alcohol limits: blood and/or breath concentration as evidence of impairment. *Alcohol, Drugs and Driving* 4:99–112, 1988.

Jones, A.W. Biochemistry and physiology of alcohol: Applications to forensic science and toxicology. In: Garriott, J.C (ed.), *Medicolegal Aspects of Alcohol,* 3rd ed. Tucson, AZ: Lawyers & Judges Publishing Company, Inc., 1996.

Kaplan, H.L. et al. Is there acute tolerance to alcohol at steady state? *J. Stud. Alc.* 46:253–256, 1985.

Kiplinger, G.F., Sokol, G. and Rodda, B.E. Effect of combined alcohol and propoxyphene on human performance. *Arch. Int. Pharmacodyn. Ther.* 212: 175–80, 1974.

Klitzner, M. Application of a systems approach to DWI and fatal crashes. *Alcohol Drugs and Driving* 10:217–226, 1994.

Kruger, H.P. Effects of low alcohol dosages: A review of the literature. In: Utselmann, H.D., Gerhhaus, G. and Kroj, G. (eds.), *Alcohol, Drugs and Traffic Safety–T'92, Proceedings of the 12th International Conference on Alcohol, Drugs and Traffic Safety, Colonge, 28 September–2 October, 1992.* Cologne: Verlag TUV Rheinland, pp.763–778.

Kruger, H.P., *Niedrige alkoholkonzentrationen und fahrverhalten.* Bergisch, Gladbach: Unfallund Sicherheitsforschung Strassenverkehr, Heft 78, 1990a.

Kruger, H.P. et al. *Auswirkungen geringer alkohol-mengen auf fahr-verhalten und verkehrssicherheit* (Problemstudie), Bergisch. Gladbach: Forschungs-berichte der Bun-desanstalt fur Strassenwesen, Band 213, 1990.

Laurell, H., McLean, A.J. and Kloeden, C.N. *The Effect of Blood Alcohol Concentration on Light and Heavy Drinkers in a Realistic Night Driving Situation,* research report 1/90. Adelaide: NH&MRC Road Accident Research Unit, University of Adelaide, South Australia, 1990.

Laves, W. Mass und Zahl in der medizinischen Begutachtung der Fahruchtigkeit. (Measure and number in medical expert testimony on ability to drive.) *Mediziniche Klinik* 50:9–12, 1955.

Levine, J.M., Krammer, G.G. and Levine, E.N. Effects of alcohol on human performance: An integration of research findings based on an abilities classification. *J. App. Psych.* 60:285–293, 1975.

Lewis, E.M., Jr. and Sarlanis, K. *The Effects of Alcohol on Decision–Making with Respect to Traffic Signals*, Research Report ICRL-RR-68-4. U.S. Dept. of Health, Education and Welfare, 1969.

Lewis, E.M., Jr. *Interaction of Age and Alcohol on Dark Adaptation Time*, DHEW Publication No. (HSM) 72-10023. U.S. Dept. of Health, Education and Welfare, 1972.

Lewis, E.G. Influence of test length and difficulty level on performance after alcohol. *Quart. J. Stud. Alc.* 34:78–88, 1973.

Linniola, M. et al. Effects of alcohol on accident risk. *Pathologist* 40:36–41, 1986.

Lundgren, N. Alkolhol och Tungt Kroppsarbete. Konditionsforandringar efter Vanlight Forekommande Spritbruk. (Alcohol and hard labor. Physical changes after the usual consumption of alcohol). *Tirfing* 41:9, 1947.

Manno, B.R and Manno, J.E. Epidemiologic basis of alcohol psychomotor performance impairment. In: Garriott, J.C. (ed.), *Medicolegal Aspects of Alcohol Determination in Biological Specimens*. Littleton,

MA: PSG Publishing Company, 1988, pp. 245–273.

Manno, B.R. and Manno, J.E. Epidemiological basis of alcohol-induced psychomotor performance (PMPI). In: Garriott, J.C. (ed.), *Medicolegal Aspects of Alcohol*, 3rd ed. Tucson, AZ: Lawyers & Judges Publishing Company, Inc., 1996.

Manno, B.R. and Manno, J.E. Epidemiological basis of alcohol-induced psychomotor performance (PMPI). In: Garriott, J.C. (ed.), *Medical-Legal Aspects of Alcohol*, 4th ed. Tucson, AZ: Lawyers & Judges Publishing Company, Inc., 2003.

Marquis, D.G. et al. Experimental studies of behavioral effects of meprobamate in normal subjects. *Ann. N.Y. Acad Sci.* 67:701–711, 1957.

Martin, C.S. et al. Development and validation of the biphasic alcohol effects scale. *Alcoholism: Clinical and Experimental Research* 17:140–146, 1993.

McLellan, D.R. The effects of alcohol in driving skill. In: Snively, G.G. (ed.), *Pre-Crash Factors in Traffic Safety*. American Association for Automotive Medicine, 1968.

Mellanby, E. *Alcohol: Its Absorption into and Disappearance from the Blood under Different Conditions*. Medical Research Committee, Special Report Series, No. 31, 1919.

Mellanby, E. Alcohol and alcoholic intoxication. *Br. J. Inebriety* 17:157–178, 1920.

Miles, W.R. *Alcohol and Human Efficiency*, Carnegie Institute publication No. 333. Pittsburgh, 1924.

Mitchell, M.C. Alcohol induced impairment of the central nervous system function: Behavioral skills involved in driving. *J. Stud. Alc.*, Suppl. 10:109–116, 1985.

Modell, J.G. and Mountz, J.M. Drinking and flying: The problem of alcohol use by pilots. *NEJM* 323:455–461, 1990.

Mortimer, R.G. Effect of low blood-alcohol concentrations in simulated day and night driving, perceptual and motor skills. *Perceptual and Motor Skills* 17:399–408, 1963.

Moskowitz, H. Alcohol influences upon sensory motor function, visual perception, and attention. In: *Alcohol, Drugs and Driving*. National Highway Traffic Safety Administration, U.S. Dept. of Transportation publication No. (HSM) 80-1096, Mar. 1974.

Moskowitz, H., Burns, M.M. and Williams, A.F. Skills performance at low blood alcohol levels. *J. Stud. Alc.* 46:482–485, 1985.

Moskowitz, H. and Robinson, C.D. *Effects of Low Doses of Alcohol on Driving-Related Skills: A Review of the Evidence*. SRA Technologies, Incorporated, DOT-HS-208-280. Springfield, VA: U.S. Department of Commerce, National Technical Information Service, 1988.

Moskowitz, H. and Fiorentino, D. *A Review of the Literature on the Effects of Low Doses of Alcohol on Driving Skills*. U.S. Department of Transportation, National Highway Traffic Safety Administration, publication No. DOT-HS-809-028, Washington, D.C., 2000.

Mueller, B. Alkoholgenuss und Fahrfahigkeit. Bericht uber modellversuche (Ingestion of alcohol and ability to drive. Report of model experiments), *Hefte z Unfallheilk, Heft* 47:188, 1954.

Nagoshi, C., Noll, R. and Wood, M. Alcohol expectancies and behavioral and emotional responses to placebo vs. alcohol administration. *Alcoholism: Clinical and Experimental Research*, 16:255–260, 1992.

Nagoshi, C.T. and Wilson, J.R. Long-term repeatability of human alcohol metabolism, sensitivity and acute tolerance. *J. Stud. Alc.*, 50:162–169, 1989.

Nagoshi, C.T., Wilson, J.R. and Rodriguez, L.A. Impulsivity, sensation seeking, and behavioral and emotional responses to alcohol. *Alcoholism: Clinical and Experimental Res.* 15:661–667, 1991.

National Highway Traffic Safety Administration. .08 BAC illegal per se level, *State Legislative Fact Sheet*, January 2002.

National Transportation Library (NTL), *The Highway Safety Desk Book*. http://ntl.bts.gov/DOCS/deskbk.html; printed 3/12/2003.

Naville, F., Herrmann, R. and DuPan, R. L'Intoxication Alcoolique Aigue ct Les Accidents d'Automobile III. Les Effets de l'Alcool Chez Les Automobilists (Acute alcoholic intoxication and automobile accidents), part 3: Effects of alcohol on automobile drivers). *Schweiz. Med. Wschr.* 76:446, 1946.

Newman, H.W. and Fletcher, E. The effect of alcohol on driving skill. *JAMA* 115:1600, 1940.

Newman, H. and Fletcher, E. The effect of alcohol on vision. *Amer. J. Med. Sci.* 202:723–731, 1941a.

Newman, H.W. and Fletcher, E. The effect of alcohol on vision. *Amer. J. Med. Sci.* 202:723–731, 1941b.

Parrott, A.C. Performance tests in human psychopharmacology, part 1: Test reliability and standardization. *Human Psychopharmacology* 6:1–9, 1991a.

Parrott, A.C. Performance tests in human psychopharmacology, part 2: Content validity, criterion validity, and face validity. *Human Psychopharmacology* 6:91–98, 1991b.

Parrott, A.C. Performance tests in human psychopharmacology, part 3: Construct validity and test interpretation. *Human Psychopharmacology* 6:197–207, 1991c.

Perrine, M.W. Alcohol influences upon driving-related behavior: A critical review of laboratory studies of neurophysiological, neuromuscular, and sensory activity. In: Perrine, M.W. (ed.), *Alcohol, Drugs and Driving*, technical report DOT HS 801-096, National Highway traffic Safety Administration, 1974.

Perrine, M.W., Peck, R.C. and Fell, J.C. Epidemiologic perspectives on drunk driving. In: *Surgeon General's Workshop on Drunk Driving*, background papers. Washington, DC: U.S. Department of Health and Human Services, Public Health Service, Office of the Surgeon General, 1988.

Pihkanen, T.A. and Kauko, O. The effects of alcohol on the perception of musical stimuli. *Ann. Med. Exp. Fenn.* 40:275–285, 1962.

Pilchen, N.B. State and federal regulations concerning driving while intoxicated with alcohol. In: Garriott, J.C. (ed.), *Medicolegal Aspects of Alcohol Determination in Biological Specimens.* Littleton, MA: PSG Publishing Company, 1988, pp. 180–244.

Prag, J.J. The chemical and the clinical diagnosis of driving under the influence of alcohol and the use of chemical tests in traffic law enforcement. *S. Afr. J. Clin. Sci.* 4:289–325, 1953.

Robinson, A. et al. Effect of ethyl alcohol on reaction times as measured on a motorcycle simultor. *(Abst) Clin. Chem.* 36:1170, 1990.

Rosen, L.J. and Lee, C.L. Acute and chronic effects of alcohol use on organizational processes in memory. *J. Abnor. Psychol.* 85:309–317, 1976.

Ross, L.E. and Mundt, J.C. Multiattribute modeling analysis of the effects of a low blood alcohol level on pilot performance. *Hum. Factors* 30:293–304, 1988.

Ryback, R.S. Effects of alcohol on memory and its implications for flying safety. *Aerosp. Med.* 41:1193–1195, 1970.

Schmidt, I. and Bingel, A.G.A. *Effect of Oxygen Deficiency and Various Other Factors on Color Saturation Thresholds.* U.S.A.F. School of Aviation Medicine Project Reports: Project No. 21-31-002, 1953.

Schmiedeberg, O. *Grundriss der Pharmakologies*, 4th ed. Vogel Leipzig, 1902, pp. 45–46.

Sidell, F.R. and Pless, J.E. Ethyl alcohol: Blood levels and performance decrements after oral administration to man. *Psychopharmacologia.* 1971; 19(3): 246–61.

Spence, A.P. and Mason, E.D. *Human Anatomy and Physiology.* Menlo Park, CA: Benjamin Cummings Publishing Co., 1987.

Stuster, J. and Burns, M. *Validation of the Standardized Sobriety Test Battery at BACs below 0.10 percent,* publication No. DOT HS 808 839. Washington, DC: U.S. Department of Transportation, National Highway Traffic Safety Administration, 1998.

Stuster, J.W. *The Detection of DWI Motorcyclists,* publication No. DOT HS 807-839. Washington, DC: U.S. Department of Transportation, National Highway Traffic Safety Administration, 1993.

Subbotin, V. Ueber die physiologische Bedeutung des Alkohols fur den thierischen Organismus. *Z. Biol.* 7, 361–369, 1891.

Talland, G.A., Mendelson, J.H. and Ryack, P. Experimentally induced chronic intoxication and withdrawal in alcoholics, part 5: Tests of attention. *Quart. J. Stud. Alc. Suppl.* No. 2:74–86, 1964.

Tang, P.C. and Rosenstein, R. Influence of alcohol and dramamine, alone and in combination, on pilot performance. *Aerosp. Med.* 38:818–821, 1967.

Tharp, V., Burns, M., and Moskowitz, H. *Development and Field Test of Psychophysical Tests for DWI Arrest,* publication no. DOT HS 805-864. Washington, DC: U.S. Department of Transportation, National Highway Traffic Safety Administration, 1981.

U.S. Department of Transportation, National Highway Traffic Safety Association. *Field Evaluation of a Behavioral Test Battery for DWI,* DOT HS 806-475. Washington, DC: U.S. Department of Transportation, National Highway Traffic Safety Administration, 1983.

Vogel-Sprott, M., *Alcohol Tolerance and Social Drinking.* NY: The Guilford Press, 1993, pp.1–197.

Vogel-Sprott, M.D., Chipperfield, B. and Hart, D.M. Family history of problem drinking among young male social drinkers: Reliability of the family history questionaire. *Drug and Alcohol Dependence* 16:251–256, 1985.

Vogel-Sprott, MD. and Chipperfield, B. Family history of problem drinking among young male social drinkers: Behavioral effects of alcohol. *J. Stud. Alc.* 48:430–436, 1987.

Wallgren, H. and Barry, H., III. *Actions of Alcohol,* vol. 1: *Biochemical, Physiological and Psychological Effects.* NY: Elsevier, 1970.

Warren, G.H. and Raynes, A.E. Mood changes during three conditions of alcohol intake. *Quart. J. Stud. Alcohol* 33:979–89, 1972.

Watson, W.A. and Garriott, J.C. Alcohol and motorcycle riders: A comparison of motorcycle and car/truck DWI's. *Vet. Hum. Toxicol.* 34:213–215, 1992.

Wechsler, D. The effect of alcohol on mental activity. *Quart. J. Stud. Alc.* 2:479, 1941.

Widmark, E.M.P. Alcoholic excretion in urine and a simple clinically applicable method for diagnosing alcoholic intoxication in drivers. *Upsala Lakaref. Forh.* 19:241, 1914.

Widmark, E.M.P. A micromethod for the estimation of alcohol in blood. *Biochem. Z.* 131:473, 1922.

Wilkinson, I.M.S., Kime, R. and Purnell, M. Alcohol and human eye movement. *Brain*, 97:785–792, 1981.

Wilson, J.R. and Nagoshi, C.T. One-month repeatability of alcohol metabolism, sensitivity and acute tolerance. *J. Stud. Alc.* 48:437–442, 1987.

Chapter 16

Alcohol and the Law: The Legal Framework of Scientific Evidence and Expert Testimony

Boris Moczula

There is hardly anything, not palpably absurd on its face, that cannot now be proved by some so-called *experts*.

    —*Keegan v. Minneapolis & St. Louis R.R. Co. (1899)*[1]

Your piece, *The Meaning of Junk*, (Science, March 22) noted the recent court rulings limiting admissible scientific testimony to that based on research published in peer-reviewed journals. It then pointed to the problems that such an index of "good science" overlooks. But if an "expert" witness is unable to persuade his peers to accept his or her theories as mainstream science, that witness shouldn't be allowed to present such theories to a jury. Judges have no business second-guessing the wisdom of established science in this regard. Our courts are capable of inflicting enormous harm on society by allowing every charlatan to be an "expert" witness. Sure, it's always possible that today's crackpot will be part of tomorrow's establishment, but that would be an exception. The courts should accept only proven scientific theories.

    —Letter to the Editor, April 19, 1993
    Newsweek magazine[2]

The debate over the nature and permissible use of scientific evidence and expert testimony has spanned decades. In an ideal situation, this evidence is offered to assist the judge or jury in resolving issues arising in litigation. But the injection of false experts and pseudo-science into trials, rather than serving as a guide in the trier of fact's search for the truth, functions to obfuscate and distract from relevant questions. The phenomenon of improper use of scientific evidence and expert testimony occurs all too regularly in litigation. Drunken driving cases are not immune to this wasteful and disruptive trend.

This chapter outlines the basic requirements for presentation of scientific evidence and expert testimony in court. Since debate over these prerequisites occurs in a legal setting, the discussion in this chapter relies upon court cases from different jurisdictions, state and federal, as informational and illustrative guides for legal and scientific practitioners. However, the requirements governing the admission of expert testimony vary across geographic lines. For this reason, consultation of local evidence rules and case law is an essential follow-up to a reading of the more general principles contained herein.

16.1 General Requirements for Admission of Expert Testimony

A. Beyond the ken of the average layperson

The first prerequisite for the admission of expert evidence is that the witness's testimony must be distinctly related to some scientific, technical or other specialized knowledge beyond the ken of the average layperson. If the proffered subject is a matter of common knowledge or is otherwise unexceptional, then a jury or judge need not hear an "expert" on the issue. Two examples of knowledge which the courts determined was *not* beyond the ken of the average layperson and, thus, for which the presentation of expert testimony was not justified: *People v. Johnson* (1993) (Proposed testimony of "expert liar" that prison inmates sometimes lie was properly excluded. "The proposition that prison inmates may lie certainly is not outside the common understanding of jurors . . .")[3]; *Kahn v. D.M.V.* (1993) (At issue was a certain "preeminent curse word." According to the court, this epithet "is commonly understood by a substantial segment of the population to be a demeaning, degrading and therefore offensive term . . . There was no need for evidence on this commonly known point . . . .")[4].

In contrast, the following opinions addressed subject matter which the courts determined was necessarily the subject of expert testimony: *Seattle v. Personeus* (1991) (Trial court excluded proposed defense expert testimony as to alcohol burn-off based on the rationale that "anyone can understand that alcohol burns off." The appeals court reversed, noting that the proposed testimony was not limited to the *fact* of burn-off, but also addressed the *rate* of burn-off. "While the former is arguably a matter of common knowledge, the latter is not.")[5]; *Carroll v. Otis Elevator Co.* (1990) (The appeals court, in a personal injury case, upheld a trial court's ruling allowing a clinical psychologist to testify, as an elevator

design expert, that red buttons attract small children, despite the defense's claim that this information was not beyond the ken of the average juror: "While it is true that one needn't be B. F. Skinner to know that brightly colored objects are attractive to small children . . . given our liberal federal standards, the trial court was not 'manifestly erroneous' in admitting this testimony . . . .")[6].

While, as evinced by the recent cases cited above, "knowledge beyond the ken of the average layperson" continues as a basic reference point for determination of the evidentiary use of expert testimony, there is no requirement that an average person be completely ignorant of a particular topic before an expert is permitted to testify about it. If a juror has some comprehension of the subject matter, but the testimony of an expert in the area would nevertheless enhance the juror's understanding of the issues in the case in which the juror is participating, the expert testimony is normally admitted. For example, the Federal Rules of Evidence expressly contemplate the admission of expert testimony that "will assist the trier of fact to understand the evidence or to determine a fact in issue."[7] Thus, scrutiny of the admissibility of expert testimony focuses not only on the juror's comprehension of the subject, but also on whether the proffered testimony will be helpful to a jury in resolving a fact in issue.[8] But the fundamental point of both inquiries remains the same: a witness with specialized knowledge, irrespective of his or her degree of experience, is simply not needed in a case where that specialized knowledge is of no use to the judge or jury.

It is also important to remember that scientific training is not the exclusive basis for expert testimony—other forms of specialized or technical knowledge may be of equal or greater value. As explained by the Sixth Circuit Court of Appeals in *Berry v. City of Detroit* (1994), the basic subject of the proposed expert testimony may be identical, but the reason the evidence is being offered often will be determinative of whether a scientific or other expert should be called:

The distinction between scientific and non-scientific expert testimony is a critical one. By way of illustration, if one wanted to explain to a jury how a bumblebee is able to fly, an aeronautical engineer might be a helpful witness. Since flight principles have some universality, the expert could apply general principles to the case of the bumblebee. Conceivably, even if he had never seen a bumblebee, he still would be qualified to testify, as long as he was familiar with its component parts. On the other hand, if one wanted to prove that bumblebees always take off into the wind, a beekeeper with no scientific training at all would be an acceptable expert witness if a proper foundation were laid for his conclusions. The foundation would not relate to his formal training, but to his firsthand observations. In other words, the beekeeper does not know any more about flight principles than the jurors, but he has seen a lot more bumblebees than they have.[9]

It may very well be that the fact finder is more likely to be convinced by the testimony of an individual whose expertise lies exclusively in practical experience with an issue, as opposed to the testimony of an expert whose background is long on educational degrees, but short on actual day-to-day exposure to a particular subject.

B. Meets legal threshold of reliability

The second and most critical prong of the admissibility test requires scrutiny of the reliability of the evidence which forms the foundation for the proposed expert testimony. In the course of this process, counsel must satisfy the court that the proposed testimony meets the jurisdiction's standard of acceptability for scientific evidence. Failure to reach this threshold results in the exclusion of the proffered evidence. Two federal court cases which are extremely relevant to the creation of fundamental jurisdictional standards for admissibility of scientific evidence are detailed below.

In the early 1920s, the predecessor to today's United States Court of Appeals for the District of Columbia Circuit considered a case which would largely set the standard for admissibility of scientific evidence for the next seventy years. In *Frye v. United*

States (1923),[10] the court was faced with the appeal of a convicted murderer who raised a single issue: the trial court's allegedly erroneous preclusion of a defense expert who was to testify as to the results of a "systolic blood pressure deception test" (a primitive form of the lie detector test) administered to the defendant. Defense counsel invoked the first prong of admissibility discussed above, stating that since the operation of the systolic blood pressure deception test was beyond the comprehension of the average juror, expert testimony should have been allowed to interpret the results.[11] The three-judge appellate panel focused on a more basic question—the degree of reliability of the proposed scientific evidence. The court thus framed the issue:

> Just when a scientific principle or discovery crosses the line between the experimental and demonstrable stages is difficult to define. Somewhere in this twilight zone the evidential force of the principle must be recognized, and while courts will go a long way in admitting expert testimony deduced from a well-recognized principle or discovery, *the thing from which the deduction is made must be sufficiently established to have gained general acceptance in the particular field in which it belongs.*[12]

Having briefly expressed its view of the relevant legal analysis, the court concluded that the systolic blood pressure deception test fell short of "general acceptance" to warrant its evidential use.[13] James Alphonzo Frye's murder conviction was affirmed.

It is doubtful that the federal appeals court realized in 1923 that its opinion, consisting of all of two pages, completely barren of citations to any legal precedent or scientific publications, and containing essentially no written analysis of the relevant issue beyond the one-paragraph excerpt quoted above, would become the bedrock standard for admissibility of scientific evidence for nearly three-quarters of a century. The court's sentence regarding "general acceptance in the particular field in which [the evidence] belongs" was quoted in subsequent judicial opinions throughout the country as the legal requirement which proponents of scientific evidence had to satisfy.[14]

The *Frye* decision, while initially garnering broad judicial acceptance, was not without its detractors. One distinct difficulty of the *Frye* test is the inherent circularity which it creates: the scientific evidence is not admissible unless it is generally accepted, but, practically speaking, the evidence is not generally accepted until admitted into evidence by a court. More to the point, *Frye* does not allow consideration of new scientific theories which, while not yet having attained the "general acceptance" level, are nonetheless credible. This creates the problem of "what to do with new scientific devices, processes, and methods the first time around. Every scientific device or method must have its first day in court."[15]

Thus, while many courts chose to blindly rely upon *Frye*, others in the legal community believed that departure from this conservative test was appropriate.[16] In 1983, lawyers and scientists participating in a workshop sponsored by the National Conference of Lawyers and Scientists determined that the *Frye* rule was unworkable and argued against its retention, but cautioned that *Frye* should not simply be replaced by an overly expansive rule of relevance governing scientific evidence.[17] The legal-scientific workshop also concluded that courts should have a more meaningful role in screening novel scientific evidence.[18]

There also arose a discernible judicial move toward a broader standard of admissibility. This trend manifested itself most evidently in toxic tort litigation. See, e.g., *Rubanick v. Witco Chemical Corp* (1991).[19] Under this alternative standard, the admissibility of expert testimony is governed by whether the basis for the testimony consists of "facts or data . . . of a type reasonably relied upon by experts in the particular field," and whether the expert's technique or methodology in using the facts or data is well founded.[20] In determining whether the facts or data are admissible, "[t]he proper inquiry is not what the court deems reliable, but what experts in the relevant discipline deem it to be." *In re Japanese Electrical Products* (1983).[21] Then, as judicial focus on relaxed standards of admissibility became more prevalent, the United States Supreme Court agreed to review a case the ultimate resolution of which largely mooted

(at least at the federal judicial level) the debate as to the substantive correctness of *Frye*.

In *Daubert v. Merrell Dow Pharmaceuticals* (1993),[22] the Supreme Court considered a civil lawsuit brought in federal court on behalf of two children who had suffered physical birth defects. The plaintiffs' claim was that the children's mother's use of Bendectin, an anti-nausea drug manufactured by defendant Merrell Dow Pharmaceuticals, caused the birth defects. The plaintiffs presented eight experts who, while conducting no studies of their own, relied upon others' animal and test tube studies, as well as their personal reevaluations of written literature, to conclude that there was a direct link between the ingestion of Bendectin and the birth defects.[23] The defendant presented an expert who concluded that no such causation existed.[24] The trial court, relying upon the *Frye* standard, granted summary judgment to Merrell Dow because the plaintiffs' causation theory was not "generally accepted" in the scientific community.[25] The plaintiffs ultimately appealed to the United States Supreme Court.

The Supreme Court sidestepped the question of whether *Frye* was a good standard—in the Court's view, this issue had become irrelevant. Rather, the Court ruled that the *Frye* general acceptance standard had been superseded by the standard of admissibility set forth in the Federal Rules of Evidence (FRE), which were adopted in 1973, fifty years after the *Frye* opinion.[26]

Ironically, until pointed out by the United States Supreme Court, this implicit modification of evidentiary standards had for the most part existed either unnoticed or ignored by the judicial community in the twenty years since the advent of the federal rules.

C. The *Daubert* standard: Reliability

The FRE standard of admissibility, as interpreted by *Daubert*, contains two prongs: reliability and relevance.[27] In its opinion, the Supreme Court to some extent fleshed out these concepts for the guidance of lawyers and judges.

The Court defined reliable scientific evidence as "scientific knowledge," that is, evidence having a "grounding in the methods and procedures of science."[28] Proposed expert testimony must be supported by appropriate validation: inferences or assertions must be derived by a scientific method and the evidence must be "trustworthy."[29] Mere subjective belief or unsupported speculation is insufficient.[30]

The Supreme Court instructed that, to evaluate reliability, a trial court should conduct a preliminary assessment of whether the reasoning or methodology underlying the proposed testimony is scientifically valid.[31] The *Daubert* opinion provided an illustrative list of factors for courts to consider:[32]

1. **Whether the scientific theory can be (and has been) tested**. The "testability" of a theory and the results of those tests yield important information as to the soundness of the theory.

2. **Whether the scientific theory has been subjected to peer review and publication**. Discussion and analysis of a theory among peers in the proponent's field also provides valuable information as to the theory's reliability. The Supreme Court cautioned, however, that publication alone did not automatically determine admissibility. Even a published, peer-reviewed theory may be judicially precluded.[33]

3. **The known or potential rate of error of the scientific technique**. The greater the actual or possible rate of error, the lesser its basic reliability.

4. **Whether the theory has received "general acceptance" in the scientific community**. If this factor sounds familiar, it should. It embodies the *Frye* test. As one court describes it, "The decision in *Daubert* kills *Frye* and then resurrects its ghost."[34] But the *Frye* test, instead of being solely determinative of admissibility, is now relegated to being just one of many components to consider.

Even before *Daubert*, legal commentators[35] suggested that other elements be thrown into the judicial mix:

1. The nature and breadth of the inference adduced.

2. The existence and maintenance of a standard governing the inference's use.

3. Analogy to other scientific techniques the results of which are admissible.

4. The clarity and simplicity with which the technique and its results can be explained.

5. The extent to which the basic data are verifiable by the court and jury.

See also *Emerson v. State* (1994)[36] (listing additional factors, including: (1) the availability of other experts to test and evaluate the technique and (2) the experience and skill of the person who applied the technique on the occasion in question).

Application of these analytical components would allow a judge to determine whether the evidence presented is of sufficient validity to warrant even basic consideration in a courtroom setting. But a finding of reliability is not enough—the court must also consider the relevance of the evidence.

D. The *Daubert* test: Relevance

The Supreme Court instructed that, in evaluating relevance, the second part of the *Daubert* test, trial courts consider whether the particular reasoning or methodology offered can properly be applied to the facts in issue.[37] There must be a valid scientific connection to the pertinent inquiry. Expert testimony which does not relate to any issue in the case is not relevant and, therefore, inadmissible.[38] In other words, "[t]he courtroom is not a classroom to be used to educate the jury on an entire field only tangentially related to the issues at trial." *Flanagan v. State* (1993).[39]

The Supreme Court described the process of determining relevance as a question of "fit."[40] "Fit" is not always obvious. Scientific validity for one purpose is not necessarily scientific validity for other, unrelated purposes.[41] To illustrate this concept, *Daubert* refers to the study of the phases of the moon—according to the Court, this evidence would be relevant and useful if the issue at trial is whether a specific night was particularly dark, but the identical evidence would not "fit" if the relevant question is whether an individual is likely to have behaved irrationally that night.[42] The Court's insistence on a "relevance" analysis underscores the precept that even scientific evidence of indisputable quality does not receive admission to the jury unless it is meaningful in the context of the particular case at hand.

What is a party's burden of proof with respect to the reliability and relevance prongs established by *Daubert*? In a footnote, the Court identified the applicable standard as "by a preponderance of proof."[43] This standard is relatively low, contemplating a mere tip of the evidentiary scales (51 percent to 49 percent), as opposed to the more burdensome "clear and convincing" (75 percent of the evidence) and "beyond a reasonable doubt" (95 percent of the evidence) standards of proof commonly used in litigation.

E. The *Daubert* parties' contentions

In fashioning its test of evidentiary admissibility, the United States Supreme Court had to deal with extreme arguments from both defendants' and plaintiffs' camps. Arguing in support of the *Frye* test, Merrell Dow claimed that abandonment of the "general acceptance" standard would result in a courtroom "free for all" which would confuse juries with "absurd and irrational pseudoscientific assertions."[44] The Supreme Court responded that "vigorous cross-examination, presentation of contrary evidence and careful instruction on the burden of proof are the traditional and appropriate means of attacking shaky but admissible evidence."[45] The Court also stressed that a judge who is evaluating a proffer of scientific evidence should be mindful of other evidentiary rules capable of limiting admissibility:[46]

1. Expert opinions based on otherwise inadmissible hearsay may be admitted only if the facts or data are "of a type reasonably relied upon by experts in the particular field in forming opinions or inferences upon the subject." Federal Rule of Evidence 703.
2. The judge has the discretion to hire his or her own expert. Federal Rule of Evidence 706.
3. The court can deny admission of prejudicial, confusing or misleading evidence. Federal Rule of Evidence 403. (The Court noted that due to the more "powerful" nature of expert evidence, a judge exercises more control over experts than over lay witnesses in this regard).

From the other corner of the litigational ring, the *Daubert* plaintiffs claimed that any evidentiary screening role for the judge would be "inimical to the search for truth."[47] Rejecting this claim, the Supreme Court noted that there is a difference between the search for truth in the courtroom and the quest for truth in a laboratory:

> Scientific conclusions are subject to perpetual revision. Law, on the other hand, must resolve disputes finally and quickly *** The Federal Rules of Evidence [are] designed not for the exhaustive search for cosmic understanding but for the particularized resolution of legal disputes.[48]

The Court's comment touches upon a basic difference between science and the law that is often overlooked by legal advocates. The accuracy and precision so often required in science, and the notion that there rarely can be an absolute answer in recitation of scientific findings, are not essential prerequisites in a legal arena which, in the interest of finality, requires definite answers on a case-by-case basis. The law is in some instances more flexible and may, in the public interest, reach decisions which science would not necessarily endorse. Differing policies produce different results.

A good example of this dichotomy is case law which disposes of "margin of error" challenges to breath test instruments. Typically, these challenges assert that the margin of error inherent in the instrumentation must be deducted from the defendant's reading, so that, in "borderline" cases involving 0.1 percent (gram per deciliter) blood alcohol readings (BAC), the prosecution has not shown beyond a reasonable doubt that the *per se* law was violated. Courts rejecting this argument do not dispute the scientific postulate that a margin of error exists and, unless accounted for, leaves uncertainty as to whether a defendant is "really a 0.1 percent." Rather, these courts hold that this potential error's evidentiary significance, or more appropriately, the lack thereof, is strictly a legislative, public safety judgment and that if a legislature, cognizant of the inherent margin of error, nevertheless sets the statutory BAC at 0.1 gram per deciliter, then a 0.1 percent (or 0.1 gram per 210 liters [See Chapters 7 and 12 for discussion of blood and breath conversion units]) breath test instrument reading is sufficient to convict. *State v. Rucker* (1972); *State v. Lentini* (1991).[49] While no one doubts the interrelationship between science and law, the two areas diverge in this respect due to the differing policies which undergird them.

F. *Daubert* II: The case on remand

In light of *Daubert*'s enunciation of a new standard of admissibility for scientific evidence pursuant to the Federal Rules of Evidence, the Supreme Court ordered that the case be returned to the Ninth Circuit Court of Appeals, which had used the *Frye* test in affirming the trial court's decision to grant summary judgment to Merrell Dow.[50] The federal appeals court's second chance at this case resulted in a very telling interpretive application of the Supreme Court's *Daubert* opinion. *Daubert v. Merrell Dow Pharmaceuticals* (1995).[51] The court released a cynical opinion which vented more than a little frustration with the role that *Daubert* had imposed upon it:

> As we read the Supreme Court's teaching in *Daubert* . . . though we are largely untrained in science and certainly no match for any of the witnesses whose testimony we are reviewing, it is our responsibility to determine whether those experts' proposed testimony amounts to "scientific knowledge," constitutes "good science," and was "derived by the scientific method." The task before us is more daunting still when the dispute concerns matters at the very edge of scientific research, where fact meets theory and certainty dissolves into probability . . . Our responsibility, then, unless we badly misread the Supreme Court's opinion, is to resolve disputes among respected, well-credentialed scientists about matters squarely within their expertise . . . .[52]

Having uttered these cryptic statements, the appeals court announced its intention to "take a deep breath and proceed with this heady task."[53] The court then set forth its own suggestions as to factors to consider in determining whether an expert's opinion has been, in the words of *Daubert*, "derived from the scientific method."

The appeals court started its review by reiterating two important parallel concepts contained in the Supreme Court's *Daubert* opinion: the illegitimacy of an expert's mere personal attestation of the reliability of his or her own work and the need for some form of independent verification of the reliability of the evidence. The court issued the reminder that "the expert's bald assurance of validity is not enough.[54] Rather, the party representing the expert must show that the expert's findings are based on "sound science," and this will require some objective, independent validation of the expert's methods.[55]

> [S]omething doesn't become "scientific knowledge" just because it's uttered by a scientist, nor can an expert's self-serving assertion that his conclusions were "derived by the scientific method" be deemed conclusive.[56]

In the absence of independent research, continued the court, the party proffering the expert testimony "must come forward with other objective verifiable evidence" (e.g., peer review and publication) that the testimony is based on 'scientifically valid principles.'"[57]

Additionally, in its most significant new contribution to the *Daubert* analysis, the Court of Appeals discussed the difference between independent research and litigational research as a critical factor in evaluating the validity of scientific evidence:

> One very significant fact to be considered is whether the experts are proposing to testify about matters growing naturally and directly out of research they have conducted independent of the litigation, or whether they have developed their opinions expressly for purposes of testifying. . . . [I]n determining whether proposed expert testimony amounts to good science, we may not ignore the fact that a scientist's normal workplace is the lab or the field, not the courtroom or the lawyer's office . . . [E]xperts whose findings flow from existing research are less likely to have been biased toward a particular conclusion by the promise of remuneration . . . That

the testimony proffered by the expert is based directly on legitimate, preexisting research unrelated to the litigation provides the most persuasive basis for concluding that the opinions he expresses were "derived by the scientific method."[58]

Having set forth its vision and enhancement of what *Daubert* required, the Court of Appeals analyzed the facts of the Bendectin case before it and found plaintiffs' case still failed to pass muster, even under the relaxed rules of admissibility extracted by the Supreme Court from the Federal Rules of Evidence. The judges noted that "[t]he opinions proffered by plaintiffs' experts do not, to understate the point, reflect the consensus within the scientific community."[59] "[A]part from the small but determined group of scientists testifying on behalf of the Bendectin plaintiffs in this and many other cases, there doesn't appear to be a single scientist who has concluded that Bendectin causes limb reduction defects."[60] "Personal opinion, not science, is testifying here."[61]

The appeals court also stressed the absence of peer review of the plaintiffs' experts' causation theories:

> Bendectin litigation has been pending in the courts for over a decade, yet the only review the plaintiffs' experts' work has received has been by judges and juries, and the only place their theories and studies have been published is in the pages of federal and state reporters.... It's as if there were a tacit understanding within the scientific community that what's going on here is not science at all, but litigation.[62]

The court also found a lack of statistically significant causation between Bendectin ingestion and birth defects. Indeed, according to the court, the numbers cited by plaintiffs' experts not only did not show a sufficient statistical connection, but actually tended to disprove legal causation.[63]

In the end, the trial court's grant of summary judgment in favor of the defendants, originally affirmed by the appeals court under the *Frye* standard,

was again affirmed by the appeals court under *Daubert*.[64] The United States Supreme Court subsequently denied the plaintiffs' petition to review *Daubert* a second time.[65] Perhaps the United States Supreme Court will once again weigh in on this evidentiary dispute in a future case.

G. The effect of *Daubert*

Because of the substantial longevity of the *Frye* "general acceptance" standard, the *Daubert* case, which announced a clean break with the *Frye* tradition, quickly became an oft-cited decision of great significance in the legal field. But scientists and attorneys must take caution not to view *Daubert* for more than it means. While a pronouncement of the nation's highest tribunal must necessarily be studied and reckoned with, *Daubert* deals strictly with the Federal Rules of Evidence and their affect on *Frye*. As such, the Supreme Court's opinion is determinative and binding only insofar as it pertains to admissibility standards in the federal court system. The individual states are not bound by the Federal Rules of Evidence. Consequently, the Supreme Court opinion does not directly resolve, or even address, the admissibility of scientific evidence in state courts. Individual states may employ different criteria and have the discretion to reject the *Daubert* rationale in favor of continuing their own alternative evidentiary tests. A relevant factor in this consideration will likely be whether, and to what degree, the state jurisdiction has elected to adopt the provisions of the Federal Rules of Evidence as its own rules of evidence.

Predictably, state courts which have considered the issue have come to varied conclusions based upon these jurisdictions' historical treatment of the admission of expert testimony. For example Iowa, Louisiana, Massachusetts, Montana, New Mexico, Oklahoma, South Dakota, Texas, Vermont and West Virginia have accepted *Daubert* as their own test of admissibility.[66] In contrast California, Florida, Nebraska, New York and Utah have elected to adhere to the *Frye* test notwithstanding *Daubert*.[67] Court opinions in the state of Washington suggest the potential for two standards of admissibility, one for civil cases and one for criminal cases.[68] Still other jurisdictions, to the extent that only an intermediate appellate court has considered this issue, merely iterate the fundamental truth that their current standard of evidentiary admissibility continues unless and until their state Supreme Courts expressly determine what, if any, impact *Daubert* should have in those jurisdictions.[69] As this disparity in judicial treatment makes evident, while an understanding of the principles of *Daubert* is important, if for no other reason than the manner in which the Supreme Court's opinion has rapidly permeated this country's jurisprudence, the only judicial body with the authority to determine whether *Daubert* is binding in a particular state is the highest appellate court of that jurisdiction.[70]

H. Criticism of *Daubert*

Daubert was decided in an atmosphere of increasing criticism of *Frye*, but critics of *Daubert* have surfaced as well (Tamarelli Jr., 1994).[71] For instance, it is readily apparent from a review of terminology alone that *Daubert* replaced the concrete, straightforward standard of *Frye* with a more vague and complex form of evaluation. In this sense, the *Daubert* test has already been labeled as "excessively cumbersome and too variable."[72] Furthermore, *Daubert* creates a much greater risk than *Frye* that litigation will be decided based on scientific evidence the validity of which will not stand the test of time and further research: "[*Daubert*] almost certainly will lead to an increase in the amount of novel, scientific testimony that parties attempt to introduce into trials."[73] See *People v. Kelly* (1976) ("The primary advantage of *Frye* lies in its essentially conservative nature. For a variety of reasons *Frye* was deliberately intended to interpose a substantial obstacle to the unrestrained admission of evidence based upon new scientific principles").[74] For these reasons, certain courts have declined to adopt the *Daubert* approach. *People v. Leahy* (1994)[75] (noting that *Daubert*, which avoided the issue of *Frye*'s "merits," presents no justification for reconsidering California's *Frye*-based test). Ironically, one court has suggested that *Daubert* and *Frye* may not be very different: "[d]espite the criticisms levelled at *Frye*, this standard is not far removed from [the] evaluation required under F.R.E. 702 . . . Nor does the *Frye* test exclude evidence from a relevancy weighing." *Lindsey v. People* (1995).[76]

Given the brief, three-year existence of *Daubert* to date, any conclusion in this respect may be premature. Real-life experience with both evidentiary standards in the years to come will be the best gauge of the extent of *Daubert*'s impact and whether that impact is positive or negative.

I. Methods of proving "general acceptance"

As noted above, the "general acceptance" test manifests itself under both the *Frye* and *Daubert* standards, constituting the dispositive question in *Frye* jurisdictions and one of various relevant analytical factors in *Daubert* states. Proof of general acceptance can be accomplished by way of three independent yet related tracks.

The most obvious way of proving the general acceptance of scientific evidence is through expert testimony attesting to general acceptance among those in the profession of the premises on which the proffered expert witness based his or her analysis. A good example of this approach is found in *State v. Klawitter* (1994),[77] the first published court opinion addressing the admissibility of the Drug Evaluation and Classification (DEC) program. In *Klawitter*, the Minnesota Supreme Court, analyzing in detail the testimony of a variety of experts presented at a trial court hearing, determined that the drug evaluation and classification protocol satisfied the *Frye* "general acceptance" standard. In an interesting sidenote, the court directed that "drug recognition expert," the title commonly given to the individual successfully completing and administering the DEC program, be changed to "drug recognition officer" for purposes of court testimony, since the term "expert" in the witness's official designation ran the risk of inappropriately enhancing the jury's perception of the credibility of the witness.[78]

Another manner of demonstrating a scientific theory's general acceptance is by use of authoritative scientific or legal writings indicating that the scientific community accepts the premises underlying the proffered testimony. This concept reflects *Daubert*'s recognition of the importance of peer review and publication in determining basic reliability.

The third method of proof involves presentation of judicial opinions that indicate the expert's premises have gained general acceptance. In a jurisdiction considering the admissibility of certain scientific evidence for the first time, other courts' dispositions of the same evidentiary issue are an extremely relevant and often compelling factor in the court's analysis. For example, if forty states have already accepted the validity of a scientific principle, then a judicial body in the forty-first state considering the same legal question is likely to be convinced of the principle's evidentiary fortitude.

An important caveat: an advocate's reliance upon a "numerical display" of jurisdictions which have legitimized the principle he or she offers, without a true understanding of the reasons for this judicial legitimization, diminishes the impact of this method of proof and runs the risk of complete backfire. Often, court opinions merely cite to other court opinions, but offer no independent explanation as to *why* they have chosen to adopt the approach of other jurisdictions. This makes older opinions vulnerable to attack by a court which, in freshly considering the issue, is not impressed by mere numbers, conducts a thorough and up-to-date substantive analysis of the available literature, and ultimately concludes, contrary to the flood of judicial authority presented to it, that the evidence compels a different result. Such was the case in *State v. Witte* (1992), where the Kansas Supreme Court rejected the State's claim that the acceptance of horizontal gaze nystagmus (HGN) by many other jurisdictions compelled the court to make a similar finding for Kansas.[79] The Kansas Supreme Court instead evaluated the available literature anew and decided that "the reliability of HGN evidence is not currently a settled proposition in the scientific community."[80] Pointedly, the court directly confronted the Arizona ruling in *Blake v. Superior Court*, a seminal case admitting HGN in drunken driving prosecutions, by listing articles not considered by the *Blake* court: "If the Arizona Supreme Court had had this evidence before it, it may not have held that HGN evidence satisfies the *Frye* admissibility requirements."[81]

There is no substitute for a detailed substantive presentation of the validity of scientific evidence to the court. The weight of favorable judicial authority serves as an important component of an advocate's presentation, but should not be counted upon to single-handedly sway the court to admit scientific evidence and expert testimony.

In certain circumstances, an evidentiary shortcut to judicial approval of a scientific theory is available. A particular principle may be so well established in the scientific community and so generally accepted as to authorize a court to take "judicial notice" of it.[82] The reliability of such scientific knowledge need not then be re-proven in every subsequent court case in that jurisdiction. Instead, the primary issue becomes the correct application of this scientific knowledge.

Breath alcohol testing instrumentation has been the subject of judicial notice, notwithstanding the periodic attacks which are mounted against it. As noted by the New Jersey Supreme Court when first applying judicial notice to the Breathalyzer, "neither unanimity of opinion nor universal infallibility is required for judicial acceptance of generally recognized matters." *State v. Johnson* (1964).[83] However, if a particular subject is not sufficiently ingrained in society's general consciousness so as to no longer be subject to serious question, judicial notice is not warranted. Effectuating this principle, the District of Columbia Court of Appeals, in *Poulnot v. Dist. of Columbia* (1992)[84] ruled that the trial court improperly took judicial notice of alcohol absorption and elimination rates since this information was not a matter of common knowledge in the general community and there were too many variables associated with such calculations.

J. Skill, knowledge or experience of the witness

Assuming that the proffered scientific evidence is beyond the ken of the average layperson and further assuming that the evidence satisfies a jurisdiction's threshold of admissibility, the third prong of evidentiary analysis of scientific evidence shifts the focus from the evidence itself to the qualifications of the witness through which the evidence will be offered. There is no absolute rule as to the degree of knowledge required to qualify a witness as an expert in a given field. Of course, the witness must be shown to be competent in the subject about which he or she will testify. A witness may be qualified by demonstrating knowledge, skill, practical experience, training, education or a combination of these factors. If the basic requirement of competency is satisfied, the extent of the expert witness's knowledge of the subject matter affects not the admissibility of the witness's testimony, but the weight that a factfinder may give to it during deliberation of a verdict.

Prior judicial recognition of an expert's qualifications is normally a significant factor in the court's evaluation, but even this axiom can be stretched too far. Recall *People v. Johnson* (1993), the case of the "expert liar":

> Although defendants suggest the trial judge overstepped her bounds here, when she frankly noted her incredulity at the attempt to call an expert liar to testify, we share the trial judge's skeptical and indeed caustic reaction. The fact that, as defendants contended, this witness had apparently been allowed to testify as a paid expert liar in numerous other cases was definitely not an argument for admission here.[85]

And, unfortunately, given the varying perceptions and predilections of those who judge, the threshold of admission of an expert can sometimes be rather low. In the case of *Mt. Vernon v. Cochran* (1993), a Washington state appeals court affirmed a court commissioner's appointment of a DWI defense expert in the face of the commissioner's less-than-ringing endorsement of the proposed expert's qualifications:

> I have listened to [defense expert] . . . he's testified several times. I've seen a lot of his information. By in (sic) large, most of what he proposes is preposterous . . . I know he testifies a lot, I know he writes a lot of articles, I know a lot of people with very preposterous ideas that write a lot of articles and get them published, but I'm not really sure that the *Frye* standard is not being met because I think there's (sic) enough people listening to what [defense expert] says . . . .[86]

A novel "under the influence" theory, and the qualifications of an expert witness to testify in rebuttal of that theory, arose in the California case of *People v. Coyle* (1994).[87] In *Coyle*, involving a prosecution for vehicular manslaughter, the State's ex-

pert testified that the defendant had a 0.22 gram per deciliter blood alcohol concentration and was under the influence of cocaine at the time of the automobile collision.[88] The defendant did not deny ingesting alcohol and cocaine. In fact, he acknowledged regular use of these two drugs for the past ten years. Rather, he testified that, based on his personal consumption and experience, the alcohol and cocaine, when ingested together "equalize each other out" resulting in a perfectly acceptable condition for operating a motor vehicle.[89]

To rebut the defendant's rather unique claim, the State called an expert with training and experience as to the individual effects of alcohol and cocaine on the human body. The expert was then asked about the combined effects of these two substances. Since the witness had no direct experience with the combined reaction, she stated that while she could only draw an inference based upon her studies of the separate effects of the two drugs, she was of the opinion that the alcohol and cocaine would not counteract each other.[90]

On appeal, defendant raised an objection to the admission of the State's expert's testimony on the ground that she was not qualified to testify as to the combined effects of alcohol and cocaine. The appeals court rejected defendant's argument, holding that, based on the expert's independent experience with each drug, it was completely appropriate for the court to allow the expert to draw an inference as to their combined effect:

> The jury could properly weigh her testimony that cocaine would not counteract the noxious effects of alcohol against defendant's rather incredible testimony that, in the words of the People, "his twice-the-legal-limit alcoholic haze was magically and precisely reversed by snorting cocaine."[91]

Finally, in conjunction with insuring that a proposed expert witness has the requisite experience and/or training to testify about scientific evidence, the advocate always should be cognizant of another basic requirement: as with any other witness, the expert must have sufficient facts or data upon which to validly form an opinion. If an expert witness, no matter how qualified, is not familiar with the particular facts of the case in which his or her testimony is being offered, the expert cannot form a relevant opinion useful to the trier of fact and should not be taking the witness stand.

K. The independent role of the court

Beyond the three prerequisites discussed above—knowledge beyond the ken of the average layperson, meeting the jurisdictional threshold of reliability and sufficient expertise of the witness—the admission of scientific evidence and expert testimony is subject to additional, generally applicable evidentiary rules.

For example, determinations as to the admissibility of evidence and witnesses' qualifications as experts are left to the sound discretion of the trial court. The court's decision in this regard will not be reversed on appeal unless it constitutes a clear abuse of that discretion. The judge also retains discretion to exclude otherwise admissible evidence if the judge finds that the probative value of the evidence is substantially outweighed by the risk that its admission will create a substantial danger of undue prejudice, confusing the issues or misleading the jury.[92]

Furthermore, expert testimony need not be given greater weight than other evidence nor more weight than it otherwise deserves in light of everyday experience. Typically, a judge will specifically advise the jury that, notwithstanding the court's qualification of a witness as an expert, the jurors are free to accept or reject all or part of that witness's testimony. It also bears emphasis that (contrary to a frequent, misguided argument made by attorneys) a factfinder, whether judge or jury, is not required to accept the testimony of a witness simply because no evidence to the contrary has been presented. While the absence of conflicting evidence is obviously a factor to consider in evaluation of a witness's statements, the factfinder has a more basic credibility judgment to make: Does the witness's demeanor make him or her believable? Does what the witness is saying make sense in light of common knowledge and practice? If the witness does not pass these fundamental inquiries, then the witness's testimony may properly be rejected even in the absence of rebuttal evidence.

Another evidentiary principle manifests itself specifically in the context of the use of expert testi-

mony in a criminal trial. Rules of admissibility of expert evidence must not impermissibly infringe upon a defendant's constitutional right to testify on his or her own behalf. In *Rock v. Arkansas* (1987),[93] the United States Supreme Court considered an Arkansas rule requiring exclusion of all hypnotically refreshed testimony. The rule was implemented in furtherance of the state's interest in barring unreliable evidence. The Supreme Court held that, absent clear evidence by the State repudiating the validity of all posthypnosis recollection, such a *per se* bar was an arbitrary restriction on defendant's right to testify on her own behalf.[94] However, the Court noted that a state is entitled to establish procedural safeguards which reduce or eliminate potential inaccuracies in the process (e.g., mandating that hypnosis be performed only by psychiatrist with special training as to the use of this technique).[95]

Rock did not deal with the issue of restriction of hypnotically refreshed testimony of witnesses other than the defendant. But the case illustrates that standards of admissibility may be different in situations where they directly affect a criminal defendant's right to present a defense.

L. Expert witness compared to lay witness expression of opinion

In contrast to the requirements applicable to expert witnesses, a lay witness need only have knowledge, acquired through his or her own senses, of the matter to which he or she will testify. Lay witness opinions are limited to such opinions and inferences as the judge finds are (1) rationally based on the perception of the witness and (2) are helpful to a clear understanding of the witness's testimony or to a determination of a fact in issue.[96] An argument can be made that these two factors are simply more subtle forms of the reliability and relevance standards applied to scientific evidence by *Daubert*.

Various subjects have been determined by the courts as properly being the subject of lay witness testimony. Some examples include:

speed of a motor vehicle. An ordinary witness can state a conclusion as to whether a motor vehicle was traveling fast or slow and give an estimate of the vehicle's speed. This conclusion can be based on visual observation, auditory perception or both. *Pierson v. Frederickson* (1968).[97]

intoxication. An average person of ordinary intelligence, although lacking special skill, knowledge and experience, may testify based upon his or her observations as to whether another person was sober or intoxicated. *State v. Pichadou* (1955).[97] In this case, a police commissioner, who was at the police station at the time defendant was brought in, testified as to his opinion of her sobriety: "I would say she was plastered."[99]

assessment of one's own sobriety. A defendant may testify as to his or her sobriety, or lack thereof, at the time of operation of a vehicle. *People v. Tucker* (1990).[100]

performance of field sobriety tests. Some court cases have held that an ordinary police officer cannot testify as to whether a suspect "failed" a field sobriety test or performed the test in a "normal" fashion. The rationale for this approach is that such conclusory expressions are not admissible if provided by lay witnesses, as distinguished from persons such as physicians, who have had training in the use of these tests and in normal and abnormal reactions thereto. However, it is entirely proper for a police officer to describe the tests administered to the defendant and testify as to the defendant's physical reaction during the performance of the tests. The reaction should be described in terms of what was observed when the tests were undertaken by defendant (e.g., lay witness testimony that defendant "was slow, swayed and stepped to the side" during the heel-to-toe test was admissible). *State v. Morton* (1963).[101] Other courts appear to have no problem with police officers' use of the pass/fail terminology.[102]

performance of breath tests by other individuals as an indicator of defendant's BAC. In a Texas case in which the defendant had refused to submit to breath testing, the State, in an effort to show the defendant's condition, called a police officer who was not qualified to administer an Intoxilyzer test, nor was a chemist, nor knew anything about the operation of the Intoxilyzer.

This witness testified that he had in the past observed persons he had arrested who "failed" the breath test and appeared to be in less of an intoxicated state than was defendant on the date of her arrest. The clear implication of this testimony was that, while no breath test reading existed to confirm this fact, the defendant's BAC must have been over the statutorily proscribed level. The Texas Criminal Appeals Court held that, given the officer's lack of qualifications and the complete lack of evidence to support the assumption that Intoxilyzer results could be predicted solely from a person's appearance, admission of the officer's testimony was reversible error. *Graham v. State* (1986).[103]

use of magnifying glass by jury. A jury properly could use a magnifying glass to examine a photograph during deliberations without first hearing expert testimony regarding the magnifying glass. *Boland v. Dolan* (1995).[104] "The focus should be first on whether such [expert] testimony is needed or whether common knowledge suffices for use of the instrument in issue. Failure to address that preliminary question would allow the use of experts for the most mundane of human events, which jurors easily understand without expert testimony. The fact that a magnifying glass is no longer used daily by the average person does not make it a highly complex scientific instrument."[105]

Those involved in litigation should be keenly aware of the distinction between lay and expert testimony. The time, expense and complexity often accompanying presentation of evidence through experts is simply unjustified when the testimony of a laywitness is sufficient.

M. Compelling an expert witness to testify at trial

As a general rule, the opinion of an expert, as opposed to lay testimony describing things perceived, may not be compelled against the wishes of the expert. Courts which take this position recognize a proprietary interest in a person's "expertise" which the person cannot be compelled to relinquish. However, this rule is not universally adopted. The minority view is that, in appropriate circumstances and with appropriate safeguards, the professional opinion of an expert witness can be compelled in the discretion of the court.[106]

N. The range of expert witness testimony

Unless the court orders otherwise, the expert may give an opinion without first revealing the underlying data for the opinion.[107] However, the expert may be required to reveal the underlying facts during cross-examination.[108] Of course, the value of an expert's opinion depends upon the evidentiary soundness of the assumptions upon which the opinion is based.

Also, expert testimony is generally not inadmissible solely because it includes an opinion on the ultimate issue of the litigation.[109] However, where an expert witness is permitted to offer an opinion as to an ultimate issue in the case, it is critically important that the judge not give the jurors the impression that they must defer to a witness's expertise and abdicate the responsibility to form their own independent judgment on the issue.

16.2 Breath Alcohol Testing
A. Admissibility of test readings

The variety of rules regarding admissibility of scientific evidence and expert testimony come into play in the prosecution of drunken driving cases, particularly as they relate to the use of a defendant's breath test readings. Some of these implications are explored below.

Before the advent of breath testing and *per se* laws, a defendant arrested for drunk driving was examined by a medical expert—a "police doctor" or "police physician"—to determine whether the defendant was under the influence of alcohol. At trial, this medical expert would be the primary source of intoxication evidence against the defendant. In the late 1950s and early 1960s, when breath testing instruments such as the Breathalyzer were first being considered by the courts in DWI prosecutions, judicial standards of admissibility in certain jurisdictions required the production of expert testimony to describe the instrument's theory and operation. As the courts became more familiar and comfortable

with the validity of these instruments, the evidentiary requirements were relaxed.

Three court decisions by the Tennessee Supreme Court illustrate this point. In 1955, in *Fortune v. State*,[110] the court determined that breath test results, to be admissible in evidence, must be introduced through professional experts who interpret these results. A decade later, in *Pruitt v. State*,[111] the court allowed some dilution of *Fortune*'s "professional expert" rule in that the actual operator of the instrument could testify as to the test results. However, the court still ruled that, although a trained operator knows the steps involved in proper operation of the instrument, the witness must further have "knowledge of the reasons for such operation and the scientific principle that reflects the results as an accurate reading of blood alcohol content."[112] Finally, in the 1992 case of *State v. Sensing*,[113] the Tennessee Supreme Court, recognizing, as had many other jurisdictions before it, that breath alcohol testing is now commonplace and of generally accepted reliability, ruled that it is no longer necessary for a certified operator of a breath testing instrument to know the scientific technology involved in the function of the instrument for admission of the readings into evidence. The State need only establish the competency of the operator, the proper working order of the instrument and compliance with testing procedures.[114]

Tennessee's thirty-seven-year legal evolution with regard to breath test admissibility, as reflected in the *Pruitt-Fortune-Sensing* trilogy (the transformation likely occurred much sooner in actual trial court practice), can be contrasted with the experience of Oklahoma, where, in the 1950s, a court had determined that presentation of expert scientific evidence was not a prerequisite to the admissibility of breath test readings. In *Alexander v. State* (1956),[115] the court held that a police officer qualified to administer Harger Drunkometer tests to the defendant could testify as to the test readings even though he did not understand and could not work the formula by which the instrument produced the readings. The court compared the situation to the ability of a witness to testify as to the time of day by looking at a clock, the temperature by reference to a thermometer or the speed of a car by looking at the speedometer, testimony which was admissible despite a witness's lack of understanding of the internal workings of these devices.[116]

There is also no serious question regarding the admissibility of alcohol test readings on constitutional grounds. The United States Supreme Court long ago established that a governmentally "compelled intrusion into the body for blood to be analyzed for alcohol content" is a search to be analyzed under the Fourth Amendment's proscription against unreasonable searches and seizures.[117] In a drug-testing case, the United States Supreme Court recognized that "[s]ubjecting a person to a Breathalyzer test, which generally requires the production of alveolar or 'deep lung' breath for chemical analysis, implicates similar concerns about bodily integrity and, like [a] blood-alcohol test . . . should also be deemed a search." *Skinner v. Railway Labor Executives Ass'n* (1989).[118] However, the Supreme Court also recognized that breath tests are far less intrusive than blood tests: "Unlike blood tests, breath tests do not require piercing the skin and may be conducted safely outside a hospital environment and with a minimum of inconvenience or embarrassment."[119] Upon evaluating the totality of relevant circumstances, the Court concluded that the administration of a breath test does not implicate significant privacy concerns.[120]

The distinction recognized by the Court all but eliminates Fourth Amendment challenges to breath testing. The Court essentially held that, barring extraordinary circumstances, breath testing is *per se* constitutionally reasonable. In reaching this conclusion, the Court apparently was driven not only by the inconsequential level of intrusion, but by its own convictions as to the accuracy of this form of testing. See, e.g., *California v. Trombetta* (1984)[121] ("A dispassionate view of the Intoxilyzer and the California test procedures can only lead one to conclude that the chances are extremely low that preserved samples [of a defendant's breath] would have been exculpatory"); *Skinner v. Railway Labor Executives Ass'n* (1989)[122] ("Respondents have provided us with no reason for doubting the FRA's conclusion that the tests in issue here are accurate in the overwhelming majority of cases").

B. Defense attacks on breath alcohol testing

1. Out-of-court experiments by defense experts

DWI defendants have relied upon defense experts' simulated out-of-court experiments in an attempt to undermine the prosecution's breath test results. Courts have not been very receptive to this tactic on the ground that the out-of-court test could not replicate, and therefore was not relevant to, the conditions which existed at the time of the defendant's evidential breath test.

In *City of Columbus v. Taylor* (1988),[123] defendant's breath test result was 0.118 percent (grams per deciliter). Approximately three months after the police-administered testing, defendant underwent simulated testing on the same instrument (BAC Verifier). The appeals court affirmed the trial court's exclusion of the report and testimony of the defense expert who conducted the simulated testing. The court determined that the conditions of the police-administered breath test could not reliably be duplicated by the simulated testing and that such evidence would both mislead the jury and be unfairly prejudicial. The court also noted that the expert's attempt to duplicate the conditions of the night of defendant's arrest were based solely on defendant's recollection, which introduced additional reliability problems.[124]

In *Burks v. State* (1990),[125] a police-administered breath test showed that defendant had a BAC of 0.11 gram per deciliter. The defense sought to have an expert testify concerning an experiment the expert had conducted with the defendant on the morning of trial, when the defendant registered a 0.00 percent (gram per 210 liters) reading on the Intoximeter, then registered a reading of 0.05 gram per 210 liters after ingesting acetone. The appeals court sustained the trial court's exclusion of this evidence on the basis that "the original test conditions, including [defendant's] own physical condition, could not have been duplicated."[126]

In *State v. Nelms* (1990),[127] the trial court permitted, over the State's objection, the testimony of a pathologist who administered a controlled alcohol consumption test to defendant to determine various blood alcohol levels. The court of appeals noted that "evidence of controlled tests regarding the issue of intoxication is of questionable relevancy due to the numerous factors which may result in an individual's intoxication. The facts and circumstances present at a controlled test may be markedly different from those that led up to and were in existence at the time of the commission of an offense involving intoxication."[128]

In a variation of this theme, courts have also blocked defense attempts to independently examine or test the evidential breath test instrument with which the defendant's test was administered. *Blanos v. State* (1989); *Stinson v. State* (1992).[129] After first rejecting the argument that due process requires that the defense have access to the State's breath testing instrument, the courts noted that independent testing of the instrument subsequent to the date of defendant's offense could not duplicate the conditions present at the time of defendant's test and would therefore be of no value.[130]

2. The legal relevance of the subject of expert testimony

Even if the witness is qualified as an expert and the topic the witness proposes to address is properly the subject of expert testimony, the witness should be precluded from testifying if the subject matter of the testimony is *legally* irrelevant to the elements of the offense for which the witness is being prosecuted.

For example, the most qualified extrapolation expert in the world (assuming that true "extrapolation experts" even exist) has no business testifying in a state where extrapolation is banned as a matter of law. *State v. Tischio* (1987)[131] (The court interpreted the DWI statute to mean that the BAC at the time of testing, not the time of operation, is the critical element. Consequently, prosecution of this offense neither requires nor allows extrapolation evidence to demonstrate what the defendant's BAC was during driving).

Similarly, expert evidence as to the defendant's alleged lack of impairment is properly excluded in a situation where the State is prosecuting the defendant under the *per se* DWI law, the elements of which focus exclusively on the quantity of alcohol in a defendant's system as opposed to the effect of that alcohol on defendant's behavior. See *State v. Allex* (1992)[132] (trial court correctly rejected defense at-

tempt to countervail properly administered breath tests with medical testimony evaluating defendant's performance on field sobriety tests. Under *per se* statute, subjective evidence of intoxication was irrelevant); *State v. Tran* (1989)[133] (under *per se* statute, a trial judge is precluded from utilizing additional observational evidence to counter results of a validly performed Intoxilyzer test showing a reading of 0.12 gram per 210 liters); *State v. Horning* (1993)[134] (defendant charged under the *per se* statute was properly precluded from presenting evidence of his alleged lack of impairment).

Some courts have held, however, that the *per se/* observational evidence distinction is too fine of a judicial line to walk. E.g., *City of Bowling Green v. Andrews* (1989)[135] (Defendant proffered the testimony of a chemist who calculated the concentration of alcohol in the defendant's system based upon factors such as the amount of drinks consumed or defendant's weight. The trial court held this evidence was not relevant since the state was prosecuting the defendant under the traditional "under the influence" offense, not for driving with a specific BAC. The appeals court held that testimony regarding defendant's BAC should have been admitted because it could have been used to rebut the accuracy of the police officer's observations regarding the alcoholic influence defendant was under).

A defense expert may also be prevented from testifying in a DWI case on the ground of *factual* irrelevance. In this scenario, a defendant's conduct at the time of the offense precludes the proposed expert testimony. *State v. Andrus* (1990),[136] (Defendant who was arrested for drunk driving refused to submit to a breath test. At his DWI trial, defendant sought to introduce evidence, through an expert witness interpreting an alcohol consumption chart, that his BAC at the time of driving was less than 0.1 gram per deciliter. The appeals court held that "[i]f a defendant has refused the police request for an alcohol concentration test and the State proceeds under general proof that he was impaired by the influence of alcohol, the defendant may not later attempt to establish by direct proof, expert testimony, hypothetical example or otherwise what his alcohol concentration was or could have been"); *Lucas v. State* (1989)[137] (A defendant who refused to submit to breath test could not produce expert testimony on purported inaccuracy of breath testing. Such evidence was irrelevant.).

3. The need for a nexus between the scientific theory being proffered and the evidence at trial

Even assuming that a witness is qualified as an expert and his or her testimony is both legally and factually relevant, there must also be some showing of the actual effect of the witness's theory on the validity of the evidence which the witness disputes. Recall the *Daubert* principle that testimony which merely speculates as to potential effect is unworthy of a finding of reliability. Courts in the following cases found an insufficient nexus between a defense witness's testimony and the reliability of the breath test readings.

City of Columbus v. Ziegler (1992).[138] Defendant claimed he suffered from a stomach acid problem which caused him to belch more than the average person. At trial, he produced a defense expert who testified as to the effects of belching on a breath test. The court held that the expert's testimony lacked sufficient specificity to demonstrate that defendant's belching, as opposed to his alcohol consumption, produced a breath test reading greater than 0.1 gram per 210 liters.

State v. Benas (1995).[139] This case involved the issue of depletion of simulator solution. The appeals court rejected the defense expert's testimony:

We note first that [defense expert] never explained how a less concentrated simulator solution used in the testing of the machine (sic) could distort actual test results . . . As we understand [defense expert's] testimony, the alcohol depletion of the simulator solution could produce an inaccurate reading, resulting in the certification of a defective machine (sic), only if there were some other unidentified and purely speculative different problem with the machine, undetected by the coordinator, and having the capacity, in combination with a depleted alcohol content, to yield a higher reading than the actual alcohol content of the simulator solution.

[Defense expert] did not, however, suggest what those problems could possibly be. Thus we view his testimony as entirely speculative.[140]

D.O.T. v. Wilhelm (1993)[141] A physician's testimony that the defendant's advanced pulmonary disease rendered him incapable of performing an Intoxilyzer test because defendant had only 50 percent breathing capacity was insufficient to undermine validity of breath test results since physician admitted that he had never seen an Intoxilyzer and did not know the specific amount of breathing capacity required to properly perform the test.

State v. Downie (1990)[142] The court rejected the defense of blood/breath ratio variability:

Biological factors such as mouth temperature, gender, body temperature, medication, menstrual cycle, and oral contraceptives may have some theoretical effect on Breathalyzer readings. In addition, hematocrit, or the ratio of the volume of blood cells to the total volume of blood, expressed as a percentage, may have some theoretical effect . . . No scientist during the remand hearing could establish that these theoretical effects were sufficiently concrete as to be significant. Moreover, these factors would not always inflate Breathalyzer readings. Even defense witnesses admitted that some of these factors would actually lower Breathalyzer readings.[143]

Finally, of need of reemphasis is the rule that even when expert testimony is admitted, the trier of fact ultimately determines how much weight the testimony is entitled to and whether that weight is sufficient to create the reasonable doubt which overcomes the prosecution's case. A good example of this principle is found in *Kehl v. Commonwealth* (1993).[144] In this case, defendant's Breathalyzer test produced a reading of 0.17 percent (gram per 210 liters) one hour and twenty-eight minutes after the defendant's vehicle was stopped. A defense expert testified that, given the lapse of time between the stop and the test, it was impossible to determine with any certainty what defendant's BAC was at the time of the stop. The expert admitted, however, that it was just as likely that the defendant's BAC at the time of driving exceeded 0.17 gram per deciliter as it was that his BAC was below 0.17 gram per deciliter. In the expert's words, his "feeling" was that defendant's BAC "was below a .10" but that his "stronger feeling" was that he did not think "anybody can say what it was." The appellate court held that evidence of this nature was insufficient to rebut the statutory presumption that the defendant's BAC at the time of testing was the same as his BAC at the time of driving.

4. Impeachment of expert witnesses

As any other witness, an expert witness may be impeached on various grounds: bias, prejudice, interest, motive, reputation, prior inconsistent or statements and so forth. Additionally, expert witnesses are subject to "impeachment by treatise," in which an expert is asked to confirm that a particular treatise is an authoritative publication in the field, then is challenged by reference to specific areas in the document which tend to cast doubt on his or her testimony. The expert's affirmation of the authoritative status of the treatise is an essential prerequisite to the use of this strategy. See *Jacober v. St. Peter's Medical Center* (1992),[145] concerning the expert who refused to be impeached by treatise:

Q: Do you accept your own writing as authoritative?
A: Only for me.
. . .
Q: [I]f I were to ask you if anything that was written in medical literature is authoritative on the subject which it addresses, you would have to say no?
. . .
A: I think those textbooks are one man's opinion.[146]

In the specific context of impeachment of DWI defense expert witnesses, the following areas would appear to be pertinent: the expert's fee arrangement; whether the expert has ever been arrested or convicted of drunken driving (this explores potential

bias); and the number of cases, of the total number of cases in which the expert has been consulted, that the expert has determined that a defendant's BAC was below a 0.1 gram per deciliter even though defendant's evidential breath test readings were above 0.1 gram per 210 liters (if the two numbers are identical, an argument can be made that the expert may well be testifying *for* a particular result instead of providing impartial testimony *about* a test reading).

Of course, if a witness is simply incomprehensible, a court cannot even begin to evaluate the probative worth of the "expert's" testimony and the testimony effectively impeaches itself. Witness the frustration of an appeals court in *State v. Mitchell* (1994):[147]

We do not understand what [the defense expert] meant by his testimony and defendant offers us no explanation that gives it meaning. [The expert] first addressed the topic on direct examination . . . Defendant's attorney did not try to clarify the answer with the witness. The municipal prosecutor tried to clarify the answer moments later at the beginning of his cross examination . . . Defendant's only reference to the testimony in his brief provides no clarification . . . Defendant's attorney gave us no further enlightenment in response to our questions at oral argument. We conclude that [the expert's] testimony on the point is at best a net opinion and cannot be given any weight.

5. Conclusion

A genuine expert witness is one whose primary mission is not to seek out court cases, but who conducts research and analysis outside the confines of litigation. When the need for the expert's courtroom involvement arises as a result of, yet independent of, the person's daily work, a judge and jury are assured of receiving information which genuinely aids in the search for the truth. But commentators lament that the legal arena often seems equally accessible to "experts" great and small:

Expert testimony is now reaching comic proportions. In the first Menendez trial, [a professor] offered her "scientific" opinion that research on snails could explain why the brothers killed. She reportedly claimed that Erik and Lyle killed their parents "in a reaction of fearful, almost primordial survival." She offered the general conclusion that child abuse had led to the "rewiring" of Erik's brain, leaving him "highly sensitive to imminent violence." If the stakes were not so high, [the professor's] pretentious babble would be laughable. But there is a serious risk that when an expert takes the stand, recites her qualifications, and the judge "qualifies" her as someone who can speak with authority, she can influence a jury's deliberations. The consequences are comic and tragic at the same time.[148]

There are other actors in the process who contribute to the accommodating fashion in which contrived expert testimony is greeted at the courtroom door. Many of these participants lack a basic understanding of science, yet are called upon to make or guide decisions applicable thereto which have the potential for considerable impact on people's lives. Professor Moenssens sees the "appalling scientific illiteracy that exists among the bench and bar" as the root of this problem:

> Expert witnesses notoriously stray outside the fields of their expertise. It should be recognized, however, that frequently this is not the expert's fault because lawyers often ask questions on issues beyond the witness's experience. The opposing attorney then fails to object because neither lawyer knows any better!
> . . .
> Some experts blatantly misstate and exaggerate their qualifications, to the point of perjury—a great embarrassment to the lawyers who called them as witnesses. (Moenssens 1993)[149]

This, of course, is not to say that the legal use of scientific evidence should be banned altogether. The wide range of issues being typically considered in today's courtrooms precludes such a drastic course. But the exposition is quite often flawed. Recently, the California Court of Appeals had this observation to make concerning the presentation of scientific evidence in a court of law:

> In reviewing cases dealing with new scientific theories, a discouraging pattern appears. Often both the scientific and legal proponents of new techniques seem ill-prepared for the inevitable courtroom clash over the admissibility of the technique. Presentations are made with few or marginal experts, techniques are offered before a reasonable time has passed for the procedure or its forensic application to become familiar to scientists, no effort is made by proponents to encourage or expedite peer review, institutional proponents, such as prosecutors, seldom appear to take a coordinated approach to qualify a new technique by, for example, choosing appropriate cases as test vehicles and combining lawyers intimately familiar with the new technique with experts qualified to discuss the procedure and its acceptance in the scientific community. Often the process followed seems a haphazard one resulting in more mischief than illumination. We encourage proponents to be more selective in choosing the time and manner in which they first offer a new technique and encourage trial courts to be more active by, for example, calling their own experts to testify on new techniques.[150]

In an attempt to make judges more conversant with scientific evidence and the legal principles attendant to its use in court, the Federal Judicial Center has published a reference manual which provides the judiciary with an overview on managing scientific evidence in the courtroom, as well as individual chapters on a number of areas of science. See Federal Judicial Center, *Reference Manual on Scientific Evidence* (1995).[151] Practical reference materials are also available for the litigator in this respect. (See, e.g., Imwinkelried 1995,[152] providing sample foundational questions for admission of scientific evidence under both *Frye* and *Daubert*.)

These are good first steps. Knowledge of the law as it applies to specialized, expert testimony is an indispensable component of curbing abuse in this area. Regular training seminars for judges and attorneys on scientific evidence should also be instituted to insure at least a basic level of familiarity with the contours of its use. Indeed, the problem is not so much the unavailability of educational materials on the subject as the lack of interest on the part of practitioners in becoming familiar with these resources. This casual, uncaring attitude must change. Then, and only then, will genuine expert testimony and its evidentiary bases realize their true potential on the witness stand.

Endnotes

1. 78 N.W. 965, 966 (Minn. 1899).

2. Churchill, M.A. (President and General Counsel, Mid-America Legal Foundation, Chicago). Letter to the Editor, *Newsweek*, April 19, 1993.

3. 23 Cal. Rptr.2d 703, 709 (Cal. App. 1993).

4. 20 Cal.Rptr.2d 6, 8, 12 (Cal. App. 1993).

5. 819 P.2d 821, 823 (Wash. App. 1991).

6. 896 F.2d 210, 212 (7 Cir. 1990).

7. Federal Rule of Evidence 702. The text of this rule and other federal evidentiary rules and rules of criminal procedure relevant to expert testimony is set forth in Appendix A to this chapter.

8. See, e.g., *State v. Berry*, 658 A.2d 702, 705 (N.J. 1995) ("[E]xpert opinion is admissible if the general subject matter at issue, or its specific application, is one with which an average juror might not be sufficiently familiar, or if the trial court determines that the expert testimony would "assist the jury in comprehending the evidence and determining issues of fact").

9. 25 F.3d 1342, 1349–1350 (6 Cir. 1994).

10. 293 F. 1013 (D.C. Cir. 1923).

11. 293 F. at 1014.

12. 293 F. at 1014 (emphasis supplied).

13. 293 F. at 1014.

14. See, e.g., Strong, J.W. (ed.), *McCormick on Evidence*, 4th ed., vol. 1. West Publishing, 1992, at 869–870.

15. James, B.L. Fryed expert witnesses: The 5th circuit takes charge of scientific testimony. *The Review of Litigation*, vol. 12, 1992, at 178.

16. Strong, *McCormick*, at 871–872. Vu, H.Q. and Tamor, R.A. Of *Daubert*, Elvis and precedential relevance: Live sightings of a dead legal doctrine. *U.C.L.A. Law Review* 41:487, 496–497 (1993).

17. Moenssens, A.A, Inbau, F.E. and Starrs, J.E. *Scientific Evidence in Criminal Cases*, 3rd ed. NY: Foundation Press, 1986, at 12.

18. *Ibid*.

19. 593 A.2d 733 (N.J. 1991).

20. 593 A.2d at 746. See also *United States v. Downing*, 753 F.2d 1224, 1237 (3 Cir. 1985).

21. 723 F.2d 238, 276 (3 Cir. 1983), reversed on other grounds by *Matsushita Electrical v. Zenith Radio*, 106 S.Ct. 1348 (1986).

22. 113 *S.Ct.* 2786 (1993).

23. 113 S.Ct. at 2790.

24. 113 S.Ct. at 2789.

25. 113 S.Ct. at 2789-2790.

26. 113 S.Ct. at 2793-2794.

27. 113 S.Ct. at 2795.

28. 113 S.Ct. at 2795.

29. 113 S.Ct. at 2795.

30. 113 S.Ct. at 2795. The Supreme Court's pronouncement on the insufficiency of "speculative" evidence was echoed in a Texas case involving another lawsuit against Merrell Dow. In *Merrell Dow Pharmaceuticals, Inc. v. Havner*, 907 *S.W.*2d 535, 541-544, 548 (Tex. App. 1994), a state appeals court issued the following admonition:

> [E]ven when an expert expresses his opinion using the magic words, "reasonable probability," the entire substance of the expert's testimony must be examined to determine if the opinion is based on demonstrable facts and does not rely solely on assumptions, possibility, speculation and surmise.
> . . .
> Reasonable probability cannot be created by the mere utterance of magic words by someone designated an expert.
> . . .
> Casting unsubstantiated aspersions on the work of others cannot be considered a substitute for real scientific data.

Another court offered this more succinct rhetorical description of the relevant theme: "In this case, we consider the question whether it is so if an expert says it is so." *Viterbo v. Dow Chemical Co.*, 826 F.2d 420, 421 (5 Cir. 1987).

For an example of a court's application of this principle, see *Joy v. Bell Helicopter Textron, Inc.*, 999 F.2d 549, 567–570 (D.C. Cir. 1993) (testimony of plaintiff's expert as to future earning capacity of decedent who had owned small toy store, particularly testimony that decedent, if he had lived, would have moved into expansive consulting and wholesaling, was based on "guesswork, speculation and conjecture" and was therefore unreliable).

31. 113 S.Ct. at 2796.

32. 113 S.Ct. at 2796-2797.

33. One court recently drew a distinction between scientific articles and legal articles which address scientific issues: "[E]ach of the articles cited is from a legal, not a scientific publication. While such articles may be useful as educational and research devices for the bench and bar, and while they may alert a court to the need for a full review of a technique, they are generally not authoritative materials either on primary scientific issues or on the ultimate issue of consensus in the relevant community." *People v. Joehnk*, 42 Cal.Rptr.2d 6, 17 (Cal. App. 1995).

34. *In re Joint Eastern & Southern Asbestos Litigation*, 827 *F.Supp.* 1014, 1033 (D.C.N.Y. 1993), reversed and remanded 52 F.3d 1124 (2 Cir. 1995).

35. Freckelton, I.R. *The Trial of the Expert: A Study of Expert Evidence and Forensic Experts.* Oxford: Oxford University Press, 1987, at 169.

36. 880 S.W.2d 759, 764 (Tex. Crim. App. 1994).

37. 113 S.Ct. at 2795.

38. 113 S.Ct. at 2795.

39. 625 So.2d 827, 829 (Fla. 1993).

40. 113 S.Ct. at 2796.

41. 113 S.Ct. at 2796.

42. 113 S.Ct. at 2796.

43. 113 S.Ct. at 2796 n.10.

44. 113 S.Ct. at 2798.

45. 113 S.Ct. at 2798.

46. 113 S.Ct. at 2797-2798.

47. 113 S.Ct. at 2798. In a recent case decided by the Texas Supreme Court, the attack on the judge's evidentiary screening role was taken to a constitutional level. In *E.I. Du Pont De Nemours and Co., Inc. v. C.R. Robinson*, 64 U.S.L.W. 2047, 1995 Westlaw 359024 (Tex. 1995), the plaintiffs contended that allowing the trial judge to act as a gatekeeper in this respect violated their right to a trial by jury because it infringed upon the jury's inherent authority to assess the credibility of witnesses and weigh their testimony. Id., 1995 Westlaw 359024 at 10. The Texas court was not persuaded, finding that adoption of the *Daubert* standard would not change the jury's primary role of evaluating weight and credibility. Id.

48. 113 S.Ct. at 2798–2799.

49. *Rucker*, 297 A.2d 400, 403 (Del. Super. Ct. 1972)("[E]vidence that the type of tests already approved by the [legislature] when properly conducted are still subject to possible variations in results is not a matter which is here left to the trier of facts"); *Lentini*, 573 A.2d 464, 467 (N.J. App. 1990) ("In the present case, defendant seeks to blunt the legislative resolve by giving new vigor to the probative value of expert testimony in the interest of eliminating a possible deviation of 1/100 of a per cent. If defendant's contention is adopted, the . . . *per se* bright line of 0.10% would have to be adjusted in derogation of the statutes' objective standards").

50. 113 S.Ct. at 2799.

51. 43 F.3d 1311 (9 Cir. 1995).

52. 43 F.3d at 1316.

53. 43 F.3d at 1316.

54. 43 F.3d at 1316.

55. 43 F.3d at 1316.

56. 43 F.3d at 1315–1316.

57. 43 F.3d at 1317–1318.

58. 43 F.3d at 1317. Pending legislation in the current Congress, in an apparent response to the perception that "junk science" is being admitted in the courtroom, proposes to amend Federal Rule of Evidence 702 to expressly require "a valid scientific connection" between the evidence and the fact that it is being offered to prove. (One Hundred and Fourth Congress, House of Representatives Bill No. 988, Section 3). This terminology is quite similar to that used in *Daubert*. H.R. 988, Section 3 would also disqualify the testimony of any witness whose compensation is contingent upon the specific outcome of the case.

59. 43 F.3d at 1314.

60. 43 F.3d at 1314.

61. 43 F.3d at 1319.

62. 43 F.3d at 1318.

63. 43 F.3d at 1321.

64. 43 F.3d at 1322.

65. 116 S.Ct. 189 (1995).

66. See *Hutchison v. American Family Mutual Ins. Co.*, 514 N.W.2d 882 (Iowa 1994) (noting that *Daubert* merely reaffirms Iowa's "liberal rule on the admission of opinion testimony"); *State v. Foret*, 628 So.2d 1116 (La. 1993); *Commonwealth v. Lanigan*, 641 N.E.2d 1342 (Mass. 1994); *State v. Moore*, 885 P.2d 457 (Mont. 1994); *State v. Alberico*, 861 P.2d 192 (N.M. 1993); *Taylor v. State*, 889 P.2d 319 (Okla. Crim. App. 1995); *State v. Hofer*, 512 N.W.2d 482 (S.D. 1994) (addressing blood/breath ratio); *E.I. du Pont Nemours & Co., Inc. v. Robinson*, 64 U.S.L.W. 2047, 1995 Westlaw 359024 (Tex. 1995); *State v. Brooks*, 643 A.2d 226 (Vt. 1993) (addressing admissibility of Datamaster breath testing instrument); *Wilt v. Buracker*, 443 S.E.2d 196 (W. Va. 1993).

67. See *People v. Leahy*, 34 Cal.Rptr.2d 663 (Cal. 1994) (adhering to *Frye*-based test in evaluating admissibility of horizontal gaze nystagmus); *Flanagan v. State*, 625 So.2d 827 (Fla. 1993)(adhering to *Frye* despite *Daubert*); *State v. Dean*, 523 N.W.2d 681 (Neb. 1994); *State v. Carter*, 524 N.W.2d 763 (Neb. 1994); *People v. Wesley*, 611 N.Y.S.2d 97 (N.Y. 1994); *Dikeou v. Osborn*, 881 P.2d 943 (Utah App. 1994).

68. *Reese v. Stroh*, 907 P.2d 282, 287–288 (Wash. 1995) (Johnson, J. concurring) (advocating *Daubert* for civil cases); *State v. Riker*, 869 P.2d 43 (Wash. 1994) (adhering to *Frye*, but also citing *Daubert* factors with approval, in criminal cases).

69. See, e.g., *State v. Alt*, 504 N.W.2d 38 (Minn. App. 1993), remanded 505 N.W. 2d 72 (Minn. 1993) (while Minnesota rules of evidence are modeled after the federal rules, appeals court declines to resolve issue until the Minnesota Supreme Court decides *Daubert*'s impact in Minnesota); *People v. Mehlberg*, 618 *N.E.*2d 1168 (Ill. App. 1993); *State v. Donner*, 531 N.W.2d 369 (Wis. App. 1995). In a recent dissenting opinion, a member of the Court

of Appeals for the District of Columbia (where *Frye* originated at the hands of this court's federal circuit appellate counterpart in 1923) urged the court to "join the Supreme Court's rejection of *Frye*[.]" *Taylor v. United States*, 661 A.2d 636, 651–652 (D.C. App. 1995) (Newman, S.J., dissenting).

70. For other examples of judicial application of the *Daubert* standard, see *Cantrell v. GAF Corp.*, 999 F.2d 1007 (6 Cir. 1993) (federal appeals court, emphasizing the "flexibility" of the Federal Rules of Evidence, affirms the admissibility of "expert" testimony on association between asbestos exposure and laryngeal cancer despite the fact that medical literature did not link asbestos exposure to cancer and the "expert" tested only three individuals employed at the site of asbestos exposure (all three of whom were also smokers); *U.S. v. Bonds*, 12 F.3d 540 (6 Cir. 1993) (court applies *Daubert* relevance and reliability prongs to admit evidence of DNA test results); *People v. Coyle*, 28 Cal.Rptr.2d 488 (Cal. App. 1994)[review granted by California Supreme Court, 31 Cal.Rptr.2d 125 (June 2, 1994), review dismissed 43 Cal.Rptr.2d 679 (July 20, 1995) (allowing testimony of State toxicologist on combined effects of alcohol and cocaine ingestion); *State v. Hofer*, 512 N.W.2d 482 (S.D. 1994) (affirming admissibility of Intoxilyzer test results despite defendant's claims that 2,100:1 blood-breath ratio was not generally accepted in the scientific community); *State v. Foret*, 628 So.2d 1116 (La. 1993) (court finds that proposed testimony of State's expert as to child sexual abuse accommodation syndrome failed to meet even the liberal *Daubert* standard due to, among other factors, the extremely high probability of error).

71. Tamarelli, A.W., Jr. *Daubert v. Merrell Dow Pharmaceuticals*: Pushing the limits of scientific reliability: The Questionable wisdom of abandoning the peer review standard for admitting expert testimony. *Vanderbilt Law Review* 47:1175, 1994.

72. *Ibid.*, at 1198.

73. *Ibid.*, at 1197.

74. 34 Cal.Rptr.2d 663 (Cal. 1994).

75. 34 Cal. Rptr.2d at 673.

76. 892 P.2d 281, 289 n. 23 (Colo. 1995).

77. 518 N.W.2d 577 (Minn. 1994).

78. 518 N.W.2d at 585-586.

79. 836 P.2d 1110 (Kan. 1992).

80. 836 P.2d at 1121.

81. 836 P.2d at 1120-1121.

82. See, e.g., Federal Rule of Evidence 201.

83. 199 A.2d 809, 823 (N.J. 1964).

84. 608 A.2d 134 (D.C. App. 1992).

85. 23 Cal.Rptr.2d 703, 712 (Cal. App. 1993).

86. 855 P.2d 1180, 1182 (Wash. App. 1993).

87. 28 Cal.Rptr.2d 488 (Cal. App. 1994) [review granted 31 Cal.Rptr.2d 125 (June 2, 1994), review dismissed 43 Cal.Rptr.2d 679 (July 20, 1995).

88. 28 Cal. Rptr.2d at 489.

89. 28 Cal. Rptr.2d at 490.

90. 28 Cal. Rptr.2d at 490.

91. 28 Cal. Rptr.2d at 491. In the course of its analysis, the court quoted the following sentence from an earlier California appellate court opinion: "[W]ork in a particular field is not an absolute prerequisite to qualification as an expert in that field." These words must be considered in the context of the *Coyle* case for, if viewed in the abstract, they establish a most alarming measuring stick for the evaluation of expert testimony.

92. See, e.g., *Federal Rule of Evidence* 403 ("Although relevant, evidence may be excluded if its probative value is substantially outweighed by the danger of unfair prejudice, confusion of the issues, or misleading the jury, or by considerations of undue delay, waste of time, or needless presentation of cumulative evidence").

93. 107 S.Ct. 2704 (1987).

94. 107 S.Ct. at 2714.

95. 107 S.Ct. at 2713-2714.

96. See, e.g., Federal Rule of Evidence 701.

97. 245 A.2d 524 (N.J. App. 1968).

98. 111 A.2d 908 (N.J. App. 1955).

99. 111 A.2d at 909.

100. 550 N.E.2d 581 (Ill. App. 1990).

101. 189 A.2d 216 (N.J. 1963).

102. E.g., *State v. Hurd*, 877 S.W.2d 644, 645 (Mo. App. 1994); *Schade v. Dept. of Transportation*, 857 P.2d 1314, 1315 (Ariz. App. 1993).

103. 710 S.W.2d 588 (Tex. Crim. App. 1986).

104. 657 A.2d 1189 (N.J. 1995).

105. 657 A.2d at 1196.

106. For a compilation of caselaw on this subject, see "Right of Independent Expert to Refuse to Testify as to Expert Opinion," 50 *American Law Reports* (4th) 680 (1986); "Compelling Testimony of Opponent's Expert in State Court," 66 *American Law Reports* (4th) 213 (1988).

107. Federal Rule of Evidence 705.

108. Federal Rule of Evidence 705.

109. See, e.g., California Evidence Code sec. 805; Nevada Revised Statutes Annotated sec. 50.295. But see Federal Rule of Evidence 704 (creating exception to general rule of admissibility of opinion evidence, which precludes an expert witness from offering an opinion as to whether a defendant in a criminal action had the requisite mental state constituting an element of the crime or of a defense thereto.

110. 277 S.W.2d 381 (Tenn. 1955).

111. 393 S.W.2d 747 (Tenn. 1965).

112. 393 S.W.2d at 752.

113. 843 S.W.2d 412, 416 (Tenn. 1992).

114. 843 S.W.2d at 416. See also *State v. Lowther*, 740 P.2d 1017, 1020 (Haw. App. 1987) (prior judicial acceptance of the Intoxilyzer as a reliable device relieves the State of the burden of presenting expert testimony regarding the scientific reliability of the Intoxilyzer in every DUI prosecution where the prosecution seeks to use the test readings. The "reliability prong" of admissibility is satisfied). And see, generally, "Qualification As Expert to Testify as to Findings or Results of Scientific Test to Determine Alcoholic Content of Blood," 77 *American Law Reports(2d)* 971 (1961).

115. 305 P.2d 572 (Okla. Crim. App. 1956).

116. 305 P.2d at 588.

117. *Schmerber v. California*, 86 *S.Ct.* 1826, 1833–1834 (1966).

118. 109 S.Ct. 1402, 1413 (1989).

119. 109 S.Ct. at 1418.

120. 109 S.Ct. at 1418.

121. 104 S.Ct. 2528, 2534 (1984).

122. 109 S.Ct. at 1421 n.10.

123. 529 N.E.2d 1382 (Ohio 1988).

124. 529 N.E.2d at 1385.

125. 394 S.E.2d 136 (Ga. App. 1990).

126. 394 S.E.2d at 139.

127. 1990 Westlaw 183753 (Tenn. Crim. App. 1990) [unpublished opinion].

128. 1990 Westlaw 183753 at 2.

129. 386 S.E.2d 714 (Ga. App. 1989); 416 S.E.2d 765 (Ga. App. 1992).

130. 386 S.E.2d at 715; 416 S.E.2d at 766.

131. 527 A.2d 388, 397 (N.J. 1987).

132. 608 A.2d 1 (N.J. App. 1992).

133. 542 So.2d 648 (La. App. 1989).

134. 511 N.W.2d 27, 30-31 (Minn. App. 1994) [review granted 3/31/94].

135. 572 N.E.2d 786, 787 (Ohio App. 1989).

136. 800 P.2d 107, 110 (Idaho App. 1990).

137. 384 S.E.2d 438 (Ga. App. 1989).

138. 605 N.E.2d 1360, 1362-1363 (Ohio App. 1992).

139. 657 A.2d 445 (N.J. App. 1995).

140. 657 A.2d at 446.

141. 626 A.2d 660, 661-662 (Pa. Comwlth. 1993).

142. 569 A.2d 242 (N.J. 1990).

143. 569 A.2d at 248.

144. 426 S.E.2d 127, 129 (Va. App. 1993).

145. 608 A.2d 304 (N.J. 1992).

146. 608 *A.*2d at 308. See also "Propriety of Questioning Expert Witness Regarding Specific Incidents or Allegations of Expert's Unprofessional Conduct or Professional Negligence," 11 *American Law Reports (5th) 1* (1993).

147. Docket No. A-570-93T5 (N.J. App. 1994) [unpublished opinion].

148. Fletcher, G.P. *With Justice for Some.* Boston: Addison-Wesley Publishing Co., 1995, at 234.

149. Moenssens, A.A. Novel scientific evidence in criminal cases: Some words of caution. *Journal of Criminal Law & Criminology* 84(1):7, 1993.

150. *People v. Joehnk*, 42 Cal. Rptr.2d 6, 17 n.10 (Cal. App. 1995).

151. *The Reference Manual on Scientific Evidence* is available through a number of publishing companies in both hardcover and soft-bound editions.

152. Imwinkelried, E.J. *Evidentiary Foundations*, 3rd ed. Charlottesville, VA: Michie Company, 1995, at 90–106.

Appendix
Federal Rules of Evidence and Criminal Procedure Relating to Expert Testimony

F.R.E. 701. Opinion Testimony by Lay Witnesses

If the witness is not testifying as an expert, the witness' testimony in the form of opinions or inferences is limited to those opinions or inferences which are (a) rationally based on the perception of the witness and (b) helpful to a clear understanding of the witness' testimony or the determination of a fact in issue.

F.R.E. 702. Testimony by Experts

If scientific, technical, or other specialized knowledge will assist the trier of fact to understand the evidence or to determine a fact in issue, a witness qualified as an expert by knowledge, skill, experience, training, or education, may testify thereto in the form of an opinion or otherwise.

F.R.E. 703. Bases of Opinion Testimony by Experts

The facts or data in the particular case upon which an expert bases an opinion or inference may be those perceived by or made known to the expert at or before the hearing. If of a type reasonably relied upon by experts in the particular field in forming opinions or inferences upon the subject, the facts or data need not be admissible in evidence.

F.R.E. 704. Opinion on Ultimate Issue

(a) Except as provided in subdivision (b), testimony in the form of an opinion or inference otherwise admissible is not objectionable because it embraces an ultimate issue to be decided by the trier of fact.

(b) No expert witness testifying with respect to the mental state or condition of a defendant in a criminal case may state an opinion or inference as to whether the defendant did or did not have the mental state or condition constituting an element of the crime charged or of a defense thereto. Such ultimate issues are matters for the trier of fact alone.

F.R.E. 705. Disclosure of Facts or Data Underlying Expert Opinion

The expert may testify in terms of opinion or inference and give reasons therefor without first testifying to the underlying facts or data, unless the court requires otherwise. The expert may in any event be required to disclose the underlying facts or data on cross-examination.

F.R.E. 706. Court Appointed Experts

(a) **Appointment**. The court may on its own motion or on the motion of any party enter an order to show cause why expert witnesses should not be appointed, and may request the parties to submit nominations. The court may appoint any expert witnesses agreed upon by the parties, and may appoint expert witnesses of its own selection. An expert witness shall not be appointed by the court unless the witness consents to act. A witness so appointed shall be informed of the witness' duties by the court in writing, a copy of which shall be filed with the clerk, or at a conference in which the parties shall have opportunity to participate. A witness so appointed shall advise the parties of the witness' findings, if any; the witness' deposition may be taken by any party; and the witness may be called to testify by the court or any party. The witness shall be subject to cross-examination by each party, including a party calling the witness.

(b) **Compensation**. Expert witnesses so appointed are entitled to reasonable compensation in whatever sum the court may allow. The compensation thus fixed is payable from funds which may be provided by law in criminal cases and civil actions and proceedings involving just compensation under the fifth amendment. In other civil actions and proceedings the compensation shall be paid by the parties in such proportion and at such time as the court directs, and thereafter charged in like manner as other costs.

(c) **Disclosure of appointment**. In the exercise of its discretion, the court may authorize disclosure to the jury of the fact that the court appointed the expert witness.

(d) **Parties' experts of own selection**. Nothing in this rule limits the parties in calling expert witnesses of their own selection.

F.R.E. 803. Hearsay Exceptions; Availability of Declarant Immaterial

The following are not excluded by the hearsay rule, even though the declarant is available as a witness:

(18) **Learned treatises**. To the extent called to the attention of an expert witness upon cross-examination or relied upon by the expert witness in direct examination, statements contained in published treatises, periodicals, or pamphlets on a subject of history, medicine, or other science or art, established as a reliable authority by the testimony or admission of the witness or by other expert testimony or by judicial notice. If admitted, the statements may be read into evidence but may not be received as exhibits.

F.R.E. 201. Judicial Notice of Adjudicative Facts

(a) **Scope of rule**. This rule governs only judicial notice of adjudicative facts.

(b) **Kinds of facts**. A judicially noticed fact must be one not subject to reasonable dispute in that it is either (a) generally known within the territorial jurisdiction of the trial court or (2) capable of accurate and ready determination by resort to sources whose accuracy cannot reasonably be questioned.

(c) **When discretionary**. A court may take judicial notice, whether requested or not.

(d) **When mandatory**. A court shall take judicial notice if requested by a party and supplied with the necessary information.

(e) **Opportunity to be heard**. A party is entitled upon timely request to an opportunity to be heard as to the propriety of taking judicial notice and the tenor of the matter noticed. In the absence of prior notification, the request may be made after judicial notice has been taken.

(f) **Time of taking notice**. Judicial notice may be taken at any stage of the proceeding.

(g) **Instructing jury**. In a civil action or proceeding, the court shall instruct the jury to accept as conclusive any fact judicially noticed. In a criminal case, the court shall instruct the jury that it may, but is not required to, accept as conclusive any fact judicially noticed.

Federal Rules of Criminal Procedure

F.R.C.P. 16 Discovery and Inspection

(a) GOVERNMENTAL DISCLOSURE OF EVIDENCE

(1) Information Subject to Disclosure

(E) EXPERT WITNESSES. At the defendant's request, the government shall disclose to the defendant a written summary of testimony the government intends to use under Rules 702, 703, or 705 of the Federal Rules of Evidence during its case in chief at trial. This summary must describe the witnesses' opinions, the bases and the reasons therefor, and the witnesses' qualifications.

* * *

(b) THE DEFENDANT'S DISCLOSURE OF EVIDENCE

(1) Information Subject to Disclosure

(C) EXPERT WITNESSES. If the defendant requests disclosure under subdivision (a)(1)(E) of this rule and the government complies, the defendant, at the government's request, must disclose to the government a written summary of testimony the defendant intends to use under Rules 702, 703 and 705 of the Federal Rules of Evidence as evidence at trial. This summary must describe the opinions of the witnesses, the bases and reasons therefor, and the witnesses' qualifications.

Chapter 17

Prosecuting Driving-under-the-Influence Cases

Jerry Landau

17.1 Introduction

In discussing the prosecution of DUI cases, what immediately comes to mind is the blood alcohol or drug test, be it a breath test from a certified instrument, a blood or urine test.[1] It is easy to get into the mindset that the "lab results" will make the case. That, however, is far from the truth. The effective prosecution of a DUI case should not center on the alcohol or drug test or analysis. That is only one of a number of components of the successful DUI case.

What does DUI stand for? Driving, or in some circumstances *actual physical control*,[2] under the influence. Therefore, the first and most important part of your case is the *driving*. From there we need to look at officer contact with the driver, field sobriety tests and finally the alcohol or drug test, be it breath, blood or urine and possibly soon to be saliva.[3] This last component will serve, not to form the only basis for the prosecutor's case, but to corroborate the other evidence gathered. Utilizing such an approach will lend credibility to the blood alcohol test and sever at

the knees some defense arguments regarding the accuracy of the instrument and test. When prosecuting a DUI case, do not concentrate on the blood alcohol or drug test to the exclusion of the driving behavior. Accentuate the defendant's driving, as well as the officer's contact with the suspect and the field sobriety tests. It is probably fair to admit, however, in the DUI-drugs case since there is no known universal correlation between a certain amount of drugs in every person's body and impairment the laboratory analysis takes on greater significance.

17.2 Preparation

Let's start at the top, however. Even before discussing the driving there is one important part of the approach we need to deal with—preparation. There is an old saying from somewhere, its origin is unknown but its words are important. Preparation is nine tenths of a trial. Trying the DUI case is much easier than might otherwise be with the proper preparation.

The importance of preparation cannot be overemphasized. Below is an outline of some hints you might want to follow.

A. Interviewing and preparing witnesses

Adequately preparing witnesses for trial is one of the most critical of all steps in the prosecution's effort to achieve a DUI conviction. This preparation includes preparing the witness not only for direct examination, but for cross-examination as well. The prosecutor should consider the following witness preparation steps:

- Review with the witness all of the events important to both the prosecution and the possible defense case.

- Read through all statements or reports in the case file with the witness and check them for accuracy. Add any notes that can be useful to the prosecution's case and build questions that the witness will be asked at trial.
- Clear up any contradictions, inconsistencies, and questions that may have arisen from a thorough reading of the witness report or statement.
- If the witness will be testifying from a diagram, be sure that the diagram is prepared prior to the trial and that the witness knows exactly how the diagram and the events fit together. Accuracy of the diagram and understanding the concepts are essential.
- If the witness' testimony is important as to estimates of time, distance, speed, or unusual circumstances, be sure that each element is thoroughly discussed in advance; all such details are firmly planted in the witness' mind and are unshakable by challenge.
- Understand the meaning of all laboratory reports and the terms contained therein.
- Review with the witness any opinions held as to the defendant's state of sobriety or impairment and be certain that the witness can articulate a sound basis for any opinions expressed.
- Prepare the witness for direct examination by reviewing all of the questions to be asked. Prepare also for all of the questions the defense may ask on cross-examination.

In addition to what is said by the witness at trial, the manner in which testimony is given during direct and cross-examination will contribute greatly to witness credibility. The following recommendations for additional trial preparation will help to insure witness credibility:

- Advise witnesses to dress appropriately for their role and responsibility. The police officer witness should be asked to wear a uniform. Lay witnesses should wear what they normally wear to work. (Do not, for example, have a garbage hauler show up in a three-piece suit or any other out-of-character apparel.)
- Urge the witnesses never to compete with the defense attorney on cross-examination. Some

will try, though most will lose in the attempt. Witnesses should not answer defense questions in a different manner from that of a prosecutor.
- Caution the witnesses always to testify to facts and events personally observed. (This does not apply to expert witnesses.)
- Advise witnesses to avoid memorizing what they intend to say at trial or sounding like what they think a witness should sound like. Encourage them to talk in plain language, using their own words. They should not try to impress, make speeches, nor do anything other than respond to questions posed in as direct and unaffected manner as possible. The statement that Bob walked over to the defendant's car is preferable to a lay witness saying Bob then proceeded to the defendant's vehicle.
- Advise the witnesses to be concise and expressive. They should measure their words and never volunteer information to either to the prosecutor or to the cross-examining defense attorney.

B. Driving

Now that we have the preparation down, let's get back to the driving. What will convince the trier of fact that a person is driving under the influence is the comparison of the person's driving to the perceived norm. If a witness, most likely an officer, is able to articulate specific differences between the defendant's driving and that of others on the roadway and also between the defendant's driving and how we all drive on an everyday basis, the prosecutor is on the way to proving the case.

These driving clues produce some powerful evidence:

- turning with a wide radius,
- straddling the center of lane marker,
- weaving,
- driving too slowly compared to the normal traffic flow,
- driving too fast compared to the normal traffic flow,
- striking or nearly striking a vehicle or object,
- stopping or backing for no apparent reason,
- following too closely,

- drifting within one lane or to other lanes,
- erratic breaking,
- slow response to traffic signals,
- slow response in accelerating after change in traffic signal,
- stopping inappropriately,
- abrupt or illegal turns,
- rapid acceleration or deceleration,
- slow or no response to police emergency lights, and
- headlights off after dark.

Officers are undoubtedly taught to look for these and other similar clues. It is the role of the prosecutor, by proper questioning, to elicit testimony from the witness at trial on these points. In addition, for each clue recognized in the defendant driver, the prosecutor should ascertain whether other drivers observed by the witness or even the witness himself exhibited similar driving action. For example,

Prosecutor:	Officer Jones, please describe what you observed about the vehicle when you first saw it.
Officer Jones:	The vehicle was in front of me in the middle lane. However, it would drift into the left lane, come back to the middle lane, drift into the right lane and back into the middle lane. This weaving action continued for approximately one mile.
Prosecutor:	Prior to and while you were observing the defendant's car did you see other cars on the roadway?
Officer Jones:	Yes.
Prosecutor:	Did any of the other cars you observed have trouble staying within its own lane?
Officer Jones:	No.
Prosecutor:	Did you have any trouble keeping your vehicle within its own lane?
Officer Jones:	No.
Prosecutor:	Was there any debris on the roadway or any problem with the road that could cause a car to weave from lane to lane?
Officer Jones:	No.

This scenario can be used for almost any clue. In addition to emphasizing the defendant's driving conduct, the prosecutor is pointing out to the trier of fact distinct comparisons between the defendant's driving and that of others on the roadway. (Was there any debris on the roadway or any problem with the road which would cause a car to weave from lane to lane?) Fully exhaust observations of driving.

C. Observing the driver and vehicle

The next step is to elicit objective signs of impairment by either drugs, alcohol or both. Many times it will be both. Notice, though, I do not say intoxication. The prosecutor is now beginning to build the blocks by bringing in additional evidence. Eventually, all these various components will be used to corroborate one another.

What else besides the defendant's driving leads us to believe the driver ingested alcohol or drugs and is impaired?

- problems with balance, such as swaying, staggering, stumbling,
- poor coordination,
- problem with speech, such as slurring words,
- talking a great deal or talking very fast or slowly,
- bloodshot eyes,
- watery eyes,
- abnormal pupil size,
- odor of an intoxicating beverage or a drug, such as marijuana,
- unkempt clothing, soiled, messy appearance, clothes inside out,
- urine or vomit on clothes,
- abnormal skin coloration,
- slow reaction and response,
- insensitive to hot or cold,
- lack of awareness,
- attitude and emotional condition,
- out of it,
- injection sites,
- abnormal blood pressure,
- abnormal respiration, and
- abnormal temperature.

Also as important are observations of the vehicle. This would include evidence of recent alcohol or drug consumption, such as beer cans, liquor bottles, roach clips, syringes, silver foil and so forth.

We now have three building blocks; preparation, driving and observations.

D. Field sobriety testing

The next component of the DUI case is the field sobriety testing. These, at least in part depending upon the jurisdiction, consist of standardized test based upon the concept of divided attention. They are designed to recognize impairment in the ability to complete complex tasks, of which driving is one. The National Highway Traffic Safety Administration has conducted extensive research on field sobriety testing and has validated three. It is recommended these tests be utilized as standard procedure in all DUI investigations. Many jurisdictions will employ others in addition to the three NHTSA tests. It is definitely not recommended that the three NHTSA-validated tests be deleted from the protocol. The three tests are:

- walk-and-turn,
- one-leg stand, and
- horizontal gaze nystagmus.

Field sobriety testing certainly has a place in the DUI investigation. However, it is, again, only one piece of the entire case. A pattern should be forming here. A person has trouble driving. The clues are extensively ferreted out and discussed. Clearly, the driving is abnormal. The person shows psychomotor deficiencies, fine and gross muscle control, both in the driving as well as observations by the officer. The officer smells an odor of an alcoholic beverage, or possibly a drug, such as marijuana on the person's breath. Evidence of alcohol or drug consumption may be found. Validated field sobriety tests that have been shown to bear a direct relationship to impairment and along with other evidence,[4] have been administered with results noted. Opinions can now be drawn from these three components; the driver's ability to drive a vehicle is impaired. By this time the officer should be forming an opinion as to whether the impairment is caused by alcohol or drugs, or

both. If the officer suspects drugs a drug recognition exam would be administered, if the jurisdiction is part of the drug recognition program. All this now is corroborated by the blood alcohol or drug test, which leads us to a discussion of the expert witness.

E. Expert witness

Ordinarily, witnesses can testify only as to what they have personally observed relating to a particular case. But an expert witness, an individual who has superior knowledge of a subject, is given the opportunity to share that special knowledge with the court.[5] Thus, the one characteristic that distinguishes experts from other witnesses is that an expert is not required to testify from personal observation, experts may offer opinions.

Expert opinion is usually admissible only on matters requiring some special skill, experience or education. If the trier of facts can reasonably be expected to arrive at the proper conclusion from facts admitted at trial, then expert testimony is not admissible.

Expert witnesses in DUI cases are usually those individuals who have knowledge about alcohol or drug impairment and the effects of alcohol or drugs on the body. Their special knowledge can be the result of training or experience. Experts commonly called at trial include a toxicologist, drug recognition expert, collision reconstructionist if a collision is involved—and yes, the officer. More is discussed about the officer as an expert later.

It is important that the prosecutor interview the expert witness before the trial. The prosecutor should have a copy of all relevant case reports available for the State's expert well before trial. (It is realized this may not be possible in high-volume courts). Often the expert may be able to point out any special problems or recommend preferred presentation methods that not have occurred to the prosecutor.

It is imperative that the prosecutor checks the chain of custody of evidence prior to trial, and obtains the opinion of the expert witness as to its adequacy or completeness. The expert should never be put in a position of having to make spot judgments as to identify, form, or substance of the evidence while in the courtroom. The expert may well claim never to have seen such materials before and, therefore, to be unable to venture an opinion. In addition the expert witness will be very unhappy with the prosecutor.

The expert witness will predominantly provide evidence relating the presence of alcohol or drugs in the driver's blood or urine and the effects of alcohol or drugs on driving. Your first expert, however, is the arresting officer.

The police officer is not many times thought of as an expert witness. However, the law enforcement officer is specifically trained in DUI detection. If a breath test is administered, it will be an officer giving that test. (Some police agencies use non-sworn personnel to administer breath tests. For our discussion, I will refer to the person administering the test as an officer.) In probably every state the officer is required to be certified by an applicable state agency to operate a breath-testing instrument and administer a test. This certification will include some sort of training and proficiency testing. The officer administering the test and testifying regarding the operation, procedures, result and so on should be presented to the trier of fact as an expert. Do not give the officer short shrift solely because that officer is not a scientist.

If the investigation included a drug recognition examination then the drug recognition expert, a police officer, is clearly an expert. In fact, the drug recognition expert, or drug recognition technician as the officer is referred to in some jurisdictions, possesses more training than the average officer. Whenever a drug recognition expert is testifying be sure to fully present that officer's qualifications to the trier of fact.

In many DUI trials, the officer is the only expert the prosecutor may call at trial. There are many jurisdictions where a criminalist or toxicologist is just not available or is not needed to admit breath test results. In presenting the blood alcohol evidence portion of your trial, the officer's expertise in the breath testing instrument and DUI detection is the only expert testimony to be introduced. The prosecutor will base a great deal of the case on this expertise. In a DUI-drugs case where blood or urine is analyzed by a toxicologist, most jurisdictions will require that person to testify. Admission of the test result without the person who conducted the analysis would be considered. The prosecutor should never stipulate to

an expert's qualifications, at least not the State's expert. Many times the defense attorney "in the interest of being friendly or in the interest of judicial economy" will offer to stipulate to the qualifications of the state's expert.

The defense attorney is in reality saying, "I don't want the trier of fact to hear how qualified the State's expert really is." Lay it out, especially in front of a jury. The trier of fact needs to hear the qualifications from the expert's mouth. The trier of fact needs to know the qualifications, as credibility and believability are based in part upon the expert's qualifications. Of course, if the expert's qualifications are not particularly impressive, agree to the stipulation.

Once qualifications are established, the prosecutor must lay the proper foundation to admit the expert testimony. For instance, areas of foundation needed to ultimately admit evidence of the defendant's impairment and the effect of the impairment on the defendant's ability to drive might include:

- materials the expert reviewed in arriving at an opinion,
- facts relied on by the expert in reaching an opinion,
- testimony of previous witnesses,
- field sobriety tests (remember that HGN is a field sobriety test),
- time of ingestion of alcohol or drugs,
- time of ingestion of food,
- observation or deprivation period,
- calibration of the instrument used to analyze the substance,
- tests or examinations conducted by the expert in arriving at an opinion, and
- factual hypothesis.

The prosecutor may have to provide the expert with the necessary foundational requirements. This does not mean just solely at trial, but during pretrial preparation as well. The expert going into trial blind could be very damaging.

In order to reap the optimum benefit from expert testimony, the prosecutor should possess a working knowledge of the subject matter to be discussed. In other words, educate yourself before you educate the judge and jury. The prosecutor will not be as knowledgeable as the expert; however a basic understanding of the scientific principles involved is extremely beneficial. Learning a scientific principle can be on an ad hoc basis before each trial. However, the preferred manner is to take steps in order to become educated in the relevant areas of expertise.[6]

A prosecutor trying a vehicle homicide case should attend traffic collision investigation or reconstruction school. A person prosecuting DUI cases should attend the HGN schools, DRE school, if applicable, and courses designed to teach subjects such as the effects of alcohol and drugs on driving, absorption and elimination rates and the pharmacology of alcohol and drugs. In many jurisdictions the local crime laboratory is only too happy to assist.

Keep in mind the defense expert. If an expert is honest and credible, the state may be in a position to obtain valuable testimony from the defense expert. While the defendant probably will score some points from its own witness there are ways the prosecution can benefit.

The prosecutor should be prepared to present its theory of the case to the defense expert, such as the toxicologist. Include in a DUI-alcohol case such facts as how many drinks the defendant consumed, the start and stop time, weight of the defendant etc. In a DUI-drugs prosecution include evidence of the type of drug ingested, manner of ingestion, time of ingestion, effect on the central nervous system and evidence of impairment are all areas of inquiry. This chapter is not meant to encompass a course on cross-examination; it is worth mentioning that with the right facts an affirmative, as well as a destructive cross-examination of the defense toxicologist can be very beneficial to the State's case. The defense toxicologist may offer an opinion based upon a particular set of facts suggested by the defendant, the toxicologist may offer another opinion based upon the facts described by the state. Both opinions may be honest and accurate, what is different are the facts. If the prosecution convinces the trier of fact to adopt its theory, the defense expert becomes a beneficial expert for the prosecution.

17.3 Sample Questions

The following are sample question dealing the introduction of breadth and blood tests. They are not meant to be all-inclusive as they will vary from state to state. However, these questions will provide a good framework for the introduction of this evidence.

A. Introduction of breath-test results

If the arresting officer did not administrator the breath test, it may be necessary to call on a person, be it a sworn officer or a civilian, to the accuracy of the instrument used. This person is an expert as well. Qualifications must be established and foundation lay. In some instances the person responsible for ensuring the accuracy and the instrument may be the person who gave the test to the driver. The following questions, at a minimum, should be asked of the person who administered the breath test.

Q. What type of testing instrument was used? (Note: Have the officer include model number, serial number and so on as appropriate.)

Q. Have you been trained and certified by the appropriate state agency? (The officer should provide date of certification (or recertification), and name of certifying agency.)

Q. Was the instrument used checked for accuracy in accordance with required state procedures?

(The person with this responsibility should testify to the maintenance schedule, providing the date of the last calibration, maintenance and so forth as appropriate. As mentioned above, the person responsible for periodic checks and maintenance on the instrument might be a person other than the officer administering the test.)

Q. (Introduce appropriate documentation, as required in your jurisdiction.)

Q. Was the defendant constantly observed for the required period of time prior to the administration of the test (to be asked of the person who observed the defendant)?

Q. Did the defendant take anything by mouth, vomit, smoke, or place anything in his or her mouth during this period?

Q. Did you follow a checklist while administering the test?

Q. How many steps are on the list? Did you perform all steps in sequence? (Offer the checklist into evidence.)

Q. What was the result of the test?

B. Qualification of the toxicologist (or other expert) who analyzed the blood sample (can also be used in a DUI-drugs case with a few modifications).

The following are sample questions for the expert witness in a DUI-alcohol case. They include questions qualifying the expert as an expert, those needed to introduce blood alcohol results, questions to elicit the physical effects of alcohol, the hypothetical question and, finally, questions to elicit information about the expert's opinion on the defendant's intoxication.

Q. Would you please state your name?

Q. What is your profession?

Q. Generally, what does the field of toxicology (or other) cover?

Q. Do you have a specialty within the field of toxicology (or other)?

Q. What is that specialty? Please describe it.

Q. What is your educational background?

Q. What, if any, particular studies did you pursue with respect to toxicology (or other area of expertise)?

Q. After completion of your training, how have you been employed?

Q. Where are you currently employed?

Q. What are your duties?

Q. Have you had an occasion to analyze blood for alcohol (or drug) content?

Q. How many such tests have you performed?

Q. Have you testified in courts before as an expert in the field of toxicology?

Q. What courts?

Q. How many times have you testified as an expert?

Next, the prosecutor should offer the witness as an expert in the field of toxicology, or of a more narrowly defined field if the witness prefers. Note, that in many states the witness is not "offered" as an expert, the prosecutor will simply continue on with the questioning. If the defendant objects for lack of qualifications the judge will rule on the objection.

In discussing the expert's educational background be sure to include both general education and more particularly, those courses of study that give special understanding to the area under discussion and investigation. In driving under the influence cases, the expert will probably be a toxicologist. Since the general public does not commonly understand toxicology, the qualifications of the expert can also be used to educate the jury as to the role and function of a toxicologist.

C. Introducing blood (or urine) test results

First, the prosecutor should present the evidence, the vial with the defendant's blood to the witness.

Q. I am handing you what has been marked for identification as State's Exhibit _____. Can you identify it?

Q. What is it?

Q. Is this your signature (or initials) on the label?

Q. What, if anything, did you do with Exhibit _____, as marked (e.g., blood tubes in kit)?

Q. How did you receive the sample?

Q. When did you receive the sample?

Q. What was the condition of the labels on the tubes? (The seals should not be broken. This is to establish the complete chain.)

Q. What was the condition of the seal on the kit? (The prosecutor needs to show that the sample has not been tampered with in any way.)

Q. Did you ultimately break the seals on the kit?

Q. What was in the kit?

Q. What did you do with the tubes?

Q. Did you make any notations on the tubes?

Q. Is there a police report number on the tubes (match the report to the case at trial?)

Q. Did you perform any sort of an analysis on Exhibit _____, the blood (or urine) specimen?

Q. What analytical method did you use in determining the blood alcohol (or drug) content of this blood (or urine) specimen? (The expert should identify the method used and provide a brief description of that method to the jury.)

Q. Were the instruments that you used to determine the blood alcohol (or drug) alcohol content working properly?

Q. How do you know? (The prosecutor should move to admit the maintenance records, if necessary, into evidence.)

Q. What were your findings with respect to this blood (or urine) specimen? (The prosecutor wants the expert to describe the test results.)

Q. Are your facilities certified by the applicable agency, such as the Association of Crime Lab Directors)?

If this series of questions is properly asked and answered, the prosecutor will have established appropriate chain of custody (i.e., the tracing of the path of the particular piece of evidence from the defendant through any intermediate parties to the witness on the stand). Sometimes all people who have handled an exhibit must be called to testify, though in many states that is not necessary. For example, it has been held that calibration records of breath test results are admissible into evidence as business records.[7]

D. Opinion as to the effects of alcohol on the body and effects of alcohol on driving

Although most states have statutes which establish a presumption of intoxication in DUI cases where the percentage of alcohol in the blood is at or exceeds a certain BAC or an illegal-per-se statute, the prosecutor should attempt to elicit testimony from the toxicologist establishing how a defendant would act with a specific percentage of alcohol in his blood. The prosecutor should also obtain testimony as to the effects of alcohol at certain ranges of blood alcohol content on driving.

The toxicologist also should be asked to determine the approximate number of ounces of alcohol that the defendant may have consumed to obtain the established blood alcohol reading. Such testimony will often conflict with the defendant's claim of having had only two beers.

Be careful—the jury can become confused if the testimony of the expert is allowed to become too specific and bogged down in detail. The expert should in general terms, explain methods of deter-mining intoxication, concentrating the testimony on explaining the effects on the body that the blood alcohol content would produce.

The following foundation questions have been developed to help the prosecutor qualify the toxicologist or other medical expert further in regard to the witness' expertise and opinion on the effects of alcohol on the body. It is a matter of preference whether the prosecutor asks these questions together or splits them up as is done here. The prosecutor can do either, that is, qualify the witness right away in all areas, or qualify first for blood analysis and then later for the effects of alcohol. Similar questions tailored to drugs can be framed as well. Facts needed to assist in optimizing the benefits of these questions include:

- effects of alcohol on driving,
- officer's observations of defendant,
- officer's observations of driving,
- roadside field sobriety tests, and
- other pertinent facts from the reports as filed.

The following questions can be then be asked after the blood alcohol results—either a blood test or breath test—are admitted.

Q. Do you have an opinion, based on a reasonable degree of scientific certainty whether or not a person having a blood alcohol level of _____ percent would be capable of safely driving a car?

Q. What is that opinion?

Q. How would such a person normally behave behind the wheel?

Q. Throughout the world, have there been any studies to substantiate the opinion you have just expressed?

Q. What have these studies shown?

Q. Do you personally have any training, education, or experience in the study of the effects of alcohol on the human body? State what that is, please.

Q. Have you personally participated in any studies relating to driving and the consumption of alcohol? (Many toxicologists working in the law enforcement arena have participated in these studies. Go into a great deal of detail as this shows the trier of fact that the toxicologist had specific first hand knowledge).

Q. Based upon your experience as a toxicologist do you have an opinion to a reasonable degree of scientific certainty as to whether there is a recognized correlation between the alcohol content of the blood and intoxication?

Q. What is your opinion?

Q. In your opinion, what is the minimum concentration of alcohol in the blood at which all persons are considered intoxicated? (The generally recognized concentration is 0.08 BAC.)

Q. What is your opinion?

Q. How does alcohol in the blood system affect certain functions of the brain, such as . . .

    perception?
    reaction?
    loss of inhibitions?
    fine muscle control?
    gross muscle control?
    visual acuity?
    memory and so on?

Q. Is alcohol a central nervous system depressant?

Q. Would you describe how the depressive effects of alcohol affect the central nervous system?

Q. Would you describe specifically what parts of the brain are affected by alcohol?

Q. Can a person compensate for the effects of alcohol that you have just described?

Q. At (defendant's blood alcohol concentration), what are the effects of alcohol in the body?

Q. At (defendant's blood alcohol concentration), what are the effects of alcohol on driving?

The expert is discussing both the visible and invisible effects of alcohol. The prosecutor may prefer to split this question so that visible and invisible effects can be separately addressed. The point is to show the jury what alcohol does and how it relates to driving.

Now take each sign of impairment, such as the effect on perception, reaction and so forth and correspond it to the defendants driving. This is where the prosecutor should spend a significant period of time with the toxicologist. For instance, relate loss of fine muscle control with weaving between lanes, loss of

inhibitions to speeding, memory to driving at night with no headlights and so on. The prosecutor is building a strong argument through such questions that can be used in the closing argument.

E. Time-of-test laws

About half the states have what is known as "time-of-tests" laws. The offense of DUI per-se is not based upon blood alcohol content at the time of driving, but within a given number of hours of driving, usually two or three depending on the state.[8] Other states require the prosecutor to prove blood alcohol content at the time of driving. In order to do that a technique known as retrograde extrapolation must be used.

Using the blood alcohol content at the time of the test along with when the defendant drove, the defendant's drinking and eating history and a "burn-off rate," a toxicologist might be able to offer an opinion as to what the driver's blood alcohol content was at the time of driving. If you are attempting to relate the blood alcohol content at the time of the test to the time of driving, the expert would first need to know what the history of the defendant's drinking was on the date in question including

- the time the defendant was observed driving,
- time of test,
- how much alcohol was consumed,
- over what period of time was the alcohol consumed,
- when the defendant first started driving,
- when, precisely, the last drink was consumed,
- what the defendant ate, when and how much, and
- accepted average burn off rate.

After obtaining the above information the prosecutor may ask:

Q. Do you have an opinion as to what the defendant's blood alcohol content would have been at (time of driving)?

Once you have that information you can, knowing the defendant's weight, determine how many drinks would have been in the defendant's system.

Q. Do you have an opinion as to the number of drinks of (beer, wine, hard liquor and so on) that would have been in the defendant's system at (time of driving)?

Of course, the above question can be asked for time of test as well. It is wise for the prosecutor always to have the expert describe how many drinks are actually in the body with that blood alcohol result. The jury relates better to numbers of drinks than to percentages, ratios, body weight-to-drinks, the scale of passing time and so forth. Such testimony also undermines the credibility of the statement on record by the defendant who said, "Officer, I only had two beers."

Be aware, however, that retrograde extrapolation comes with risks. Many toxicologists will not perform a retrograde extrapolation—or as it is commonly called, relate back—because some assumptions must be made. If the defendant does not provide information about his drinking and eating history, it may be very difficult to relate back. Also, while there is an accepted average burn-off rate of .015–.018, that rate does vary in individuals. Such a variance can be exploited by the defense attorney. Problems associated with relation back have caused may state legislators to adopt the "time-of-test" law.

17.4 Conclusion

It has been said that it is easier for a prosecutor to try a murder case than a DUI. That might be an overstatement but as you can see a DUI trial, from preparation to verdict, is not simple. All state laws provide for significant sanctions upon a DUI conviction. Jail time is mandatory in many states, driver license will be suspended, fines will be levied and insurance rates go up. DUI defense is a big business. Virtually every case involves scientific testimony. Experts abound. Preparation, knowledge and organization are a must.

References

Portions reproduced, with permission, from *The Prosecutor's Trial Manual for DWI*, produced by the Arizona Prosecuting Attorney's Advisory Council.

The National Highway Traffic Safety Administration.

Endnotes

1. Many jurisdictions are now opting for blood tests instead of the traditional breath test in a DUI case. Mesa, Scottsdale, Arizona. Urine samples should be obtained in DUI-drugs cases.

2. "Actual physical control" is defined peculiar to state statute or case law. Its meaning will vary somewhat from state to state.

3. Urine is of no benefit in a purely DUI alcohol case, but could be very important in a DUI-drugs case.

4. Drug Recognition Examination.

5. See, Fed. Rules of Evidence, Rule 701

6. The author, as a prosecutor, attended collision reconstruction schools, HGN classes and drug recognition training.

7. See. Fed. Rules of Evidence, Rule 803(6)

8. For instance, in Arizona a person can be charged with DUI if the person's blood alcohol content is .08 within two hours of the time of driving based upon alcohol consumed before or during driving. A.R. S. §28-1381.

Chapter 18

Defending Driving-under-the-Influence Cases

William C. Head

18.1 Introduction

This chapter focuses on strategies, tactics and methods utilized by a defense attorney in handling drunk driving (DUI) cases. Because the "science" involved in these criminal prosecutions poses the greatest difficulty for most criminal defense lawyers, this summary is devoted to addressing recurring issues relating to blood and breath testing. Forensic blood testing (or breath testing) is an attempt to measure the amount of alcohol within a subject's blood at a given point in time. The "standards" for quality assurance and precision of the analytical device utilized for testing vary widely from state to state. A general maxim for defense attorneys in the investigation of a blood test case is "the test is only as good as the lab and the chain of custody of the sample." In dealing with breath testing, a good general maxim is "the test

is only as good as the device and the state's quality assurance program to assure that the machine can render accurate and reliable results."

States use the breath alcohol concentration (BrAC) blood alcohol concentration (BAC) as circumstantial evidence of whether an individual is impaired to the point that his mental and physical faculties are diminished. Furthermore, since the advent of so-called "per se" laws in the 1970s, all but one state now uses BAC results to support a prosecution for a second type of offense: driving with an unlawful blood alcohol level. Attorneys typically refer to these offenses as "per se" offenses or "driving UBAL" (driving with an unlawful blood alcohol level).

In many jurisdictions, blood tests are rare in DUI prosecutions that do not involve accidents, because state law mandates a breath test, not a blood test (e.g., South Carolina). In other states (e.g., Georgia) the arresting officer is permitted to choose which type of test or tests to be administered. In others, breath tests are the "standard" but the DUI suspect may opt for a blood test at state expense, so as to have access to independent testing (e.g., California).

Fortunately, for many accused persons, *blood* alcohol results may not be accurate or reliable for several reasons:

- there is great potential for error in the blood collection process;
- people are inherently different and an "across-the-board" standard for measurement of *level of impairment* of every subject is necessarily flawed;
- hidden or unknown factors (such as disease) which may cause an erroneous reading;

- medications taken by or given to the arrest suspect may alter impairment results;
- humans are conducting and performing the analytical testing, so the possibility of human error always exists (in the analysis of printouts and graphs from testing equipment, refrigeration, preservation, reporting, handling the sample and so on);
- machines are measuring the results, and machines malfunction or sometimes are not maintained with exacting standards;
- because testing of blood *plasma* or *serum* blood is quicker and easier for hospital laboratories to perform, variations in results (when compared with testing *whole* blood) can occur. False high readings will result when blood plasma or serum is tested rather than whole blood, unless an "adjustment" is made in the final results;
- infusion of intravenous fluids may affect BAC results when a hospitalized subject is being tested;
- trauma to an accident victim may cause a delay or cessation of gastric motility (stomach contents being processed out of the stomach). This will significantly alter the true BAC results *at or near the time of driving*, which is the relevant "time" of interest to a court or a jury; *and*
- because most blood tests are taken at local hospital facilities, the competence of the nurse or phlebotomist can vary widely, and samples can be improperly sealed, or might not be "inverted" properly in order to mix anticoagulant and preservatives with the blood in the sample, or might be missing critical documentation needed for the chain of custody within the collection kit packaging.

As opposed to a breath test, which is often performed by the arresting officer, blood samples can often involve three to seven *different,* additional people handling or processing the "evidence." This is especially true if different technicians in the crime lab perform separate testing for alcohol and for drugs.

This chapter will address the fallibility of blood alcohol tests, will identify areas where "reasonable doubt" can be shown, and will point out how this in-

herent unreliability can be used at a criminal trial to attack the blood alcohol results. In addition, breath tests have many more limitations on both accuracy and reliability, and can be rendered all but useless by identifying a plethora of environmental, contamination and electrical glitches that occur on a daily basis.

Finally, urine tests are not being addressed in this chapter due to the inability of urine tests for alcohol concentrations to provide meaningful *quantitative* numbers for a subject's BAC level. Due to "pooling" of urine in the bladder, and wide swings in alcohol concentration levels unless two bladder "voids" are observed *before* collecting the sample, urine testing is really only usable for determining "the presence of" alcohol in the test subject. Any expert witness with a real degree in medicine, human chemistry or pharmacology will not stake his or her professional reputation on the accuracy and reliability of urine testing to obtain quantitative results.

18.2 Statutory or Regulatory Controls

State statutes and regulations generally govern all forms of chemical testing for blood alcohol content. Reference to your jurisdiction's laws is an essential starting point in researching and investigating a DUI case. The manner of testing, the procedure by which the tests are given, the qualification of individuals performing those tests and even the methods of reporting the test results are typically governed by statutes, regulations, or both. In many jurisdictions, regulations may be so sketchy as to violate due process for persons accused of DUI. *Mayo v. City of Madison,* 652 So.2d 201 (Ala. 1994); *State v. Ripple,* 637 N.E.2d 627 (Oh. 1994); *State v. Tanner,* 457 So.2d 1172 (La. 1984); *State v. Rains,* 735 N.E.2d 1 (Oh.App. 6th Dist., 1999).

Often, case law (appellate decisions) has been required to determine the meaning of legislation relating to blood testing. Prosecutors have been successful in getting "short cut" evidentiary foundational matters approved by the state legislature, only to see the courts strike down laws that circumvent the rule of law. *Miller v. State*, 472 S.E.2d 74 (Ga.1996) (due process violation).

A careful analysis of the applicable statutory and regulatory language as well as an examination of any applicable case law construing them can lead to a successful motion to suppress. Because driving under the influence is a *criminal* offense (in all but a few states) and because the chemical test result will either lead to an *inference* of guilt, or *per se* guilt (where the state permits prosecution for operating a vehicle while having an unlawful blood alcohol level), the state must prove beyond a reasonable doubt that the statutory and regulatory procedures for chemical testing have been met. Pertinent statutes and court decisions in your jurisdiction should be carefully reviewed.

Case law

In *State v. Blanchard*, 498 So.2d 211 (La.App. 1 Cir. 1986), the court held that a report that simply reflects the name of the scientist conducting the testing is not sufficient. To comply with statutory requirements, the state must show that the individual who performed the analysis possessed a valid permit issued by the Department of Public Safety or similar Department of Motor Vehicles, crime lab agency and so forth.

Inquiry

- What are the specific requirements of the statute?
- Was the person who drew the blood "approved" to do so?
- Are regulations in place that restrict who or what facility may analyze the blood?
- Is the laboratory periodically inspected under federal law and is it in compliance with federal regulations?
- Does the state have all the necessary people (involved in the chain of custody of the blood) available in court? Were all of these names provided in a timely fashion as part of the pretrial discovery?

18.3 Qualifications to Draw or Analyze Blood

Particular attention should be paid to qualifications and certification of personnel who perform the tests and operate the blood testing equipment. Track down the name, identity and qualifications of each and every person in the chain of custody for blood

sample (Barnard, 1985). Some states have held that the qualification of a mere phlebotomist (as opposed to a registered nurse) is a fact-specific determination.

When the State offers testimony of the operator of the testing device as evidence that there was compliance with the prescribed methods of conducting the chemical test, defense counsel should cross-examine that person *in detail* to determine his or her familiarity with the rules and regulations in question. Furthermore, additional questioning should address compliance with each rule or regulation. That additional inquiry must be made concerning compliance with all medical due diligence by the hospital collecting the blood and the laboratory analyzing the blood.

Case law

In *Weavers v. City of Birmingham*, 340 So.2d 99 (Ala.App. 1976) (overruled on other grounds), the court reversed and remanded a conviction of driving while under the influence stating that, while the officer who administered the chemical sobriety test testified that he had attended an approved course on the operation of the photo electric Intoximeter (PEI) machine, that he held a valid permit to operate it, and that he followed a checklist given to him by the state board of health, such testimony was no substitute for a copy of the regulations.

In *Kent v. Singleton*, 457 So.2d 356 (Ala. 1984), the Alabama Supreme Court held that blood test results were inadmissible in a wrongful death case absent evidence that the blood was drawn by a qualified person or tested using scientific methods.

Inquiry

- Whether the blood test was administered according to state statute.
- Whether the operator of the testing device successfully completed a training program for the specific device.
- When the phlebotomist's training program was undertaken, and has the person taken any required "update" or proficiency courses.
- How long the training program lasted.

- Whether the operator of the device had the requisite permits from the appropriate state agency.
- How well the operator understood the theory and operation of the device.
- How many tests the operator had conducted up to the time he or she performed the test on the defendant.
- Whether the blood collection witness correctly inverted the sample tubes to "mix" the blood (refer to the manufacturer's directions in the kit, which generally specify that gently inverting the tubes ten to fifteen times is the proper practice).

18.4 Procedure

State statutes generally provide for specific procedures for laying an evidentiary foundation for conducting a chemical sobriety test. Where the state fails to present adequate evidence of compliance with the statute, on proper objection, the courts will generally exclude evidence of the test result.

Similarly, where an accused party has issued a proper subpoena seeking detailed disclosure of testing protocol and procedure, and the state seeks to quash the subpoena, such evidence should not be denied by the court. *Eason v. State*, 396 S.E.2d 492 (Ga. 1990).

Case law

In *State v. Miles*, 775 So.2d 950 (Fla. 2000) the Florida Supreme Court held that the State was not entitled to any presumptions of impairment when quality assurance relating to the blood test was not followed.

In *State v. Deimeke*, 500 S.W.2d 257 (Mo.App. 1973) the State failed to carry its burden imposed on it by statute which made admissible into evidence the results of the chemical analysis of blood only where the test was performed according to methods approved by that State's division of health. The statute called for strict compliance with the operating procedures established by the manufacturer.

In *Patton v. City of Decatur*, 337 So.2d 321 (Ala. 1976) it was not shown in the record that daily adopted methods or regulations of the state board of health were followed in administering a chemical sobriety test, nor did the trial court have before it certified methods promulgated by the board of health for administering a test. The court held that evidence relating to performance of the chemical test in accordance with methods approved by the state board of health was a condition precedent to admissibility, and that a proper evidentiary predicate is necessary.

In *State v. Fairleigh*, 490 So.2d 490 (La.App. 4 Cir. 1986), the State failed to show strict adherence to promulgated methods and procedures of chemical analysis in arriving at blood test results. Thus, the State was precluded from offering such results in evidence at a trial where defendant was charged with causing the death of another while operating a motor vehicle under the influence of alcoholic beverages. The evidence revealed that the person who withdrew the blood sample from the defendant was not identified by her full name, and was not established to be a physician or doctor of medicine or otherwise qualified to withdraw the blood sample from the defendant. Further, no evidence was introduced to show that replicate analysis was performed in accordance with applicable regulations.

A Florida appellate court also reversed a conviction where a "high probability" existed that the blood sample's integrity was compromised due to noncompliance with state regulations. *Rafferty v. State*, 799 So.2d 243 (Fla. 2001).

Inquiry

- What is the procedure in your state for obtaining blood for alcohol analysis according to the statute?
- Were the procedures outlined in the state statute followed to the letter?
- Is the person who collected the blood identified fully and properly?
- Did the person who collected the blood sign the vials and all packing forms?
- What are the person's qualifications, insofar as drawing blood?
- What is the educational background or certification of competency of the person who tested the sample?
- Who are *all* the people who handled the evidence from the time of the blood draw until analysis and written reports were completed?

- Was the blood *always* under lock and key to assure no tampering occurred, or was the evidence in an unlocked refrigerator or in a police car for some period of time?

18.5 Breath Tests and Blood Alcohol Concentration

Statutes in some states specify blood alcohol concentration (BAC) because the subject of the inquiry in a DUI prosecution is *blood* alcohol levels. Most states have enacted other laws that specifically proscribe impaired driving by virtue of a *breath* alcohol test. Usually, these dual standards are found within the definitional section of the state's criminal laws. Most tests on defendants are made on breath alcohol concentration (BrAC) due to the convenience and instant results obtained when measuring breath alcohol. In the United States, a standard conversion (partition) ratio of 2,100:1 has been used to estimate BAC based on BrAC (Wade, 1990; Dubowski, 1961).

Statutes have erroneously assumed that the same partition ratio applies to everyone. Scientific studies have shown ACTUAL partition ratios to be as low as 1,100:1 and higher than 2,700:1. A true average for all persons may more accurately be stated at 2,300:1 and 2,350:1. All breath testing devices used in America *assume* that the test subject's breath will be *exactly* 2,100 times greater than the concentration of alcohol in the person's blood. Statutes also erroneously assume that alcohol is absorbed and eliminated at identical rates by every person, when *in vivo* testing thoroughly refutes this assumption. (See Chapters 8 and 12 for current breath alcohol standards).

Basic human physiology renders this "legal" assumption erroneous. First, the ratio used for breath testing devices is set most closely to a *male* standard than a female. Hence, the machine is biased slightly against females, on average. Second, a person's ratio *changes*, sometimes radically over the course of a typical long day for a person drinking alcohol at night after a day at work. Thus, any "fixed" ratio that the law mandates is nothing more than a legal fiction to help facilitate the use of breath testing devices.

The function of the stomach is digestion. Absorption of alcohol into the bloodstream takes place primarily in the small intestines. Only 5 to 20 percent of the alcohol consumed by an individual is absorbed in the mouth, esophagus and stomach (Fitzgerald, 1999). Not until the food is digested is it emptied into the intestines, where the remainder of the alcohol is absorbed into the bloodstream.

The time it takes the stomach to digest its contents depends, in part, on the kind of food eaten; carbohydrates are digested fairly rapidly; protein takes longer; and fat may take up to twenty hours (Davenport, 1971). In addition, trauma, such as may result from an accident and possibly even stress from being arrested, can cause a detainee's stomach to retain its contents for hours or even days.

Once in the body, alcohol is eliminated primarily through several stages of metabolic breakdown in the liver. A person's rate of elimination will vary based upon numerous factors. Most individuals eliminate from 0/.04 g/dL to 0.006 g/dL BAC per hour (Wade, 1990; Bogusz, 1961). Many police training courses and state breath testing manuals teach that the "standard" average rate of elimination is .015 percent per hour (Wade, 1990). Thus, it may take some people more than twice as long as the "average" to eliminate the same quantity of alcohol. In addition, food that was consumed before or with the alcohol can affect elimination of alcohol as well as its rate of absorption into the bloodstream.

Consequently, any significant delay between the driving incident and BAC measurement typically will render the result meaningless as far as ascertaining the *true* BAC *at the time driving occurred*. Despite some statutory language stating that a BAC measurement made within two or three hours of an incident is "competent" evidence to prove that a subject was driving with an unlawful blood alcohol level at the time of arrest, there is *no scientific support* for the assumption that a later BAC reveals the BAC at the time of the incident.

On the "traditional" or common law impaired driving charge, the issue of the person's BAC level at the time of driving is *always* relevant. The defense will need its own expert witness to challenge the states offer of proof. See *Mata v. State*, 46 S.W.3d 902 (Tx.Crim.App., 2001). These statutes are—once again—merely a statutory "fudging" to give prosecutors an edge in obtaining convictions at trial.

Case law

Case law in many jurisdictions requires that expert testimony be used to "extrapolate" (give an educated guess) of the BAC level *at the time of driving*. Case law in other states has excused the prosecution of any such proof, thereby making the job of the prosecutor much easier.

In *Desmond v. Superior Court*, 179 P.2d 1261 (Ariz. 1986), the Arizona Supreme Court held that some evidence relating the BAC to the time of driving must supplement the breath test results.

In *State v. Ladwig*, 434 N.W.2d 594 (S.D. 1989), the Supreme Court of South Dakota held that, absent evidence enabling the jury to related test results back to the time of driving, blood test results do not constitute sufficient evidence to support conviction.

The highest courts of other states have taken a contrary position. Even where undisputed evidence exists that the driver's BAC was *lower than* the *per se* limit at the time of driving, if the results obtained at a subsequent blood or breath test reveals a BAC over the legal limit, the *per se* charge can be supported. *cf. Bohannon v. State*, 497 S.E.2d 552 (Ga.1998).

Inquiry

* What time was the client stopped and taken into custody?
* What time was the blood or breath sample taken?
* How much time lapsed between the client's arrest and when the blood or breath sample was taken?
* What did the client say to the arresting officer about "number" of drinks?
* What was the drinking "pattern" of the client?
* Did the arresting officer gather any such evidence relating to the time of drinking before or after arrest?
* What was the chronology of the drinking and food intake?
* If an accident is involved, did the client have *any opportunity* to consume alcohol *after* driving ended? (Remember, the state must *prove* all elements of each offense.)

Note: Obtain from the client a complete listing of his or her dietary intake within the twenty-four hours before the arrest. Food mixes with and slows down the rate of absorption of alcohol. Depending on when, what, and how much the client had eaten prior to and during drinking, tremendous variations in the shape of a client's BAC curve and the client's peak (highest) BAC level can be expected.

18.6 Limitations of Breath Testing Devices

This chapter is not intended to provide a full training course for all breath test devices. Whole books and multi-day training courses on specific breath testing devices are a good place to learn much more about these evidential analysis devices. For a listing of courses and written materials relating to these topics, see www.duiseminars.com or www.ncdd.com/sessions for details on programs restricted to *defense attorney* training.

The author has developed a checklist of potential challenges to breath tests. The list covers a variety of defenses or strategies. Not all defenses are applicable to every device, or for every test subject, or in every state (due to pro-prosecution laws designed to eliminate certain defenses).

In the United States and Canada (as well as numerous other countries in Europe), the following breath testing machine (instruments) are currently in use.

* **Intoxilyzer® 5000**. The most widely used breath testing device in America in 2003, having held that position since the mid-1980s. Older models, such as the "64 series," have been phased out. The subsequent generation, the "66 series" is still in use in several states in 2003, but has now been replaced with one of three newer models. The 64 and 66 series had only three filters (to help the device identify SOME possible interfering substances). The "68 series" originally reached the market around 1992. The original version (the "68-00" series) was the first five-filter device made by CMI. IN 1998, a new edition of the "68" series, the "68-01" or "68EN" series was created. This new "68" has been so radically changed from the 68-00 devices that a new cover and case had

to be manufactured to house the unit. New solenoids, a new breath path, a new bio-directional printer and a more reliable light source (as opposed to the "instant on" source in the 68-00) are some of its features (See Figure 8.5, Chapter 8 and Figure 18.1).

- **Intoxylizer® 8000**. The CMI's latest attempt to keep its market share by creating a duel wavelength device (against the Drager® 7110 and the Intoximeter® EC-IR). This eight-filter device checks for alcohol at two wavelengths. Florida and other states began approving these devices in 2002 and 2003 (see Figure 8.7).

- **Drager® 7110**. German manufacturer's dual wavelength device that checks (verifies) that alcohol is being detected at two wavelengths (at the 3.4-micron range and at the 9.5-micron range). This device also is equipped with a breath temperature adjustment capability in order to help avoid arguments of possible "elevated" breath temperatures. However, in the USA, only Alabama has implemented the temperature adjustment feature as of April 2003. New Jersey, New York, and other states have embraced the Drager as their breath-testing instrument, but have opted to *not* use some of its innovative "reliability" functions (see Figure 8.14).

- **BAC Datamaster.®** Manufactured by National Patent in Mansfield, Ohio, these devices have been in use for about twenty years. Using a quartz prism and a folded breath path with reflective surfaces (to lengthen the path for analysis), this single-wavelength device is in use in South Carolina, Ohio, Arkansas, California and the state of Washington, to name a few (see Figure 8.3).

- **Intoximeter® EC-IR**. Used in Tennessee, Wisconsin and other states, this device utilizes infrared (IR) analysis (from the former Intoxilyzer 3000 device) and a fuel detector analyzer that "counts" molecules of ethanol on an electronically charged plate (EC). The technology utilized is old, but this is the only currently available breath-testing device using two different forms of analysis (see Figure 8.9).

Because many defense attorneys lack adequate scientific training or experience at trial fighting breath tests, the author has put together a brief checklist of ways to challenge breath tests. This list

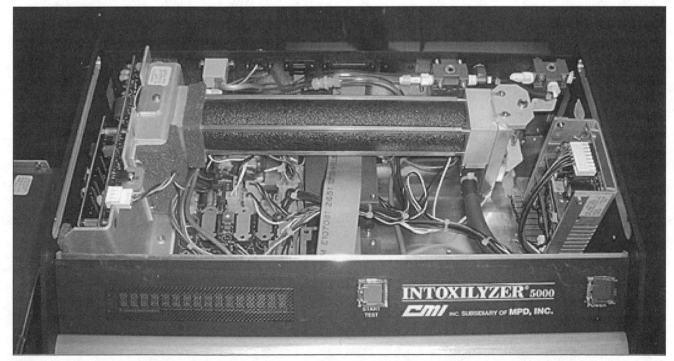

Figure 18.1 *Intoxilyzer 5000 (cutaway)*

is merely a suggestion and is not intended to be exhaustive.

Breath testing devices currently in use in America share several common characteristics:

- All have onboard computers that are capable of recording a wide range of operational data. This data can be analyzed and evaluated by the state (and defense counsel) if the state uses readily available software to gain access to this vital information. Failure to do this is tantamount to destruction of potentially exculpatory evidence.
- All devices are subject to "contamination" by mouth alcohol that can come from a burp, gastric reflux, denture adhesives or foreign objects in the mouth cavity.
- All devices are subject to possible "RFI" (radio frequency interference) that can be generated from police radio equipment, telephones. Pagers or nearby electromagnetic fields created by a variety of different types of equipment (microwaves, copy machines, computers, walkie-talkies, elevator motors, electric jail door latches and closure motors and so forth).
- All devices can be fitted with a "simulator" (see Figure 8.2). The simulator can be a "wet-bath" simulator or a "dry gas" simulator. A simulator is nothing more or less than a reference to a known "standard" to check to see if the machine is properly calibrated. A typical wet-bath simulator is a peanut-jar sized glass container with a sealed lid. Inside it has a rudimentary heating element, a thermometer and a stirrer. A mixture of de-ionized (or distilled water) and ethyl alcohol is poured into the "jar," which is sealed and started (see Figure 8.2). When properly heated, stirred (mixed) and assuming that the "known alcohol concentration" solution inside is really at the *true* value being tested, the simulator's vapor solution can be checked along *with each test subject's* sample, to assure that the device is operating correctly. Some states use this in *every* test (e.g., Colorado) and others *never* use it on arrestee's tests (e.g., Georgia).
- All breath-testing devices need periodic maintenance and re-calibration. These functions are most often performed at the factory, but some states have opted to establish in-state repair and maintenance facilities. Records of all repairs, parts replacements and re-calibration work should be maintained by your state breath test instrument agency charged with upkeep.
- Beyond repairs and re-calibration, periodic "calibration checks" are required to be done by all states based on concepts of "due process". Since breath tests are given a "shortcut" legal foundation by each state legislature, the state must put into place some reasonable plan for assuring that the devices work correctly. Plans vary widely from state to state in their "due process" characteristics.

18.7 Fifty Potential Challenges to Breath Tests

1. Manifestations and actions of defendant don't match test (use third party witnesses to establish the contrary facts).
2. Officer untrained or marginally trained and cannot explain anything about how breath testing works.
3. Officer fails to follow breath test training manual protocol, just like a cook not following a recipe or a doctor skipping steps in performing an operation.
4. Officer fails to follow own training protocol from breath test school (e.g., not waiting the fifteen- or twenty-minute deprivation period).
5. Defendant has a physical problem or health limitation, which officer did not ask about or request alternative type test (e.g., emphysema, dentures and spongy adhesives adhering them in subject's mouth and so on).
6. Testing room or circuitry has a problem (RFI; recently painted walls or trim; certain cleaning solutions, smoking in or near machine; shared power supply with heater or other appliance—must be dedicated "clean" electrical source; machine may have been "malfunctioning").
7. Defendant has had environmental exposure to volatile chemicals and will have cumulative reading of any ethanol plus readings from these other volatiles. (See *National Law Journal*, New

drunken-driving defense causes a stir, April 18, 1988, p. 7.)

8. Defendant unable to blow sufficient sample due to lung capacity or size, respiratory health or high alcohol level (e.g., many Intoxilyzer 5000 machines are equipped with pressure switches and require sufficient *time, pressure* and a proper *"slope"* of the alcohol curve to deliver a valid reading).

9. Improper or inadequate inspections by state inspectors (example: no linearity proven, or single tests being run at the target alcohol concentrations).

10. Use of machine after factory repair is made but before new calibration check is done by inspector or breath instrument supervisor at police department site.

11. Air bag defenses—"the Tyndall effect"—diffusion of light; propellant exposure; cut lips; lung and airway irritation and fluid buildup from caustic gas propellant. See *DWI Journal: Law & Science,* vol. 15, No. 10, October 2000.)

12. Videotape refutes the high reading, supports sobriety, based on voice, demeanor and ability to perform field tests reasonably well.

13. High test result, yet defendant never urinates for three to four hours or more—physiological impossibility [*Young v. City of Brookhaven,* 693 So. 2d 1355 (Miss. 1997)].

14. Unintentional alcohol, from Nyquil®, Vicks Formula 44®, lip balms, toothache drops, chewing gum and so on. (Some states have legislated away this defense.)

15. Something in person's mouth containing alcohol (ex: Breath Drops® with SD alcohol).

16. Something in mouth that contains interfering or contaminating substance (Skoal® snuff—wintergreen; Altoids® curiously strong mints).

17. Dentures, gingivitis, bridgework, "pockets" (video or photo of this and dental records).

18. Vomiting, belching within fifteen to twenty minutes of test and no rinsing of mouth permitted, or inadequate deprivation period before retest is started.

19. Insufficient observation period, as per breath test training manual (some states—Tennessee for example—say error excludes test; others—Georgia, among them—say goes to weight and credit).

20. Actual improper or out of "agreement" tests, without follow-up tests to correct (e.g., both results must be within 0.02 of each other, as per the law of many jurisdictions).

21. Police report supports sobriety, or lack of investigation of alternative causes.

22. Rising BAC showing time of driving BAC would have been lower than time of testing (if available in your state).

23. Elevated breath temperature caused by fever, hot tub, sauna, detention in hot sun or back of patrol car in summer, dancing, menstrual cycle, menopause (hot flashes) and so forth (only Drager and the Intoxilyzer 8000 are *supposed* to catch this). (See newsletter, *International Association for Chemical Testing,* vol. 9, number 2, July 1998 for article explaining the state of Alabama's inhouse testing of random subjects that proved the Intoxilyzer 5000 produced significant error due to inability to adjust to the subjects' body temperature variations.)

24. Failure to verify simulator temperature remains constant and within tolerance; otherwise, results cannot be accurate. (See recommendations of The National Safety Council, Traffic Safety Division, Subcommittee on Technology's *NSC/CAOD Simulator Solution Guidelines,* 10/25/1989.)

25. Assumed breath-blood ratio (2,100:1) not proven to be defendant's ratio; show how minor error gets multiplied by an algorithm of 1,000 to 3,000, depending on type of machine used. Example: on an Intoxilyzer 5000, an indicated 0.12 result, if accurate, contains only 17/10,000,000th of an ounce. The algorithm for the Intoxilyzer results in a multiplier of 2,592 (derived from the 81-cc size of the sample chamber as compared to 210 liters of air). Any minor error can skew results dramatically. (Some states have case law or statutes that eliminate this defense.)

26. Show defendant has abnormally *low* blood or breath conversion ratio through testing or experts. (Some states have case law or statutes that eliminate this defense.)

27. If BatMOBILE, wiring issues and electrical configuration; AC/DC issues; low voltage spikes; police radios inside the van (like a BB bouncing around inside a boxcar).

28. No proper periodic calibration checks using quantities of commonly occurring interfering substances (e.g., toluene, acetone, acetaldehyde) likely found in a living subject, to assure machine's ability to distinguish alcohol from other volatiles.

29. Improper or incomplete computer data or breath technicians use secret "function key" tests to *hide* error reports, to assure that faults of the device do not get recorded (e.g., as was being done by the state of Arizona's breath testing program in the year 2000 and subsequent years; see *State v. Hentges,* CV-01-0311-SA, where 1,400 breath test cases were dropped by Arizona courts due to the State's manipulation and "hiding" of error reports for the Intoxilyzer 5000).

30. Burp, belch that is silent (client may need to testify here).

31. Gastric reflux or hiatal hernia, preferably diagnosed and treated before arrest occurred (bring the "scope" photos taken during endoscopic surgery by a physician).

32. Officer refuses to permit second, independent test sought by defendant, or at the chosen test location or by physician of defendant's choice. *Joel v. State*, 538 S.E.2d 847 (Ga.App. 2000). *State v. Braunecker*, 566 S.E.2d 409 (Ga.App. 2002).

33. Mouthpiece not examined (plastic extrusion blocking tube eliminates or refutes refusal).

34. Certified pre-mix or laboratory-mixed simulator solutions not kept for subsequent re-analysis, to assure accuracy of mixture.

35. Random vials of simulator solutions not checked by GC-mass spec analysis upon receipt from company that sells them, therefore, no assurance of precision for target alcohol concentrations.

36. Inherent "sampling variability" or "margin of error" issues (e.g., 0.088 reading in an 0.08 state, and manual acknowledges ± 0.01 or ± 0.02 precision problem).

37. Blowing pattern irregularities (blubbering and crying causing artificially high water vapor problem; mucus buildup from a cold, sinus infection can trap alcohol and increase BrAC).

38. Prosecutor fails to lay a proper evidentiary foundation for admission of the test. *Mullinax v. State*, 499 S.E.2d 903 (Ga.App. 1998).

39. Defendant on strict high protein diet, then ingests carbohydrates, thereby triggering auto-generated alcohol production when ketones (accumulated from the diet) are converted to isopropyl alcohol (some state statutes prohibit alcohol being in the person's system *by any means*—e.g., Wisconsin—whereas others provide that the impairment must come from "alcohol ingested before the driving ending"—e.g., Georgia).

40. Discovery not provided in a timely or complete manner; results excluded. *Kyles v. Whitley*, 514 U.S. 419 (1995).

41. Failure to give timely, complete or "correct" (e.g., failed to read the correct warning for a minor) implied consent warning. No matter how high the test results, the test must be excluded. *Daniel v. State,* 488 S.E.2d 129 (Ga.App. 1997); *Kitchens v. State,* 574 S.E.2d 451 (Ga.App. 2003). *Also see* the landmark case of *Nelson v. City of Irvine,* 143 F.3d 1196 (9th Cir. 1998), where officers were requesting blood, rather than giving the California arrestees the *option* of asking for blood, as mandated by California's implied consent law.

42. Defendant has diabetes, is "borderline" diabetic or is hypoglycemic and consumes alcohol in *any* amount, causing conversion of high acetone levels into isopropyl alcohol.

43. Officer obtains first set of BAC results, which will not support a *per se* case, then waits a few more minutes and retests, obtaining a reading *above* the *per se* limit—illegal.

44. Officer gives implied consent, but then goes too far by threatening dire license suspension issues for which there is no factual basis (misstating consequences or misleading the test subject about his or her options). Officer gives implied consent, but then makes improper, coercive statement to subject, thereby obtaining the test result by violating the law. *State v. Boger*, 559

S.E.2d 176 (Ga. 2002); *State v. Leviner*, 443 S.E.2d 688 (Ga.App. 1994).

45. State fails to prove that results were obtained with the statutorily imposed time limit (typically, two or three hours after driving ended). *Yarbrough v. State*, 527 S.E.2d 628 (Ga.App. 2000).

46. State fails to prove the alcohol was consumed either *during* driving or *before* driving ended (most states).

47. State fails to prove *venue*, beyond a reasonable doubt. *Jones v. State,* 537 S.E.2d 80 (Ga. 2000).

48. Officer fails to get his or her annual or periodic updates in training, thereby disqualifying the test operator from administering tests.

49. In handling case, officer commits crime (e.g., obstruction of justice or perjury) in an effort to conceal evidence; prosecutor cannot proceed to trial *or* (more commonly) makes an illegal, warrantless stop or arrests person without probable cause.

50. "FIRD" defense. Officer gets fired, indicted, retires (and moves away) or dies (from DUI defense guru Reese Joye of North Charleston, SC).

18.8 Intravenous Blood Samples

Typically, a sample of blood is drawn and tested for alcohol content in two DUI/DWI situations: when requested by law enforcement officers in connection with a suspected drunk driving case, or at the request of hospital medical personnel in connection with diagnosis and treatment of a patient who has been brought in after an accident. In the former situation, the blood is sometimes referred to as "legal blood" and whole blood is typically collected; in the latter, it is sometimes called "medical blood" and is typically serum. The methods used to draw, prepare, track, and test *legal* blood often differ from those used for *medical* blood.

A strong argument exists that serum blood samples, due to the problems with accuracy, show lack of trustworthiness as forensic evidence of the actual blood alcohol reading of a patient. Firstly, every individual has a different serum or whole-blood ratio that varies from 1.90 to 1.35 (Frajola, 1993). Furthermore, an arbitrary or average conversion ratio does not give an accurate result for a particular individual.

Second, when medical staffers draw "legal" blood, they follow procedures promulgated specifically for blood alcohol testing. Often, state regulations or statutes will specify a particular type of "kit" that has alcohol-free swabs in the package, as well as a series of labels, seals, and "packing" forms to assure that all necessary steps are taken to obtain a sample that can be admitted in evidence.

In order to challenge the admissibility of a "legal" blood sample into evidence, the attorney must question the medical personnel involved to determine whether the blood was drawn and tested in compliance with state regulations. The defense attorney should also determine whether the regulations that were designed to ensure accuracy and reliability were followed. These regulations often specify that the vials shall contain anticoagulant and a preservative and be "stopped" and capped (or sealed) to prevent loss of contents through evaporation. These tamper-proof seals also will reveal any tampering with or compromise of the vials. Also, some jurisdictions mandate that all vials be marked with certain essential tracking information. Regulations or statutes may even specify the method of cleansing the subject's skin before blood is drawn (i.e., with soap or Betadine, not alcohol).

Blood vials that are to be used for *legal* samples generally contain an anticoagulant and a preservative, and generally have a gray-colored septum (indicating that vials have these two chemicals inside the vacuum tube). Other vials, used for various medical or laboratory purposes, may have red, yellow, purple or other colors signifying whether the vial contains certain chemicals.

Vials used in collecting medical blood samples may *lack anticoagulant and preservatives*. These vials generally have red septums, meaning that the blood collected is pure blood without anticoagulant or preservative added to the vial. A red-stoppered vial will become clotted (due to lack of an anticoagulant) and will "deteriorate" much more quickly than those with gray stoppers, due to lack of a preservative.

The attorney should ascertain the condition of the tube used, because an improperly capped or filled tube may result in an incorrect BAC value. If the hospital (or police) sends blood to an outside private lab or the state crime laboratory for testing, counsel should check to see if the blood was continuously refrigerated, because the red-stoppered vials used by hospitals typically lack preservatives, and the alcohol content in the sample might actually increase if left at room temperature for an extended period of time (Kaye, 1980). Jurors are shocked to learn that normal blood (with no alcohol in it at all) that decomposes actually *creates* ethyl alcohol as a by-product of the decomposition.

The party seeking to admit a blood alcohol result into evidence usually does so by introducing the hospital record that contains the result. Different states have varying rules of evidence concerning when and how such result may be admitted into evidence. Some jurisdictions have passed laws to permit abbreviated proof of blood technician's credentials without putting the witness on the stand at trial. Uniform Evidence Code section 803(6) allows information kept in the course of a regularly conducted business activity to be admitted as an exception to the hearsay rule when authenticated by the records custodian. However, there is one significant exception to the admissibility of a business record. A business record is not admissible when the "sources of information or other circumstances show *lack of trustworthiness.*"

Through use of expert witnesses, the party opposing the admission of blood test evidence should attempt to bring out evidence of the unreliability of the blood test results in the current case. First and foremost, emphasize that every individual has a different serum or whole-blood ratio and the use of an arbitrary or average conversion ratio does not give accurate results for a particular individual. If an incorrect color cap was used on a vial, or if an anticoagulant or preservative was omitted, this may offer "reasonable doubt" about the integrity of the blood test results, particularly if gaps exist in the chain of custody.

During a 1995 visit to an Atlanta-area hospital, the author checked the lab technician's Vacutainer® vials. The hospital was using vials that were out of date. The vials that were being used in August of 1995 had expired in April of 1995 (see photocopy of

actual vial, Figure 18.2). Almost all blood collection vials have an expiration date. Manufacturers claim that this is only relevant to the warranty on the vacuum within the vial. Jurors may see the issue differently, if defense counsel analogizes to milk or bread sold after an expiration date.

Inquiry

- Who requested the sample and for what purpose?
- Did the suspect actually "consent" to the test?
- What type of vial was the specimen collected in?
- Was the vial properly capped, and with what color cap?
- Did the vial have a preservative in it?
- Did the vial have an anticoagulant in it?

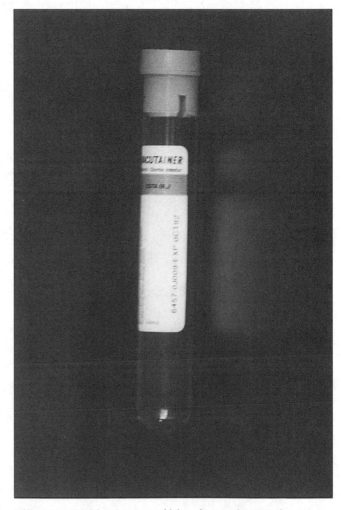

Figure 18.2 *Photocopy of blood-sampling vial, showing expirartion date*

- Was the vial continuously refrigerated after the sample was collected?
- What is the expiration date on the vial?
- Was the suspect given all proper implied consent advisements?

18.9 Blood Sample Kits

The blood testing regulations of your state may require that only a certain kind of blood kit may be used. The defendant may have been taken to a hospital or medical center where a "regulation" kit was not used. In the event this happens, you should move to suppress the test results, based on unreliability and noncompliance with quality assurance regulations.

In addition, sealing and labeling the ampoule immediately after collection is essential to proving "chain of custody." Look carefully at the handwriting on the vials to see if the nurse or phlebotomist marked the vials. In some cases, the police officer gets overzealous and performs functions that the certified blood drawer is *required* by law to perform. Check all state and federal guidelines concerning proper procedures for labeling and sealing a sample.

Case law

In *Wilson v. State*, 536 A.2d 1192 (Md.App. 1988), the court held that testimony by the technician that she drew blood using the "legal alcohol police kit" sufficiently linked the blood sample to the actual kit used in taking the sample.

Inquiry

- Does your state require that a "regulation" blood kit be used?
- Was the "regulation" blood kit used?
- Are the kit and the various "seals" still available for inspection?
- Was the sample sealed and marked properly so that a chain of custody can be established?
- What is the expiration date on the contents of the kit?
- Who provided the kit—the police or the hospital?
- What does the kit manufacturer say about inverting the vials to mix the blood and the chemicals contained in the vial? (Some say to gently invert—not shake—the vials ten to fifteen times. Look at the written insert in the kits used in your state.)

18.10 Contamination

A problem might occur with the contamination of the specimen. For example, the antiseptic used to cleanse the area may contain alcohol in amounts sufficient to produce measurable amounts of alcohol on a gas chromatograph. In emergency room settings, it is routine to use an alcohol-based antiseptic to clean the skin. It may also be routine to use Vacutainers and vials that are *not* in compliance with state regulations and statutes.

Any antiseptic that was provided in blood alcohol collection kits (or otherwise used to draw blood specimens) should be analyzed by an independent laboratory to determine whether the antiseptic contains alcohol in sufficient amounts to produce measurable amounts of alcohol. While many jurisdictions have regulations and procedures governing blood testing, and despite the fact that most specifically prohibit using any alcohol solution as a skin cleanser, some of the swabs that are used in blood collection kits contain a substance known as benzalkonium chloride as an active ingredient. This compound contains approximately 2 percent or more ethanol concentration (Taylor, 2000; Nichols, 1990).

Ethanol in measurable quantities also has been found in three types of disinfectants: Clinipad® brand antiseptic towelette, PDI® brand towelette and Triad® brand towelettes (Taylor, 2000). Swabbing the skin with ethanol before taking a blood sample for measuring blood ethanol concentration may increase the apparent blood ethanol level by up to 0.018 percent (g/dL) (Nichols, 1990), even if the skin is allowed to dry before the sample is taken. When a "wet" site is used, and a "wet" swab is held over the site to withdraw the needle (which has a vacuum to draw in the blood from the suspect's vein), the potential additive effect is much greater.

Defense attorneys frequently succeed in convincing a jury that a percent of alcohol that was found in the blood sample was added to the test result because the person who withdrew the blood improperly used alcohol on the skin. In one jury trial, for example, the questioning went as follows (Heise, 1959).

Q. Doctor, suppose just one drop of alcohol was added to 100 drops of normal blood, what percentage of alcohol would you find?

A. If the drop of alcohol were the same size as a drop of blood, I would expect to find 1.0 percent by volume, or 0.80 percent by weight.

Q. What state of intoxication would you expect to find with 0.80 percent alcohol in the blood?

A. That person would be dead.

Q. Now, if only half a drop of alcohol was added to the 100-drop sample, what would you expect to find in the blood test?

A. Approximately 0.40 percent by weight.

Q. And what stage of intoxication would that percent correspond?

A. Marked intoxication, probably unconsciousness.

Q. Now supposed that one one-tenth drop of alcohol got into the 100 drops of blood, how would that affect the blood test?

A. The reading would be approximately 0.08 percent.

The attorney then successfully argued to the jury that a mere fraction of a drop of extraneous alcohol that had been applied to the skin had been responsible for a possible miscarriage of justice, and his client was acquitted.

The blood taken from a DUI suspect involved in an accident may also be contaminated if there was an intravenous fluid being administered at the time the blood was drawn. The specimen may be inaccurate either because of the increased volume of fluid in the circulatory system changes the blood alcohol level (lowers it) or the blood may have been drawn from the same extremity that the IV is in and therefore the sample is contaminated with the intravenous fluids. If there was injury to the defendant, and the paramedics responded, it is very likely that an IV was started *en route* to the emergency room.

Contamination can also occur if the equipment used to draw the blood is not sterile (Taylor, 2000). This may not pose as big a problem today as it did years ago before pre-wrapped disposable needles became the standard. However, in some emergency room settings, nurses "set up" their trays and carts anticipating an emergency. That is, the needles have been removed from the package and placed on the table along with other routinely used items so that these items will be readily available when an emergency comes in. If this is the case, a needle or syringe may have been left exposed for an undetermined amount of time and is no longer sterile (Shilling, 1987). Check your state regulations concerning the propriety of using such items, in a non-sterile situation.

Case law

In *State v. Hanners*, 774 S.W.2d 568 (Mo.App. 1989), the trial court's order sustaining the motion to suppress was confirmed where the review of the transcript of the hearing revealed that an alcohol swab was used in the area from which blood was drawn. Also, while it was likely that the needle assembly used to draw the blood was sterile, this probability never ripened into fact because the medical personnel were never asked if the equipment used was sterile. Further, the container provided by the officer was also not proven to be sterile as required by the statute.

In *Kyhl v. Commonwealth*, 135 S.E.2d 768 (Sup.Ct.App.Va. 1964), the court held that in the absence of showing that the instrument used to withdraw blood was sterile, the prosecution had not met its burden.

In *State v. DeBerg*, 288 N.W.2d 348 (Iowa 1980), the court found that the state failed to carry its burden of proof that it complied with a statute requiring "only new, originally factor wrapped, disposable syringes and needles, kept under strictly sanitary and sterile conditions." The court would not infer that these conditions were met merely because the test was performed at a hospital.

In *Gibson v. State*, 503 So.2d 230 (Miss. 1987), the court held that testimony by the nurse drawing the blood was sufficient to establish that there was no contamination where she stated that she "regularly used iodine as a skin preparation prior to collection of a blood sample for the police, *being aware of the need to avoid an alcohol-based mixture*."

Inquiry

- Was alcohol used to cleanse the site?
- Was a towelette or chemical used which contains alcohol?
- Was the area cleansed *at all*?
- Whether intravenous fluids were infusing when the blood was drawn. If so, where was the intravenous catheter located and from what location was the blood drawn?
- What types of fluids were infusing?
- Whether the equipment was taken from its sterile package and "set up" in advance?

18.11 Plasma or Serum Blood or Whole Blood

To challenge a serum blood alcohol result, attorneys must know the differences between whole and serum (or plasma) blood readings. The admissibility of a blood alcohol test as evidence at trial will depend on the specific language of the relevant state statute and on the ability of the attorney opposing the test result to identify all the ways in which it is unreliable. In some states (i.e., Georgia) no published regulation controls how serum or plasma blood readings will be "adjusted" to reflect approximate whole blood alcohol levels.

A potential source of error involves reporting plasma or serum values that are assumed to be whole blood values. The defense attorney should try to discover whether whole blood, serum or plasma was analyzed. Some studies indicate that plasma and serum alcohol levels are as much as 16 to 21 percent higher than whole blood levels (Taylor, 2000; Fitzgerald, 1999).

After the blood is drawn, it is often centrifuged (spun in a mechanical device) and separated into its "solid" and "liquid" components for analysis (Taylor, 2000). What is being analyzed by the toxicology lab may *not* be whole blood, but serum or plasma and, therefore, an analysis of plasma or serum will produce a higher percentage of alcohol than would actually be present in whole blood. Hence, the results must be mathematically "adjusted" or truncated to show the approximate true BAC.

Some police departments and state forensic laboratories analyze whole blood. Many hospitals and clinical laboratories routinely analyze only se-

rum. Evidence of a client's blood alcohol level indicating a result of 0.10 percent (g/dL) BAC may, in fact, reflect a true BAC of 0.08 to 0.09 g/dL if serum was used (Winek et al., 1987).

In addition to the distorted reading, the testing may be challenged on the grounds that a serum alcohol concentration test is not a blood test for the purposes of the statute. Therefore, carefully review the chemical sobriety test statutes and definition sections of the criminal code.

Case law

In *Commonwealth v. Wanner*, 605 A.2d 805 (Pa.Super. 1992), State's evidence of defendants intoxication based upon test performed on defendants blood plasma, and not on whole blood was insufficient to support convictions for driving while under the influence of alcohol. Statutes prohibiting driving under the influence of alcohol require blood alcohol count from *whole* blood, and results from tests performed on blood plasma will not suffice.

Inquiry

- Does the statute specify "whole blood" or "serum?"
- Was the proper component of blood tested?
- If the "type" test is not shown in the state's reports, can you obtain a sample of the blood for independent analysis?
- Is there a second vial of blood still sealed, from which you can seek an independent analysis of whole blood?

18.12 Variations in Blood Testing

Due to variations in body chemistry plus the chemical changes that the blood undergoes while in the glass ampoules, the specimens may become unrepresentative of the person accused. The difference is due to what occurs *in vivo* (those which occur inside the body) and *in vitro* (those which occur while the blood is in glass ampoules). *In vivo* changes occur because of normal fluctuations in the blood from moment to moment after the blood's ability to hold and release alcohol (Chang et al., 1984).

It is not an uncommon practice to let the blood specimen sit for days before analyzing it due to delay in getting it to the laboratory, or due to simple neglect. Because the carousels on most gas chromatographs hold fifty or 100 vials, many laboratories wait until a full carousel can be obtained before running the tests. Defense counsel may be surprised to learn how long a sample was not refrigerated.

Because blood is an organic material, it will decompose as a result of enzyme activity and bacterial action. One of the results of this decomposition is that ethyl alcohol is *created from* the breakdown of the blood. This is sometimes referred to as "endogenous" alcohol production. In a sample originally containing *no alcohol*, decomposition can cause an alcohol content reading of 0.25 g/dL or even higher depending on the stage of decay (Taylor, 2000).

Usually the specimen will be refrigerated to prevent degradation of the sample. However, refrigeration will only *slow down* the decomposition process, not prevent it. To stop this decaying of the blood and the resultant formation of alcohol, a preservative such as sodium fluoride solution should be added. Blood without sodium fluoride is reliable at normal room temperature for about two days. Without sodium fluoride, the BAC may rise to a maximum concentration in about fifteen days and then fall (Kaye, 1980).

Failure to add sodium fluoride or potassium oxalate (and this is not uncommon) should provide counsel with sufficient ammunition to discredit the test results, if not prevent their admission into evidence. In a criminal trial, *raising reasonable doubt* only requires that a sufficient factual basis for questioning the reliability and accuracy of the test results be raised by the defense.

18.13 Medication and Disease

Certain medications and the "disease process" can affect the level of BAC. Any medication that alters the rate of metabolism can affect blood alcohol levels. For example, an article in the *Canadian Society of Forensic Science Journal* has reported that women taking oral contraceptives appear to eliminate ethanol significantly faster than women not taking oral contraceptives (Papple, 1982). Also, *Candida albicans* is a yeast-based medical problem that can cause alcohol to be created *inside* the vial, after being drawn from the subject's arm.

The human body eliminates the amount of alcohol by oxidation of the "poison" (alcohol) in the liver. Like any other foreign compound, alcohol is broken down by enzymes in the liver and gradually reduced until 100 percent is eliminated. Therefore, any disease process affecting the liver, such as hepatitis, will impair results. Also, any condition that causes "extracellular" water retention (heart disease or many forms of high blood pressure or diabetes, for example) will alter results. Alcohol is "water miscible" meaning that it mixes easily with water. Alcohol also "migrates" to any water source, whether in the human body or in a test tube. Also, many women retain water on and around the time of menses. Therefore, defense counsel in the investigation of the case should obtain this information.

Inquiry

- Was the blood sample properly sealed?
- Did the vials remain in a police cruiser in an unrefrigerated condition?
- How long was the specimen left unrefrigerated?
- What was the temperature of the refrigerator where the specimen was stored?
- Was a preservative added to the specimen prior to its storage?
- What is the subject's medical history and medication history and was any abnormal condition present when the blood sample (or breath sample) was taken?

Note: a complete medical history should be obtained from your client. Information regarding illnesses and both prescribed and non-prescribed medications should be solicited. In cases where the test subject has a significant medical history, an expert witness should be consulted to determine the effect of the person's history on the indicated BAC results. Many cases can be won using an expert to explain why the client was "not a proper subject" for breath or blood testing.

18.14 Chain of Custody

The State must also establish the proper chain of custody of its blood sample (Shilling, 1987). The American Medical Association has established certain procedures that must be used to insure the integrity of the samples and to insure an accurate analysis. Without an appropriate chain of custody, it will be difficult for the prosecution to establish that these appropriate and proper procedures were utilized.

Defense counsel should note, however, that the issue of the propriety of the chain of custody is a matter of "weight and credibility" for the trier of fact (judge or jury) to decide. Don't expect a trial judge to throw out a blood test at pretrial motion, no matter how questionable the chain of custody may be. *Swanson v. State,* 545 S.E.2d 713 (Ga.App. 2001).

For example, the chain of custody must establish that at various stages, not only was the blood sample obtained, but that an appropriate anticoagulant was added to the Vacutainer in order to prevent the sample from clotting inside the vial. In addition, the party proposing to use the sample must be able to prove that a preservative was added to prevent yeast growth that may cause the blood to ferment and to thereby increase the concentration of ethyl alcohol in the sample. Next, the party offering the blood test must show that the sample was stored in a cold or frozen condition to retard microbial action. Also, the state must be able to show that microorganisms were not allowed to grow, thereby inhibiting glycolysis and potentially affecting results.

The chain of custody should demonstrate not only *who* handled the blood sample, but also *how it was handled* and *for what purposes.* For example, the quantity of sodium fluoride, when used in the sample, can be reliably tested when stored *at room temperature* for only two days. On the other hand, if the sample is *refrigerated or frozen*, it may be reliably tested for a longer period of time. The trunk or glove compartment of an automobile is an unsatisfactory storage location for a blood sample, even for a short period of time.

In cross-examining state witnesses on chain of custody issues, reasonable doubt can be established if anyone who is not properly licensed or certified withdrew the sample, tested the sample, stored the sample, or took custody of the sample. Technically, a break in the chain of custody can occur at any time the sample is stored in a location that was accessible to an individual who is not a proper custodian for the sample. A serious chain of custody problem can result in a dismissal of all charges, or at least result in a verdict of acquittal. If the person who *analyzed* the blood is no longer available to come to court, the State may be unable to provide a proper evidentiary foundation to get the results admitted at trial.

Defense counsel should always use motions to exclude and should object to admission of test results without a complete showing of chain of custody, if only to establish a record for appeal. Usually, a number of individuals have handled the sample, including the arresting officer, the medical technician, nurse or physician, the transporting officer, a mail intake staff member at the crime lab, the individual in charge of labeling and refrigerating evidence at the laboratory, and or the state's laboratory technicians or chemists. Technically, a break in the chain of custody can occur at any time the sample is stored in a location accessible to individuals who are not proper custodians of the sample.

Counsel should consider subpoenaing each such individual who came in contact with the sample. However, defense counsel's strategy may be just the opposite: tell the jury that the state intends to prove the reliability of the blood sample by putting up only two of the seven people who handled or transported the blood. Let the "missing links" be your closing argument graphic in explaining why reasonable doubt exists concerning the BAC results being touted by the State.

Case law
In *State v. McDonald*, 697 P.2d 1328 (Mont. 1985), the Supreme Court of Montana held that the trial court erred in allowing into evidence a blood alcohol test report and testimony on the report without a proper foundation where the report did not contain the name or initials of the person who withdrew the blood for the purpose of determining the blood alcohol content. In the *McDonald* case, the officer could not recall the person who drew the blood sample at the hospital but only testified that she was wearing a tag that said "registered nurse."

In *State v. Williams*, 392 S.E.2d 181 (S.C. 1990), the chain of custody for defendant's blood test was rendered fatally defective by the fact that no one in the emergency room could identify the person who sealed and labeled the blood sample utilizing the defendant's patient number. Furthermore, neither the emergency room nor laboratory personnel could recall who transported the blood sample to the laboratory. Finally, the defendant's emergency room record was initially mislabeled as that of another person.

In *State v. Nygaard*, 426 N.W.2d 547 (N.D. 1988), the results of the blood alcohol test were inadmissible in a driving while intoxicated prosecution where the officer failed to seal the vial with one layer of tape and label the vial with the name of the subject. Moreover, no testimony was provided by the state to verify that the blood sample tested was the same blood collected from defendant.

In *People v. Sansalone*, 208 Misc. 491, 146 NYS 2d 359 (1955), the court held that blood alcohol evidence was inadmissible where the vial of blood was taken home by an officer, kept in his refrigerator overnight, and then mailed to the laboratory for analysis.

Compare *Sansalone* to *Gibson v. State*, 503 So.2d 230 (Miss. 1987), where the officer also took the sample home over the weekend and placed it in his refrigerator. There the court determined that his actions were an "instance of his dedication to his profession, properly preserving evidence for analysis, with no indication or reasonable inference of probable tampering, sufficient to break the chain of possession."

In some appellate courts, clear evidence of problems with a blood sample is ignored. For example, in *Lewis v. State*, 451 S.E.2d 116 (Ga.App. 1994), the intermediate appellate court found the chain proper when the technician drawing the blood testified that two samples were taken and placed in vials, one with a gray top and the other with a red top. The samples were then given to the officer who placed the samples in evidence locker number 19. An evidence technician testified that she removed the samples from locker 13 (not 19) and placed them in the refrigerator. Finally, the chemist who received the blood for testing said he received two vials, one with a gray stopper and the other with a yellow and black stopper. Despite these facts, the court determined that there was no evidence of tampering or broken chain of custody. Also, see *Swanson v. State*, 545 S.E.2d 713 (Ga.App. 2001).

Inquiry

- What "path" did the blood specimen take after leaving the hospital?
- How was the specimen delivered to the lab?
- Who received the specimen?
- Did the person who received the specimen "mark" the container or put his or her initials on it?
- Was a barcode assigned to the sample? By whom and when?
- Did *only* authorized personnel handle the blood?
- Where and how was the specimen stored prior to testing?
- If the specimen was stored in the refrigerator, was the refrigerator unlocked and accessible by unauthorized persons?
- Does the description of the vials (as testified to by the person who drew the blood) match the police officer's description? The laboratory's description? Color of the stoppers? What was written on the vials?
- How many "missing links" does the State have in its "chain"?

18.15 Destruction of Blood Samples after Discovery Request

In some states, the law relating to destruction of the State's samples after a defense request for preservation of the evidence for later independent analysis can result in exclusion of the State's chemical test results. *State v. Blackwell*, 537 S.E.2d 457 (Ga.App. 1997). See also *State v. Rains*, 735 N.E.2d 1 (Oh.App. 1999) and *People v. Newberry*, 652 N.E.2d 288 (Ill. 1995).

The landmark decision of the United States Supreme Court, *California v. Trombetta*, 467 U.S. 479 (1984), dealt with the issue of the state not preserving test evidence. In any case involving the state's destruction of a blood or breath test sample, re-read *Trombetta* carefully. California's law had a built-in protection for DUI suspects that most states do not: you have an absolute right to request blood, not breath tests, and at State expense. This assured that the defendant could make an independent analysis at a later time, if the 'blood' test option had been made. Your state's laws may violate due process laws, if similar protection of the "sample" is not available under your statutory scheme.

18.16 Documentation Errors

A source for locating possible chain of custody errors is in the paper trail of the laboratory. The defense attorney should try to establish the complete time line for the samples within the record, apart from what the technician or laboratory supervisors might say was done. The defense attorney must challenge each assertion and confirm what was done in the laboratory with the blood sample, and what occurred prior to the receipt of the sample by the testing facility. Errors in the chain of custody or testing protocol will be uncovered only by checking each item of evidence, including the vials that were used to collect the blood.

Case law

In *State v. Cribb*, 426 S.E.2d 306 (S.C. 1992), two nurses attended to defendant upon his admission to the emergency room. One of the nurses testified that the other nurse administered an intravenous (IV) solution to defendant and it was customary for blood to be drawn by the person administering the IV. The nurse who administered the IV did not recall drawing blood, but assumed she did when she started the IV because that was her standard procedure. The lab technician did not know who drew the defendant's blood or how it was transferred to the lab. Neither defendant's medical records nor the label on the blood sample disclosed the person who drew the sample and transported it to the lab. The evidence was suppressed.

Inquiry

- Do the records themselves reflect a careful handling of the sample?
- Does the record reflect a time, date and signature for the sample's minute-by-minute "passage" from initial blood draw, through testing and analysis, and then to its final destination in a locked and refrigerated storage unit?
- Does the record reflect how the test result was initially recorded and by whom? (Check all handwriting on all vials and documents)

- Does the medical record reflect the utilization of checklists and procedures or the omission of such procedures, which would increase the chance that false values might be reported due to mislabeling, careless reporting, confusion or switching samples?
- As to the internal procedures of the laboratory to assure reliability, does the record reflect what regular calibrations or checks were conducted on the equipment or chemicals used for the test?
- Does the lab meet federal NIDA standards? Does the lab have proof of periodic "proficiency" inspections by outside testing organizations?
- Did the hospital or its laboratory keep a ledger or log of all samples collected, including "time of the blood draw"?

18.17 Consent

In most cases, the defendant will be taken to a hospital to have his or her blood drawn. Medical records confidentiality statutes, or state physician-patient privilege statutes may provide confidentiality of medical records. Other states do not follow this rule, except for psychiatric records. Where confidentiality statutes exist, the police cannot obtain the results of the blood test unless the defendant signs a waiver form releasing the results to the police or a search warrant issued by a judge or magistrate is issued. If no such waiver is signed or no warrant exists, the defense may have a good argument for suppression of the results.

In 2000, the Georgia Supreme Court rendered a landmark ruling that extended a "right of privacy" to a person's "hospital" blood test results. In *King v. State*, 535 S.E.2d 492 (Ga. 2000), Georgia's highest court found that a patient had a "reasonable expectation of privacy" in the information contained therein. See *King v. State*, 577 S.E.2d 764 (Ga. 2003), where a different result was obtained once a search warrant for the blood was issued. Some states permit no exceptions to their physician-patient privilege. Other states have special conditions on its use. Check the statues in your jurisdiction.

Case law

In *State v. Cribb*, 426 S.E.2d 306 (S.C. 1992), the South Carolina Supreme Court held that the implied consent statute did not apply to a hospital patient suspected of being an intoxicated motorist whose blood sample was drawn for medical purposes *before* the patient was arrested. The officers went to the hospital to discuss the accident with the patient, but did not charge him with a crime. They met with the physician and asked him to draw a vial of blood to be tested for alcohol by the State Law Enforcement Division. Rather than drawing a second sample, the doctor ordered a blood alcohol test on the sample that had been drawn earlier for medical diagnosis purposes. Officers later obtained arrest warrants for the defendant based upon the test results. The court held that the results were inadmissible because the police did not comply with provisions of the implied consent statute.

In *State v. Vandergrift*, 535 N.W.2d (S.D. 1995), another appellate court ruled that a defense attack on a blood sample taken strictly for medical purposes would not succeed, based upon noncompliance with South Dakota's implied consent statute.

Inquiry

- What is covered in your state's implied consent law?
- Was the implied consent statute complied with?
- What was the exact wording of the implied consent advertisements given to the client?
- Taken in its entirety, were the advisement and any "explanation" of the advisement by the police officer misleading or coercive?
- If your client was unconscious at the time blood was drawn, was the sample collected by the state taken from a "medical purpose" vial, or from a separate "legal" collection of a specimen?

18.18 Refusal

Even where a defendant has refused to take the state's chemical sobriety test, the refusal to allow a sample to be taken can be excluded. Examples of this occur when the state gives improper implied consent warnings to the defendant, the defendant has a fear of needles, the defendant was "deaf." Further-

more, if the defendant was asked to sign hospital "liability waiver forms," but refused to do so, this may *not* be a "refusal." If the officer considered this a *refusal* to take the state's test, the addition of a nonstatutory requirement (that is mandated by the hospital's staff, in trying to shield itself from medical negligence) may run afoul of the implied consent laws of your state.

Case law

In *State v. Leviner*, 443 S.E.2d 688 (Ga.App. 1994), the court held that "the obfuscatory version of the implied consent law read to the defendant rendered meaningless the intent and spirit of the implied consent law." The implied consent rights were found to be misleading, inaccurate, and contained extraneous information that confused the defendant. The defendant's refusal to submit to the state's test was rendered inadmissible. *See also State v. Boger*, 559 S.E.2d 176 (Ga.App. 2002).

Other problems with implied consent warnings may affect the admissibility of evidence that a suspect refused a state-administered chemical sobriety test. For example, the warning given may be impermissibly coercive and false relating to the "true and legitimate" consequences of refusing the test. *State v. Renfroe*, 455 S.E.2d 383 (Ga.App. 1995); *State v. Coleman*, 455 S.E.2d 604 (Ga.App. 1995).

Beyond excluding evidence of refusal, deficient or misleading advisements may result in test results being excluded from evidence at trial. *Causey v. State*, 449 S.E.2d 639 (Ga.App. 1994); *Deckard v. State*, 436 S.E.2d 536 (Ga.App. 1993); *Hulsey v. State*, 225 S.E.2d 752 (Ga.App. 1976). Also, a person who is "hearing impaired" can't be expected to comprehend verbal implied consent advisements. *Yates v. State*, 545 S.E.2d 169 (Ga.App. 2001).

18.19 Summary of Potential Blood Test Errors

- Failure to follow the state testing or blood collection regulations
- Individual drawing blood not properly qualified
- Procedures set out in state statute not followed
- Failure to use regulation blood kit

- Introduction of ethanol in the specimen by the operator (perfume or lotion on hands may introduce error)
- Subject's arm swabbed with disinfectant containing alcohol
- Were intravenous (IV) fluids running at the time of the blood draw?
- Blood sample left to sit for any significant period of time
- Blood sample not refrigerated or treated with preservatives
- Expired blood-drawing equipment or vials
- Improper vial used for collection of blood sample (red top/gray top)
- Omissions or discrepancies in the medical record
- Equipment used to draw blood was not sterile.
- State unable to account for the chain of custody of the blood.
- Disease or condition altering blood alcohol levels
- Medication interference with blood alcohol levels
- Incorrect component of blood tested (whole blood or serum)
- State unable to produce all required witnesses at trial.
- Officer or hospital personnel obtaining or attempting to obtain a written waiver or patient's permission sheet when implied consent law does not require same
- Inaccurate, coercive or misleading implied consent warnings cause results or refusal to be excluded from evidence at trial.

Additional Reading

This chapter merely outlines issues for defense counsel to consider. Other chapters of this book further illuminate critical issues on forensic science relating to blood testing.

For the best comprehensive national research resources for criminal defense attorneys specializing or emphasizing DUI defense, consider the following books and newsletters.

Books

Taylor, L. *Drunk Driving Defense,* 5th ed. NY: Aspen Law & Business, 2002.

Nichols, D.H. and Whited, F.K., III. *Drinking/Driving Litigation Criminal and Civil,* 2nd ed. West Group, 2001.

Fitzgerald, E. *Intoxication Test Evidence,* 2nd ed. West Group, 2001.

Tarantino, J.A. *Defending Drinking Drivers,* 2nd ed. Costa Mesa, CA: James Publishing, 2003.

Newsletters

Drinking Driving Law Letter (Donald H. Nichols and Flem K. Whited III, ed.). Published 26 times per year by West Group, 620 Opperman Drive, St. Paul, MN.

DWI Law & Science Journal (John Tarantino, ed.). Published monthly by Whitaker Newsletters, 313 South Avenue, P.O. Box 192, Fanwood, N.J. 07023.

References

Barnard, J. Proof of hospital-performed blood alcohol tests in evidence. *American Journal of Trial Advocacy* 9:43–52, 1985.

Bogusz, M. Comparative studies on the rate of ethanol elimination. *J. Forensic Sci.* 22:446–451, 1977.

Chang, R.B. et al. The stability of ethyl alcohol in forensic blood specimens. *J. Anal. Toxicol.* 8:66–67, 1984.

Davenport, H.W. *The Physiology of the Digestive Tract.* Chicago: Yearbook Medical Publishers, 1971.

Dubowski, K.M. *Alcohol and Traffic Safety,* Public Health Service Publication No. 1043. U.S. Dept. of Housing, Education and Welfare, 1961.

Fitzgerald, E.F. *Intoxication Test Evidence.* West Publishing, 2001, §2.2.

Frajola, W.J. Blood alcohol testing in the clinical laboratory: problems and suggested remedies. *Clin. Chem.* 39:377–379, 1993.

Heise, H.A. How extravenous alcohol affects the blood test for alcohol. *Am. J. Clin. Pathol. 32:169-170, 1959.*

Kaye S. The collection and handling of the blood alcohol specimen. *Am. J. Clin. Pathol.* 74:743–745, 1980.

Landis, D.T. *Necessity and Sufficiency of Proof that Tests of Blood Alcohol Concentration Were Conducted in Conformance with Prescribed Methods.* 96 ALR 3d 745, 751.

Nichols. Disinfectant Swabs may compromise blood-alcohol tests. *Chicago Daily Law Bulletin* 136:2 Feb. 12, 1990.

Papple. The effect of oral contraceptive steroids (O.C.S.) on the rate of post-absorptive phase decline of blood alcohol concentration in the adult woman. *Can. Soc. Forensic Sci. J.* 15:17, 1982.

Shilling, D. *Winning Defenses in Drunk Driving Cases: Admissibility of Chemical Test Results.* NY: Prentice-Hall, 1987, pp. 56–60.

Taylor, Lawrence. *Drunk Driving Defense*, 5th ed. Boston, MA: Aspen Publishing Co., 2000, §8.3.2.

Tarantino, J.A. *Defending Drunk Drivers.* Costa Mesa, CA: James Publishing Co., 2002, §200-240.

Wade, T.C. DUI Statistics often don't add up: Here's how to challenge them in court. Section of *Criminal Justice of the American Bar Association*, Spring 1990. pp. 18–20, 37–39.

Winek, C.L. and Carfagna, M. Comparison of plasma, serum, and whole blood ethanol concentrations. *J. Anal. Toxicol.* 11:267–268, 1987.

Chapter 19

The Role and Responsibilities of an Expert Witness

Theodore F. Shults, J.D. and Yale H. Caplan, Ph.D.

19.1 Introduction

A. The need for expert witnesses

Science and technology have a profound impact on society and social policy. The law, along with society at large, is constantly assimilating new technology and evolving scientific theory and practice. The courts have always struggled with the interpretation of technical data and with establishing the standards of practice in professional fields. This struggle is on-going. The need for competent and effective expert witnesses who can help the courts and "finders of fact" effectively do their job is growing.

The expert witness plays an important role in society. If the court accepts bad guidance or flawed technical analysis or fails to understand the facts or principles involved, the ripple effect goes beyond the simple case at hand. When bad science becomes incorporated into legal opinions, the nature of legal precedence can perpetuate it for a long time. The consequences of bad expert testimony are bad law followed by bad policy decisions.

Thus, the role of an expert witness is an important part of each professional's profile and contribution. It is true that the legal process can go on with or without your help as an expert; however, to the degree that you can help shape good decisions based on the limits of sound scientific principle, you will be making a valuable contribution.

The focus of this chapter is to provide you, as an expert witness, with an overview of the legal process, and to provide guidance for developing your skills and competency in this important task. The material assumes you have little experience testifying as an expert. Even if you are experienced, this information may serve as a good review or provide added insight to help you be more effective.

B. What is an "expert witness"?

There are two types of witnesses: a fact witness and an expert witness. Fact witnesses will testify as to what they personally did, or saw or heard. Expert witnesses are used when information is expected to be of a scope beyond what the layman would likely know. At the time of testifying, the expert's special qualifications will be explained to the jury. The expert witness can offer opinions based upon his or her training, scientific knowledge and experience.

If you work in the area of forensics, then by definition part of your job is being an expert witness. An essential part of the forensic laboratory "product" is the ability to present the findings in an adversarial setting. No matter how elegant the laboratory method, no matter how small the co-efficient of variation, no matter how good the proficiency testing, accuracy and precision, if the data cannot be introduced into evidence or the significance explained clearly by a credible expert, it is forensically of little value-if not worthless.

The standard in federal court is whether the expert's testimony will be helpful to the jury. The Federal Rules of Evidence (Fed. Rules Evid.), which are used in federal courts and are a model for other jurisdictions, defines the basic parameters of expert witnesses.

UNITED STATES CODE ANNOTATED
RULES OF EVIDENCE FOR UNITED
STATES COURTS AND MAGISTRATES
ARTICLE VII. OPINIONS AND EXPERT
TESTIMONY
4-2-01

Rule 702. Testimony by Experts

If scientific, technical, or other specialized knowledge will assist the trier of fact to understand the evidence or to determine a fact in issue, a witness qualified as an expert by knowledge, skill, experience, training, or education, may testify thereto in the form of an opinion or otherwise, if (1) the testimony is based upon sufficient facts or data, (2) the testimony is the product of reliable principles and methods, and (3) the witness has applied the principles and methods reliably to the facts of the case. (As amended Apr. 17, 2000, eff. Dec. 1, 2000.)

C. Expert witness fees

First things first: there is a distinction between witness fees and expert witness fees. Witness fees are established to take care of the ordinary expenses that citizens who are subpoenaed would incur by going to court to testify, such as travel and attendance in court. These fees are determined by statute, are often nominal, and generally do not include compensation for loss of productive work and time. Government employees such as police officers and laboratory analysts for crime or toxicology laboratories are generally not entitled to any additional fees above their normal pay and compensation.

A person who is called by a party to a lawsuit to testify as an expert witness is, however, normally entitled to an expert witness fee. The amount of the fee is subject to an arrangement between the expert witness and the attorney who engages his or her services. Unless your job description includes acting as an expert witness, you are entitled to a reasonable fee for the time you spend reviewing data, researching, preparing reports and preparing to testify, and for telephone consultations with the attorney, out-of-pocket expenses, overhead expenses, travel time and expenses (hotels, meals, parking), and so on. In complex cases, you may be spending considerable time, and thus the fees can be significant.

Develop an hourly rate that takes into account your time away from your office or laboratory. This amount is negotiable between you and the attorney. It is a good idea to keep a log, tracking the time you spend reviewing records, developing demonstrative evidence, research writing, and forming opinions. For trial days, you may want to negotiate a flat daily rate, or per diem. Some expert witnesses are concerned that receiving a hefty hourly rate will appear to color their testimony. That is certainly the case where the reimbursement is unreasonably high, but in most cases, paradoxically, most jurors will think that the more you make, the better witness you are.

It is interesting to note that when you are called to testify in a deposition, your reimbursement is paid by whoever subpoenas you. (Subpoenas and depositions are discussed in more detail below.) Your deposition fees are typically the same as the fees you charge for the other services listed above. Often an attorney will prepare a letter of agreement retaining your services for a particular case, or he or she will ask you to provide a letter outlining your professional fees and expenses for assisting in the development of a specified case. The expert witness fee must be reasonable and may not be contingent on the outcome of the case. Contingency fees for an expert witness are unethical, often illegal, and at a minimum void, as a matter of public policy.

D. Retainer and billing issues

It is a good idea for you as an expert witness to receive some funds up front that you can bill against. This is called a retainer. After the retainer is expended, you can submit monthly invoices. It is preferable to itemize the invoice on an hourly basis, briefly explaining each activity listed on the invoice.

Try not to let an outstanding bill accrue. Once a case is over, either by verdict, dismissal or settlement, it may suddenly get harder to get paid. (A thumb rule of criminal attorneys is to receive payment before trial. It is hard to get paid after your client is found guilty, and it is surprisingly hard to get paid even if your client is found not guilty, since they may not like the idea of having to pay to "prove" their innocence!)

Use your time efficiently and keep your attorney apprised of the amount of time you need and are spending on a case. On the other hand, do not let the attorney overly constrict your reasonable efforts to review all of the relevant records and materials in preparation of or in support of your opinion.

19.2 The Law of Evidence
A. Overview

In a civil proceeding, the issues in a lawsuit are defined by the pleadings (the complaint and answer), any formal stipulations or admissions, and the applicable law. Sometimes the parties agree on all or most of the facts but disagree on what the facts mean in respect to the law. Usually, the law is clear, but the parties disagree on the facts.

Today's legal process is the product of thousands of years of evolution regarding how to make the best determination of what the "facts" are in a particular controversy, and then applying the facts to the applicable law to determine a fair outcome. Following the principles of the English common law and jurisprudence, the American legal system is set up in an adversarial manner, where each side to a controversy strives to prove their case zealously but ethically. This adversarial approach is designed to generate some heat with the hope that it will also generate some light, so that a "finder of fact" may determine the facts and arrive at a just resolution.

Establishing facts that are in controversy requires the production of evidence. Your testimony is evidence. In fact, this chapter really deals with the law of evidence. The law of evidence is a body of legal rules and procedures that defines what is admissible and what is not, what is prejudicial, and what is fair practice and procedure.

B. Burden of proof

Whether it is a simple shoplifting case, a homicide, a regulatory violation, a products liability class action, or a malpractice case, there are essential elements which need to be established by the party who carries the burden of proof. The burden of proof rests upon the parties to an action to persuade the trier of facts, also referred to as the finder of facts (such as an administrative law judge or arbitrator, or a jury), that a proposition or element of the case asserted by a party to the action is true. It is necessary for the attorneys and ultimately the judge to determine which party has the burden of proof with respect to each issue.

Thus, the burden of proof as to each issue is determined before trial and remains upon the same party throughout the trial. The burden of going forward is a related but different concept, and it does shift from one party to the other in the course of the trial.

To quickly illustrate how this works, consider a DUI/DWI prosecution. The prosecutor in the criminal trial initially has the burden of going forward first. Under most state laws, the introduction of a breath alcohol test result above the state law BAC threshold, which has been performed in accordance with the applicable statutory requirements, gives rise to a presumption of impairment. At this point the burden of going forward shifts to the defendant, who can introduce evidence that the BAC was incorrect, or argue that there is a reasonable doubt, or even put on evidence that he or she was not impaired. The prosecutor still has the burden of proof, but the burden of going forward on any issue can shift back and forth. This seesaw shifting of the burden of going forward is more evident in civil cases where there is a lower degree of evidence required to sustain or establish an issue.

C. Degree of evidence required to sustain the burden of proof

1. Beyond a reasonable doubt

In a criminal case, the State has the burden of proving "beyond a reasonable doubt" that a defendant committed a crime. Reasonable doubt has been defined in a number of ways, and every prosecutor and defense attorney has a pat speech that discusses what it is and what it is not. Each jurisdiction has jury instructions that define what is meant by a reasonable doubt. It boils down to an honest and reasonable uncertainty about the guilt of the defendant.

In practice, this standard is often very hard to meet. A defendant's most common defense is often to argue that there is reasonable doubt-that is, that the prosecutor hasn't done a sufficient job of proving that the defendant is guilty.

This does not mean that the testimony of an expert witness in a criminal trial must be beyond a reasonable doubt, unless that evidence is the only evidence against the criminal defendant. This is a relatively rare situation. Usually expert testimony is only part of all the direct and circumstantial evidence that is introduced to show the guilt or innocence of a defendant. Each piece of evidence is a piece of a puzzle. No one piece will show the total picture. When added together, the evidence may show a very clear picture-at least, that is what a prosecutor would like to achieve.

2. Preponderance of the evidence

In a civil case, the plaintiff (the party who has instituted the action against a "defendant") has the burden of proving their case by a preponderance of the evidence. The legal dictionaries define the preponderance of the evidence as the standard of proof in which the party bearing the burden of proof must present evidence which is more credible and convincing than that presented by the other party or which shows that the fact to be proven is more probable than not. The standard is often described as presenting greater than a 50% probability of the fact being true.

If the evidence is equally balanced, or if it leaves the jury in such a doubt as to be unable to decide the controversy either way (the 50-50 split), judgment must be given against the party which has the burden of proof.

3. Clear and Convincing Evidence

In the now-ancient legal text *Richardson on Evidence*, tenth edition, published back in 1973, the author Jerome Prince (and law professor for one of the authors here) wrote that the meaning of the term "proof by clear and convincing evidence" is none too clear. Not much has changed in thirty years.

The standard of clear and convincing evidence is theoretically an intermediate standard between preponderance of the evidence and beyond a reasonable doubt. It is the level of proof required for some civil cases or motions in which the party bearing the burden of proof must show that the truth of the allegations is highly probable. This standard is used in many administrative proceedings (such as proving violations of environmental pollution by a regulatory agency).

In respect to a technical element of a case, the clear and convincing standard is often described as a standard of a high degree of scientific certainty. This does not mean that you cannot offer an opinion on an aspect of the case unless you have a certain level of scientific certainty, only that at the end of the proceeding the party with the burden of proof has established the case with this heightened level of evidence.

D. Reconciling statistical confidence levels and legal proof

In the universe of science, statistical tests and confidence levels are used to provide information concerning the probability that an observation is not merely the result of chance but rather an effect caused by the specific factor being studied. As you can appreciate by now, the process of scientific proof is vastly different from the judicial establishment of facts, conclusions and final decisions.

In the judicial universe, the primary tools are the adversarial system in conjunction with the laws of evidence, finders of fact, and the deliberation process. The law's approach is a quasi-scientific one at best, so it is important for the expert witness to understand how to qualify technical observations and professional opinion in an appropriate legal contest.

Attorneys who deal with expert witnesses have often noted (or complained) that many scientific experts have not been willing to state any opinion unless the weight of the evidence overwhelmingly favors the conclusion. Some scientific experts have adopted qualitative measures of the weight of proof necessary (e.g., "strong evidence," "to a high degree of scientific certainty," "clear and convincing," among others) and others use quantitative measures (95% or 99% level of certainty).

These characterizations of the weight of proof communicate an overwhelming sense of the probability that the conclusion is correct. A 95% or 99% level of certainty, however, is not necessary in litigation. Admissible and useful scientific opinion need not stand alone as conclusive scientific evidence.

The level of proof required for civil or criminal litigation is not the same as the confidence level used in a statistical evaluation of data. In civil litigation, a scientist only needs "50.1% certainty," a judgment that with a reasonable degree of scientific certainty, it is "more likely than not" that something is true or there is a causal association.

Even in a criminal case, each piece of evidence the prosecutor introduces need not be beyond a reasonable doubt. It is after the presentation of all the evidence that the jury must decide whether all of the evidence paints a picture that is beyond a reasonable doubt proof of guilt for each element of the alleged crime.

Even when a particular piece of evidence is statistically significant, the mere statistical evidence of a relationship may not be conclusive, scientifically or legally. For example, the relationship between the illumination of the Fasten Seatbelt sign on a passenger aircraft enjoys a statistically significant relationship with the occurrence of air turbulence. However the pilot's turning on the light does not cause the turbulence. Legal causation often requires other elements of proof.

Obviously, expert conclusions should be worded as strongly and clearly as possible. If there is a strong statistical confidence level supporting a particular piece of evidence, this should be stated.

19.3 Categories of Evidence

There are four traditional types of evidence: real, documentary, testimonial, and demonstrative. (Many of the examples below may also be described as physical evidence, which consists of articles, records, exhibits, and other things that the court or the jury can see and inspect.)

- **Real evidence** is the thing or object itself: a body, a weapon, clothing, laboratory samples (blood, urine, DNA materials and so on), laboratory instruments, reagents, other chemical substances, or drugs.
- **Documentary evidence** is derived from conventional symbols (such as letters) by which ideas are represented on material substances: writings, inscriptions, tax records, laboratory logs, copies of accounts or billings, tapes (audio or visual), medical records, laboratory manuals, quality assurance procedures and records, and laboratory operating manuals and procedures (SOPs). These can be considered real evidence as well.
- **Testimonial evidence** is the most basic form of evidence and the only kind that does not usually require another form of evidence as a prerequisite for its admissibility [Fed Rules Evid. 602]. It consists of what is said in the court, or at a deposition under oath, or at the proceeding in question by a competent witness.

In general, a fact witness is competent if he meets four requirements: (1) he must, with understanding, take the oath or a substitute (Fed. Rules Evid. 603); (2) he must have personal knowledge about the subject of his testimony—in other words, the witness must have perceived something with his senses that is relevant to the case (Fed. Rules Evid. 602); (3) he must remember what he perceived; (4) he must be able to communicate what he perceived (Evid. Code §701(a)(1)).

- **Demonstrative evidence** is visual or auditory evidence (i.e., perceived by the senses), such as charts, diagrams, photographs, copies of laboratory analyses, models, radiographs, illustrations, and equipment prepared by the attorney or his expert to help the judge or jury understand the testimony.

A. Expert reports

You may be asked to prepare an expert report on your analysis of the presenting case. You may also be specifically asked not to prepare a written report until later in the case. This is a tactical question for the attorney. An expert report can be useful to settle a case; on the other hand, your expert report can be discovered and turned over to the opposing party at an early point in the case.

Naturally, if the opposing party has an expert who has written a report, it would be a good idea to evaluate it.

B. Diagrams and demonstrative evidence

You may be asked or you may want to offer to prepare pictures, diagrams, records, or slide presentations that will help you present and explain technical information. It is common in big cases to see experts use video presentations, animated PowerPoint presentations, models and other types of "demonstrative" aids. When properly prepared and presented in court, these materials can be powerful aids in helping the jury understand the points you are trying to make.

The admissibility of such evidence is within the sound discretion of the judge. Many times this evidence is shown to the jury but not admitted into evidence. Acceptance of the evidence is reversed only when abuse on appeal or indiscretion is demonstrated and its acceptance is determined to be preju-

dicial to the jury. Demonstrative evidence may be highly technical, and consultation with the attorney is absolutely essential, even prior to preparing it.

19.4 The Threshold Question of Admissibility

The touchstone of the law of evidence is authenticity, reliability and veracity of information and material presented in a proceeding. The primary rule of evidence is admissibility. In general, if evidence is shown to be relevant, material, and competent, and is not barred by an exclusionary rule, it is admissible. [Fed. Rules Evid. 402.] Evidence, which includes expert testimony, is relevant when it has any tendency in reason to make the fact that it is offered to prove or disprove either more or less probable. [Fed. Rules Evid. 401.]

To be relevant, a particular item of evidence need not make the fact for which it is offered certain, or even more probable than not. All that is required is that it has some tendency to increase the likelihood of the fact for which it is offered. It is a question of law as to whether any evidence is admissible, which is to say that the judge or court must determine admissibility.

The adversarial system does have its limitations, particularly dealing with science and distinguishing it from what is referred to as "junk" science. You may believe that household mold causes global warming, and you may be right, but until it meets certain standards of admissibility, your expert opinion will not be admitted into evidence. Neither the court nor society at large is well served by the "expert witness" who brings to the proceedings bad data, bad science, unsubstantiated observations, and a paid opinion with a view toward deciding the outcome of a case for the unenlightened.

Since 1985 the federal courts and many other jurisdictions have developed a body of case law and rules that define the minimum "entry level" evidentiary requirements of admissibility. This is known generically as the *Daubert* rule, named for the leading Supreme Court case on this issue, *Daubert v. Merrell Dow Pharmaceuticals, Inc.* 509 U.S. 579 (1993). Rule 702 of the Federal Rules of Evidence, which was quoted earlier in the chapter, incorporates this admissibility standard.

Daubert rules and the various admissibility tests and standards used by the courts are not a perfect filter. Junk science can look just like real science. At times real science, particularly new theories and observations, may be characterized or labeled as "junk science." Thus, good science is sometimes inadmissible, and sometimes junk gets in. When junk does get in, and assuming you are not the one introducing it, your role becomes more critical. You may be cast in the role of challenging the validity of the opponent's opinion or providing an alternative opinion. Your effectiveness is not merely developing your theory and testimony, but educating the jury and selling it to them.

The operative issue is that you must draw your expert testimony, conclusions and opinions from facts or data that are reasonably relied upon in the field. These are facts that you can articulate, and which are applied to scientific theory that is in at least some minimal way established in your field. And your field cannot be astrology.

19.5 Discovery and the Expert Witness

A. The discovery process

The essence of the old-fashioned TV court drama is the courtroom surprise. The audience can usually count on a surprise witness, a hidden video recording, and the ultimate moment when the witness, confronted with overwhelming evidence and trapped in his own lies, confesses on the stand. That is what makes the classic TV court cases fun. Art does imitate life, and today there are fewer surprises in TV renditions of court cases. Now everyone (usually) knows what happened. The focus of the production is on the pathos, ethics and drama of human events-this is what captures our attention.

The basic idea behind the legal discovery process in the real world is that there should be no surprises or ambushes of witnesses. The discovery process is designed to identify what facts everyone agrees to and what is in dispute. Discovery is a formal legal procedure used in both civil and criminal trials to help both sides of a controversy determine what will be presented in a trial. Hopefully, the process will help the parties resolve their controversy.

There are a few noteworthy differences in discovery between criminal, civil and administrative proceedings. In criminal proceedings, there is an affirmative legal duty of the prosecutor to turn over "exculpatory" evidence to the defendant. The prosecutor has the burden of proof beyond a reasonable doubt to establish each element of the crime alleged. There is no symmetrical rule requiring a criminal defendant to turn over either incriminating or even exculpatory evidence to the prosecutor. The constitutional protection against self-incrimination also precludes prosecutors from most of the discovery process. (Prosecutors do have the ability to investigate cases through the police and grand jury proceedings.)

The discovery process in civil proceedings is extensive. All parties to a civil proceeding have the right to submit formal written questions, called interrogatories, to opposing parties. These questions have to be answered in writing. All of the parties can request the production and inspection of records or other evidence in the control of opposing parties. Witnesses and parties can be questioned under oath in a pretrial deposition. As the stakes in any particular case go up, so does the amount of time spent on discovery.

The evidentiary and discovery process in administrative proceedings are generally more relaxed and informal. The operative word here is "generally." The attorney who is calling you as an expert should be knowledgeable with both the formal and informal procedural requirements of the forum in which the case is being litigated. There are numerous reference books available to counsel providing model questions and guidance on how to question different types of experts.

B. If you are contacted by the opposing attorney

In many jurisdictions, the lawyer is prohibited from making an *ex parte* communication with another party's expert witness. *Ex parte* communication is any communication to a judge, witness or adverse party in the absence of the opposing party's attorney.

Despite the expansive philosophy of modern discovery, with few exceptions it is not a good idea to discuss your ideas about a case or expected testimony with the opposing party without the consent or presence (or both) of the attorney who will be calling you. The exception to this rule is a seasoned forensic expert who testifies on a regular basis in criminal cases on "routine" laboratory findings (e.g., fingerprints, blood type, and cause of death). Even here the expert should understand what the local rules and customs are in this regard, and should be cleared by his or her office and the prosecutor's office to discuss the matter informally with defense counsel.

In all other cases, the appropriate response is to tell the opposing counsel that you would be happy to discuss the case, but that he or she must set up an informal interview with the attorney who is going to call on you to testify.

Remember, the opposing party will have the opportunity to cross-examine you, examine copies of reports you have prepared, and will probably have a good idea of what you are going to say from speaking with the attorney who is going to call you.

C. Informal interviews

Although it seems like a useful practice, "informal interviews" are not that common. More often, discovery is achieved through discussions between opposing counsel and the somewhat controlled formal discovery procedure of interrogatories and depositions. Nevertheless, an expert witness interview can be arranged with either attorney.

It is a good idea to ask who is going to pay for your time. Sometimes your attorney wants to show the opposing side what they are dealing with, and will be happy to pay for your time. It is rare where the other side will pay for an interview, but it is possible.

The interview may take place in either attorney's office, the office or laboratory of the expert, or by telephone. The person being interviewed determines the location and time, since it is an informal, two-party discussion. The attorney who has called you and for whom you are expert witness should always be present at this type of meeting.

The interview may be taped. If so, it is a good practice for both parties to make their own tapes or hire a third party to do the taping. If a tape is made, copies must be obtained in order to review them prior to deposition or trial.

Request a tape or transcript of your interview and review it for correctness. If you need to correct or clarify, do so immediately in writing. It is much easier to do this before testifying in the courtroom. Review and familiarize yourself with the answers prior to testifying. Request a transcript while recording is occurring so that your request becomes part of your interview. Then if you are cross-examined about your interview and have not seen the transcript, that will be an embarrassment to the cross-examining attorney who did not provide it as formally requested.

If a question arises that you cannot answer at the time, delay your answer until you have discussed it with your attorney or have had time to research it.

D. Written interrogatories

A great deal of the preliminary discovery is done with written interrogatories. Typical interrogatories directed toward expert witnesses are intended to establish what your position is and what your credentials are. The interrogatories will ask whether you have testified before, and what you have testified about. They will ask what records you have examined, and whether you have prepared any expert reports or opinions.

Your written answers to these questions should be developed in conjunction with the attorney who has called you as an expert. The answers are often used to develop questions that you will be asked at a deposition or trial.

E. Affidavits

An affidavit is a written or printed declaration or statement of facts, made voluntarily, and confirmed by oath or affirmation of the party making it. The form an affidavit takes is defined by state law. It is usually executed before a person having authority to administer such an oath or affirmation, such as a notary public. (Again, state law varies on the technical requirements.)

As a "sworn statement," an affidavit is used to establish some or all of your opinion or testimony in a case. If both parties agree, an affidavit can be used in legal proceedings as an alternative to live testimony. A common example is the affidavit of a "custodian of records" of physical evidence, stating that he or she is the custodian of that evidence. Affidavits can be used in what attorneys call "motion practice."

These are the legal proceedings used to establish jurisdiction of a court or seeking the dismissal of a case or controversy. Affidavits of experts are often used as the basis of a settlement agreement.

The attorneys will determine the time and location for taking the affidavit. The affidavit process may seem casual in some cases, but be aware that an affidavit is treated as sworn testimony—such as might be given in a deposition. It can and will be used against you in court if it differs from your trial testimony. Obtain and keep a copy of your affidavit for your review.

F. The subpoena

A subpoena is a court order to appear at a certain time and place to give testimony upon a certain matter. There are several versions of a subpoena, but one important type for an expert witness is a *subpoena duces tecum*. The *subpoena duces tecum* is a court order issued at the request of a party, which orders a witness to appear at a location to testify and to bring with you specified documents or other physical evidence that are in your possession. A *subpoena duces tecum* may require you to produce books, papers, research materials, billings, statements or other materials that are the basis for your opinion.

In civil cases, the *subpoena duces tecum* is often "bundled" with a discovery request for a deposition. It is basically requiring your appearance with relevant documents in hand at the agreed-upon site of the deposition.

If you are subpoenaed:

- Remember that a subpoena is a court order. Do not fail to comply without approval of the court. The failure to respond to a subpoena will be considered contempt of court. A warrant could be issued for your arrest or a fine could be levied against you. Generally, this is not a good way to start as an expert.
- Notify the attorney who has requested your services that you have received a subpoena. (He or she has probably already received a copy of the subpoena, but never assume this has happened.) This attorney can decide whether to challenge the legality of the subpoena. Although all subpoenas are court orders, in most jurisdictions

attorneys involved in the case or controversy simply draft and issue subpoenas without the court's oversight. Your attorney can decide to challenge the scope of the subpoena's request, or even move to quash the subpoena, with the court.

- Understand and know the requirements stated in the subpoena. If you have any questions regarding the contents of the subpoena, consult with the attorney who has requested your services.
- If it is not already clear, or if the subpoena raises additional issues for you to deal with, such as the production of records, now is the time to discuss financial aspects of your response: time, research efforts, travel and accommodations when away from your residence or office, and the costs of demonstrative evidence that might be used in an interview or trial.
- Sometimes, particularly in criminal cases, "your" attorney may subpoena you to appear. There are some tactical reasons for this move. From the attorney's perspective, it gives good assurance that you will be there. It also helps give the appearance that you are not there because it is your job or that you are being compensated (both of which may be true).

G. The deposition

The deposition is a critical point in the life of a lawsuit or controversy. A deposition is the process of obtaining testimony of both expert and fact witnesses. A deposition is a legal proceeding conducted in accordance with state or federal court rules. It is taken under oath and before a court reporter rather than in open court.

Even though the deposition is not courtroom testimony, it will be treated as such by the court. It is a discovery device by which one party asks oral questions of the other party or its witness. The person being deposed is called the deponent.

- The deposition can be taken in either civil or criminal cases.
- The setting may be informal or formal. It is usually in an attorney's office or conference room.

Occasionally the deposition will be taken at the court reporter's office.

- The persons present usually include the deponent, the attorneys, a court reporter or a notary; the latter will swear you in. It is best to have attorneys from both sides present, and on occasion there may be multiple attorneys representing all parties present.

- Depending on the case, a deposition can last for hours or days. Court rules may limit the amount of time spent on a deposition. In general, if the deposition requires several sessions, you are not sworn in each time but warned that you are still under oath.

- The transcript is a word-for-word account of the deposition made by a court reporter. The deposition may be recorded on audiotape, videotape, or in writing by the court reporter. In some cases, more than one method may be used.

- You are entitled to a copy of the transcript to clarify an answer or correct misspellings. This right should not be waived, because this document may be used to discredit your court testimony. As with informal interviews, make your request for a copy as part of the records.

Depositions are used for:

- Preserving the testimony of a deponent who is moribund, terminal, or unavailable at the time of the trial.

- Determining opposing counsel's case or the expert's opinion. Consider it a fact-finding or information gathering mission by the opposing counsel. Your testimony at the deposition is the primary basis for preparing opposing counsel's cross-examination of you at trial.

  One key strategy of the opposing party is to have you as the expert identify and produce every piece of physical evidence and every document that you have relied upon to form your opinion. The good adversary will also mark each item you produce as evidence, so there is no question about what you had knowledge of at the time of the deposition. If you rely on something new when you testify at trial, expect the attorney object vigorously on the grounds that it was not disclosed during discovery.

- Determining the qualifications of the expert and the possibility of discrediting the witness. All essential elements that you have used to establish your credentials will be questioned. Have your CV up to date. In addition, know all things used to form your opinion: experience, practice, research, texts, journals, and consultations with colleagues.

- Converting any or all of your opinion to opposing counsel's case and agreement with his expert.

The rules of the road, so to speak, will be explained to you at the beginning of the deposition. Although the proceeding is somewhat more relaxed in that it usually occurs in an attorney's office, it is a critical part of the process. Testimony taken is under oath and being transcribed, and in more and more cases it will be videotaped as well.

When a deposition is videotaped and can be introduced as substantive evidence at the trial in lieu of calling the witness to the stand, the witness must balance the original desire for terse answers with the desire to enhance his or her credibility.

The opposing attorneys cannot ask you the same question numerous times. If this happens, one of the most common objections your attorney may make is, "Asked and answered." Upon completion of the deposition, your attorney may ask additional questions to clarify testimony or to avoid confusing statements.

A very important aspect of a deposition is to see how effective you are as a witness. It is not unheard of for an attorney to try to shake up an opposing witness by embarrassing, intimidating, angering, or harassing you, and if that does not work, by being extremely friendly. Your testimony may determine the focus of the case for both sides depending on how strongly you present it and how difficult it seems to attack your opinion.

19.6 Elements of testimony

A. Direct examination or examination-in-chief

During the direct examination, the witness is examined by the party who called him or her. It is designed to introduce evidence, educate the judge or jury, and introduce facts or opinion to build or support the case. It may be used to weaken the opponent's case, or to strengthen or weaken the credibility of other witnesses.

B. Cross-examination

In the cross-examination, the opposing side questions a witness. The cross-examination, as everyone who has ever watched the television show *Perry Mason* knows, is a critical part of the adversarial process. Cross-examination is confrontational and is supposed to be the test of credibility. Here is where Perry shows that the star eyewitness cannot see who is standing in the back of the courtroom. The purpose of the cross-examination is to introduce alternative explanations, weaken the credibility of the witness, find support for the opponent's theory, and clarify (or confuse) the issues.

The law allows for much more latitude in the questioning of an adversarial witness. Here the opposing counsel can ask what are called "leading questions." To an expert witness, many of the questions may seem misleading. (Example: "Please answer yes or no—Is it possible that the earth can stop spinning on its axis?")

Cross-examination is generally the worst part of giving evidence. A good cross-examiner can make the most truthful witness appear uncertain and confused. Counsel on cross-examination may attempt to confuse you, have you argue with him, or have you lose your temper. A vigorous cross-examination may occasionally seem like a personal attack on the witness, but remember that it is the evidence that the cross-examiner is attacking, not the witness. Keep calm, and do not argue with the challenging attorney.

C. Re-direct

Following the cross-examination, there is the opportunity to re-direct or re-examine the witness. Here is where the witness can further explain the basis for a yes-or-no question and expand on issues raised.

19.7 Credibility and Communication

Your efficacy as a witness will depend on personality, experience, training, and demeanor. The key is your ability to communicate, both verbally and nonverbally, and your ability to relate to strangers. The communication skills of both attorneys and expert witnesses can be improved and polished. Your job is to get your message across.

With guidance from the attorneys calling on you to testify in a particular case, even a beginner witness can begin to master the practice. The best advice you will get is from the attorney who is calling you to testify. However, that attorney may be somewhat new, or overloaded with other case preparation. In such cases, the following guidance and advice may be useful.

A. Credibility determinations and the jury

Juries are presented with the rather difficult task of finding facts, a process that involves the determination of credibility. Whom do you believe? There are numerous variables in this process, and there are many examples of the fallibility of the process. However, juries, despite their limitations, are remarkable judges of human nature. There is a lot of combined wisdom and discernment embedded in a jury panel.

B. Credentials and your testimony

Many experts, even those with sixty-page CVs and multiple graduate degrees to their credit, feel insecure about their credentials. Sometimes this is actually expressed by overconfidence or arrogance. There is always the fear that there is someone with one more paper, one more set of initials after his or her name. Know who you are, and don't worry about how you may compare to others.

Experience and credibility are two different but interrelated issues. Credentials are important, but not as important as they used to be. We live in a very skeptical world. The credentials of an expert are only as important as that person's credibility as a witness. What is critically important is not to exaggerate or overstate your credentials. A national headhunting firm has recently found that about 75 percent of the resumes submitted from job seekers in both management and technical fields contain "overstatements."

As an expert, you have to assume that opposing parties will carefully research your background. They may also scrutinize your prior testimony, answers to interrogatories, your criminal record, and even your credit history. In today's wired world, it is easy to look up how an expert witness has detailed his or her professional experience in prior testimony. When you testify, you are building your own trial record of credibility.

The trial transcripts are full of examples of experts who were "defrocked" by what may have been in their minds harmless exaggerations. What is the difference between actually graduating and being one credit hour short? Probably nothing—if you do not lie about it.

A question that experts are often asked is "Have you done research in this area?" If you have, that's fine. If you have not, that is fine, too. Studying the issue in high school biology is not what they mean. If you are not the right expert to testify, that is not your fault-but this determination should be made with the attorney calling you before you testify.

19.8 Keys to Effective Testimony

Shakespeare's insight that the whole world is a stage is most evident in the courtroom. The architecture of the court, like a stage, is quite intentional. It is designed to communicate the importance of the judge and the importance of the process that is taking place. The ambiance of the courts will vary greatly-from the quiet, intimidating atmosphere of a federal district court, to the chaos of a big city criminal trial court.

Your role in all of these venues is an important one. You have to play yourself in the role of the expert witness. It is usually a leading role in a case or controversy. You need to be prepared. No matter how prepared you or your attorney may be, there will be an element of uncertainty. Remember, as a scientist you are at home in the laboratory, but as a witness you are playing in someone else's ballpark. Here are some fundamentals that will be helpful to you in carrying out your role effectively.

A. Before you get to the witness stand

- **Educate your attorney**. Your first job is to educate your attorney on the technical aspects of the case, your expected testimony and testimony that you anticipate from other experts. You will be surprised at how knowledgeable at-

torneys can be in respect to the narrow issues that are relevant to their cause of action.

- **No secrets**. From the beginning, you should inform the attorney about potential weaknesses in his or her theory or case. Include potential weaknesses in your own theory or data. Also keep the attorney up to date on any new or unfavorable findings from your review or research regarding the opponent's case.
- **Do your homework**. Be prepared. Be organized. In the best situations, you will have the opportunity to go over the questions that the attorney will be asking you and to prepare your answers. If you see potential problems in any area of the case, you should point them out to your counsel.

You may have read documents in preparation for testifying. Review them a day or two before coming to testify. Organize your materials; know where to find material that you are going to use. Refresh your recollection of what the case is all about. Review your reports and any prior testimony you may have given in the case. Review the opposing expert reports and testimony if available.

- **Pretrial practice sessions**. Discuss the details of the case and have at least one practice session with your attorney to cover the questions that are going to be asked. In a complex case this should involve a substantial amount of role-playing, in which the attorney will illustrate the kind of attack the examiner is expected to mount through actual questioning.
- **Be familiar with courtroom surroundings**. Become familiar with the courtroom and trial procedure. If at all possible, attend a trial to get a feel for the court in action.

B. In the courtroom

- **Show up**. Be on time for all meetings and court appearances. Courts and most attorneys will work with you to arrange your appearance at a time that will work with your schedule. Showing up is an important part of testifying. If you are going to be late, or if you have a schedule change, contact your counsel as soon as you can. Obtain a cell phone number for your attorney or the attorney's assistant, so that you will be able to call if you are delayed. Give your cell phone number to the attorney, so if the case is "continued" or the deposition is cancelled at the last moment, you can be contacted.

- **Dress appropriately**. The legal system has not adopted casual Friday. This does not mean that you have to put on a pinstriped suit, but remember the first impression that the fact-finder will have of you stems from your appearance. When you testify, all eyes are on you. If you have any question regarding what is appropriate, ask. Grooming is also relevant. The disheveled look worked for Einstein, but it will not work for most others. Wear conservative clothing and be neat in dress and demeanor.

- **Be careful of casual conversations** while waiting to testify or during breaks in the proceedings. These can come back to haunt you if overheard by opposing counsel. It is best to avoid any discussion of the case, your work, or your opinions while in court-related areas. Listen, but do not engage in trial-related topics.

C. On the stand

- **Courtesy and manners are important**. Common courtesy and good manners are invaluable assets to an expert witness. Say good morning or good afternoon to the judge when you approach the witness stand. Nod or say good morning to the jury before the first question is asked. Assume that one or more members of the jury or a potential jury member will probably be observing you from the moment you arrive at the courthouse steps, because it is probably true. Your behavior is under surveillance by someone involved in the case all of the time you are involved in preparing for and testifying in the case.

  Have a pleasant demeanor and have a good attitude during the presentation of testimony. Do not show any visible signs of displeasure regarding any testimony with which you are in disagreement.

Always be courteous to the attorneys, especially during the cross-examination. This is an absolute must when the cross-examining attorney harasses or provokes you in any manner. Do not be argumentative, sarcastic, caustic, or pompous. By keeping your cool, you only increase in stature in the eyes of the jury and you gain the jurors' respect, and perhaps their sympathy as well.

- **Body language has an impact**. Remember that body language often communicates more than verbal language. Be yourself and relax. Never slouch on the stand or hold on to the rail. Sit comfortably in the chair, and rest your arms on the sides of the chair or keep them folded in your lap or placed casually on the desk. Lean slightly forward to give the impression of confidence and capability.

- **Answer questions facing the jury**! This may be the most important tip you can get on being an effective witness. Look at the attorney while the question is asked and then turn to the jury to present your answer. One step better is to try to make eye contact with all of the members of the jury.

  In some jurisdictions, attorneys are required to stay seated. In others, the attorney has to ask questions standing at their desk or behind a podium. Others allow the attorney to wander around while questioning witnesses. Opposing counsel may try to direct your responses away from the jury by standing opposite them or even blocking your view of the jury. If this happens, simply ask the examining attorney to allow you to reply to the jury.

- **Be confident and attentive**. Present information or evidence with assurance and confidence. Confidence is not arrogance; never answer in a cocky manner. Do not exaggerate or bluff. You should appear interested in the courtroom proceedings and your testimony. Never appear bored or exasperated, no matter how obvious or redundant questioning becomes.

- **Educate**. Use terminology that will be understood by the jury. Be careful about the use of acronyms. Explain what they stand for. Scientific terms should be defined in lay terms.

You may disagree with other authorities or so-called authorities, but it is important to disagree on a sound basis. You must give impartial testimony and your opinion must be based on accepted scientific principle and data or on firsthand knowledge of the facts of record.

- **Be succinct.** Answer only the questions asked with only the necessary elaboration to explain the answer. Never volunteer information when it is not requested. Try to keep your answers short, particularly on cross-examination. Do not ramble on or volunteer information. Do not assume you know the next question and thereby answer it. The attorney may not fully understand the questioning, and by giving more information, you may be answering follow-up questions that they would never have known to ask. What you think is harmless may be the downfall of the case.
- **Refresh your memory.** If you need to, refer to notes to refresh your memory. These documents may be admitted as evidence.
- **Be careful in your testimony.** Your reputation as an expert witness can be ruined by just one serious mistake on the witness stand, such as being caught in a lie or even a contradiction in your testimony. The success of an expert witness depends in great measure on building and maintaining a good reputation for veracity in the minds of the jurors. Be straightforward with counsel. Any answers designed to cover up or cloud an issue or fact will, if discovered, serve only to discredit any previous testimony you may have given.
- **Listen carefully to questions.** This is harder than it sounds. You want to say something and you may not be listening carefully. Listen carefully to every question and be sure you understand it before answering. Be sure to ask for clarity in any ambiguous questions. Do not assume that you know what they mean.
- **Answer questions clearly.** Speak distinctly and loudly enough for the jury to hear each word and make no mistakes in understanding the testimony. Use words, not gestures. Never mumble or slur. If there is a microphone, move

it to a comfortable position so that you can talk into it and still be looking at the jury.

Give clear and direct answers to every question whenever possible. If you honestly cannot fairly answer "yes" or "no" to a question, say so and explain your answer. If the judge asks you to answer, leave it to your attorney to rehabilitate you during the re-direct process (i.e., "You answered yes to such and such a question; would you like to clarify your response?").

- **Be honest when you cannot answer a question.** Do not hesitate to refuse to answer a question outside the scope of your expertise. You may not know all the details of the physics or chemistry of the instrument you are using. Be comfortable in knowing what you do not know. Never be afraid of saying the three hardest words in the English language for any expert: "I don't know." Saying these simple words may make you appear more human and more credible to the jury. Say them without embarrassment.

Do not look at the judge or your attorney when a hard question stumps you.

If you can't remember an answer to a question, say, "I can't recall" or "I can't remember." If you can only approximate dates, times and distances, give only your best approximation.

- **Listen to objections.** If either side makes an objection to any question or answer, stop. Wait for the judge to rule. If he overrules the objection, answer the question. If he sustains the objection, simply wait for the question. Never try to squeeze in an answer when an objection has been made.

D. The "don'ts"

- **Do not put on an act.** The most important advice lawyers learn about being in court is to be themselves. If you are trying to be cool, or act the sophisticate, or generally put on an act, you are usually transparent.
- **Do not underestimate your audience** and do not prove how smart you are. The jury may not have any formal technical background in the subject matter you are testifying about, and

there will be members on the jury panel who do not have college or advanced degrees. This makes it all the more important for you to respect their intelligence and educate them. Never talk down to the jury. They can get even with you.

Never underestimate the knowledge of the opposing counsel, the judge, the jury or even the attorney who calls you. Playing dumb is a relatively effective strategy for an opposing attorney dealing with an expert witness (even if they are not playing).

Most scientists feel that scientific reasoning is more disciplined and logical than that of the law. It is also often easy for the technical expert to see how muddled a technical issue can become in court. The expert witness who has mastered the field may think that his or her sophistry and logic will carry the day. They may feel that it is reasonable and appropriate to engage in an antagonistic exchange between opposing counsel, opposing experts or even their own counsel! There is a very thin line between being correct and looking arrogant and condescending.

The demonstration of intellectual prowess and winning a technical point may feel good, but it may not be as redeeming to a fact-finder who is listening to all this or reviewing deposition tapes at a later date to determine what actually happened and to decide an important legal case.

- **Do not dramatize**. Do not over-dramatize the facts, or your opinion. Never give the impression that your testimony is memorized or routine.
- **Do not deny**. Never deny discussing the case or certain issues with your attorney when questioned about such a practice.
- **Do not advocate**. Do not act as an advocate or exhibit partiality. During breaks, do not be too "chummy" with your attorney, the client, the court officials, or other witnesses. Be fair in cross-examination.
- **Do not wear out your welcome.** At the conclusion of your testimony, you will be given permission to leave; if not, you may ask for permission from the judge. When you are given permission, leave the courtroom, and if possible, the courthouse. Your attorney may want to have you available, but do not hang around with the spectators unless you are specifically asked to listen to further testimony.

E. Final pointers

- **Admitting authoritative references**. Under modern evidence codes, expert witnesses not only battle with each other before the jury, but in theory, an expert can end up battling the entire corpus of scientific thought. The vast body of science may be introduced by expert witnesses through their testimony about articles, treatises and data upon which they reasonably rely and which are authorities in their particular field of expertise. A few magic words by an expert are all that it takes.

  Attorneys may present you with citations from textbooks or other scientific literature and ask if the source is authoritative. Be careful on cross-examination to avoid the phrase, "This is authoritative." These words are a blanket endorsement of the entire text. Ask to see and read the original source, book, document, or paper, before commenting on phrases taken out of context.

  Remember, if you agree that something is authoritative, anything stated therein, whether quoted to you or not, will be deemed to be accurate. Rather, reply that the author is well known and has published many articles in the literature, or that the textbook contains much useful information. Another approach is to qualify your response by saying, "I do not believe that everything in this text is authoritative." See Fed. Rules Evid. 703 and 803(18).

- **"Isn't it true" questions**. If the examiner begins his question with "Won't you agree," or "Isn't it true," never use "yes" as the first word of your answer, even if your answer eventually confirms the examiner's leading question.

19.9 The Nature of Litigation

A. Hurry up and wait

As an expert witness, you will probably experience two phenomena of litigation: the slowing of time during the proceeding and the random spontaneous resolution of a case.

Juries and expert witnesses are not part of all the action in a case. Even on a good day, the legal process is often a slow and tedious one. A few minutes of good *Court TV* are often the highlights of days of process and testimony.

Legal actions have a great tendency to resolve with or without (and sometimes despite) your help. The law, or at least the majority of judges, will view all settlements as a success. The very discovery process that you have been involved in is designed to help the parties resolve their differences and disputes.

Although a high percentage of legal actions are resolved prior to trial, and even after the trial has commenced, the expert should never anticipate settlement. The odds of going to trial and actually testifying are in direct inverse proportion to how well you are prepared. If you want good odds on being called and having a grueling cross-examination, simply be unprepared. (That is junk science, but it is true.)

B. Variables in litigation

The science and the facts may be on your side, and they may not be, but there is more to litigation than that. You are not going to be on the winning side of every case. The adversarial process is nowhere near a perfect one. There are a lot of variables in litigation, such as who are the parties, who are the attorneys, who is the fact-finder, what is the law, and who is the judge. Do the best you can, and do not take it personally if you do not like the results. It may take some time and distance to get a clear perspective and to do a "post-game" analysis.

Always remember that you are not there to "win" the case. You are there to lend your expertise to aid the jury (or judge) in understanding your work, the results, and the science. It is the lawyers who will win or lose the case.

Selected Reading

Brodsky, S.A. *The Expert Expert Witness: More Maxims and Guidelines for Testifying in Court*, illus. ed. Washington, DC: American Psychological Association, 1999.

Froede, R.C., M.D. *The Scientific Expert in Court: Principles and Guidelines*. Washington, DC: American Association for Clinical Chemistry (AACC) Press, 1997.

Furst, A. *The Toxicologist as Expert Witness: A Hint Book for Courtroom Procedure* NY: Taylor & Francis, 1996.

Poynter, D. *Expert Witness Handbook: Tips and Techniques for the Litigation Consultant*, 2nd ed. Santa Barbara, CA: Para Publishing, 1997.

Smith, C. and Bace, R.G. *A Guide to Forensic Testimony: The Art and Practice of Presenting Testimony as an Expert Technical Witness*. Boston, MA: Addison-Wesley, 2002.

Chapter 20

Alcohol Testing in the Workplace

Kurt M. Dubowski, Ph.D. and Yale H. Caplan, Ph.D.

20.1 Introduction

Efforts to prevent alcohol[1]-related problems in the workplace have a long history in the United States. Testing of workers and job applicants for alcohol has more recently been adopted as a tool for the recognition and reduction of alcohol-related problems in the workplace. It has been estimated that one in every ten people in the United States has an "alcohol problem" (U.S. Department of Labor, 1990), and the total direct and indirect economic costs of alcohol abuse were estimated as $70.3 billion for 1985 (Eighth Special Report, 1993a). Problems of such magnitude clearly affect the workplace as well as other components of society. Further, under the impetus of several highly publicized accidents and incidents involving the operation of commercial transport aircraft, marine tankers, railroad trains, and subway trains by persons allegedly under the influence of alcohol, the Congress in 1991 enacted the Omnibus Transportation Employee Testing Act of 1991 (Public Law 102-143, 1991). In a preface to the Act, the Congress stated seven findings, including these: (1) "alcohol abuse and illegal drug use pose significant dangers to the safety and welfare of the Nation;" (4) "the use of alcohol and illegal drugs has been demonstrated to affect significantly the performance of individuals, and has been proven to have been a critical factor in transportation accidents;" and (5) "the testing of uniformed personnel of the Armed Forces has shown that the most effective deterrent to abuse of alcohol and use of illegal drugs is increased testing, including random testing;" (Public Law 102-143, 1991). The Act mandates testing for alcohol, under U.S. Department of Transportation (DOT) regulations, of covered persons performing safety-sensitive functions in aviation, railroading, commercial motor vehicle operation, and mass transit operations. Under other existing federal statutory authority, DOT's Research and Special Programs Administration, which regulates pipeline and liquefied natural gas facilities and operations, also mandated workplace alcohol testing of covered workers. It thus came about that the great majority of persons required to undergo alcohol testing in the workplace work in transportation industries which fall under DOT jurisdiction. The U.S. Coast Guard was originally included in the DOT mandate but in 2003 was transferred to the new Department of Homeland Security.

A. Industries and workplaces affected by alcohol

Because of the pharmacological action and effects of alcohol, covered in detail elsewhere in this publication (see Chapters 2, 13 and 15), alcohol-induced impairment of mental and physical capabilities and functions can adversely affect work performance in most, if not all, industries and business activities (*Eighth Special Report*, 1994b). Some workplace activities obviously entail greater actual or potential hazards than others, and involve substantial risks to the worker, the workplace, and other parties if carried out by alcohol-impaired workers. In particular, the transportation workplace in all transport modalities entails basic safety hazards which are increased by the effects of alcohol on workers performing particular safety-sensitive functions. The Department of Transportation in 1994 provided an estimate of the number of workers in safety-sensitive positions in six of the transportation methods it regulates (U.S. Department of Transportation, 1994). Current figures are shown in Table 20.1 (U.S. Department of Transportation, 2003).

If applicants for safety-sensitive jobs in the DOT-regulated transportation industries are tested for alcohol, as federal law allows but does not require, the number of persons subject to testing for alcohol is obviously greatly increased.

Many nontransportation industries and workplaces involve transport of people, goods and materials as a core element. In others, transportation is absent or only incidental to other activities and operations which are inherently hazardous (e.g., mining) or associated with potential risks (e.g., energy production) which are increased when alcohol is present in workers engaged in safety-sensitive functions. Table 20.2 lists ten such nontransportation industries and workplaces which are affected by alcohol. Other commercial activities could be appropriately added to those listed (e.g., health care and medical services and communications).

Table 20.1
Commercial Transportation Employees Subject to DOT-Regulated Workplace Alcohol Testing

Industry (DOT Operating Administration)	Number of Covered Workers	Safety-Sensitive Employees
Aviation (FAA)	525,000	Flight crew, attendants and instructors; air traffic controllers; aircraft dispatchers; maintenance, screening and ground security coordinator personnel
Commercial Motor Vehicle (FMCSA)	10,941,000	Drivers (commercial vehicle driver's license holders)
Railroad (FRA)	97,000	Hours of Service Act employees: engine, train and signal services, dispatchers, operators
Mass Transit (FTA)	250,000	Vehicle operators, controllers, mechanics and armed security personnel
Pipeline (RSPA)	190,000	Operations, maintenance and emergency response personnel
Total	**12,003,000**	

DOT operating administrations:**FAA**. Federal Aviation Administration; **FMCSA**. Federal Highway Motor Carrier Safety Administration; **FRA**. Federal Railroad Administration; **FTA**. Federal Transit Administration; **RSPA**. Research and Special Programs Administration

Table 20.2
Some Nontransportation Industries and
Workplace Affected by Alcohol

- agriculture, forestry and fishing
- construction and demolition
- energy production and distribution
- manufacturing
- mining
- petroleum production and refining
- pipeline operations
- professional sports
- public safety and security
- warehousing and distribution

B. Regulated and nonregulated testing for alcohol

The universe of alcohol testing in the workplace is readily divided into governmentally regulated testing for alcohol, and nonregulated testing (i.e., testing for alcohol which is not required or controlled by law). Until recently, regulated testing was mostly performed under federal mandates. However, an increasing number of states have enacted laws that regulate the testing for alcohol and other drugs of workers within the state, under other than federally-regulated testing schemes. In the professional sports arena, such organizations as the National Football League and the National Basketball Association control and regulate testing for alcohol and other abused drugs of professional athletes in their respective franchise clubs. The current situation is shown

schematically in Figure 20.1. Some shifting among the several forms of regulation of workplace alcohol testing can be anticipated as the system matures and as the states further enlarge their oversight over workplace testing for alcohol and other drugs, which is not federally regulated. As is expectable, the majority of testing in the workplace occurs under mandate of law. A much smaller number of employers who are not mandated to do so by law carry out alcohol testing on selected members of their work force under employer policies reflecting the employment-at-will doctrine or labor agreements.

20.2 Some Legal Aspects of Alcohol Testing in the Workplace
A. In general

The legal background of workplace alcohol testing includes the federal and state regulatory environment, a substantial body of labor case law—mostly at the federal level—and a full array of policies imposed by employers or developed through collective bargaining. Many but not all recent legal aspects of the more fully developed system of workplace testing for drugs of abuse other than alcohol apply to the alcohol testing situation (e.g., constitutional issues and confidentiality and privacy considerations) (Dubowski and Tuggle, 1990). Workers fall into three major categories with respect to alcohol and drug testing: government employees, private-sector employees covered by union-negotiated or other contractual relationships, and private-sector employees

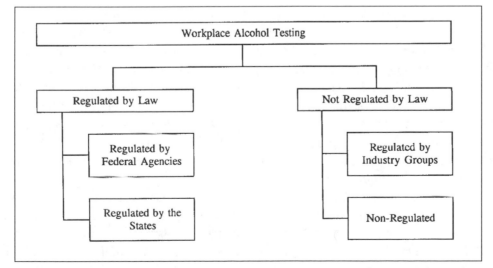

Figure 20.1 *Scheme for regulated and nonregulated workplace testing for alcohol*

in employment-at-will settings. In the future, students and perhaps other classes of people may be merged into one of these categories, or form a separate group. Workers, students, and others differ with respect to what constitutional, statute and administrative laws apply to them.

Traditionally, such constitutional rights as those against unreasonable searches and seizures, to due process of law, and to equal protection under the laws have been held to be applicable to only actions of the federal government and state governments. More recently, these constitutional issues have also been raised concerning nongovernmental workers in highly regulated industries, especially those federally regulated, such as the transportation industries. Two constitutional issues which have been raised concerning testing for alcohol and other drugs are search-and-seizure and due process. Several U.S. Supreme Court decisions undergird the legality of testing for alcohol and other drugs in the law enforcement and workplace settings, and have circumscribed such testing. In 1966, the High Court addressed the constitutional search-and-seizure issue in *Schmerber v. California* (384 U. S. 757 [1966]). The Court decided that the extraction of blood from an uncooperative driver under arrest on drinking-driving charges was a search-and-seizure under the Fourth Amendment,[2] but was reasonable in the particular circumstances of that case. The doctrine and impact of *Schmerber* have since been substantially extended since 1966. In *Skinner v. Railway Labor Executives' Association* (489 U.S. 602 [1989]), the High Court recognized that collection of breath or urine should also be deemed a search, upheld Federal Railroad Administration regulations governing drug and alcohol post-accident and reasonable-cause testing of covered railroad employees, and concluded that issuance of a warrant or the existence of probable cause or individualized suspicion is not a minimum essential requirement in establishing the reasonableness of such a search under an administrative testing program. In a companion case, *National Treasury Employees Union v. Von Raab* (489 U.S. 656, 1989), the Supreme Court again upheld a urine drug testing program for certain federal customs officers, and ruled that neither probable cause, reasonable suspicion, nor a warrant is required to collect

body fluids under this kind of governmentally sponsored drug-testing program, although such collection does constitute a search (National Treasury Employees Union, 1989). A 1993 U.S. District Court ruling affirmed that suspicionless random testing of commercial motor vehicle operators for alcohol and controlled substances, as mandated by Section 5(b) of the Omnibus Transportation Employee Testing Act of 1991, comports with the Fourth Amendment of the U.S. Constitution and is not an unreasonable search-and-seizure (*Owner-Operator Independent Driver Association, Inc. v. Peña*, No. 93-1427, U.S. District Court for the District of Columbia, November 1, 1993). Likewise, random breath-alcohol testing of transit system operating employees was upheld by a federal appeals court (*United Transportation Union v. Southeastern Pennsylvania Transportation Authority*, 884 F. 2d 709 [1989]).

Consistent with these court decisions, the alcohol testing mandated by Congress under the Omnibus Transportation Employee Testing Act of 1991 is constitutionally permissible, where the Congress determined that (1) there is a need for properly administered alcohol testing to ensure that employees in transportation industries are not adversely affected by alcohol while performing safety-sensitive functions, and (2) that need outweighs the privacy interests of these employees.

The Fifth Amendment and the Fourteenth Amendment of the U.S. Constitution guarantee that due process of law will be afforded to all persons subject to the actions of the federal, state and local governments.[3] In recent years, there has been a trend to extend due process guarantees to an ever-enlarging universe of quasi-governmental and private actions and issues, especially those of an adverse nature, including "academic due process," disciplinary proceedings of membership organizations, and employer-employee relations involving discharge and so on. The extension of the due process guarantees to the nongovernmental arena has usually been through case law, involving both substantive and procedural due process issues. An essential due process element in all of these situations is the incorporation of adequate procedural safeguards into applicable policies and practices. In the context of workplace alcohol testing, those prime procedural safeguards include (1) actions to assure the reliability and validity of the testing process and its results, and (2) the opportunity for the tested person to challenge a result and an adverse action based on a test result. A meaningful opportunity to challenge a test result requires timely notice detailing the reasons for a proposed adverse action, such as termination of employment, full access to all relevant information about the testing process and its outcome in issue, and a forum in which to contest the result, typically a timely hearing. Due process issues have been raised mostly in workplace drug-testing rather than alcohol-testing cases because of the much longer experience with the latter, but the same legal principles are applicable. Procedural due process challenges have been aimed at both the testing process (*Banks v. FAA*, 687 F. 2d 92 [5th Cir. 1982]) and its aftermath, such as employee termination (*Shoemaker v. Handel*, 619 F. Supp. 1089 [1985]). It has been stated in the drug testing context that due process has been equated to "fundamental fairness" (Kwong, 1988; *Superintendent v. Hill*, 105 S. Ct. 2768 [1985]), which generally involves a balancing of competing interests.

There is also a High Court decision on the reliability of forensic breath-alcohol analysis in traffic law enforcement. In *California v. Trombetta* (467 U. S. 479, 1984) the Supreme Court in 1984 dismissed challenges to the reliability of breath-alcohol analysis by means of automated infrared spectrometry, under the due process clause of the Fourteenth Amendment to the U.S. Constitution (California, 1984). The Court also held that "the Due Process Clause of the Fourteenth Amendment does not require that law enforcement agencies preserve breath samples in order to introduce breath-analysis tests at trial." It, however, is relevant to workplace alcohol testing that the High Court also acknowledged that "State courts and legislatures, of course, remain free to adopt more rigorous safeguards governing the admissibility of scientific evidence than those imposed by the Federal Constitution," and further, and pertinently, stated that "Respondents could also have protected themselves from erroneous on-the-scene testing by electing to submit to urine or blood tests . . . ." (*California*, 1984). The federal workplace alcohol testing regulations in effect at the time of this publication do not allow tested subjects to choose those

tests as either alternatives or in addition to employer-performed alcohol testing. Other constitutional issues that have been raised in federal and state courts in connection with workplace drug testing are equal protection and privacy (Farmer, 1987). Space limitations and the complexity of these issues prevent their discussion here. A comprehensive body of literature does exist on these matters (e.g., Cornish, 1988). Employers planning to carry out workplace alcohol testing need and should be guided by appropriate legal advice on these and related issues.

B. The regulatory environment

The primary regulatory control of alcohol testing in the workplace is by federal agencies. Federal regulations universally preempt and supersede state laws and regulations except for those concerning traffic law enforcement. In addition, most states have enacted laws providing for state regulation of workplace alcohol (and drug) testing in circumstances other than those subject to federal control. Lastly, rudimentary regulation of alcohol (and drug) testing exists in some specialized workplaces (e.g., professional sports under the aegis of the respective sports leagues or associations). Generally, information about the latter is not public, while the federal and state regulated testing regulations are, of course, fully disclosed and widely publicized. Table 20.3 lists programs for workplace alcohol control and alcohol testing established by several federal agencies, with the respective primary regulatory reference in the Code of Federal Regulations (CFR). The provisions of CFR have the force of federal law and generally supersede any conflicting state laws or regulations. The federal agencies listed in Table 20.3, and others, have in aggregate promulgated hundreds of regulations pertaining to control of alcohol use and abuse and workplace alcohol testing of those members of the federal workplace and employees of federally-regulated industries who perform safety-sensitive functions. Because of their volume and the frequent revisions in these rules, it is impracticable to enumerate and discuss them in this chapter. Current rules are available on the DOT website at www.dot. gov/ost/dapc.

The alcohol misuse prevention testing rules of the several federal agencies are based on universal

Table 20.3
Some Federally Regulated Workplace Alcohol Control and Testing Programs

Agency		Regulatory Reference
National Aeronautics and Space Administration		14 CFR Part 1272
Nuclear Regulatory Commission		10 CFR Parts 2 and 26
U.S. Department of Energy		10 CFR Part 707
U.S. Department of Transportation		49 CFR Part 40
	Federal Aviation Administration	14 CFR Parts 61, 121, 135 et al.
	Federal Motor Carrier Safety Administration	49 CFR Part 382 et al.
	Federal Railroad Administration	49 CFR Part 219
	Federal Transit Administration	49 CFR Part 655
	Research and Special Programs Administration	49 CFR Part 199
U.S. Department of Homeland Security		
	U.S. Coast Guard	33 CFR Part 95; 46 CFR Parts 4, 16 et al.

CFR = Code of Federal Regulations

public safety considerations and the general safety authority of the individual agencies. In addition, the Omnibus Transportation Employee Testing Act of 1991 (P.L. 102-143, Title V) is a direct federal statutory mandate for alcohol testing in the aviation, motor carrier, rail, and mass transit industries. Employees and employers in some industries are subject to multi-agency coverage of alcohol misuse and testing regulations; possibly with different definitions of such terms as accident, covered employee, and safety-sensitive function. Most federal agency programs are deterrent-oriented with minor fitness-for-duty components. In contrast, the drug and alcohol control programs of the Nuclear Regulatory Commission (NRC) are primarily fitness-for-duty programs and are so titled, with a minor deterrent component. The NRC's rationale for its fitness-for-duty program was set forth as follows in its final rule adoption (Nuclear Regulatory Commission, 1989):

> The general objective of this program is to provide reasonable assurance that nuclear power plant personnel are reliable, trustworthy, and not under the influence of any substance, legal or illegal, or mentally or physically impaired from any cause, which in a way adversely affects their ability to safely and competently perform their duties. A fitness-for-duty program developed under the

requirements of this rule is intended to create an environment which is free of drugs and the effects of such substances.

The Americans with Disabilities Act (ADA) of 1990 is frequently cited as imposing limitations on adverse employer actions taken against certain workers who yield tests positive for alcohol or other drugs (Public Law 101-136, 1990). The Congress declared that among the purposes of the ADA are: (1) "to provide a clear and comprehensive national mandate for the elimination of discrimination against individuals with disabilities;" and (2) "to provide clear, strong, consistent, enforceable standards addressing discrimination against individuals with disabilities." Various provisions of Title I of the ADA relate to workplace alcohol and drug testing. The ADA broadly prohibits discrimination by any covered entity (employer) against a qualified individual with a disability. Court decisions interpreting Section 504 of the Rehabilitation Act of 1973, with which ADA employment provisions are intended to be consistent, have established that alcoholism can be a disability that may call for the reasonable accommodation required by ADA, unless providing that reasonable accommodation creates an undue hardship. The ADA specifically authorizes covered entities to comply with workplace standards of the Department of Defense, the Nuclear Regulatory

Commission, and the Department of Transportation relating to alcohol control and alcohol testing of employees. The ADA, however, also prohibits covered entities from conducting a medical examination or making disability-targeted inquiries until after an offer of employment has been made to a job applicant, and subject to certain additional restrictions. It is presently apparently unsettled whether such alcohol testing of job applicants, which is authorized by DOT regulations or otherwise outside of the DOT, constitutes a medical examination or inquiry under ADA.

In addition to the federal laws and regulations addressed above, there are many state regulations, typically administered by the state Department of Health, which mirror the federal regulations in many, but not all, respects. Because of the preemptive provisions of the Omnibus Transportation Employee Testing Act of 1991 and other federal laws and agency regulations, state laws and regulations only affect alcohol and drug testing which is not federally regulated and is carried out within a given state by entities of that state and its political subdivisions or by private sector employers within the state. Law enforcement applications of alcohol and drug testing are typically excluded. In workplaces or with respect to workers not covered by federal or state laws and regulations, alcohol testing may be, and is, carried out under employee policies that may, in some circumstances, be subject to labor agreements. Such private sector testing, like regulated testing, is also subject to applicable federal laws and regulations that impinge on alcohol and drug control and testing programs, such as the ADA.

20.3 Features of Alcohol Testing in the Workplace

From the overwhelming amount of information about the effects of alcohol and about alcohol abuse and misuse in the workplace and elsewhere (*Eighth Special Report*, 1994b; Forney, 1987; *The Existing Safety Problem*, 1994; Pawlowski, 1992; U.S. Department of Labor, 1991), some principles and various recommended policies and practices emerge. Those discussed in this section of this chapter apply generally to unregulated workplace testing for alcohol. They may also be partly applicable to regulated

alcohol testing situations; to the extent that differences exist, the pertinent regulations will prevail and control.

The recommended overall general principle is simple: Workers should be free of alcoholic influence at work. The various elements of workplace alcohol control and testing programs are intended to bring about conformance with that principle. In the implementation of the overall principle, three additional recommendations predominate:

- Workers should abstain from alcohol intake for twelve to twenty-four hours before undertaking critical and safety-sensitive tasks.
- An appropriate program of alcohol testing should be implemented, with on-site and off-site components.
- Breath-alcohol concentrations (BrAC) less than 0.01 g/210 L, and blood and saliva-alcohol concentrations less than 0.01 g/dL should be deemed "alcohol-free status."

A. Special features of workplace testing for alcohol

During the past three decades, testing for commonly abused drugs other than alcohol in the military environment and the civilian workplace has been widely practiced and has become commonplace in many settings. In contrast, testing for alcohol has been very widely performed in the United States in connection with traffic law enforcement for more that fifty years; but has only recently been introduced into the workplace as a tool for prevention and control of alcohol abuse.

The special aspects of alcohol control and testing in the workplace include these: Alcohol purchase, use and testing for alcohol are specially regulated by the federal government and the states. Alcohol impairs work performance at all measurable concentrations. The technology of alcohol testing is highly advanced and is well understood.

There are also several key differences between alcohol and other abused drugs and between testing for alcohol and other commonly abused drugs. First and foremost, alcohol is a licit drug and consumption of alcoholic beverages by adults is lawful, with limited exceptions, such as while driving motor vehicles. The mere presence of alcohol in the body and in body fluids (e.g., breath or saliva) does not imply a violation of law, as would be true for presence of Schedule-I controlled dangerous substances, the possession and use of which is an illegal act. Alcohol in the body has a short half-life,[4] meaning that its elimination from the body is significantly faster than that of other commonly abused drugs (i.e., measured in hours rather than days or weeks). This, in turn, affects the timing of specimen collection for alcohol testing and militates for on-site testing. The relationship between alcohol concentration in such body fluids as blood and breath and alcoholic impairment is well-established. That relationship is, in fact, much better understood and documented than is true for any other drug-of-abuse. Various specific statutory and regulatory prohibitions exist for stated alcohol concentration thresholds; those pertaining to motor vehicle operation are the most widely recognized and applied. Statutory and regulatory limitations on use of alcohol typically address such issues as where, when, under what circumstances, and by whom possession and consumption of alcoholic beverages is prohibited or restricted; and typically also establish thresholds of alcohol concentrations in human body fluids at and above which particular actions are interdicted or become unlawful. Finally, in contrast to drug-use testing in urine specimens, review and interpretation of testing results by a medical review officer (MRO) is unnecessary and uncommon.

One additional, universal feature of alcohol testing in the workplace deserves recognition. The majority of workplace alcohol testing is carried out under mandate of law. Moreover, reliance upon workplace alcohol test results in disciplinary proceedings, formal challenge of some test results, and their involvement in arbitration, litigation and other adversary proceedings are expectable and predictable consequences of workplace alcohol testing: Therefore, alcohol testing should be, and is, considered to be a forensic toxicology activity;[5] and should be carried out with due consideration for that status and in accordance with all of the applicable principles, procedures, and safeguards of forensic toxicology.[5]

B. Purpose of alcohol testing in the workplace

In regulated industries and workplaces such as transportation, testing for alcohol is mandated, and the principal reason for instituting and conducting an alcohol-abuse control and testing program is to comply with the pertinent regulatory mandates. The regulations, of course, are typically justified as necessary to minimize the risks of alcohol in the workplace and to deter inappropriate alcohol use by covered workers.

There remain a number of industries and workplaces with inherent hazards and increased risks (e.g., construction and mining) to which regulated workplace alcohol testing is of only incidental and of limited applicability—usually in connection with commercial motor vehicle operation. In these and other workplaces for which alcohol testing is not mandated, policy decisions to implement testing are safety-based. The National Safety Council's Committee on Alcohol and Other Drugs in 1995 developed "A Model Program for the Control of Alcohol in the Workplace" (Committee, 1995). That document was developed chiefly to assist employers and others required to establish alcohol testing programs in response to the Omnibus Transportation Employee Testing Act of 1991 and its implementing regulations, and suggests that the purpose of alcohol testing programs is "to help prevent accidents and injuries resulting from the misuse of alcohol by employees who perform safety-sensitive functions in . . . industry . . . ." That statement succinctly summarizes the principal goal of alcohol testing programs in general.

There are, of course, other indications for workplace alcohol testing as a fact-finding tool in accident investigation, determination of fitness-for-duty, and other specified situations, as further discussed below.

C. Alcohol testing categories and indications for alcohol testing

There are several classifications in use for testing categories, mostly derived from the long experience in applying alcohol testing to traffic law enforcement and to a lesser extent from the current practices in drug-use testing. The simplest classification is by test class:

- initial test and
- confirmatory test.

Initial tests, sometimes referred to as screening tests or preliminary tests, are intended and useful primarily to establish whether the tested person is alcohol-free or not. Alcohol-free status obviates the need for any further testing for alcohol. Screening tests to be most practical must be simply and rapidly performed with minimal training. They do not possess the necessary validity for evidential use. Confirmatory tests are those performed with evidential-grade testing devices or systems, after an initial test has indicated the presence of alcohol in the tested person. The results of the confirmatory tests are those relied upon for such immediate safety-related personnel actions as removal from current safety-sensitive duties, and for any subsequent disciplinary or other employment consequences.

A more comprehensive scheme of classification is by testing categories, shown in Table 20.4.

The testing categories are largely self-explanatory. DOT-regulated testing lacks a requirement for applicant testing, but substitutes a "pre-employment" testing requirement as authorized for employees newly hired for or transferred to safety-sensitive duties before they first perform those duties. Reasonable suspicion and reasonable cause testing are the workplace equivalent of the probable cause required for a valid arrest on an alcohol-related traffic offense or other criminal charge. In law enforcement situations, alcohol testing involves search-and-seizure incident to a lawful arrest, while the lesser probative value indication of reasonable suspicion or reasonable cause suffices to initiate a workplace alcohol test. The random testing category in principle encompasses on-duty testing of all covered employ-

Table 20.4
Workplace Alcohol Testing Categories

- applicant testing
- reasonable-suspicion and reasonable-cause testing
- fitness-for-duty testing
- post-accident testing
- return-to-duty and followup testing
- random testing

ees. It is usually represented as the key deterrent component of a workplace alcohol-misuse control program. Covered employees are subject to unannounced random, patternless testing based purely on a nondiscriminatory class characteristic. It is the only category of testing not triggered by or conducted in response to another event. Random testing rates are prescribed by industry for regulated testing and vary between 10, 25 and 50 percent of the covered work force annually. The various federal regulations provide for annual review and adjustment of the industry's random alcohol test rate, based on a performance standard related to its random alcohol violation rate. The selection mechanism for random testing must be by means of a scientifically valid, unbiased method such as a computer-generated random number that is matched with employees' social security or employee identification numbers. The controlling principle is that every covered employee must have an equal chance of being tested. It is equally important for the deterrent effect that random tests be spread reasonably throughout the year and not follow a predictable pattern (e.g., always on a given weekday). Typically, random testing is also by far the largest portion of a workplace alcohol testing program.

Nonrandom tests are triggered by a particular event. Post-accident testing is largely self-explanatory, but requires that the employer policy clearly define the triggering accident event in such respects as fatalities, personal injury, property damage of a particular kind or above a fixed dollar amount, connection of the covered employee to the accident apart from later determination of causation, time frames relative to occurrence or discovery of the accident and so on. In regulated testing, these matters are fully covered in the pertinent regulations.

D. Reasonable suspicion testing

This testing occasion is triggered when an employer, though the employer's agent such as a designated and qualified supervisor, has reasonable suspicion or reasonable cause to believe that an employee has violated the employer's alcohol abuse control policy, or violated the provisions of agency rules in regulated testing environments. Commonly, that reasonable suspicion is grounded in the employee's behavior and appearance indicating alcohol misuse. The determination of policy or rule violation must be contemporaneous with the conduct, behavior or appearance involved, be based on specific articulable observation and findings by a trained supervisor, and must occur during, or just preceding or just after the safety sensitive function in issue. The usual determinants will be appearance, behavior, speech, performance, or alcohol beverage odor emanating from the employee. The key is short-term, contemporaneous and articulable observations, rather than such secondary events often associated with chronic substance abuse as a pattern of absenteeism, constant lateness, or abuse of sick leave. In this context, the term "articulable" observations are derived from the case law of evidence in criminal offenses and means observations and findings which can be described with particularity. They encompass but are not limited to the indications that persons are under the influence of or impaired, or apparently intoxicated by alcohol. Because these observations and conclusions are subjective, the reasonable suspicion or reasonable cause determination must be followed by testing for alcohol as soon as possible. The behavior, appearance and results of observation of a covered employee which are considered to give rise to reasonable suspicion testing should not per se be considered to be prohibited conduct that triggers the full consequences of policy or rule violation, without confirmation of alcohol misuse by a positive test result. The acute effects of alcohol, short of obvious intoxication, which can be a guide to the triggering of reasonable suspicion or reasonable cause alcohol testing, may include slurred speech, dilated pupils, neuromuscular incoordination, and sensory and perceptual alterations.

Diagnostic features of alcoholic intoxication have been developed by the American Psychiatric Association, as shown in Table 20.5 and in the following excerpted description from the APA's *Diagnostic and Statistical Manual of Mental Disorders*, DSM-IV (Diagnostic and Statistical Manual, 1994).

> . . . The essential feature of Alcohol Intoxication is the presence of clinically significant maladaptive behavioral or psychological changes (e.g., inappropriate sexual or ag-

gressive behavior, mood lability, impaired judgment, impaired social or occupational functioning) that develop during, or shortly after, the ingestion of alcohol (Criteria A and B). These changes are accompanied by evidence of slurred speech, incoordination, unsteady gait, nystagmus, impairment in attention or memory, or stupor or coma (Criterion C). The symptoms must not be due to a general medical condition and are not better accounted for by another mental disorder (Criterion D) . . . The levels of incoordination can interfere with driving abilities and with performing usual activities to the point of causing accidents. Evidence of alcohol use can be obtained by smelling alcohol on the individual's breath, eliciting a history from the individual or another observer, and, when needed, having the individual undertake breath, blood, or urine toxicology analyses.

Table 20.5
American Psychiatric Association Diagnostic Criteria for Alcohol Intoxication (*Diagnostic and Statistical Manual*, 1994)

A. Recent ingestion of alcohol.
B. Clinically significant maladaptive behavioral or psychological changes (e.g., inappropriate sexual or aggressive behavior, mood lability, impaired judgment, impaired social or occupational functioning) that developed during, or shortly after, alcohol ingestion.
C. One (or more) of the following signs, developing during, or shortly after, alcohol use:
  (1) slurred speech
  (2) incoordination
  (3) unsteady gait
  (4) nystagmus
  (5) impairment in attention or memory
  (6) stupor or coma
D. The symptoms are not due to a general medical condition and are not better accounted for by another mental disorder.

E. Testing locations: On-site versus off-site

The decision whether to conduct workplace alcohol testing at the employee's work site location ("on-site") or at another location ("off-site") hinges on a variety of factors—economic, time-related, test volume and locations of work sites and so forth. Testing conducted under Nuclear Regulatory Commission or Department of Transportation regulations must generally be carried out on-site, except for post-accident testing which may of necessity be performed on injured workers at a hospital or similar healthcare facility. The purpose of the testing is also dispositive. If the employer policy calls for alcohol-free status of designated employees prior to commencing safety-sensitive functions, testing must generally be performed on-site. In contrast, return-to-duty and follow-up testing could be carried out off-site, say at a counseling clinic. Timely accessibility of test facilities will also control where reasonable suspicion testing is to be done. Random testing must (in regulated testing) or should (in nonregulated testing) immediately precede or follow a normal work period or shift. In most situations that requirement dictates on-site testing. On-site testing does not, however, require establishing and maintaining a continuously manned testing facility at every work site. Third-party consortia or a multisite employer such as an airline can provide mobile equipment and personnel to operate a temporary testing activity at preselected locations, chiefly for random testing which can be appropriately scheduled. On-site testing can be limited to initial (screening) testing for alcohol if a suitably equipped and staffed facility is available within a short distance and time-frame to conduct confirmatory breath-alcohol testing on workers who are escorted to the latter facility after an initially positive screening test result. In DOT-regulated testing, the confirmation test must be conducted within thirty minutes of the completion of the screening test (Department of Transportation, 1995). In practice, that limits the conduct of screening and confirmation tests at different sites to those at prearranged nearby locations. While covered employers always remain responsible for having the proper category of testing accomplished, they can delegate the testing function to other qualified and authorized parties such as testing consortia or third-party administrators by con-tract or similar arrangement; that includes confirmatory testing.

The foregoing considerations in workplace alcohol testing differ markedly from the situation for federally regulated workplace urine drug testing, in which on-site activities are typically limited to specimen collection and forwarding, while most actual drug testing and all confirmatory testing is performed in DHHS-certified laboratories.

20.4 Alcohol Testing Regulated by the U.S. Department of Transportation

Workplace alcohol testing regulated by the U.S. Department of Transportation is mandated by the Omnibus Transportation Employee Testing Act of 1991 (Public Law 102-143, 1991) for certain transportation methods and is authorized for others (e.g., pipeline operations), by other statutes or under the general safety enforcement authority of the applicable operating administration (e.g., RSPA). The pertinent DOT regulations, policies and practices are very comprehensive and have operating administration-specific features. Because of those differences and the inevitable periodic revisions in the regulations, the information in this section is necessarily restricted to DOT-wide provisions. A comprehensive discussion of the background of the DOT regulations and the basis for various DOT decisions on alternatives is contained in the *Federal Register* issue of February 15, 1994 and revised extensively in the *Federal Register* issue of December 19, 2000 (Department of Transportation, 2000).

A. Prohibited conduct

Performance of safety-sensitive functions by a covered employee in any DOT-regulated entity is prohibited: (1) When such person has an alcohol concentration (AC)[6] of 0.04 or greater, as indicated by a breath-alcohol test, or temporarily when such person has an alcohol concentration of 0.02 or greater but less than 0.04; (2) while such person is using alcohol; and (3) within four hours (eight hours for flight-crew members) after using alcohol. In addition, refusal to submit to testing for alcohol and use of alcohol within eight hours after involvement in an accident or until tested, for employees required to be tested, are prohibited.

B. Required alcohol testing

Under the rules issued pursuant to the act, in general the following categories of alcohol testing are required:

- **pre-duty**. Conducted before employees actually perform safety-sensitive functions for the first time, or when other employees transfer to a safety-sensitive position. This was modified pursuant to court rulings and continues to be authorized but not mandated by the revised rules issued in 2000 (Department of Transportation, 2000).
- **post-accident**. Conducted after involvement in accidents by employees whose performance could have contributed to the accident.
- **reasonable suspicion**. Conducted when a trained supervisor observes behavior or appearance in an employee which is characteristic of alcohol misuse.
- **random**. Conducted on a random unannounced basis just before, during, or just after performance of safety-sensitive functions.
- **return-to-duty and followup**. Conducted when an individual who has violated the prohibited alcohol conduct standards returns to safety-sensitive duties. Followup tests are unannounced and must include a minimum of six tests within the first twelve months after return to duty, and may be enforced for up to sixty months thereafter.

There are differences in the application of the required testing conditions and schedules among the several DOT operating administrations.

C. Features of alcohol testing under DOT regulations

Testing for alcohol under the DOT regulations has the following common features.

Alcohol is defined as "The intoxicating agent in beverage alcohol, ethyl alcohol or other low molecular weight alcohols including methyl or isopropyl alcohol." Alcohol concentration is defined as "The alcohol in a volume of breath expressed in terms of grams of alcohol per 210 liters of breath as indicated by a breath test . . . ." All alcohol testing is to be carried out on-site at the workplace, except in some post-accident situations. Breath and saliva are the only acceptable specimens for initial "screening" tests. "Screening" and "confirmation" tests are required in defined circumstances. Breath is the required and only acceptable specimen for "confirmation" tests, with some exceptions for post-accident testing. All testing for alcohol in breath or saliva must be carried out with testing and associated devices appearing on NHTSA Conforming Products Lists (NHTSA, 1997; NHTSA, 2001; NHTSA, 2002). Screening tests on breath or saliva must use breath or saliva-alcohol screening test devices appearing on the NHTSA Conforming Products List, or be performed on breath with evidential breath testers (EBTs) appearing on the NHTSA Conforming Products List. Confirmation tests must be carried out on breath and must use EBTs which are (1) capable of providing a printed result in triplicate, (2) capable of assigning a unique and sequential number to each completed test, and displaying same before the test, (3) capable of printing on each copy of the result the manufacturer's name for the device, the device serial number, the time of the test, and the test number, (4) able to distinguish alcohol from acetone at an alcohol concentration of 0.02 g/210 L, and (5) capable of testing an air blank prior to each collection of breath, and of performing an "external calibration check." Confirmation tests must be carried out within thirty minutes of the completion of a screening test which yields an alcohol concentration of 0.02 or greater. A deprivation period of not less than fifteen minutes must precede, and thereafter an air blank yielding 0.00 g/210 L result must precede breath collection in a confirmation test. Air blanks are not required before or after a screening test on breath. Testing must be performed by a breath alcohol technician (BAT) who has successfully completed a course of instruction equivalent to the DOT model course, as determined by NHTSA, and who has "demonstrated competence in the operation of the specific EBTs" which the BAT will use. Law enforcement officers who have been certified by state or local governments to conduct breath-alcohol testing with the EBT concerned are deemed by DOT to be qualified as BATs. Inability of an employee to participate in or complete a breath-alcohol test requires subsequent evaluation by a physician, with stated consequences. There is no stipulated role for a medical review officer (MRO) in conducting alcohol testing or interpreting alcohol test results.

D. Significance, interpretation and consequences of test results

The significance, interpretation, and consequences of alcohol test results under 49 CFR Part 40 are complex and vary somewhat among DOT operating administrations and with the test category and situation. In general, alcohol test results have the following significance and consequences with a bifurcated 0.02 and 0.04 alcohol concentration standard.

An alcohol concentration result (screening) less than 0.02 is considered a negative test, and no further testing is authorized. A saliva result (screening) indicating an alcohol concentration of less than 0.02 has the same significance. An alcohol concentration result (screening) of 0.02 or greater on breath or saliva must be followed by a "confirmation" test on breath within thirty minutes of the completion of the screening test. A BrAC result (confirmation) less than 0.02 g/210 L is considered a final negative test. A BrAC result (confirmation) of 0.02 g/210 L or greater requires removal of the covered employee from a safety-sensitive function. If the BrAC is 0.02 g/210 L or greater but less than 0.04 g/210 L, the employee is temporarily prohibited from performing or continuing to perform a safety-sensitive function until the next regularly scheduled duty period, but not less than eight hours after administration of the test (twenty-four hours for those regulated by FMCSA), or until a retest yields a BrAC less than 0.02 g/210 L. A final, confirmed BrAC result of 0.04 g/210 L or greater prohibits the employee from performing or continuing to perform a safety-sensitive function, and subjects the employee to other specified consequences (e.g., mandatory referral to a "substance abuse professional"). In the event that the screening and confirmation tests yield dif-

ferent results, the confirmation test result is deemed to be the final result. The rules have somewhat complex provisions for what constitutes or leads to a cancelled test. The following events, among others, give rise to cancelled tests: (1) The next "external calibration check" of an EBT yielding a result varying from the target value by more than "the tolerance stated in the QAP." In such an event, all test results of 0.02 g/210 L or greater obtained on the device since the last valid "external calibration check" are cancelled. (2) Failure to observe the minimum fifteen-minute deprivation period prior to a confirmation test. (3) Failure to perform an air blank test prior to a confirmation test, or an air blank test result greater than 0.00 g/210 L prior to the breath collection. (4) Failure of the EBT to print a confirmation test result. (5) Failure of the sequential test number or the test result displayed by the EBT to match the printed output.

A schema summarizing the foregoing DOT testing procedure and test result consequences is shown in Figure 20.2.

Extrapolation of results is not permitted. Further and in contrast to the universal practice for breath-alcohol testing in traffic law enforcement, failure of an employee to comply with the instructions of the breath alcohol technician (e.g., to refrain from smoking or ingesting any substance during the fifteen-minute observation-deprivation period prior to breath-alcohol testing) is not treated as a "refusal" to be tested with no test given. Instead, the test is given and the details of the irregularity are annotated in the record.

E. Quality assurance aspects

Evidential breath-alcohol testing (EBT) devices used for either screening or confirmation tests are subject to a quality assurance plan (QAP) developed by the respective device manufacturer. The QAP for evidential breath-testing devices must be submitted to and approved by NHTSA, and shall: (1) Designate method(s) for performing control tests termed "external calibration checks" of the instrument, us-

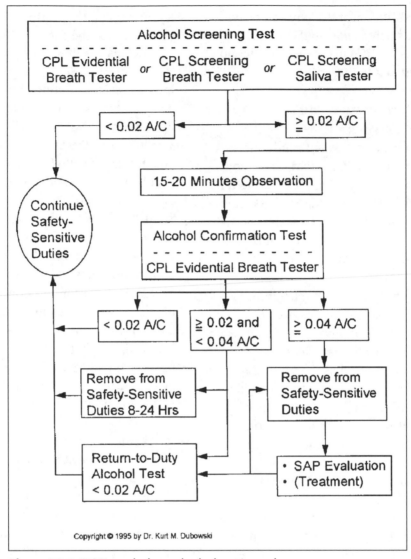

Figure 20.2 *DOT workplace alcohol testing schema*

ing calibrating devices on the NHTSA Conforming Products List of Calibrating Units for Breath-Alcohol Testers. (2) Specify the minimum time intervals for control tests of the device, and the "tolerances on an external calibration check within which the EBT is regarded to be in proper calibration." (3) Specify inspection, maintenance, and calibration requirements and intervals for the EBT. Inspection, maintenance, and calibration of EBTs must be performed by the device manufacturer or a "maintenance representative" certified by the device manufacturer or by an appropriate state agency. Employers must ensure compliance with the details of the QAP, must maintain certain QAP records for two years and records of "external calibration checks" for five years, and store EBTs in a "secure space" when not in use. The

term "external calibration check," as DOT regulations use it, contemplates performance of a control test, such as analysis of a vapor of known alcohol content produced by equilibration of air with an ethanol solution of known concentration at a fixed temperature (Dubowski and Essary, 1992), or analysis of a gas-vapor mixture of known alcohol content released from a compressed gas mixture of alcohol in an inert gas such as nitrogen, adjusted for the ambient atmospheric pressure and the temperature of the sample chamber. There are separate DOT requirements for quality assurance plans for nonevidential screening devices for alcohol.

F. Statutory and regulatory changes in transportation workplace alcohol testing

Enactment of the Omnibus Transportation Employee Testing Act of 1991 was soon followed by lobbying by transport workers unions, industry organizations and others seeking to repeal or modify various provisions of the act. Debate over the effectiveness and cost of alcohol testing of applicants for safety-sensitive duty jobs (as distinct from employees) was particularly intense. The Department of Transportation, as a consequence of litigation and its own policy questions on the interpretation of the Act, never implemented applicant or pre-employment testing for alcohol by regulation. Subsequent legislation approved on November 28, 1995, P. L. 104-59, Section 342. Alcohol and Controlled Substances Testing, finally clarified the situation. The Congress directed the Secretary of Transportation to promulgate regulations for alcohol testing which require the conduct of reasonable suspicion, random, and post-accident testing for alcohol of mass transportation employees responsible for safety-sensitive functions (as decided by the Secretary) and which permit the conduct of pre-employment testing of such persons for alcohol at the employer's option. P. L. 104-59 also requires the Secretary of Transportation to promulgate comparable regulations for alcohol testing of motor carrier and air carrier employees, and certain employees of the Federal Aviation Administration.

The statutory language "preemployment testing of such employees" seems destined for further interpretation in the courts. It appears to contemplate conduct of tests for alcohol not on applicants but on persons hired to perform safety-sensitive functions or transferred to such functions, prior to first performance of covered functions. In any event, the principal policy difference between the 1991 act and the 1995 act is that preemployment testing for use of alcohol (no longer for use of alcohol "in violation of law or Federal regulation") is now permitted at the option of the employer, but no longer required or controlled by federal law or regulation. Further, in 2000, DOT modified its rules authorizing transportation employers to conduct preemployment testing if desired, reiterating that such testing is not mandatory.

There are also provisions in the federal DOT regulations for periodic changes in the proportion of covered workers required to be randomly tested for alcohol each year, in keeping with the prior year's positive test rate. These random test requirements are industry-specific.

20.5 Testing Technology and Practices
A. Analysis and specimens

The principles underlying the analysis for alcohol in breath and other specimens are discussed in detail in other chapters in this publication. These include such considerations as duplicate testing, mouth alcohol, reporting units, and the applicability of various specimens including breath, saliva, blood and urine.

The DOT regulated program focuses on the use of breath. Breath specimens can be collected by non-invasive techniques, are representative of the dynamic circulating blood and brain alcohol concentrations, have been extensively utilized by law enforcement in drinking driving arrests, and have been successfully accepted and defended in the courts. Blood specimens require the services of a qualified phlebotomist; hence adding cost and the stigma of venipuncture to testing. In addition, blood testing is laboratory based and therefore would require certified facilities. Further, the results would be delayed and not immediately available. The DOT program permits saliva as an alternative screening-only specimen.

Urine specimens, on the other hand, are neither useful nor permitted for DOT testing. Urine is a static specimen and as such is not representative of the blood or breath. Proper collection would require collecting two sequential timed specimens. In the presence of alcohol producing microorganisms and glucose, alcohol can be produced in urine; hence, there could be both qualitative and quantitative concerns when testing at the targeted 0.02 and 0.04 AC. Additional discussion on this topic is presented in Chapter 5.

B. Testing in the DOT program

Testing in the DOT program is controlled by regulation as previously described. Screening tests permit breath or saliva, while confirmatory tests require breath. DOT regulations provide the following documents that define the criteria for evaluation and provide notice of acceptable products that meet the established criteria:

1. a. Model Specifications for Evidential Breath Testing Devices (NHTSA, 1993)
   b. Conforming Products List of Evidential Breath Testing Devices (NHTSA, 2002)
2. a. Model Specifications for Screening Devices to Measure Alcohol in Bodily Fluids (NHTSA, 1994)
   b. Conforming Products List of Screening Devices to Measure Alcohol in Bodily Fluids (NHTSA, 2001)
3. a. Model Specifications for Calibrating Units for Breath Alcohol Tests (NHTSA, 1997)
   b. Conforming Products List of Calibrating Unit for Breath Tests (NHTSA, 1997)

These notices have been published in the *Federal Register* over the years to identify equipment approved for law enforcement driving while intoxicated (DWI) programs. Such programs were traditionally focused on 0.08 and above AC as needed to sustain DWI charges. Recent emphasis in the police arena for youthful offenders targeted at 0.02 AC and commercial driver offenses focused at 0.04 AC coupled with the needs of the new DOT workplace program has promulgated a re-evaluation of all specifications. This has resulted in updating and re-publication of all documents and lists since 1993 with further revisions thereafter particularly adding new products.

C. Screening tests

Screening tests serve as initial tests; hence, are not preceded by a blank test and may be conducted on single use or multiple use breath or saliva devices meeting the model specifications. Since these tests are not designed to provide quantitative results, the model specifications require only that they can discriminate a negative based on forty tests conducted at a 0.008 concentration and a positive based on forty tests at a 0.032 concentration (NHTSA, 1995). The available saliva tests use an enzyme assay technology while the non-evidentiary breath devices are based on fuel cell technology.

Table 20.6
Alcohol Screening Devices

Akers Laboratories, Inc., Thorofare, NJ
    Alcohol
Alco Check International, Hudsonville, MI
    Alco Check 3000 DOT
    Alco Screen 3000
    Alco Check 9000
Chematics, Inc., North Webster, IN
    ALCO-SCREEN 02
Guth Laboratories, Inc. Harrisburg, PA
    Alco Tector Mark X
    Mark X Alco Checker
Han Internatonal Co., Ltd., Seoul, Korea
    A.B.I. (Alcohol Breath Indicator)
OraSure Technologies Inc., Bethlehem, PA
(formerly STC Technologies, Inc.)
    Q.E.D. A150 Saliva Alcohol Test
PAS Systems International Inc., Fredericksburg, VA
    PAS IIIa
    PAS Vr
Repco Marketing, Inc., Raleigh, NC
    Alco Tec III
Roche Diagnostics System, Branchburg, NJ
    On-Site Alcohol
Sound Off, Inc., Hudsonville, MI
    Digitox DOT

Table 20.6 provides a list of approved products as of May 2001 as listed in the Conforming Products List of Screening Devices to Measure Alcohol in Bodily Fluids (NHTSA, 2001).

D. Evidentiary tests

All evidentiary tests are confirmation tests which are preceded by a fifteen-minute deprivation period and a blank reading. Breath test devices are required. The revised model specifications include testing at new lower concentrations, 0.02, 0.04, 0.08 and 0.16 AC as well as a test for the presence of acetone. Three technologies are employed: fuel cells, infrared spectrometry and gas chromatography. These are described in detail in Chapter 8. Evidentiary breath testing (EBT) instruments as listed on the October 2002 Conforming Products List of Evidential Breath

Table 20. 7
Evidentiary Breath Alcohol Devices

Alcohol Countermeasures Systems Corp., Mississauga, Ontario, Canada
    Alert J4X.ec, PBA 3000C

CMI, Inc., Owensboro, KY
    Intoxilyzer, 200, 200 D, 300, 400, 400 PA, 1400, 5000, 5000 CD, 5000 CD/FG5, 5000 EN, 5000
    (CAL DOJ), 5000 VA, 8000, SD-2, SD-5

Drager Safety, Inc., Durango CO (also National Draeger, Inc.)
    Alcotest 7110 MKIII, 7110MKIII-C, 7410, 7410 Plus, Breathalyzer 7410, 7410-II

Galls, Inc., Lexington, KY
    Alcohol Detection System—A.D.S. 500

Intoximeters, Inc., St. Louis, MO
    Alcomonitor, Alcomonitor CC, Alco-Sensor III, Alco-Sensor IV, Alco-Sensor IV-XL, AlcoSensor
    AZ, RBT-AZ, RBT III, RBT III-A, RBT IV, Intox EC/IR, Intox EC/IR-2, Portable Intox EC/IR

Life-Loc, Inc. Wheat Ridge, CO
    PBA 3000 B, PBA 3000 C, Alcohol Data Sensor, Phoenix, FC1O, FC 20

Lion Laboratories, Ltd., Cardiff, Wales, UK
    Alcolmeter 300, 400
    Intoxilyzer 200, 200 D, 1400, 5000 CD/FG5, 5000 EN

National Patent Analytical Systems, Inc., Mansfield, OH
    BAC DataMaster, BAC Verifier DataMaster, DataMaster cdm

Seres, Paris, France
    Alco Master, Alcopro

Sound-Off, Hudsonville, MI
    AlcoData, Seres AlcoMaster, Seres Alcopro

U.S. Alcohol Testing, Inc./Protection Devices, Inc., Rancho Cucamonga, CA
    AlcoAnalyzer, 1000, 2000, 2100

Verax Systems, Inc., Fairport, NY
    BAC Verifier Datamaster

Testing Devices (NHTSA, 2002) are shown in Table 20.7.

Fuel cells are the most common and least expensive technology. They are compact and portable. They are sensitive to methyl and isopropyl alcohol to varying degrees in addition to responding to ethyl alcohol. Although accurate, they have seen limited use; however, as evidentiary devices in the law enforcement arena. Infrared instruments are generally larger, less portable and more expensive than fuel cells. They use varying wavelengths or combinations of wavelengths to enhance their specificity for ethyl alcohol. They have been the primary instrument used by law enforcement in recent years; hence, have been subjected to extensive court review. Gas chromatography units are uniquely specific for ethyl al-

cohol and no other alcohols interfere. The instruments are notably larger and the most complicated to operate, particularly requiring tanks of compressed gases for operation. Although still listed, none are generally available.

All technologies and devices on the conforming products list (Table 20.7) are approved and acceptable for DOT testing. Although there are differences in the technologies used, all are capable of making equivalent quantitative measurements for ethyl alcohol and other low molecular weight alcohols in breath.

EBT devices can be compared by cost versus the intended use or need. Screening-only devices (i.e., those which conform to EBT model specifications but do not meet other DOT documentation rules) are fuel cell-based and cost approximately $500–$600. Fuel cell devices that meet confirmation documentation requirements are those interfaced to printers. These are lightweight and portable and cost about $2,000. Their data acquisition and transmission capabilities are generally limited. At the next level are the infrared devices which are less portable and cost about $5,000–$6,000. Most are readily linked to computer systems and have more extensive data capabilities for storing, transmitting and handling information. In summary, instrument selection should be based on type and location of use, space available, data handling needs, and volume of work. The DOT program at its inception was designed with the idea that these instruments would be used by employers at their work sites to conduct the required testing. In actual practice, laboratories, third party organizations, individual consulting services, and others are providing a substantial portion of the alcohol testing for the industry. The evidentiary fuel cell printer combinations have emerged as the dominant technology for DOT testing.

E. Calibrating devices

All instruments require a means for calibration and quality control. This is achieved in one of two ways: the breath alcohol simulator or the use of dry gases. Model specifications and conforming products lists have been published (NHTSA, 1997). See Chapter 8 for further discussion. The wet bath simulators are available from a number of manufacturers. In addition, several companies provide dry gas standards. A list of these products is shown in Table 20.8.

Wet bath simulators use 500 ml of aqueous solutions of ethanol that are available as certified ready to use solutions or can be made from certified stock solutions by dilution using Class-A volumetric pipettes and flasks. Compressed gases are different from the wet bath simulators in that the gas concentrations must be adjusted for barometric pressure at the site of use.

F. Training requirements

1. Breath alcohol technicians

The breath alcohol technician (BAT) is an individual trained to proficiency in operating an EBT. Training is conducted according to the 6.5-hour BAT

Table 20.8
Alcohol Calibrating Devices

CMI, Inc., Owensboro, KY
  Toxitest II
Gateway Airgas, Inc., St. Louis, MO (formerly A.G. Specialty Gas and Acetylene Gas Company)
  Ethanol Breath Alcohol Standard
Guth Laboratories, Inc., Harrisburg, PA
  Model 34 C Simulator
  Model 3412
  Model 10-4
  Model 1214
Lion Laboratories, plc, Cardiff, Wales, UK
  AlcoCal Gas Standard
Liquid Technology Corporation, Orlando, FL
  Alcohol-in-Nitrogen Calibrating Unit
National Draeger, Inc., Durango, CA
  Mark IIA
PLD of Florida, Inc., Rockledge, FL
  BA 500
Repco Marketing Inc., Raleigh, NC
  AS-1
  Model 3402C
Scott Specialty Gases, Inc. Plumsteadville, PA
  Model EBS Gaseous Ethanol Breath Standard
US Alcohol Testing, Rancho Cucamonga, CA
  Alco-Simulator 61000

Model Curriculum provided by DOT. This includes: Introduction and Overview; EBT Methodology/Preparing for Testing; Conducting a Screening Test; Conducting a Confirmation Test; Obstacles to Completing a Test; Disclosure of Information and Record Keeping; and Proficiency. Certified BATs must complete the BAT Model Course or its approved equivalent. A *Student Handbook and Instructor Training Curriculum* are available from the DOT (Department of Transportation, 2001a, 2001b). The employer must document BAT training and proficiency. Additional training is required if the BAT performs EBT calibration checks or maintenance. Specific instrument training varies according to the instrument selected.

2. Screening test technicians

The screening test technician (STT) performs the screening functions only. Training must be conducted in accordance with the DOT Model Course or its equivalent (Department of Transportation, 2001c). Individuals who successfully complete the model course or its equivalent may perform tests if they have been deemed proficient and able to discern correctly the changes in the test that produces positive or negative results. Training and proficiency must be documented. Anyone meeting the requirements as a BAT may act as a STT.

3. Testing in the Nuclear Regulatory Commission programs

The Nuclear Regulatory Commission (NRC) had instituted alcohol testing prior to the DOT Program. Their regulations state:

> Tests for alcohol must be administered by breath analysis using breath alcohol analyses devices meeting evidential standards described in Section 2.7 (O)(3) of Appendix A of the NRC Rules. A breath alcohol content indicating a blood alcohol concentration of 0.04 percent or greater must be a positive test result. The confirmatory test for alcohol shall be done with another breath measurement instrument. Should the person demand further confirmation, the test must be a gas chromatography analysis of blood.
> (Code of Federal Regulations, 1989)

There are some similarities and differences. Both DOT and NRC principally use breath testing. DOT allows two tests on the same instrument while NRC requires two tests on two different instruments (either of the same or alternate technologies). NRC allows optional blood testing. It should be noted that many breath test devices used in NRC programs were evaluated prior to the more recent DOT induced Model Specifications and Conforming Product List updates.

20.6 Interpretation of Alcohol Test Results

In relation to alcohol testing in the workplace, an understanding of the acute effects of alcohol as reflected by the alcohol concentration of blood, breath or saliva is necessary chiefly in three regards: (1) Establishing appropriate alcohol concentration thresholds, at or above which specified work-related activities such as performance of safety-sensitive functions are prohibited by the employer's alcohol abuse prevention and control policy; (2) interpretation of alcohol test results in reasonable cause or reasonable suspicion and post-accident testing; and (3) assessment of fitness for duty. An alternative to promulgating one or more alcohol concentration thresholds is a policy requiring covered employees to be alcohol-free at work. Such "alcohol-free" status can be defined in terms of alcohol concentration as discussed below.

Interpretation of alcohol test results to workplace alcohol testing is addressed in this chapter with special reference only to the extent necessary to supplement the information found elsewhere in this publication. The workplace is not unique with respect to the significance of alcohol test results or the effects of alcohol on impairment. In the simplest form of alcohol test result interpretation, a given threshold, say zero AC[7] or any other AC, constitutes the dividing point between permissible and impermissible alcohol presence. A confirmed alcohol test result equal to or greater than that threshold, by itself, triggers the prestipulated consequence, whether standing down from safety-sensitive duties or other work-related outcome. In addition to thresholds established specifically for a given workplace by governmental regulation or by employer policy, the normal per se thresholds and presumptive interpretations of federal, state, and local statutory prohibitions remain applicable and enforceable by police and prosecuting agencies and the courts. The most common examples are the alcohol elements of motor vehicle offenses (e.g., operating a motor vehicle under the influence of alcohol, or while impermissibly impaired by alcohol or by the combined effects of alcohol and other drugs). There are also special work-related statutory prohibitions, such as that against operating a commercial motor vehicle, as defined by federal law, when the driver has any demonstrable presence of alcohol in the body.

What constitutes "zero alcohol" in a worker is subject to several considerations, including the purely technical issue of what putative alcohol concentration in breath or saliva, if any, could be obtained in a properly conducted alcohol analysis on an alcohol-free subject. As reflected elsewhere in this publication, modern methods and techniques of breath or saliva-alcohol analysis uniformly yield results of less than 0.01 AC in alcohol-free subjects. We therefore propose that a breath, blood, or saliva-alcohol concentration of less than 0.01 AC be considered as indication of alcohol-free state of the tested person at the time of the test. This proposal is substantially consistent with positions of the National Safety Council's Committee on Alcohol and Other Drugs and with the majority recommendation of the Transportation Research Board's Committee on Benefits and Costs of Alternative Federal Blood Alcohol Concentration Standards for Commercial Vehicle Operators, rendered in 1987 (Special Report 216, 1987). Any AC of 0.01 or greater would, therefore, indicate the presence of alcohol at the time of the test. An alcohol-free status requirement would appropriately apply only to a true "zero alcohol" employer policy, enforced for example on employees previously diverted to substance abuse evaluation and treatment for documented alcohol abuse, upon their post-treatment return to duty in a safety-sensitive function.

The other extreme is represented by high alcohol concentrations such as those corresponding to visible, gross alcoholic intoxication. Between these extremes are intermediate thresholds, the most common of which are 0.02, 0.04, and 0.08 AC.

A. Acute effects of alcohol

The central nervous system depressant effects of alcohol occur at any measurable alcohol concentration; and the measured concentration is a valid correlate of alcohol effects, including impairment of CNS and other body functions. Extensive reviews of the literature by Moskowitz and Robinson (Moskowitz and Robinson, 1988), exploring the evidence of alcohol effects on reaction time, tracking, concentrated attention, divided attention, performance, information processing capabilities, visual function, perception, psychomotor performance, and driving performance led to the conclusion that impairment measured by those parameters can occur at AC as

low as 0.02; and has been reported for most of these performance areas at AC between 0.01 and 0.02 . A comprehensive survey of the literature reflecting post-1984 research on alcohol effects on human behavior and performance was carried out by Holloway (Holloway, 1994). Among the workplace-relevant conclusions reached in that review were that: (1) 70–80 percent of the studies reviewed report significant effects for intoxication ratings and for controlled laboratory performance at or below 0.04 AC; (2) several task characteristics may influence the relative sensitivities of certain tasks to alcohol effects, including: task complexity, multiple tasks, directed attention or concentration, performance feedback and contingent incentives; and (3) several environmental factors or contextual parameters may influence the sensitivity of one or more alcohol effects, including time-of-day, phase of sleep-wake cycle, and social context.

The NSC Committee on Alcohol and Other Drugs in 1971 took the position that "a concentration of 80 milligrams of ethanol per 100 milliliters of whole blood (0.08 percent w/v) in any driver of a motor vehicle is indicative of impairment in his driving performance" (Committee, 1992). It follows from statistical considerations applicable to any cumulative normal (Gaussian) distribution phenomenon such as driving impairment at various alcohol concentrations that when 100 percent of the sample population is affected at 0.08 AC, 50 percent of the same population is affected at 0.04 AC. In other words, reliable experimental evidence exists that the driving ability of predictable portions of the population are demonstrably impaired at alcohol concentrations less than 0.04 AC, half are so affected at 0.04 AC and all are impaired at 0.08 AC. It is reasonable to apply the same population impairment statistical approach to other-than-driving tasks in the workplace that make comparable demands on cognition, signal processing, decision-making, psychomotor functions and so forth. In effect, that is what imposition of the 0.02 and 0.04 AC thresholds in the DOT and NRC regulations acknowledges in banning performance of safety-sensitive functions at those alcohol concentrations.

Two other workplace related truisms about alcohol and impairment are: (1) In any given individual, acute impairment increases with increasing alcohol concentration; and (2) the proportion of the population which is acutely impaired in any given respect or to any given extent increases with increasing alcohol concentration. Both of these truisms obviously have functional upper limits.

B. Combined effects of alcohol and other drugs

Consideration of interactions between alcohol and other drugs becomes relevant in several workplace-related situations. They include alcohol test results that are markedly inconsistent with observed (impaired) behavior or performance of the tested employee in reasonable cause or reasonable suspicion or post-accident alcohol testing. Another example is the decision on what alcohol concentration, if any other than zero, should be acceptable as a policy matter in workers who are taking prescribed medications chronically, as for management of diabetes or for seizure control. Clearly, some of these decisions involve medical aspects as well as workplace-alcohol issues.

Alcohol has been demonstrated to interact with a great number and variety of other drugs, both therapeutic substances and drugs-of-abuse. Such interactions are so ubiquitous that alcohol probably manifests more combined effects with other drugs than does any other single drug. The nature, extent and duration of interaction depend upon the particular combination of drugs, and fluctuate widely. The most common drug interactions are additive, others are synergistic, potentiating, and antagonistic. An additive effect indicates a summing of the individual effects of the two or more drugs in question. Synergistic effects are those in which the combined effects of two or more drugs are greater than the sum of the individual effects if the drugs were given alone. Potentiation is now usually considered as increasing the effect of a toxic substance acting simultaneously with a nontoxic one. Antagonistic effects are those constituting mutual interference of two or more drugs, thus canceling the respective effects in part or in full. Thus, the combined effects can produce increases in or diminutions of the normal individual effects or actions, including the production of toxicity. The mechanisms of these various effects are complex and cannot be considered in detail here. The interactions can be functional, chemical as in-vivo changes in one or both of a drug combination, dispositional with respect to duration of action and rate of elimination of the respective drugs, or receptor-based, in which blockage occurs at a receptor site through competition of two or more drugs for the same receptor-action site. A major concern about interaction of alcohol with other drugs is for hazardous additive or synergistic effects with other drugs which are psychoactive, particularly those which are also central nervous system depressants, like alcohol. Prolongation of sedative or other adverse psychoactive drug effects in the workplace is also a concern; the combination of alcohol and diazepam is a prime example of such prolongation of drug action as well as intensification of impairing effects.

Sources for information on interactions of alcohol with other drugs include both classical references (Forney and Hughes, 1968; Hansten, 1989) and current compilations that are frequently upgraded (*PDR Guide*, 2003; *Drug Interaction Facts*, 2003), as well as computerized listings. The combined actions can be one-way or mutual; some drugs increase the subject's sensitivity to alcohol, while the effects of other drugs are enhanced or prolonged by alcohol. A widely used reference on drug interactions lists ninety-three drugs and drug classes which have been reported to interact with ethanol, from acetaminophen to warfarin (*Drug Interaction Facts*, 2003).

C. Hangover effects of alcohol

Alcohol and some other drugs have after-effects that persist past the period of actual presence of the parent drug or its metabolites in the body. With alcohol, these residual effects include the "hangover" syndrome experienced, typically, the morning after a bout of heavy drinking. Hangover has been variously characterized as subacute intoxication (Israel and Mardones, 1971), a very mild form of alcohol withdrawal (Mendelson and Mello, 1985a), or a mini-withdrawal syndrome (Mendelson and Mello, 1985b). The term usually refers to the combination of headache, gastric discomfort, general malaise and mild anxiety. However, there may be more severe post-alcoholic effects causing a wide span of physical and physiological distress including fatigue, thirst, vertigo, nystagmus, and nausea in addition to the characteristic "pounding" headache. The syndrome was described more than twenty-five centuries ago in the Hindu medical literature (Leake and Silverman, 1966). It typically appears many hours after the peak alcohol concentration, often in the morning after an evening-long drinking episode, and is usually most severe when little or no alcohol is detectable in the body. Fortunately, the condition is temporary. Modern studies have demonstrated that the hangover form of alcohol after-effects can and does impair critical task performance, such as aircraft operation (Wise, 1992; Wolkenberg et al., 1975; Yesavage and Leirer, 1986). It is noteworthy that the pilots studied by Yesavage and Leirer could not accurately judge their own degree of flight impairment on the morning after ingesting the alcohol (Modell and Mountz, 1990).

In brief, hangover and other after-effects of over-indulgence in alcohol constitute a real and variably-extensive source of performance decrement and impairment for critical work tasks. The situation was well summarized by Kelly et al. in their seminal article: "The results of this investigation show that alcohol in the dose used caused significant impairment and changes in a variety of physiological variables not only during intoxication but also during the post-alcohol stage" (Kelly et al., 1970). Alcohol test results by themselves, of course, afford no information on the presence and intensity, or absence, of hangover and other after-effects of alcohol.

D. Abstention period

Some federal anti-alcohol abuse regulations applying to railroading and aviation impose mandatory pre-duty abstention periods (e.g., four or eight hours during which no alcohol intake is permitted). Even strict and faithful compliance with those restrictions cannot assure alcohol-free status after moderate or greater alcohol consumption, or guarantee that an alcohol concentration below the trigger thresholds of 0.02 and 0.04 alcohol concentration will be reached in every person in that time-frame because of variability in alcohol uptake and elimination patterns in the general population, in addition to beverage-related and drinking situation-specific differences

(Dubowski, 1976; Dubowski, 1985; O'Neill, Williams, and Dubowski, 1983). Of the healthy adult male subjects studied by Dubowski, those with the lowest alcohol elimination rate found would require more than twenty-four hours to become alcohol-free after reaching a 0.15 g/210 L peak breath-alcohol concentration, while those with the highest experimentally determined rate would require only about six hours (Dubowski, 1985).

There are, however, some broadly applicable guidelines. Some rule-of-thumb estimates can be derived from well established experimental data showing a mean alcohol elimination from the body of about 100 mg per kilogram of body weight per hour for men. For a typical healthy normal adult man weighing 68 kilograms (150 pounds), that corresponds to elimination of about the alcohol content of six ounces of beer per hour—or the alcohol content of about one 12-ounce container of beer in two hours. About four hours is typically needed in that situation to become alcohol-free after consuming two 12-ounce portions of beer, six hours for three 12-ounce portions and so on if the beer is consumed in increments over a reasonable time period rather than as rapidly as possible (Dubowski, 1976). Elimination of alcohol from other sources than beer is mostly comparable for equivalent total alcohol intake.

Clearly, the safest course is to abstain from alcohol intake entirely or for longer than the minimally mandated periods, if the objective is not to exceed prohibited alcohol concentration thresholds. Over-the-counter disposable alcohol test devices for self-monitoring are available to assist in guidance to alcohol-free status. For workers subject to duty calls on short notice, avoidance of alcohol intake for at least one day or so before any such on-call schedule period is the most appropriate action.

20.7 Acknowledgment

The authors acknowledge the assistance of Kenneth Edgell of the Office of Drug and Alcohol Policy and Compliance in the U.S. Department of Transportation, Office of the Secretary in reviewing the DOT-related issues discussed in this chapter.

References

Code of Federal Regulations, Title 10, Part 26, 1989.

Committee on Alcohol and Other Drugs. *Committee Handbook*. Itasca, IL: National Safety Council, 1992, p. 12.

Committee on Alcohol and Other Drugs. *A Model Program for the Control of Alcohol in the Workplace*. Itasca, IL: National Safety Council, 1995.

Cornish, C.M. *Drugs and Alcohol in the Workplace: Testing and Privacy*. Wilmette, IL: Callaghan & Co., 1988.

Department of Transportation, Office of the Secretary. Procedures for Transportation Workplace Drug and Alcohol Testing Programs; Procedures for Non-Evidential Alcohol Screening Devices, 60 *Federal Register* 19675–681 (April 20, 1995a).

Department of Transportation, Office of the Secretary. 49 CFR Part 40 Procedures for Transportation Workplace Drug and Alcohol Testing Programs, Final Rule, 65 *Federal Register* 79462–579 (December 19, 2000).

Department of Transportation. *Breath Alcohol Handbook (BAT), Training, Student Handbook*, 2001a.

Department of Transportation. *Breath Alcohol Technician (BAT) Training, Instructor Training Curriculum*, 2001b.

Department of Transportation. *Screening Test Technician Training (STT) Instructor Training Curriculum*, 2001c.

Diagnostic and Statistical Manual of Mental Disorders, 4th ed. (DSM-IV). Washington, DC: American Psychiatric Association, 1994, pp 196–197.

Drug Interaction Facts. St. Louis, MO: Facts and Comparisons, 2003.

Dubowski, K.M. Human pharmacokinetics of ethanol, part 1: Peak blood concentrations and elimination in male and female subjects. *Alcohol Technical Reports* 5:55–63 (1976).

Dubowski, K.M. Absorption, distribution and elimination of alcohol: Highway safety aspects. *J. Studies on Alcohol* Supplement No. 10:98–108, 1985.

Dubowski, K.M. and Essary, N.A. Field performance of current generation breath-alcohol simulators. *J. Analyt. Toxicol.* 16:325–327, 1992.

Dubowski, K.M. and Tuggle, R.S., III. *Drug Use Testing in the Workplace: Law and Science*. Eau Claire, WI: PESI Legal Publishing, 1990.

Eighth Special Report to the U.S. Congress on Alcohol and Health from the Secretary of Health and Human Services, September 1993. NIH Publication No. 94-3699. Rockville, MD: National Institute on Alcohol Abuse and Alcoholism, 1994a, p. 255.

Eighth Special Report to the U.S. Congress on Alcohol and Health from the Secretary of Health and Human Services, September 1993. NIH Publication No. 94-3699: "Effects of Alcohol on Behavior and Safety." Rockville, MD: National Institute on Alcohol Abuse and Alcoholism, 1994b, pp. 233–252.

Farmer, L.M. Employee privacy rights vs. business needs: Drug testing in the workplace. *New England Law Rev.* 22:413–451, 1987.

Forney, R.B. Alcohol: An abused drug. *Clin. Chem.* 33/11(B):82B–86B, 1987.

Forney, R.B. and Hughes, F.W. *Combined Effects of Alcohol and Other Drugs*. Springfield, IL: Charles C. Thomas, 1968.

Hansten, P.D. *Drug Interactions*, 6th ed. Philadelphia: Lea & Febiger, 1989.

Holloway, F.A. *Low-Dose Alcohol Effects on Human Behavior and Performance: A Review of Post-1984 Research*. DOT/FAA/Aar-94/24. Washington, DC, U.S. Department of Transportation, Federal Aviation Administration, November 1994.

Israel, Y. and Mardones, J. *Biological Basis of Alcoholism*. NY: Wiley-Interscience, 1971.

Kelly, M. et al. Effects and after-effects of alcohol on physiological and psychological functions in man: A controlled study. *Blutalkohol* 7:422–436, 1970.

Kwong, T.C. et al. Critical issues in urinalysis of abused substances: Report of the Substance-Abuse Testing Committee. *Clin. Chem.* 34:605–632, 1988.

Leake, C.D. and Silverman, M. *Alcoholic Beverages in Clinical Medicine*. Chicago: Year Book Medical Publishers, 1966.

Mendelson, J.H. and Mello, N.K. (eds.). *The Diagnosis and Treatment of Alcoholism*, 2nd ed. NY: McGraw-Hill, 1985a.

Mendelson, J.H. and Mello, N.K. *Alcohol. Use and Abuse in America*. Boston: Little, Brown and Co., 1985b.

Modell, J.G. and Mountz, J.M. Drinking and flying: The problem of alcohol use by pilots. *New Engl. J. Med.* 323:455–461, 1990.

Moskowitz, H. and Robinson, C.D. *Effects of Low Doses of Alcohol on Driving-Related Skills: A Review of the Evidence,* DOT HS 807-280. Washington, DC: National Highway Traffic Safety Administration, 1988.

National Highway Traffic Safety Administration. Highway safety programs: Model specifications for devices to measure breath alcohol. 58 *Federal Register* 48705–48710, September 17, 1993.

National Highway Traffic Safety Administration. Highway safety programs: Model specifications for screening devices to measure alcohol in bodily fluids. 59 *Federal Register* 39382–39390, August 2, 1994.

National Highway Traffic Safety Administration. Highway safety programs: Model specifications for calibrating units for breath alcohol testers: Conforming products list of calibrating units. 62 *Federal Register* 43416–43425, August 13, 1997.

National Highway Traffic Safety Administration. Highway safety programs; Conforming products list of screening devices to measure alcohol in bodily fluids. 66 *Federal Register* 22639–22640, May 4, 2001.

National Highway Traffic Safety Administration. Highway safety programs: Model specifications

for devices to measure breath alcohol. 67 *Federal Register* 62091–62094, October 3, 2002.

Nuclear Regulatory Commission. Fitness-for-duty programs. 54 *Federal Register* 24468–24508, June 7, 1989.

O'Neill, B., Williams, A.F. and Dubowski, K.M. Variability in blood alcohol concentrations. Implications for estimating individual results. *J. Studies on Alcohol* 44:222–230, 1983.

Pawlowski, A.A. et al. Symposium on life transitions and alcohol consumption: Work-related issues. *Alcoholism, Clin. & Exp. Research* 16:145–205, 1992.

PDR Companion Guide. Montvale, NJ: Medical Economics Co., 2003.

Public Law 101-136. Approved July 26, 1990.

Public Law 102-143, Title V. Approved October 28, 1991.

Special Report 216: *Zero Alcohol and Other Options. Limits for Truck and Bus Drivers*. Washington, DC: Transportation Research Board, National Research Council, 1987, p. 154.

U.S. Department of Labor. *An Employer's Guide to Dealing with Substance Abuse*. Washington, DC: U.S. Government Printing Office, 1990.

U.S. Department of Labor, Office of the Assistant Secretary for Policy. *Workplace Alcohol and Drug Abuse Training Program: Trainer's Guide*. Washington, DC: U.S. Government Printing Office, 1991.

U.S. Department of Transportation. The Existing Safety Problem, Limitation of Alcohol Use by Transportation Workers, Notice, 59 *Federal Register* 7306–7309, February 15, 1994.

U.S. Department of Transportation. *Alcohol and Drug Rules: An Overview*. Washington, DC: U.S. Dept. of Transportation, 1994, p. 3.

U.S. Department of Transportation, Office of the Secretary, Office of Drug and Alcohol Policy and Compliance, personal communication, 2003.

United Transportation Union v. Southeastern Pennsylvania Transportation Authority, 884 F. 2d 709 (1989).

Wise, L.M. Residual effects of alcohol on aircrew performance. *Safety Journal* 10:28–31, 1992.

Wolkenberg, R.G. et al. Delayed effects of acute alcoholic intoxication on performance with reference to work safety. *J. Safety Research* 7:104–118, 1975.

Yesavage, J.A. and Leirer, V.O. Hangover effects on aircraft pilots 14 hours after alcohol ingestion: A preliminary report. *Am. J. Psychiatry* 143:1546–1550, 1986.

Endnotes

1. The unmodified term *alcohol* as used in this chapter means *ethanol*.

2. The Constitution of the United States, Fourth Amendment: "The right of the people to be secure in their persons, houses, papers, and effects, against unreasonable searches and seizures, shall not be violated . . . ."

3. The Constitution of the United States, Fifth Amendment: ". . . nor shall any person . . . be deprived of life, liberty, or property, without due process of law . . . ."

   The Constitution of the United States, Fourteenth Amendment: ". . . nor shall any State deprive any person of life, liberty, or property, without due process of law . . . ."

4. The time required for the alcohol concentration in a given body compartment (e.g., the blood) to be reduced to one-half of the original peak value.

5. The American Board of Forensic Toxicology adopted the following position in November 1986: "It . . . is declared the policy of the American Board of Forensic Toxicology that drug (substance)-use testing activities by means of laboratory examinations be considered as encompassed within the scope of forensic toxicology when carried out under mandate of law, or under equivalent circumstances."

6. Alcohol concentration (AC) as that term is used in DOT regulations means the alcohol in breath, in g/210 L, or the alcohol in blood, in g/100 ml.

7. Again, for the purposes of this section of this chapter, alcohol concentration means g/210 L of breath or g/dL of blood.

About the Authors

William H. Anderson, Ph.D.
Forensic Sciences Division
Washoe County Sheriff's Office
Reno, Nevada

Barbara Basteyns
Green Bay, WI

Yale H. Caplan, Ph.D.
Director, National Scientific Services
Baltimore, MD

Kurt M. Dubowski, Ph.D.
Oklahoma City, OK

James C. Garriott, Ph.D.
Consulting Toxicologist
San Antonio, Texas

Bruce A. Goldberger, Ph.D.
Associate Professor, Departments of Pathology,
  Immunology and Laboratory Medicine
University of Florida College of Medicine
Gainesville, Florida

Patrick Harding, B.S.
Toxicology Section Supervisor, Wisconsin State
  Laboratory of Hygiene
Madison, WI

William C. Head
Attorney at Law
Atlanta, GA

A.W. Jones, Ph.D., D.Sc.
Associate Professor, National Lab of Forensic
  Chemistry, Department of Forensic Chemistry
University Hospital
Linköping, Sweden

Graham R. Jones, Ph.D.
Office of the Chief Medical Examiner
Edmonton, Alberta, Canada

Jerry G. Landau
Special Assistant County Attorney
Maricopa County District Attorney's Office
Phoenix, AZ

Barbara R. Manno, Ph.D.
Professor, Louisiana State University Health
  Sciences Center in Shreveport
Department of Psychiatry
Shreveport, LA

Joseph E. Manno, Ph.D.
Professor, Louisiana State University Health
  Sciences Center in Shreveport,
Departments of Psychiatry and Emergency Medi-
  cine (Section of Toxicology)
Shreveport, Louisiana

Morton F. Mason, Ph.D. (deceased)
Department of Pathology, University of Texas
  Health Science Center at Dallas
Dallas, Texas

Bill H. McAnalley, Ph.D.
Mannatech, Incorporated
Coppell, Texas

Boris Moczula
First Assistant Prosecutor, Passaic County
   Prosecutor's Office
Paterson, New Jersey

Herbert Moskowitz, Ph.D.
President, UCLA and Southern California Research
   Institute
Encino, California

Richard F. Shaw, B.S.
Consultant in Toxicology
San Diego, CA

Theodore F. Shults, J.D.
Durham, North Carolina

Index

A

abdominal cavity, 169

absinthe, 3, 17

absorption, 6, 24, 34, 47–49, 51–63, 65–66, 70, 74–76, 80–81, 85–86, 90–95, 115, 125–126, 128, 132–133, 135–137, 150, 152, 155–156, 164–165, 167, 169, 177, 180, 191, 245, 303, 344, 368, 377–378
    of alcohol, 47–48, 54–56, 75, 80, 91, 132–133, 135, 150, 152, 165, 191, 245, 303, 344, 368, 377–378
    phase, 52, 55, 61, 70, 90, 125–126, 136, 150, 164
    rate of alcohol, 56, 135

accident(s), 31–32, 34, 134, 178, 253–256, 258, 261, 264–266, 269–271, 273–278, 280–291, 299–304, 316–317, 321–326, 373–374, 377–378, 383, 386, 392, 411, 416, 418–422
    age-associated, 282, 286–287
    automobile, 270, 277–278, 281, 288
    incidence, 32, 274, 281, 290
    males, 286
    pedestrian, 270, 277, 281, 283, 287
    rail, 286
    socioeconomic level, 282
    statistics, 274–275, 281

accuracy, 187, 191–192, 220–221, 223, 232–233, 251, 303–304, 312, 314, 316, 319–320, 325–326, 340, 349–350, 362–364, 368, 374, 382–383, 388, 396
    method, 220–221, 232–233, 251, 326

acetaldehyde (ACH), 5, 9–10, 12, 23, 36–37, 57, 66, 68–70, 113–117, 119–123, 138, 150, 197, 213–214, 238, 242–243, 249, 382
    alcohol metabolism, 122
    blood, 69, 115, 121, 138
    breath, 115, 121–123, 197, 249
    dehydrogenase, 36, 116–117

acetate, 10, 12–13, 17, 113, 116–117, 119, 138, 217

acetic acid, 5–6, 14, 20, 68, 70, 196–197, 213

Acetobacter, 6, 14

acetone, 14, 70, 118, 120, 163, 190, 193, 195, 214, 216, 219, 232, 234–235, 243, 249, 349, 382, 422, 426
    in breath, 190

acetonitrile, 220, 249

acetyl coenzyme a, 117, 138

acrolein, 9

addiction, 23, 37, 69, 121

ADH (see alcohol dehydrogenase)

adipose tissue, 54

adrenocorticotropic hormone, 25

affirmation, 352, 402

African-American(s), ADH in, 118

agave, 4

age, 23, 29, 37, 47, 57, 64–66, 80, 94, 114–115, 118, 133, 153, 174, 197, 254–257, 264, 266, 273–275, 279–280, 282–290, 298, 307, 315, 322

aggression, 71, 253, 265, 316

aguardiente, 3

aircraft, 31–32, 253, 277, 283, 287, 314, 399, 411, 432

alanine, 5, 139

alanine aminotransferase, 139

Alco-Analyzer, 206–208

alcohol(s)
    biochemistry, 113
    drug interaction, 431
    elimination rate, 72, 432
    endogenous, 67, 170–171, 316, 388
    ethyl, 1, 3, 9–12, 14, 23–26, 29, 32, 34, 67, 163, 166, 169–171, 188, 190–191, 193, 197, 203, 206, 213–223, 249–251, 380, 384, 388–389, 422, 427
    grain, 1, 11
    half-life in body, 38
    ingested, 24, 32, 34–35, 54, 60, 79, 82, 124, 136, 139, 166, 170, 197, 264, 345, 365, 382
    kinetics, 115, 138
    lethal blood, 173
    methyl, 11, 171, 197, 214, 216, 218–220, 422, 427
    physiology, 113, 377
    postmortem formation, 154
    tolerance test, 128
    withdrawal symptom(s), 114
    wood, 11, 163

alcohol consumption, 24–25, 29, 32, 35, 37–38, 139, 242, 253–254, 264, 274, 280, 284, 288, 309, 314, 326, 349–351, 432
    evidence for, 350

alcohol dehydrogenase (ADH), 35, 47, 57–60, 67–71, 73–74, 92–93, 113–120, 127, 133–137, 153, 155, 214–216
    alcohol metabolism, 47, 113
    metabolism of acetaldehyde, 36, 121–122
    gastric, 35, 136
    molecule, 118
    polymorphic, 60, 118

alcohol screening (testing), 86, 167, 185–194, 202–203, 206–208, 217, 229, 245, 270, 287–288, 302, 315, 321,